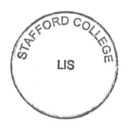

The Illustrated Veterinary Guide for Dogs, Cats, Birds, & Exotic Pets

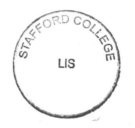

To Tracy and the kids

"God saw all that he had made,
and it was very good"
(Genesis 1:31)

The Illustrated Veterinary Guide for Dogs, Cats, Birds, & Exotic Pets

Chris C. Pinney, DVM

Illustrations by Sandra G. Pinson

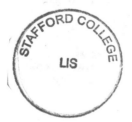
TAB Books
Division of McGraw-Hill, Inc.
Blue Ridge Summit, PA 17294-0850

Stafford
COLLEGE

NOTICES

Prescription Diet®   Hill's Pet Products Division of
Colgate-Palmolive Company

Pepto-Bismol™   The Proctor & Gamble Company

FIRST EDITION
SECOND PRINTING

© 1992 by **Chris C. Pinney**.
TAB Books is a division of McGraw-Hill, Inc.

Printed in the United States of America. All rights reserved. The
publisher takes no responsibility for the use of any of the materials
or methods described in this book, nor for the products thereof.

Library of Congress Cataloging-in-Publication Data

Pinney, Chris C.
    The illustrated veterinary guide for dogs, cats, birds, and exotic
pets / by Chris C. Pinney.
        p.   cm.
    Includes index.
    ISBN 0-8306-1986-0 (h)
    1. Pet medicine—Handbooks, manuals, etc.   2. Dogs—Diseases-
-Handbooks, manuals, etc.   3. Cats—Diseases—Handbooks, manuals,
etc.   I. Title.
SF981.P56   1991
636.089—dc20   91-28718
                                                        CIP

Acquisitions Editor: Kimberly Tabor
Book Editor: April D. Nolan
Director of Production: Katherine G. Brown
Page Makeup: Wanda Ditch
Typesetting: Jana L. Fisher
            Donna K. Harlacher
            Olive A. Harmon
            Lisa M. Mellott
Book Design: Jaclyn J. Boone
Cover design and illustration: Denny Bond, East Petersburg, Pa.

Contents

Acknowledgments

THE AUTHOR WOULD LIKE to thank the following contributors for their part in the development of this book:

Elizabeth M. Hodgkins, DVM, of Hill's Pet Products for her contributions on canine and feline nutrition.
Claudia L. Barton, DVM, for her contributions on cancer in companion animals.
Larry P. Tilley, DVM Diplomate, A.C.V.I.M. for his contributions on cardiology and heart disease in dogs.
James R. Smith, DVM for his contributions on dermatology and skin diseases.
Lon D. Lewis, DVM, Mark L. Morris Jr., DVM and Michael S. Hand, DVM of Mark Morris Associates for their input regarding canine and feline nutrition.
Michael O. Woolley, DVM for his contributions on geriatric care and behavioral problems in pets.

The author would also like to acknowledge those published resources used to verify and support much of the material contained herein:

Kirk, Robert W. ed. 1986. Current Veterinary Therapy IX: Small Animal Practice. W.B. Saunders Company. Philadelphia.
Kirk, Robert W. ed. 1989. Current Veterinary Therapy X: Small Animal Practice. W.B. Saunders Company. Philadelphia.
Mastin, M.M. ed. 1990. Quarterly Index: Information Access for the Small Animal Practitioner. Veterinary Interface. Riverbank, CA.
Mastin, M.M. ed. 1991. Quarterly Index: Information Access for the Small Animal Practitioner. Veterinary Interface. Riverbank, CA.

Introduction

IT'S A PROVEN FACT: People love pets! And regardless of whether they're furred, feathered, or finned, these companion animals serve vital roles, both physical and psychological, in our society. The popularity of dogs and cats as pets is ever on the rise; in fact, in the United States, cats have surpassed dogs in popularity.

But don't get the idea that dogs and cats monopolize the hearts of all pet owners. The appeal of less conventional pets such as birds, small rodents, rabbits, ferrets, fish, and pigs—that's right, pigs!—is growing, as well. Furthermore, households containing these birds and exotic pets are often inhabited by dogs and/or cats, too, with all the animals cohabitating peacefully (or sometimes not so peacefully!). Because of the multi-pet fancies exhibited by numerous pet owners, a need was seen for a resource that contained information on all types of pets, all condensed into one layman's volume. It was for this reason that *The Illustrated Veterinary Guide for Dogs, Cats, Birds, and Exotic Pets*, a comprehensive, up-to-date guide, was written.

The Illustrated Veterinary Guide for Dogs, Cats, Birds, and Exotic Pets is loaded with illustrations and covers important topics concerning husbandry and health care for all of the popular species of pets. It doesn't matter if you own one pet or multiple species of pets, *The Illustrated Veterinary Guide for Dogs, Cats, Birds, and Exotic Pets* covers them all. Just look at some of the subjects presented:

○ How to treat annoying behavorial problems in dogs and cats.

○ How to protect your cat from the newest threat to feline populations around the world: the Feline Immunodeficiency Virus (Feline AIDS)

○ New steroid-free treatments for canine skin allergies

○ Breakthroughs in the treatment of arthritis and cancer in pets

○ Information on the newest in vaccines for pets, including those targeted against feline infectious peritonitis, avian pox, and Lyme disease

○ Vital first-aid procedures, all of which could save your pet's life some day

○ Seven steps to increasing your pet's longevity

○ The threat of zoonotic (pet-borne) diseases to pet owners

○ Tips on bird care, husbandry, and disease prevention

○ Care and husbandry of exotic pets, including ferrets, rabbits, guinea pigs, hamsters, gerbils, mice, rats, reptiles, and tropical fish

○ Care and husbandry of the newest pet craze, miniature pot-bellied pigs

○ How to maintain high water quality in aquariums

○ . . . . and much more!

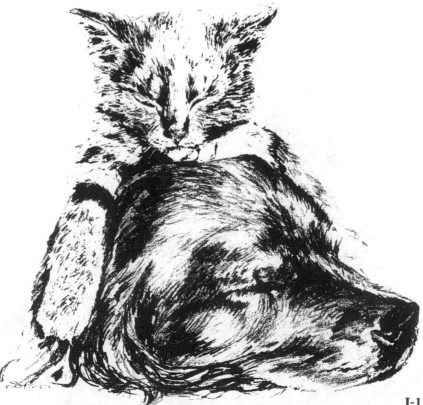

I-1

Part I deals with man's best friend, the dog. Information ranging from breed selection to all aspects of preventative health care are covered in this section. In addition, those disease conditions commonly seen in dogs are discussed, along with the latest treatments.

Part II is dedicated to—you guessed it—the cat. For centuries, this creature has been a faithful companion to man and has sparked the fancy of millions of pet owners throughout the world. In this section, you'll learn how to properly care for your own cat, with subjects again ranging from the selection process to coping with a diabetic feline. There are even tips on training these sometimes independent creatures.

As more and more people move into smaller residences that might have restrictions on pets and their sizes, the popularity of pet birds has increased. Part III of *The Illustrated Veterinary Guide for Dogs, Cats, Birds, and Exotic Pets* covers important information regarding the selection, housing, feeding, breeding, and preventative health care of pet birds, as well as on those diseases most often seen with birds. There are

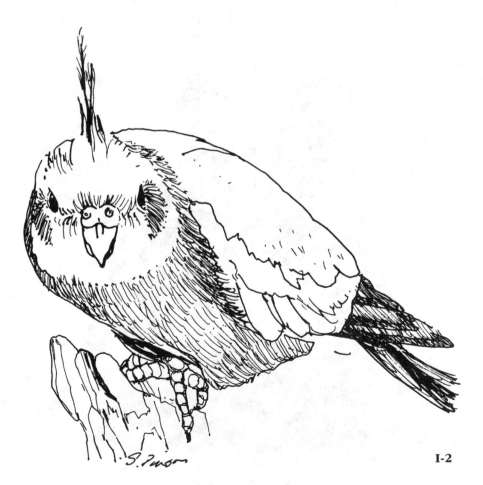

I-2

even sections on hand-raising baby birds and on emergency and first aid procedures for our feathered friends.

For those pet fanciers who prefer less conventional choices for companionship, Part IV deals with small rodents and exotic pets, including guinea pigs, hamsters, gerbils, mice, rats, rabbits, ferrets, miniature pot-bellied pigs, and reptiles. For tropical fish lovers, there is also a chapter on aquarium maintenance and disease prevention in fish.

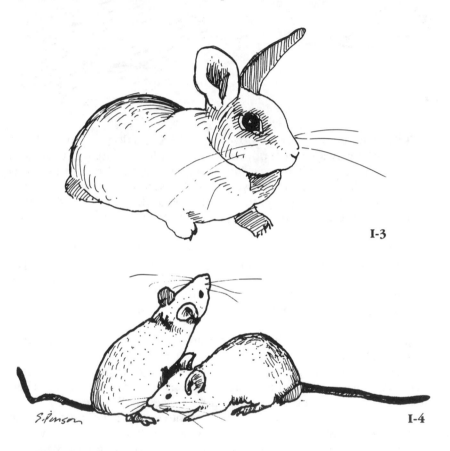

I-3

I-4

Part V concentrates on the health and longevity of your dog or cat. It not only includes a chapter on how you can help your pet live longer through preventative health care, but it also sensitively covers serious life-and-death situations, such as cancer and the euthanasia decision. Also included in this section is an eye-opening look at the zoonotic diseases, or diseases that can be transmitted from pets to people. Although the chances of such a transmission can be minimized through a good preventative health-care program, many pet owners fail to realize the importance of such care. As a result, they can be inadvertently placing the health of themselves and their families in jeopardy.

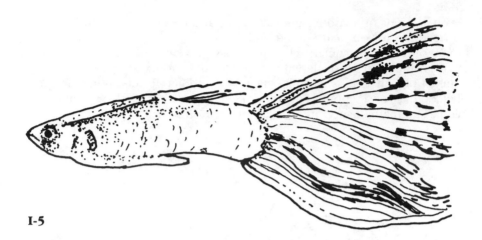

I-5

If you have ever wondered how to give CPR to a dog or a cat, or what to do if your pet swallowed a poison, the appendix will answer those and other important questions regarding emergencies and first aid for dogs and cats. In fact, this could very well be the most important section of the book, since in emergency situations, timing is of the essence. As a result, the material presented in the appendix could very well save your pet's life one day.

Finally *The Illustrated Veterinary Guide* contains two more valuable features that make it a must for any pet owners. The first is the multitude of illustrations that accompany the text of the book. Someone once said, "A picture is worth a thousand words," and we heeded this advice when preparing this book. The second special feature is the complete and comprehensive index.

Of course, despite all the above features, this book is not designed to replace quality veterinary care for pets, but rather to supplement it. If your pet is exhibiting signs of injury or illness, always consult your veterinarian. Remember: the sooner a diagnosis can be made by a qualified veterinarian, the greater the chances are for a succesful treatment.

Now get set for an informative voyage into the world of pets with the *The Illustrated Veterinary Guide* as your guide. Regardless of your pet fancy, this book is sure to enrich the relationship you have with your loving companion.

DOGS

THE DOG: what can be said about this magnificent creature? For ten thousand years, it has been an integral part of man's social and cultural development. Its blood and toil has helped man discover new lands and build civilizations; its effectiveness in war has helped topple the same. It has hunted beside man for centuries and has been hunted by man for food. As eyes for the blind and ears for the deaf, the dog has become an indispensable member of our modern society. But what really sets the dog apart from all the rest? Millions of dog lovers will agree that it's the special loyalty and devotion the dog exhibits towards members of our own species—a characteristic that has justly earned it the proper title of "man's best friend."

All dogs are thought to originate from a common ancestor called *Miacis*, a carnivorous creature that lived over forty million years ago. Many theories exist regarding the evolutionary process that concluded with the domestic dog as we know it. One popular theory is that the modern-day dog descended from the wolf, which, over time, gave rise to four separate groups of dogs.

The first group, the Dingo Group, is descended from the wolves of Asia. Its members were dispersed throughout the Asian, African, and Australian continents. Modern-day descendants of this group include Rhodesian ridgebacks, basenjis, and the dingoes of Australia. One distinguishing characteristic of this group is that they don't like to bark too much.

A second group of dogs, the Greyhound Group, is believed to have evolved from wolves in the open plains of Asia, Africa, and the Middle East. The oldest member of this group, the saluki, is thought to have been around prior to 1400 B.C. Distinguishing features of the Greyhound group include a keen eyesight and incredible speed, two characteristics the Egyptians found especially useful for hunting purposes. Besides the saluki, other modern representatives include the Afghan hound, the borzoi, and, of course, the greyhound.

The Northern Dog Group is a third group of canines that are believed to have evolved from the large grey wolf of Northern Europe. Generally regarded as one-master dogs, descendants of this group have proved especially useful to man for a variety of functions, including pulling his sleds (Alaskan malamutes, Siberian huskies), hunting his game (Norwegian elk hound), and guarding his flocks (collies).

A final group, the Mastiff Group, arose from wolves occupying the mountainous regions of Eurasia. Gifted with a keen sense of smell, members of this group were commonly used as war dogs and for hunting game. We still use retrievers, setters, and pointers for similar purposes, even today. The Mastiffs, the St. Bernard, and the Great Pyrenees are a few of the more sizable relatives in this group.

1

Choosing the Right Dog for You

BECAUSE THE ANCESTRY of the dog is so varied, all sorts of shapes, sizes, colors, coat lengths, and personalities exist. With such a multitude of groups and types from which to select your pet, how do you know which is going to be just right for you and your particular situation? Questions you should ask yourself include the following:

○ Why do I want a dog in the first place?
○ What type of dog do I want?
○ Do I want an indoor or outdoor dog?
○ How will my new dog affect my existing pets?
○ Am I willing to devote the time and money needed to be a responsible pet owner?

Your answers to these questions will have great bearing on the type of dog you'll want to choose.

WHY DO YOU WANT A DOG?

If companionship is your underlying motive for dog ownership, your selection is wide open. Regardless of breed—be they purebred, or products of more creative genetic blends—dogs make great companions. After all, they weren't coined "man's best friend" for nothing! Obviously, you'll want to focus on those breeds or blends that strike your individual fancy during the selection process (FIGS. 1-1 through 1-9).

For instance, say you want a jogging companion. You will want a larger dog whose stride length and aerobic capacity won't slow you down. Or you might just want a cute lap warmer. If so, toy breeds weighing under 10 pounds serve this function quite nicely (and, I might add, quite comfortably!). By giving such matters a little thought when selecting a canine for companionship, you won't be disappointed (FIG. 1-10).

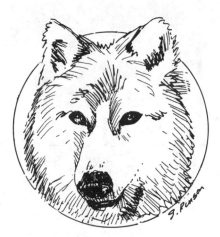

1-1 *Dogs are believed to be descendants of wolves.*

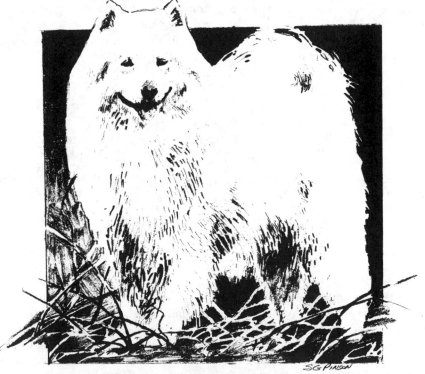

1-2 *Samoyed.*

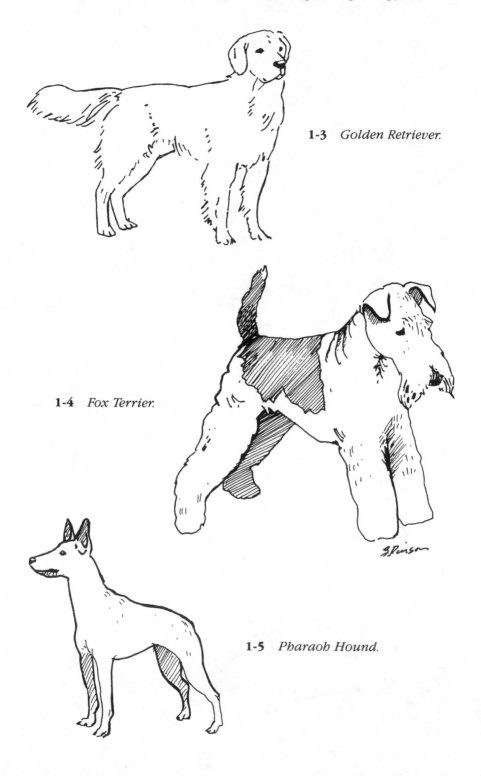

1-3 *Golden Retriever.*

1-4 *Fox Terrier.*

1-5 *Pharaoh Hound.*

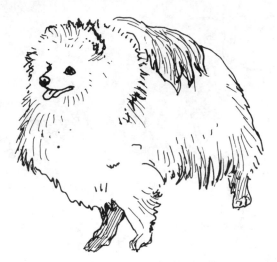

1-6 *Pomeranian.*

1-7 *Shih Tzu.*

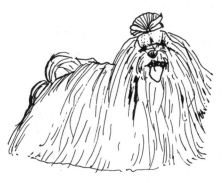

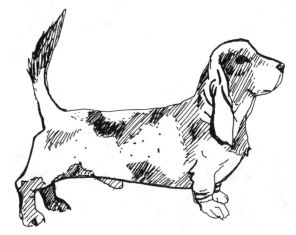

1-8 *Bassett Hound.*

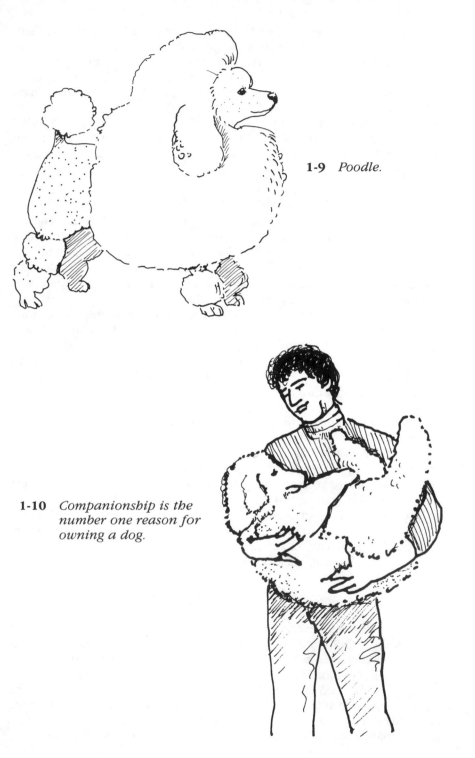

1-9 *Poodle.*

1-10 *Companionship is the
number one reason for
owning a dog.*

Though your intentions might be pure and good-hearted, **never** surprise someone with a new dog or puppy unless you are positively, absolutely sure that they want one in the first place. Think about it; your gift to them not only includes that furry bundle of energy, but also a hearty commitment to training, time, and money. Unfortunately, too many people do fail to think about it, and as a result, our nation's pounds and shelters are overflowing with unwanted pets turned in by disgruntled or disinterested gift recipients. It is best to allow other people to come to a decision about pet ownership by themselves, and not to force it upon them by your good intentions. Everyone will be happier in the long run!

Dogs as protectors

Many potential dog owners desire such a pet for protection purposes. If this is your sole reason for wanting a dog, it is a poor one. Obtaining a dog under such pretenses is only asking for trouble (and liability), and I heartily advise against it. If, on the other hand, you plan to treat such a dog as a true companion and household member as well as a protector, then your qualifications for ownership are acceptable.

It stands to reason that an 85-pound rottweiler with glistening white teeth would certainly be more imposing as a protector than an 11-pound Lhasa apso! (Not that the latter wouldn't try, mind you—Lhasa apsos were originally bred for this purpose.) However, it is instinctive that all dogs, regardless of breed or size, will actively defend pack members (that includes you!) or territory if they feel threatened. As a result, where other people are concerned, your dog, big or small, needs to know from the start who *does not* constitute a threat, especially if you plan on giving it any special protection training.

For the safety of yourself and others (including your children, visiting neighbors, etc.), your dog must be properly socialized (see chapter 2) before you undertake protection training. Police canine units are perfect examples of this approach. These dogs are trained to attack on command only. Off duty, however, most are gentle as lambs. This is how your dog should be. Not only is it the smart thing to do to avoid tragic consequences, but it also might keep you out of a lawsuit. Remember: A socialized dog can be a great protector; an unsocialized dog is downright dangerous!

Dogs and children

Dogs can provide an excellent means for educating and teaching children about responsibility and about life itself. For this reason, many parents choose to purchase a new puppy or dog for their offspring. If this is the case in your situation, keep these guidelines in mind.

First, for maximum benefit and enjoyment, consider waiting until your children are at least 5 years old before acquiring a new pet. Younger children, some of whom might just be starting to crawl or walk, stand a greater chance of being accidentally hurt by a playful puppy than do older ones. In addition, older children are better equipped to learn about and/ or undertake responsibilities associated with pet ownership, and can become active participants in its care.

Choose a pup with an outgoing personality—one that can stand up to the rigors of ownership by a child. Shy, introverted pups rarely satisfy the energy requirements of children. As a result, such dogs might be difficult to socialize.

As far as size is concerned, medium to large breeds are preferred for children (FIG. 1-11). Toy breeds, owing to their small stature, are more susceptible to accidental injury at the hands and feet of young ones. On the other hand, while one of the giant breeds can be gentle as a lamb, such a pet could still pose a significant health threat to your child due to sheer mass.

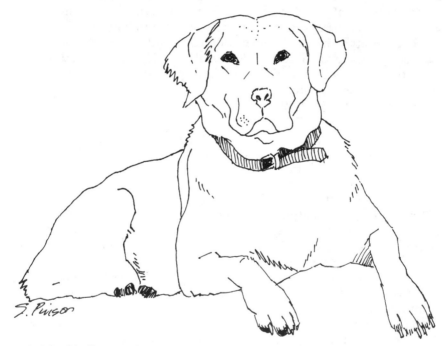

1-11 *Medium to large dogs often make the best pets for children.*

Personality features to look for include low aggressiveness, high tolerance, and low excitability. Golden retrievers are a favorite among parents, owing to their reputation for gentleness. Basset hounds, Labrador retrievers, and collies are also popular picks for children.

Where children are concerned, limit your selection of a puppy to one that is between 8 and 12 weeks old. Because socialization naturally occurs during this time, a greater bond will form between it and your child. Along the same lines, a dog older than 12 weeks of age should not be placed with children unless it is known to be correctly socialized to them. One word of caution: Be certain that your child is not allowed to abuse or hurt his new pet during this sensitive socialization period. Such an adverse interaction could just as easily ruin their relationship for years to come. It is every parent's responsibility to teach their children that their cuddly new friend is not a toy, and that it needs to be handled with loving care.

Dogs for hunting or jogging

If you are in the market for a hunting dog, there's lots to choose from. Setters, pointers, and spaniels come in a wide variety of types and sizes, as do retrievers, who are notorious for their expert swimming abilities. For tracking larger game, one of the keen-scented hound breeds might be what you require. Regardless, read up on your favorite, and, if possible, confer with a local gun club before you buy to be sure that the instinctive strengths of that particular breed match your hunting needs.

On the other hand, if you are interested in an exercise or jogging companion, stick to those breeds or mixes with the size and aerobic capacity to keep up with your marathon pace! Recognize that proper command training beforehand is essential to the safety and well-being of you and your partner in fitness.

Breeding

Unless you plan to become (or are already) a professional dog breeder, don't purchase a dog with visions of large profits from the sale of future litters. Most novices find out the hard way that breeding operations, if done correctly and humanely (and they should always be), represent a considerable investment in time and money. If you are a beginner to the dog-breeding business, be sure to become an expert on the business and on the breed or breeds you want to propagate before your first purchase.

It is wise, if you are a beginner, to confine your efforts to one of the larger, more popular breeds, such as golden retrievers or Labradors, versus those more exotic, delicate strains, such as Shar Peis and Dandie Dinmont terriers. In general, you'll be rewarded with larger litters and less problems with *dystocia* (difficult or complicated birthing). In addition, the more popular the breed, the greater the demand will be for your puppies, resulting in greater financial rewards.

But beware: When selecting your initial breeding stock, closely scrutinize the pedigree of the dog's parents. All that it takes is one genetic defect to appear in one or more of the offspring, and your reputation as a breeder could be ruined! (For more information about breeding, see chapter 3.)

AKC competition

For many, the pleasure of dog ownership is compounded by the thrill of competition in the show ring. Thousands of events are sanctioned each year by the American Kennel Club (AKC), which, as an organization dedicated to the advancement of purebred dogs, registers over a million canines each year. Often, those motivated by these events are breeders as well, for earning the reputation of producing champion-quality canines is rewarding to the ego, not to mention the pocketbook (FIG.1-12).

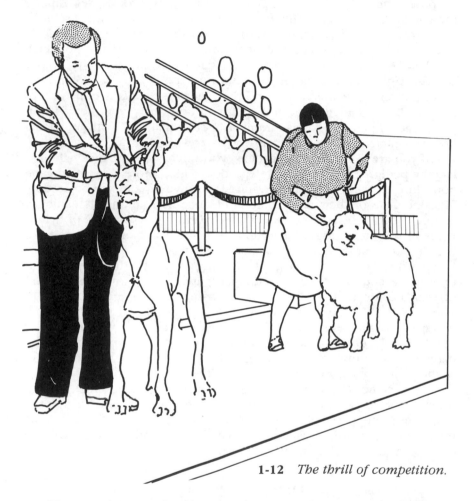

1-12   *The thrill of competition.*

If you are interested in showing dogs, many good books are available at the library or bookstore that can help you on your way. For a list of upcoming competitions, contact your local kennel club or the American Kennel Club, 51 Madison Ave., New York, NY 10010.

WHAT TYPE OF DOG DO YOU WANT?

The choice of your new dog's pedigree is entirely up to you. If you choose to go the purebred route, expect to pay more up front for your purchase. In addition, you run greater risk of facing congenital problems inherent to that particular breed or pedigree. This risk can be minimized by being very cautious and prudent in your selection process.

The AKC has set standards for purebred dogs that are recognized in the United States, Canada, Mexico, and South America. For registration purposes, the AKC divides breeds into distinct groups or classes. Among these include the *Working Breeds* (Doberman pinscher, standard schnauzer, boxer), the *Terrier Breeds* (Welsh terrier, Manchester terrier, Airedale terrier), the *Sporting Breeds* (cocker spaniel, golden retriever, pointers), the *Non-Sporting Breeds* (chow chow, dalmatian, poodle), the *Hound Breeds* (Afghan hound, beagle, dachshund), the *Toy Breeds* (Shih Tzu, Yorkshire terrier, Pomeranian), and the *Herding Breeds* (German shepherd, collie, Old English sheep dog). If you don't have your heart set on any breed in particular, there are many books that deal with individual breed characteristics that can help you narrow the field.

If you are like many dog fanciers, you might be less finicky about a lengthy pedigree and instead prefer a dog with a more diversified gene pool. In fact, there are some advantages to owning a mixed-breed dog. First, because of their diluted, colorful ancestries, mongrels exhibit a unique genetic phenomenon known as *hybrid vigor*. Because of hybrid vigor, mixed-breed dogs as a group tend to be healthier overall and live longer than their purebred parents or cousins.

Another obvious advantage of choosing a hybrid is that they cost less to purchase and to produce than do their papered pals. Because there are no standards or rules to follow when choosing a mixed-breed, it is best to ask yourself, "What type of purebred breed(s) do I like best?" Look in the newspapers or in pet stores for crosses that contain one or more of your purebred selections. In many instances, the origins or make-ups of the parents are unknown, yet you can usually guess the genetic background of the pooch by anatomic features or by its behavior.

For instance, let's say you notice that its ears stand erect, yet are folded halfway. There is a good chance that this mystery breed is part terrier. Does it enjoy lounging around in its water dish? It could have some retriever blood within. Chances are, your particular mixed-breed will be a cross between one or more of the top-ten most popular breeds (see TABLE 1-1).

DO YOU WANT AN INDOOR OR OUTDOOR DOG?

When choosing a dog, consider carefully where it will live. All dogs, regardless of whether or not you plan to keep them outdoors 100% of the time, should be first trained as indoor dogs. Why? First of all, if the need ever arises, it is easier (and certainly more sanitary) to later convert a dog accustomed to the rules of the house into an outdoor one rather than vice-versa. Secondly, dogs raised as indoor dogs respond more favorably to training and have less behavioral problems than those who are perpetu-

Table 1-1   The 10 Most Popular Dog Breeds

1   Cocker spaniel
2   Labrador retriever
3   Poodle
4   Golden retriever
5   Rottweiler
6   German shepherd
7   Chow chow
8   Dachshund
9   Beagle
10   Miniature schnauzer

Source: American Kennel Club 1990

ally banished to the backyard from day one. The reason: Dogs crave the attention and company of people, and, in most instances, a backyard existence does not fulfill this need. Problem behaviors and disobedience frequently result from such discontent.

Excitability, size, and coat length are certainly three important considerations when deciding indoor or out. In general, the more excitable the dog, the more attention that dog will crave. Isolate an excitable dog in a backyard away from human contact, and you are just begging for bark-filled nights and yards full of holes. At the same time, selecting a large dog for a house pet and failing to housetrain or command-train it properly could lead to some very interesting events. If you are not willing to devote the time to this, you should select a smaller breed of dog, primarily to limit the damage that is going to be done to your carpet and furniture!

Depending on the type of climate you live in, hair coat length becomes an important factor to consider when deciding indoor vs. outdoor (FIG. 1-13). In colder climates, dogs with long coats and dense under-

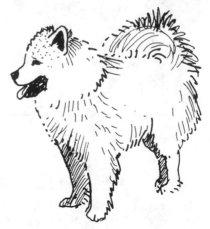

1-13   *Consider breed and coat length when deciding whether your new dog is to be kept indoors or outdoors.*

coats brave the outdoor chill much better than their short-haired counterparts. Conversely, dogs like the Siberian husky and chow chow can have a difficult time in the southern heat due to their overabundance of fur. If you live in a warm climate, plan on making that chow chow an indoor dog.

In addition, long hair coats traditionally take more time and effort to keep clean and looking nice. Consequently, if breeds with these types of coats are kept outdoors, they need to be groomed for at least 15 minutes daily to prevent tangling and matting and to keep the skin healthy (FIG. 1-14). Are you willing to devote this time each day? If not, select one with a shorter coat that is easier to maintain.

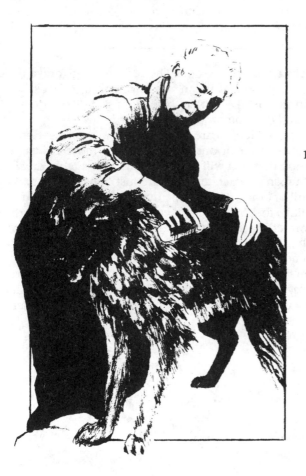

1-14 *Long-haired dogs should be groomed on a regular basis, particularly if they are kept outdoors.*

HOW WILL YOUR NEW
DOG AFFECT EXISTING PETS?

Are there other pets in your household already? Jealousies or incompatibilities could arise which need to be anticipated before the new dog is brought home. Household cats can have a particular aversion to such additions to the family.

Another important question to ask yourself if you already own a dog is, "Has it ever been socialized to other dogs?" If your existing dog is the type that attacks anything that barks or moves on four legs, it might have a big problem with your new arrival. These unsocialized dogs (and even some that are properly socialized) might refuse to accept another dog into its territory. In fact, if you try to force the issue, you often find that you have a pitched battle on your hands.

Any newcomers should be gradually introduced to the old timers, a day at a time. Keep your new dog in a separate room or yard, allowing interactions to take place only under your direct supervision. These gradual encounters should eventually help break the ice between the two and help establish a social pecking order within your furry family.

ARE YOU WILLING TO BE A RESPONSIBLE PET OWNER?

By nature, dogs are pack animals, and they crave attention from their human pack members (FIG. 1-15). Certainly one of the easiest ways to upset a dog is to ignore it outright. In fact, this lack of owner attention underlies many of the problem behaviors seen in dogs. Regardless of whether you keep your dog indoors or out, consider how much quality time you'll be able to spend with it each day. If your projections are low, sometimes two dogs are better than one. The company one provides the other while you are away can be an effective substitute for your affections.

Another factor to consider is how much time you will have to devote towards training. I cannot stress enough how important this is to your future relationship with your dog. It is definitely one aspect of pet ownership that should never be neglected.

The financial aspect of pet ownership is a major consideration if you are in the market for a dog. The actual cost of owning a dog—including food, supplies, training, and veterinary care—easily exceeds $500 per year. Are you willing to accept financial responsibility for your pet's preventative health care or for treatment in an event of an injury or illness? If not, you are not ready for the responsibility of dog ownership.

FINDING THE RIGHT DOG

Once you've decided on a particular type or breed of dog, now is the time to start your search. Newspapers, pet stores, veterinary hospitals, and word of mouth are fruitful avenues for information. If you're not interested in a registered dog, check with the local humane society or animal shelter in your area. These are excellent places to start and are often jam-packed with mixed breed and purebred dogs alike, all eager to be adopted into happy homes. Usually, one can be yours to love for only a

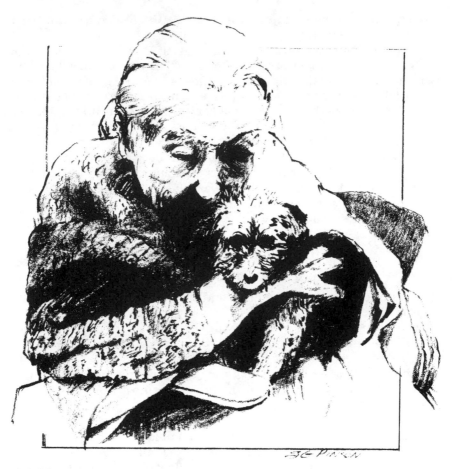

1-15 *By nature, dogs are pack animals, and they crave attention.*

nominal adoption fee. As an added benefit, you will feel good knowing that you've saved an unwanted pet from an uncertain future.

If a registered purebred fits your fancy, check pet stores or contact dog breeders within your area. Local veterinarians and groomers can often provide specific recommendations. Magazines catering to dog owners or outdoorsmen can also be excellent reference sources for purebred dogs and professional breeders. Finally, dog shows provide a means of giving you a first-hand glimpse of the cream of the crop and can give you the opportunity to meet prominent dog breeders in person.

Before you go shopping, do your homework. Find out what the going rate is for the particular breed you want. Beware of the small-time operator who advertises or offers you a great deal on a "registered" pup. These so-called "great-deals" can end up costing you more in the long run in medical bills and emotional drain. Where quality counts, stick with reputable breeders who can provide you with the complete pedigrees of both parents and references of satisfied clients. This rule holds true for pet-store purchases as well. Before buying from a pet store, ask where the pup came from and who the breeder was. Ask to see the pedigrees of both parents. Reputable pet stores will have all this information readily available for your inspection. And don't hesitate to ask for references from satisfied customers. If the store is unwilling or unable to divulge such information, look elsewhere.

Whatever you do, don't rush your decision. Remember: You are fixing to make a long-term commitment. Take your time, and pick out that special puppy or dog just right for you!

PRE-PURCHASE EXAM

Once you think you've finally found the perfect companion, now what? For starters, you want to be sure you are getting a healthy specimen. Be sure to inquire as to the dog's vaccination/deworming history. You might be told that all of the "shots" and dewormings have been given. This might be true, but don't hesitate to ask for dates and names of products used in writing. This list can then be reviewed for completeness by your veterinarian during the pre-purchase exam.

Even before your veterinarian becomes involved, perform your own pre-purchase exam on the prospect. It is easy to do on-site and will help illuminate many problems that might otherwise elude the untrained eye.

1. Environment For starters, take note of the surrounding environment the puppy or dog is being kept in. Does it look and smell clean, or is it filthy, with urine and feces lying all around? If the latter is true, you should begin to question the integrity of the seller.

Observe all of the pups and dogs in the litter or group. Do any appear sickly, depressed, or otherwise unhealthy? An infectious disease can have free run through such a congregation of canines, and it could be just beginning to rear its ugly head within the group.

2. Attitude Now focus your attention on the actual candidate. Start with overall attitude. Does it appear active and healthy, or is it lethargic and depressed? Are breathing problems evident? Does it seem friendly and outgoing to people and to the other dogs in the group, or does it seem shy and introverted?

Dogs destined to be good pets should take an instant fancy to people, and should outwardly show this affection. At the same time, avoid those individuals with overbearing and domineering personalities. Observe how your favorite treats other members of its group. Domineering personalities are usually quite evident. As a general rule, choose one that is middle of the road: Not too domineering, yet not too shy.

3. Skin and coat Once attitude and personality have been evaluated, check out the skin and coat. Any fleas or ticks present? How about any hair loss, scabs, or signs of infection? These could be indicators of diseases such as mange or ringworm, both of which can have *zoonotic* (diseases passed from pets to people) potential.

4. *Lumps, bumps, or swellings* Run your hands over the umbilical and *inguinal areas* (where the inner thighs connect with the abdominal wall). Notice any soft, fluctuant masses? These could be herniations, especially in young pups. Run you hands over the entire body surface, feeling for other types of lumps and bumps. Note the location of any.

Does the belly seem distended? If so, it could be full of food, or it could be full of worms. Check beneath the tail, looking for tapeworm segments (see chapter 7) and for evidence of diarrhea. Soiling on and around the hair in this area should tip you off to this.

5. *Other anatomical considerations* Observe leg conformation, and the way the puppy or dog walks and runs. Any obvious deformities and/or lameness should be noted.

In male dogs, check for descent of the testicles. Both testicles should be present at birth; if they aren't, be prepared to neuter at a later date, not only for health reasons, but also to prevent the passage of this inheritable trait to future generations.

6. *Head region* Now focus in on the head region. Using your eyes and your nose, check the ears for discharges or strong odors (usually a sign of infection). Both eyes should be free of matter, with no cloudiness or redness. Compare both eyes, making sure they are of the same size, and that the pupils are of the same diameter. Glance at the nose, noting any discharges or crustiness to it.

Finally, look into the mouth. The gums should be nice and pink; if whitish, the dog could be anemic. Notice any severe underbites/overbites, or any missing teeth (see chapter 11). Also look at the roof of the mouth. In young puppies, a cleft palate is a serious birth defect, and unless it is surgically corrected, it will lead to secondary aspiration pneumonia and death.

Consulting your veterinarian

Let's say you've completed the above exam and have found some potential problem areas. What do you do next? First of all, don't get discouraged. Many of these potential problem areas have quick, inexpensive solutions. This is where your veterinarian comes in handy.

Don't feel awkward asking the seller to pick up the tab for a professional pre-purchase exam by a veterinarian of your choice. Those sellers confident in the quality of their dogs should have no qualms about this. If they balk, a warning light should flash in your head. And don't get suckered into a "money-back" or "lifetime" guarantee on a pet as an alternative to a professional pre-purchase screen. Such a guarantee doesn't protect you against the emotional distress caused by returning a pet you've already grown fond of.

Follow your veterinarian's recommendations as to the purchase quality of the dog in question. If the one you have your heart set upon does have medical problems that can be easily corrected, talk to the seller and see if he or she won't deduct these costs from the purchase price. They aren't obligated but by character to do so; as a result, you must decide on your next move if they refuse or fail to compromise. The extra expense out of your own pocketbook might be worth it if you think you have truly found the dog of your dreams! You be the judge.

DOG-PROOFING YOUR HOME

If you choose to allow your new pet to have the run of the house, you should take steps to pet-proof your home.

For instance, be sure to keep all plants out of reach. Puppies love to chew on plants, and could harm themselves if they ingest a harmful ornamental variety. Dogs have an instinctive craving for vegetation, and puppies are no exception.

Also, keep electrical cords well out of reach. This might mean banishing your playful pet from certain areas of the house, but it is a minor inconvenience compared to a potentially fatal accident. Again, puppies love to chew, and electrical cords are mighty appetizing to this unrefined taste.

Puppies explore with their mouths, and will pick up anything. Keep everything that's not a toy picked up, including spare change. Pennies can have high levels of zinc in them, and could cause a severe gastroenteritis if swallowed. Also, be careful when putting out roach or rat poisons, keeping them out of reach of curious mouths.

Be sure to establish an area in the house that your dog can call its own. When you first get your dog home, begin by introducing it to its special room. Allow it 15 minutes or so to scope out the strange surroundings and to become familiar with the kennel or box you have provided for sleeping quarters.

Finally, consider confining nonsupervised puppies to noncarpeted floors until proper housetraining has been accomplished. Even so-called "stain-resistant" carpets might not uphold this claim after repeated bombardments.

Your dog's outdoor home

If you decide to keep your new dog outdoors, you need to provide it with a means of shelter from the inclement weather. True, some old-timers insist that back in their younger days, dogs did just fine by themselves braving the elements without any outside interference. Well, I'm not sure what "fine" means, but I know it doesn't mean "comfortable." Dogs get hot and cold just like we do, and they need a means of protection against extremes in the weather.

Dog houses   Your dog is entitled to a sturdy, well-insulated shelter. It should be positioned in a relatively shady area of the yard, away from major areas of activity. It should also be elevated a few inches off of the ground using bricks or wood to prevent flooding in the event of a rain storm (FIG. 1-16). Ideally, the shelter should have a short, enclosed porch that leads into the main house. This will help keep wind drafts out of the main living area. Finally, a ramp can be constructed to allow your dog easy access into its new abode.

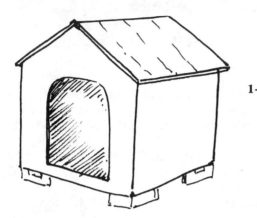

1-16 *Your outside dog should have a sturdy house that is elevated from the ground.*

If you want to build the house yourself, select sturdy building materials, remembering that they might need to be able to withstand constant punishment from teeth and claws. If you plan to use fiberglass insulation, make certain it remains well-contained and sealed within the walls and roof; such materials can wreak havoc on a dog's stomach if they are swallowed.

Dog runs   If you plan to confine your dog further to a pen or run, use a smooth concrete or quarry tile as flooring for the enclosure. Though such surfaces might not be the most comfortable for your pet, they are the most sanitary and easy to clean. Floors consisting of grass, sand, pebbles, or just plain dirt only serve to trap and accumulate filth and disease and should be avoided.

The fence surrounding the enclosure should be made of wire chain link and should be tall enough to prevent an acrobatic exit (FIG. 1-17). Exposed metal points from the chain links at the top of the fencing material should not be allowed to extend above the metal support bar, to prevent injuries if your dog does try to jump. The same rule applies for the bottom perimeter of the fence as well, just in case your dog tries to squeeze its way out.

NAMING AND INTRODUCING YOUR DOG

Naming your new pet should be fun and involve the entire family (FIG. 1-18). You can even find entire books dedicated to choosing the right

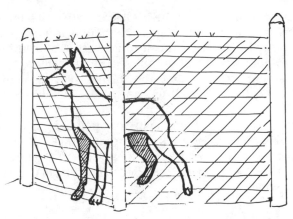

1-17 *Be sure that your dog's run or pen is safe for your dog and that it can't get out.*

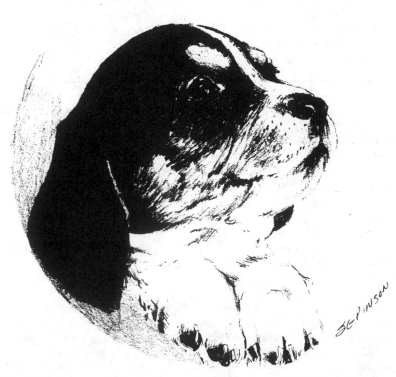

1-18 *Consider your dog's personality and its ability to distinguish commands when choosing its name.*

name for your dog at your favorite bookstore. Stick to names having two syllables; this will allow your dog easy differentiation between its name and those one-syllable commands it must learn. You can further set the name apart by adding a vowel sound to the end of it.

Be consistent when using the name. If you name your dog "Beverly," don't shorten it to "Bev." You'll only confuse your pet about its true identity.

You will want to do everything in your power to make your new dog feel comfortable and secure in its new home (TABLE 1-2). Your new dog's first encounters with the rest of your family are important. Be sure initial introductions, be they with children or other adults in the family, turn out to be positive ones.

Table 1-2   Supply Checklist for Your New Dog

☐ Food and water bowls	☐ Brush
☐ Dog (puppy) food	☐ Comb
☐ Collar	☐ Bed or dog house
☐ Leash	☐ Travel kennel
☐ Training lead/rope	☐ Nail trimmers
☐ Identification tag	☐ Ear cleanser
☐ City license (if required)	☐ Toothbrush/paste
☐ Proof of rabies vaccination	☐ Toys
☐ Heartworm preventative	☐ Flea control products

Carefully supervise child-pet interactions, and stress to your children the importance of gentle play and handling. Instruct your children and other adults on the proper way to pick up and hold a new puppy. Dogs should not be picked up solely by the front legs or by the neck; instead, the entire body should be picked up as one unit, with the hind end supported, not left dangling in mid-air.

If they had it their way, most children, and some adults for that matter, would love to play with a new puppy 24 hours out of the day. With children, you need to stress the importance of rest times for their new puppy after periods of play, and lay strict ground rules against disturbing it while in its special room or bed.

RULES OF PLAY

Puppies love to play. In fact, it's part of their normal behavioral development. However, realize that there is a right way to go about it and a wrong way. Follow specific "rules of play" to be sure yours is the correct approach (FIG. 1-19).

To begin, toys that you purchase for your dog to play with should be made of nylon, rawhide, or hard rubber. Of the three, the first is most

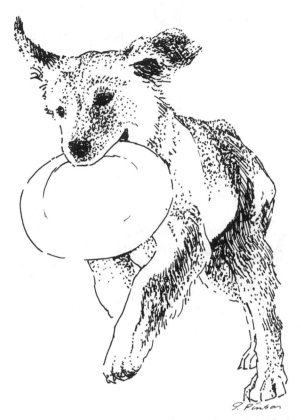

1-19   *Make sure your dog knows the rules of play.*

desirable because it is most easily digestible if swallowed. Rawhides are fine if the dog takes its time and chews slowly. For gulpers or engulfers who don't have time for chewing, avoid giving rawhides, which can cause serious stomach upset and sometimes intestinal blockages if swallowed whole. Also, some dogs have difficulty differentiating rawhide from refined leather, which could put your new pair of shoes in serious jeopardy!

Rubber chew toys should be solid so they cannot be ripped apart easily by sharp puppy teeth. Avoid chew toys with plastic "squeaks" in them. These can be easily extracted by most dogs and can be swallowed or aspirated. Regardless of the type of chew toy you pick, choose it as you would a toy for a child. If its design is such that it could cause suffocation or serious problems if swallowed, put it back and choose a safer one.

Avoid using old socks, shoes, or sweatshirts as substitute toys for your dog: It won't be able to tell the difference between old and new. Allow a puppy to chew on an old shoe or sweatshirt while still an adolescent, and you might find it fancying your expensive leather shoes or tennis warm-ups when it grows up.

It is OK to play hard with your puppy, but overt rough-housing should be avoided. If a play session progresses from a friendly romp to an all-out frontal assault, end it immediately. Your puppy needs to learn how to control its activity level to an intensity that is socially acceptable. Also, be sure your puppy gets time to rest after an especially active play period (FIG. 1-20).

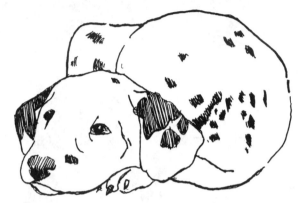

1-20   *Puppies need time to rest between play sessions.*

The same applies to chewing. It's perfectly natural for a puppy to want to explore its environment with its mouth. During play, there will be times when the pup will bite and nip; when this occurs, simply and strongly say no, and provide a chew toy as a substitute. In essence, what you want to tell your pup is that it is OK to use its mouth during play, just as long as it doesn't use it on people. You'll be surprised how quickly it will catch on.

TRAVELING WITH YOUR DOG

When transporting a dog by car, the comfort and safety of both driver and passenger must always be considered. Whether you are bringing your dog home for the first time, or simply taking it on a Sunday afternoon drive, keeping these rules in mind will make the ride easier and safer for the both of you.

For starters, when traveling by car, it is always recommended that pets be confined to travel carriers or kennels (FIG. 1-21). Not only will this help ease your pet's travel anxieties, but it will also ensure a safe trip for you. If your dog is too large to fit comfortably into one of these carriers, then the back seat will have to do. And to all truck owners, *never allow any dog to ride in the bed of a pickup truck unless it is confined to a carrier*. If you do, you are just asking for trouble!

Also, never allow your dog to hang its head out of an open car window while driving. Canines with long, floppy ears can easily suffer

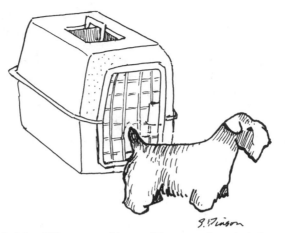

1-21   *When traveling with your dog, it is best to use a dog carrier or kennel.*

trauma to the ear flaps due to such wind resistance. Also, both ear and eye injuries from insects and flying road debris have been documented in dogs allowed such freedoms.

Regardless of trip length, keep the interior of your car well-vented and cool. Excited or nervous dogs forced to travel in hot, stuffy environments or ones filled with cigarette smoke are prime candidates for car sickness. Cigarette smoke in itself can be quite irritating to the eyes, nose, and mucous membranes of dogs, so if you have to smoke in the car, don't forget about your friend next to you. Crack the windows a bit!

Car exhaust fumes can also be nauseating to traveling canines. For this reason, don't leave a pet inside a parked car while it is still running. Instead, turn it off and crack the windows about a third of the way open. However, if external environmental temperatures exceed 80 degrees Fahrenheit, **never** leave a pet inside a parked car for more than five minutes, even with the windows partially opened. On sunny days, temperatures within the car can quickly rise to intolerable levels within minutes and predispose your pet to heat stroke.

If the car ride is going to be lengthy, be sure to take along plenty of water for your dog to drink. Dogs riding in automobiles have the potential to lose lots of body water through panting and can develop quite a thirst in a very short period of time. Keep water in the carrier itself, or plan water stops every couple of hours along the way. Freezing some water prior to the trip in the water bowl intended for the carrier provides a long-lasting source of water for those extra-long sojourns.

Finally, let's talk about motion sickness. If this becomes a problem in your dog, there are a few things you can do. First, when your pet gets car sick, observe whether there is food in the vomitus or if it is liquid? If food is present, be sure to withhold food before further travels. If, on the other hand, food is not present, try feeding your dog a small amount prior to the trip. For dogs with sensitive stomachs, this small portion of food is often all it takes to do the trick. If this doesn't work, an antihistamine, such as diphenhydramine—administered at a dose of 0.5 to 1 mg per pound thirty minutes before the trip—can be used.

For those dogs absolutely terrified of the car, actual tranquilization prescribed by your veterinarian might be needed. Though this should be used only as a last resort, it can be an effective tool for taking the edge off your phobic pooch and thereby make the ride much less stressful for everyone concerned.

2

Training Your Dog

PROPER TRAINING IS definitely the key to a happy owner-pet relationship. It establishes your dominance in the relationship between you and your pet right from the start, and it can help prevent many behavioral problems from rearing their ugly heads later on (FIG. 2-1). Not only that, solid training can also keep your pet out of troublesome situations that could threaten both its health and yours!

There is one characteristic exhibited by every good trainer: Patience. Without this virtue, you're going to have a tough time teaching your dog anything. You need to set aside time each day for training and resolve to stick to it. Keep in mind that it will only be a temporary dip into your time budget. After all, the more time you devote from the start, the quicker and more satisfying the results will be.

What about training school? Is it worth the time and the money? The answer is yes if it will motivate you to devote the time for the task at hand. You still have to be physically present during the training (you can't have someone else train your dog, then expect your star pupil to respond likewise to your commands). If you choose this route, enroll in an active-participation class in which an instructor directs you and your dog through the training session. However, keep in mind that such a class doesn't relieve you of your homework duties. You still need to practice with your dog daily on your home turf.

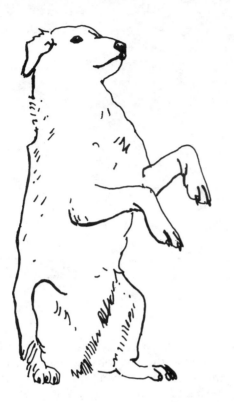

2-1   *Effective training is an excellent way to make your relationship with your dog a good one.*

MAIN PRINCIPLES OF TRAINING

For any training method to be effective, it needs to follow some basic principles to ensure its success. These principles include the following:

Consistency and repetition

The magic success formula for all training endeavors is derived from two key concepts: consistency and repetition. Consistency provides the building block; repetition is the mortar that holds the program together. Without the two, you might as well try to teach a rock how to fetch. The results will be the same!

Consistency means more than just using the same commands over and over again. It also means using the same praises and corrections each time and keeping your voice tones consistently unique for each. Even your body language and postures used during training should remain uniform between sessions. As trivial as it might seem, dogs pick up on stuff like that. Dogs like routine, so stick to it. Train at the same hour each day and for the same length of time for each daily session.

Just as important as consistency to a dog's learning process is repetition. Repeating an action or training drill over and over will help reinforce the positive response you are looking for. Furthermore, the more repetition you implement into training, the leaner and more refined your dog's learned skills become.

Verbal praise

Use verbal praise instead of physical pain in your training sessions. Dogs, especially puppies, should always be rewarded for a job well done with lots of praise and attention on your part. Food treats are fine as a reward supplement, but they should never replace verbal compliments. Punishment might be warranted if your puppy or dog purposely disobeys a command or commits an undesirable act, but this should never take the form of physical punishment. There are alternative means, each of which is just as—if not more—effective than physical violence.

Punishment

Dogs can be reprimanded effectively with a sharp verbal *no*, or by banishment into confinement. Water sprayers, air horns, a can full of coins, hand-held vacuums, and so on can all be used to gain your dog's attention quickly without inflicting any pain.

If you decide to use punishment, be sure to institute it quickly, preferably within 5 seconds of the act. If you don't apply it before this time expires, any punishment thereafter might satisfy your anger, but it will serve no useful training purpose.

Don't extend your punishment past a few seconds. Prolonged exhortations will only confuse your pet (and cause you to lose your voice).

Never use your pet's name during the negative reinforcement. If you do, your dog might start to associate its name with the bad act and eventually become a basket-case whenever the name is called. Reserve this name-calling for positive, happy experiences only.

If you do punish, always follow it up shortly thereafter with a command or drill that will lead to a praise situation. Always end your time together on a positive note, and you'll make progress in leaps and bounds. Remember: The most effective training programs rely more on praise than they do on punishment. For some dogs, simply withholding praise from them is punishment enough to modify their behavior! By rewarding your dog for doing good rather than punishing it for doing bad, you'll get the positive results you are looking for much faster.

Get the whole family involved

In any training situation, always try to involve all members of the family whenever possible. An all-too-common scenario is one in which a dog all but ignores the commands of anyone but the one person who trained it. To avoid this, get the whole family involved. Just be sure to remain consistent within the family with regards to the training methods and commands used.

Use short commands

All verbal commands you employ need to be kept short and sweet. Using slightly different voice tones for each command will help to prevent confusion. If verbal punishment is to be used, make certain that it is totally different in tone and in presentation than the other commands.

Start young

Always start your dog's training at an early age. While it is true that certain advanced training techniques can be best taught at around 6 months of age, basic training, including house training, should be started as early as 8 weeks of age. If basic command training is not taught this early in life, bad habits arise later on—some of which can put a damper on future training efforts.

Keep training sessions short

Try to keep the training sessions short and to the point. For puppies 8 to 12 weeks of age, devoting 10 minutes two to three times daily will yield excellent results. As your dog matures, the length of each of these sessions can increase. Let your dog's attitude be your judge. If it seems bored, indifferent, or has become totally unruly, you have probably exceeded its attention span.

End on a good note

Always end your training session on a good note. Doing so is very constructive in terms of your pet's mental development, and effectively sets the tone for the next session.

ASSERTING YOUR DOMINANCE

One of the purposes of training a dog is to establish your dominance in the relationship right from the start. Your dog needs to realize who's boss, who's the head of the pack. There are five effective ways to assert this dominance during your training sessions:

1. Control your dog's neck region

It is especially important in the early stages of training to maintain control of your dog's head region. The collar and leash were originally developed with this principle in mind. Dogs are naturally very protective of their neck regions because in a fight, this is often the first area that the opponent will attack. You've probably noticed that most dogs will lower their heads in a menacing gesture if they feel threatened. Puppies grasped by the scruff of the neck by their mother become limp in willful submission.

Along these same lines, when your dog allows you to put a collar on and maneuver it with leash pressure applied to the neck region, it is in essence submitting itself to your dominant position. Your dog's new collar should be fitted in such a way that you can easily slip your fingers between the buckled collar and the neck. If you've got a puppy, make certain to check the collar's tightness on a weekly basis. As the puppy grows, the collar must be loosened periodically to accommodate for an increasing neck diameter.

2. Apply pressure along the back region

As you will see, this concept comes in handy when teaching your dog to sit or lie down. In nature, a dog will assert its dominance over another by mounting the other's back with his forelegs. By applying direct pressure on the back (i.e., teaching to sit) or by simply petting your dog along the neck and back region, you are essentially doing the same.

3. Stay calm and relaxed during training

Dogs can sense nervousness or distress on your part. Overbearing and stubborn dogs might try to take advantage of such a situation and refuse to submit to authority. Exhibit an air of confidence and control around your dog, and it will catch on quickly that you mean business.

4. Avoid physical or painful punishments

As mentioned before, physical punishment really serves no purpose and could trigger retaliatory attacks, which will completely ruin your training sessions, not to mention the relationship you have with your dog. In addition, such behavior on your part could turn your pet into a sniveling, cowering mass of extreme submissiveness, which also will hinder your training efforts. Your dog will be more worried about when the next punishment is coming rather than about learning the training material.

5. Establish direct eye contact

Always establish and maintain direct eye contact with your dog when giving a command. Don't be the first to look away, for the one who wins the stare-down wins the dominance play. Use caution: An overly-aggressive dog might refuse to submit, and can see your eye contact as a direct challenge. For these dogs, it's best to avoid the confrontation.

BASIC COMMANDS

Some tools of the trade you'll want to acquire to assist you in your training efforts include a leash, a 20- to 25-foot rope with an end clasp attached, and a sturdy collar (FIG. 2-2). You can substitute a harness if you desire.

    If you decide to use a *slip* or *choke* chain collar, read the package directions and make certain you know how to use it properly; otherwise, serious damage to your pet's neck and trachea could result. Because misuse of this device is not at all uncommon, many veterinarians recommend not using them unless you are a seasoned trainer.

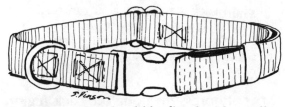

2-2 *Every dog should be fitted with a collar.*

If your new puppy or dog is not used to wearing a collar or leash, you must get it accustomed to these two devices prior to any training efforts (FIG. 2-3). Start by placing a collar on your dog and allowing it to wear the collar for several days.

Once you think your dog feels fairly comfortable wearing it, attach a leash to the clasp and allow your dog to walk around with the leash dragging behind. To protect your dog from snagging furniture or other objects

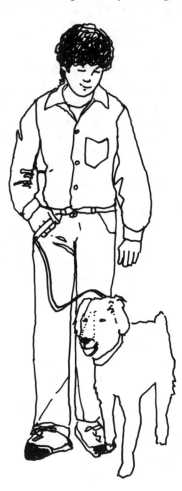

2-3 *Dogs should be taught to walk on a leash.*

with the leash and hurting itself, be sure you are around during these sessions. After about six to eight sessions of 15 minutes apiece, your dog should feel more comfortable with its leather attachment, and should be ready for further instruction.

Heel

The first command you will teach your four-legged student is to *heel*, or walk at your side. To begin, position yourself on your dog's left side facing forward, with its shoulders even with your knee. Take up the slack on the leash to prevent your dog from becoming entangled in the excess. Now, in simultaneous fashion, give a quick forward tug on the lead, say "Heel," and start forward with your left foot leading. As your dog follows, keep its head level and in control using the leash. Start out by going five yards at a time, then stopping to praise for a job well done.

If your dog refuses to move on your initial command, go back to the starting line and set up again. This time, if needed, follow the quick tug with an encouraging pull on the lead to initiate movement. Start and stop frequently, praising as you go. As your dog starts to catch on, increase the distances you go each time. The ultimate goal is to have your dog walk briskly by your side until a command is given to do otherwise.

If your dog gets too far out in front of you, a quick, backward tug on the lead should be used to correct the discrepancy. For those trainees more interested in playing rather than learning, stop the training session temporarily and ignore or confine your dog until it settles down. Don't scold or show any other acknowledgement of its antics. It will soon learn that you mean business!

Once your dog has become comfortable walking in straight lines by your side, take it through some turns both to the right and to the left. During the turns, your dog's shoulder should remain aligned with your knee.

Stop

Once your dog responds favorably to the *heel* command, it is time to teach it the command *stop*. With your dog heeling at your side, give a sharp backward tug on the leash as you say "Stop," and halt your forward motion. (The verbal exclamation differentiates this from the backward tug used to slow an overenergetic heeler.) Hold the stop for three seconds, then praise heavily for compliance. Afterwards, have your dog heel again, and repeat the process over and over again, gradually increasing the amount of time you require your pet to remain still.

Sit and stay

From the stop position, pull upwards on your dog's lead while at the same time saying "Sit," and pushing down on its rear end to achieve the sitting position (FIG. 2-4A). Have your dog maintain this posture for a good five seconds, then break into a heel. Gradually increase the sitting interval as your training progresses.

When your dog has learned what *sit* and *stop* means, it's time to teach the *stay* command. This is where your 20-foot rope lead comes in handy. Attach this to the collar and walk your dog again through the heel,

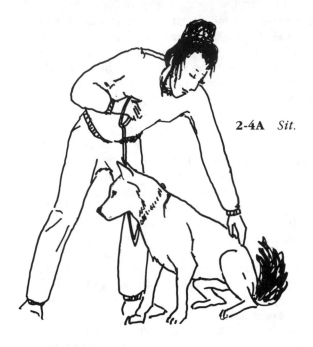

2-4A *Sit.*

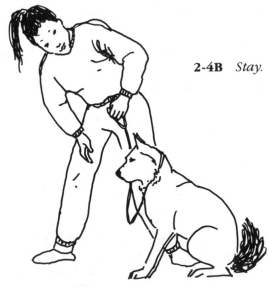

2-4B *Stay.*

stop and sit routine. Once your dog is in the sitting position, place your left hand in front of its face and say "Stay" (FIG. 2-4B). Now slowly walk about 3 yards away, keeping your back to your dog. If it breaks its stay when you move, reel your dog in with the lead, and make it immediately return to the sitting position. Then try again.

If the student stays in place even for three seconds after you walk away, heap on bundles of praise. If your dog still disobeys, walk it through your Heel-Stop-Sit routine a few more times before returning to the stay command. As your pet starts to catch on, you can begin increasing the distances you go and time intervals for it to stay put.

Other commands

Heel, Stop, Sit, and Stay are the basic obedience commands that you should start teaching your dog as early as 8 weeks of age. Two other commands that are optional, yet could come in handy in certain instances, are *down* and *here* or *come*.

Down should be included as an adjunct to the Sit command. After your dog is in the sitting position, say the command while applying downwards pressure with your free hand to its shoulder region. Note the difference from the Sit command, in which downwards pressure is applied to the hind end. Now, from this Down position, you can proceed into the Stay drill.

Come can be taught as a continuation of the Stay command. With your dog sitting or lying at rope's length, give a quick forward tug while saying the command "come." Again, use the lead to reel it in if it decides to wander off-track. Praise your dog only if it comes directly to you from its original starting position.

When, and only when, your dog has mastered these commands and responds to them consistently, you can discard the leash or lead (FIG. 2-5). For off-leash training, repeat each command sequence as before. Don't hesitate to put the lead back on if your dog fails to cooperate. At first, it is especially important to hold all off-leash training sessions in enclosed areas or fenced-in yards to prevent you star pupil from unexpectedly dashing off into the sunset!

HOUSEBREAKING YOUR PUPPY

Puppies should be housebroken at an early age, preferably when they are as close to 8 weeks old as possible. The reason: This is when that period of stable learning begins in adolescent dogs. Their minds are wide open to suggestions, and they learn quite quickly at this early stage.

If you expect to yield successful results, you must be willing to devote some quality time to the task. Recognize that puppies have four fairly predictable elimination times:

1. After waking
2. After eating

3. After exercising
4. Just before retiring for the night.

Make a concerted effort to take your puppy outside during these times, and every 3 – 4 hours in between. When you suspect that it has to go, take your pup outside and set it down in the grass. If elimination takes place, praise your puppy like it was going out of style and then take it immediately back inside the house. By doing so, you will help it associate the act with the location.

If a minute passes and your puppy hasn't gone, take it back inside. Don't leave it outside to play or roam. Puppies trained in this manner soon realize that their primary business for being outside is to eliminate, not to play.

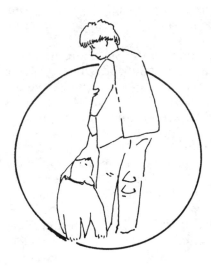
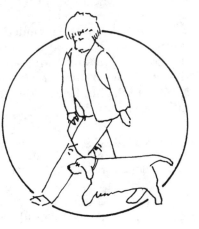
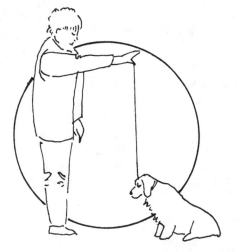

2-5 *Before attempting off-leash training, be sure your dog has mastered all commands while on the leash.*

What happens if you catch your puppy in mid-act? If this is the case, go ahead and rush it outside. The puppy might finish what it started before you make it out, but don't get upset (FIG. 2-6). Again, praise it immensely for going outside, then bring it immediately back inside.

If you happen to miss an accident altogether, don't fret. If you saw it happen, a verbal punishment is warranted. On the other hand, if you didn't see it happen, do nothing. Simply try to be more attentive next time.

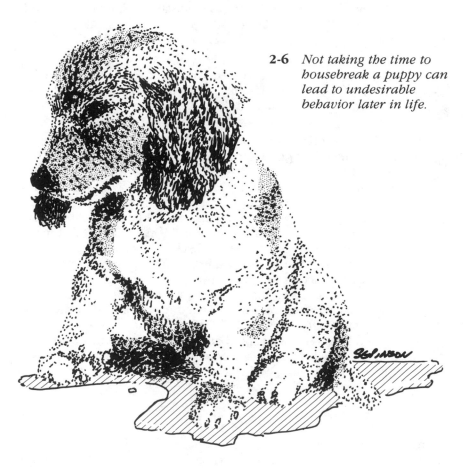

2-6 *Not taking the time to housebreak a puppy can lead to undesirable behavior later in life.*

Other housetraining tips to remember

1. Be sure your puppy is current on its vaccines (since it will be going outside) and is free of intestinal parasites. The latter is very important because the presence of worms in the intestinal tract will cause unpredictable urges to eliminate.

2. Always use lots of praise; never physically punish. Again, remember that puppies crave praise, and if they don't get it, they feel

punished. Give plenty of praise when they deserve it; hold it back when they don't. And don't ever stick a puppy's nose in its eliminations as a form of punishment. For some reason, this type of punishment is still quite popular among pet owners, even though it serves no useful purpose. In fact, if you really want to adversely affect your puppy's mental development, this is a good way to do it.

3. When verbal punishment is indicated, avoid associating your puppy's name with the reprimand. For instance, simply say "Bad," instead of "Bad dog, Sugar." By leaving names out of it, the puppy won't associate its name with the bad behavior.

4. Establish a regular feeding schedule for your new puppy. Feed no more than twice daily, and take your puppy outside after it finishes each meal. It is preferable to feed the evening portion before 6:00 p.m. in order to help reduce the number of overnight accidents that can occur otherwise.

5. To help prevent accidents, keep your puppy in a confined area at night. It should be puppy-proofed and have a floor that won't be damaged if a slip-up occurs. Utility rooms and half-bathrooms work well for this purpose, as do kitchens if they can be cornered off. If an accident occurs during the night or while you are away, don't get upset. As your training sessions progress, you'll find that this will become less and less of a problem. A natural instinct of any canine is to keep its "den" clean. These inherent instincts, combined with correct housetraining efforts on your part, will help fuel the success of your training efforts.

6. When cleaning up an accident, always use an odor neutralizer rather than a deodorizer on the area in question. These are available at most pet stores, and will usually eliminate any lingering scents that can lure your pet back to the same spot. Avoid using ammonia-based cleaners, since ammonia is a normal component of canine urine. Such cleaners might serve to attract, rather than to repel, repeat offenders.

SOCIALIZING YOUR DOG

There is no doubt that the most important time in a new puppy's life is between the ages of 3 – 12 weeks. During this short time span, a puppy will learn who it is, who you are, and who and what all of those other living, moving beings surrounding it are as well. This stage of life in which such vital learning takes place is called the *socialization period.*

If for some reason a puppy fails to be properly introduced to members of its own species or to other species (including children) during this time, then there is a good chance that it will not recognize these individuals for what they are, and it might even show aggressiveness toward them. For example, dogs intended for breeding purposes must be properly socialized to members of their own species if they are to be expected to breed with one of these members.

Good examples of dogs not properly socialized include those that show extreme aggressiveness to men only, or those aggressive to children (FIG. 2-7). Dogs see people as two species: Big people and little people. As a result, while a dog might recognize an adult person as the one who feeds and commands it, it might not recognize a small toddler as one who commands the same respect if the pet is never properly socialized to small children.

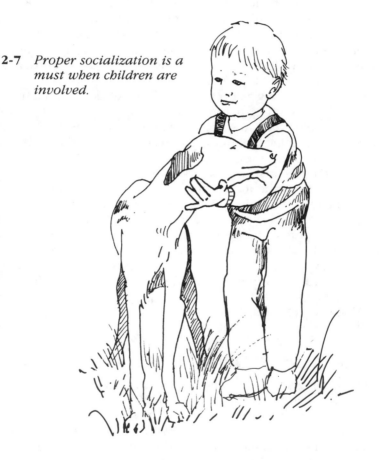

2-7 *Proper socialization is a must when children are involved.*

Some dogs aren't fit for any type of human interaction at all; these have absolutely no socialization whatsoever and could pose a threat to humans.

Another good example of the socialization principle is the relationship between dogs and cats. Dogs and cats that grow up together from the start can be best of buddies, whereas those that don't can exhibit marked animosity towards one another.

Improper or negative socialization is even worse than no socialization at all. Any traumatic experience or physical punishment that occurs between 8 and 12 weeks of age could permanently scar a dog's personality to a specific group or species for life. For instance, many dogs who fear men were actually abused by a member of this sex during the most important socialization time. This is one reason why all physical punishment should be avoided during this time in your puppy's life. Such activity could damage the pup's relationship with the punisher for life!

The existence of this socialization period is one reason you should steer towards puppies less than 12 weeks of age when choosing a new companion. If you don't, you have no way of knowing whether or not proper socialization has taken place, and you might be faced with behavioral problems in the future. Socializing a puppy is not that difficult if you remember to keep all interactions positive and to guard against any physically and emotionally traumatic situations.

Before introducing a new puppy to other dogs, it should have had at least two of its series of puppy shots and be current on its vaccination schedule to be on the safe side. In addition, always be sure that the animals you are planning to introduce it to are socialized themselves, or else you could have a fine mess on your hands.

A weekend excursion to a park or a neighborhood stroll with your puppy are some of the more opportune ways of introducing it to other animals and to other adults and children. Allow children to freely interact with your pup, but again, be sure none gets too rough. For best results, you should repeat such encounters throughout your pup's socialization period. And by all means praise your puppy for good behavior during these interactions. It will leave a lasting impression upon its personality!

One word of caution: Socialization, like any personality skill, can eventually be lost if it is not reinforced periodically. As a result, even as your dog matures, don't just discard those trips to the park or strolls through the neighborhood. Remember: You have to use it or lose it!

SOLVING PROBLEM BEHAVIORS IN DOGS

When searching for the leading cause of dissatisfaction among dog owners, problem behaviors top the list. Each year, a multitude of dogs are abandoned, evicted from their homes, or even put to sleep because of annoying behavioral activity. However, by understanding and employing special training techniques and/or therapy to correct such vices, and by allowing the veterinarian to play an active role in the treatment process, dog owners can often avert such drastic actions.

Separation anxiety

It has happened to many of us: we leave the house, sometimes for only a few minutes, and our "best friend" proceeds to chew up the furniture, bark or howl, and/or eliminate in the house. If your dog behaves this way when you leave your home, it is probably suffering from the behavioral problem known as *separation anxiety.* (**Note:** Medical problems can be the cause of such aberrant behavior; these must be ruled out before you can safely assume that you are dealing with a case of separation anxiety.) Before you can successfully treat a problem like separation anxiety, it is helpful to know what causes it.

Dogs are considered *pack animals;* that is, they prefer to associate in groups rather than (as cats prefer) individually (FIG. 2-8). Because you are its owner, a dog will consider you part of its "pack" and will constantly want to associate with you. When you leave, you separate the dog from its pack, and this creates separation anxiety. This behavior will be magnified if you tend to make a big fuss over the dog when leaving or returning to the house.

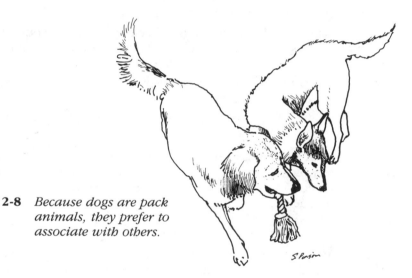

2-8 *Because dogs are pack animals, they prefer to associate with others.*

Furthermore, certain other behavioral patterns on your part, such as rattling the car keys or turning off the TV, can be associated to your departure by the dog.

When treating separation anxiety, you must remember that it is an instinctive behavior; it is not due to disobedience and/or lack of training. As a result, overt punishment for the act tends to be unrewarding. In fact, most of these dogs would rather be punished than left alone! The key to treating this problem lies in planning short term departures, then gradually lengthening them until your dog gets used to your absence.

Begin by stepping out of the house for only a few seconds (10-15) at a time for the first few days or so. Hopefully this will allow your dog to get used to you leaving the house, since it will learn that you will return soon. Vary your training session times throughout the day. The idea is to gradually lengthen your leaves of absences (30 seconds at first, then one minute, then two minutes, etc.) so that your departures soon become second nature to the dog.

Points to keep in mind when attempting to break your dog of this annoying behavior are as follows:

1. Don't make a fuss over your dog within five to ten minutes of your arrival to or departure from home. This will help keep the excitement and anxiety levels in your dog to a minimum.

2. During your training sessions, try not to re-enter the house while the dog is performing the undesirable act. Doing so will only serve to positively re-enforce the dog to repeat the act. (I realize that this last statement will be difficult to enforce in those cases where the dog chews or eliminates in the house, but do the best you can. Dogs that are properly house trained in the first place rarely have problems with the latter behavior.)

3. Eliminate any behavior that might key the dog off to your departure, such as rattling your car keys, saying goodbye to your dog, etc.

4. For the dog that likes to chew a lot, provide plenty of nylon chew bones to occupy its time.

5. Leaving the TV or radio on while you're gone seems to help in some cases.

In severe cases, veterinarians can prescribe anti-anxiety medications such as amitriptyline HCl to help assist in the treatment of separation anxiety. As a result, don't hesitate to contact your veterinarian if you are having difficulty in quelling your dog's separation anxiety problem.

Excessive (nuisance) barking

Let's face it: Some dogs just love to hear their own voice! Unfortunately, most owners and their neighbors hardly share the same adoration. There is no doubt that dogs who bark excessively are a nuisance and can cause many a sleepless night. For this reason, correction of the problem is essential to your sanity, and that of those who live around you.

A dog might bark excessively for a number of reasons. The first is boredom. Dogs that have nothing else to do might simply "sing" to themselves to whittle time away.

Another potential cause is territoriality. Outsiders, be they human or animal, will almost always elicit a bark out of a dog if threatening to encroach upon its territory. Dogs can also use the bark indiscriminately as a communique to other outsiders to stay away. In such instances, the barking episode can be started by the far-off bay of a neighborhood dog or the slamming of a car door down the street.

Separation anxiety is another common source of nuisance barking. Some dogs have it so bad that they bark continuously when their owner leaves them, even for a short period of time. Often, the owner will return home to find their dog hoarse from so much barking.

When attempting to break your dog of this annoying habit, always remember this one principle: If you respond to your dog's barking fit by yelling at it or physically punishing it, you are going to make the problem worse. Dogs that are isolated from their owners for most of the day don't give a darn about what kind of attention they receive (positive or negative), just as long as they get some. Dogs that are barking out of boredom or from separation anxiety will soon learn that their action will eventually get them attention, and they'll keep doing it. Even dogs that are barking for other reasons can catch on quickly that such vocalization will bring them a bonus of attention from their beloved owners. As a result, no matter how mad you get, or how sleepy you are, avoid the urge to punish your dog for its barking.

The first thing you need to determine is whether or not separation anxiety has anything to do with the problem. If you think it does, treat it as you would any other case of separation anxiety. In many cases, dogs that bark for this reason alone can be broken of their habit.

Keep in mind, though, that the source of the barking might involve a combination of the factors, not just one. Dogs that bark for reasons other than separation anxiety need to be given more attention throughout the day. A dog that tends to bark through the night should be given plenty of exercise in the evening to encourage a good night's sleep. A nylon or rawhide chew bone can be helpful at diverting its attention. Feeding its daily ration later in the evening can also promote contentment for the night.

For those times of the day or night that the barking seems the worst, consider bringing the dog inside the house or inside of the garage. This, of course, will not be possible if you failed to instruct your dog as to the ways of household living when it was a puppy. Nevertheless, removing your dog from its primary territory and/or increasing the amount of contact with members of its pack can help curb the urge to bark. Also, if possible, encourage your neighbors to keep their pets indoors at night, since nighttime roaming activities of neighborhood dogs and cats is a major cause of nuisance barking.

House soiling

It has happened to all of us—the early morning encounter in the family room, the unexpected (or sometimes expected) surprise awaiting our arrival home from work—house soiling. It is a dirty habit, yet one that millions of pet owners have to put up with each day. In many of these cases, the problem had an origin traceable to puppyhood; for others, it results from developmental behavioral and/or health problems. Regardless of the cause, pet owners can take an active role in most cases to minimize or stop completely this annoying habit (FIG. 2-9).

To date, I have yet to meet a dog owner who has truly broken a dog

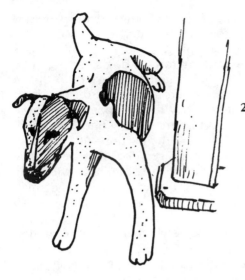

2-9 *House-soiling can have several different causes. Be sure you know what's causing your dog's bad behavior before you try to correct it.*

of this nasty habit by sticking the dog's face and nose in the excrement after the fact. Not only is this action illogical and inappropriate for the particular situation, some dogs might even enjoy it! Instead, pet owners need to take a more rational approach to identifying the cause and solving the problem. To do that, you must first determine what is causing it.

Lack of or improper housetraining   The most common case of house soiling is undoubtedly the failure of owners to housetrain the dog properly during its puppyhood. Many pet owners can't understand why their puppy has no problems going on newspaper, but just can't get the knack of going outside when the newspapers aren't there. They seem to forget that, to a puppy, newspaper and grass are two different surfaces with different smells. To paper-train a puppy and then expect it to switch easily to another type of surface is asking a lot, and this often presents a confusing dilemma to the poor creature.

Puppies need to be taught right from the start to go outside to use the bathroom instead of encouraging them to go within the confines of the home. At the same time, dogs who are going to be spending a great deal of time outside need to be housetrained as puppies, just in case the need arises later in life to bring them indoors for whatever reason. If you miss this chance when it is a puppy, you could be in for trouble later on.

Contrary to popular opinion, you *can* teach an old dog new tricks—it just takes longer! With older canines that weren't properly potty-trained, proceed with training or re-training as you would with a puppy. Along with lots of praise, a favorite treat or snack can also be used to reinforce desired behavior. For those times you can't be at home to monitor indoor activity, confine your dog to a travel kennel or small bathroom, since dogs are less likely to have premeditated accidents in such confined spaces. Just be reasonable as to the amount of time you make it wait between eliminations.

Separation anxiety Inappropriate elimination activity can, as do many other behavioral problems, result from separation anxiety. Dogs left on their own will often become frustrated and soil one or more parts of the house as a result. Some dogs can even become downright spiteful, targeting favorite furniture, bedding, and, if kept in the garage, even the roofs of automobiles. If your dog is truly suffering from separation anxiety, most of its adverse behavior will occur within 15 to 20 minutes after you leave. This predictability can assist in efforts to correct the problem. Treat as you would any other case of separation anxiety.

Desire to delineate territory The desire to delineate territory is another reason why a dog may choose to urinate (or sometimes defecate) indiscriminately. Certainly, intact (non-neutered) male dogs are more prone to this instinctive activity. Dogs have such a keen sense of smell that the mere presence of a canine trespasser around the perimeter of the home can set off a urine-marking binge. Owners who move into pre-owned homes often find out the hard way that the previous owners had a poorly trained or highly territorial pet housed within.

Neutering your pet may or may not help solve this problem, depending upon its age. In many older males, house soiling has become more habit than hormonal, and neutering does little to prevent it.

Use of a pet odor neutralizer on the carpet and baseboards is warranted if you suspect that a previous occupant is to blame. Use of fencing or dog repellent (not poison!) around the perimeter of the house may also help keep conceited urine-markers away from your house.

Extremely submissive behavior Extremely submissive behavior often results in a cowering dog that urinates whenever anyone approaches. This type of adverse elimination is not uncommon in dogs that have been abused as puppies or have spent most of their growing years in a kennel or pound facility.

Management of such behavior depends on your actions and body language when approaching or greeting such a dog. Try to avoid direct eye contact and sudden physical contact with such dogs, for by doing so, you can send them into immediate submissiveness. If you've been gone from the house for a while, avoid sudden and exuberant greetings when you get home. By ignoring your dog initially, you'll lower its excitement level, reduce the immediate threat, and give no reason to urinate.

One trick you can try is to immediately and casually walk over to your dog's food bowl and place some food or treats in it. The idea is to distract your dog's attention away from the excitement of your arrival and create a more comfortable, pleasing situation for it. Once you've been home a while, then you can (and should) offer more of your attention.

Illness or disease Finally, don't forget that some diseases or illnesses can cause a pet to urinate or defecate indiscriminately. For instance, dogs that tend to defecate inside the house should be checked for internal parasites. Diets with increased fiber content can also increase the amount of trips your pet will need to take outdoors.

Certainly if the stools are semi-formed or seem to differ in normal appearance or consistency, an underlying medical reason should be suspected. In addition, some of the conditions that can increase the frequency and/or urge to urinate include urinary tract infections, kidney disease, and diabetes mellitus. *Urinary incontinence,* characterized by the inability of the bladder to retain urine due to poor sphincter function, is not at all uncommon in older dogs. For these reasons, don't just assume that your dog's soiling problem is purely mental; have the potential medical causes ruled out first, then you can concentrate on behavioral modification.

Just a word about cleaning up an accident in the house. When using cleaners to tackle the initial mess, be sure they don't contain ammonia. Dog urine contains a form of ammonia, and such products might actually attract your dog back to the same spot later on. Along this same line, after the initial manual cleaning, your next job is to ensure that residual smell doesn't attract your pet back to the same spot. To accomplish this, you need to employ a product containing odor neutralizers specifically targeted for dogs. These products are available in grocery stores or your favorite pet supply. Deodorizers should not be used, for it is virtually impossible to completely mask or hide a scent from the keen canine nose.

Digging

Although separation anxiety can cause digging episodes, on the average, its influence is much less than with other problem behaviors. Instead, sheer boredom and/or instinctive behavior are the two common states of mind that compel a dog to dig (FIG. 2-10). Dogs with nothing else to do might opt for yard excavation just to help pass the time or to use up extra energy.

The urge to break out of confinement and roam the neighborhood can also compel a dog to start digging.

Finally, as you might have already experienced, many like to bury personal items such as bones or toys only for exhumation at a later date. Such instinctive behavior, though aggravating, can hardly be considered abnormal, and so it is difficult to eliminate totally.

Increasing your dog's daily dose of exercise could be just what the doctor ordered to help resolve its boredom and release any pent-up energy.

Diverting the attention of a chronic digger is another plausible treatment approach; for instance, some troublesome cases have responded very well to the addition of another canine playmate. Rawhide bones and other chewing devices can also be used as attention-grabbers, but only if they don't end up underground themselves.

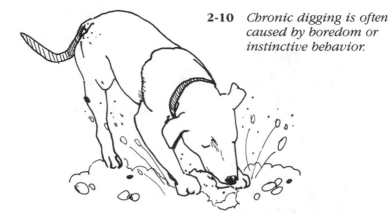

2-10 *Chronic digging is often caused by boredom or instinctive behavior.*

If most of the digging occurs at night, overnight confinement to the garage might be the answer to spare your yard from the ravages of claws. Finally, if you haven't already done it, neutering can sometimes help snuff out the strong urge to dig in those dogs wanting to roam.

Destructive chewing

Many canines are literally "in the doghouse" with their owners because of their destructive chewing (FIG. 2-11). No one wants a pet who seeks and destroys any inanimate object it can sink its teeth into. However, the urgency for dealing with such behavior is not just governed by personal property damage. Many of these chewers also end up in veterinary hospitals suffering from gastroenteritis or intestinal obstructions. Hence, such adverse activity can cost more than just replacement value of furniture or fixtures. It can even sometimes cost the life of a pet!

In puppies, destructive chewing can easily arise from lack of training and from inappropriate selection of toys. Although puppies are naturally going to explore their environment with their mouths, they need to learn at an early age what is and isn't acceptable to chew on. Solid command training is a must in these little guys.

Avoid providing normal household items such as old shoes, T-shirts, or sweatshirts as toys to play with. Puppies can't tell the difference between an old shoe and a new shoe, and they might decide to try out your new pair for a snack one afternoon!

Objects that repeatedly bear the brunt of your dog's teeth should be placed as far out of reach as possible. For furniture or immovable objects, special pet repellents should be sprayed around their perimeters to make a mischievous puppy think twice before sinking its teeth into the item.

In young to middle-aged adults, separation anxiety is probably the number one cause of destructive chewing. As with all cases of separation anxiety and the behavior it provokes, correction of the problem should focus on correction of the anxiety attack.

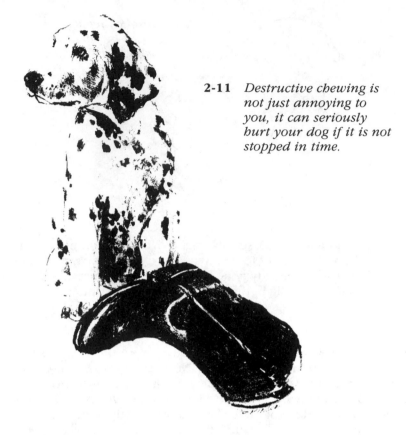

2-11 *Destructive chewing is not just annoying to you, it can seriously hurt your dog if it is not stopped in time.*

Finally, as with problem barking, boredom plays a leading role in destructive chewing in some adult dogs. If you think this might be the case, increase your dog's daily activity, and provide it with plenty of alternative targets, such as rawhides or nylon bones, on which to chew. Divert its attention, and most likely it will divert its chewing.

Jumping

Talk about annoying behavior! Jumping is right up there with house soiling and incessant barking. "Jumpers," as I shall call them, are usually right there at the door when visitors call and have this innate tendency to spoil a perfectly cordial greeting. After all, nobody wants a dog with dirty paws to jump on their nice, clean clothes, especially if the dog weighs 50 pounds or more! (FIG. 2-11).

This is one problem behavior that should never be allowed to gain a firm root in a puppy. Probably the best way to assure this is through strict command training, starting at an early age. Until it learns its commands, be sure to discourage your dog from jumping on you or family members when the occasion arises.

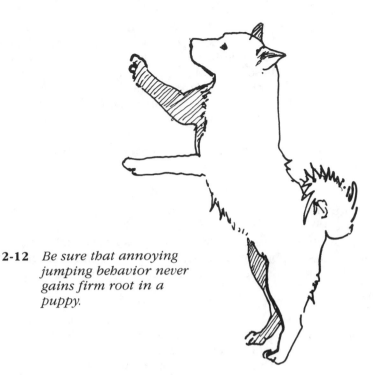

2-12   *Be sure that annoying jumping behavior never gains firm root in a puppy.*

When it does jump at or on you, quickly push it off with your hands and shout "No." Or, as an alternative, flex your knee and make sudden, but gentle contact with its chest, making it fall backwards. If your puppy insists on coming back for more, invoke the harshest punishment of all: Isolation. Most puppies will soon catch on quickly.

For adult dogs who never learned their manners, a refresher course in command training is the most effective method of curing the chronic jumper. Sometimes dogs that jump are simply trying to tell their owners that they want more attention. In such cases, a few more moments of your time devoted to your furry friend each day is an important adjunct to therapy.

Fear of loud noises

Fear induced by loud noises such as thunder or gunshots can be a common cause of aberrant behavior in canines. Many people argue that because of the ultra-sensitive hearing of dogs, pain induced by the noise might play a bigger role than fear itself. Regardless of the reason, when confronted with the disturbing sound, these dogs often become hysterical and quite destructive in their attempts to escape. Many might even injure themselves or their owners in the process.

In the case of the hunting dog who fears the gunshot, training sessions involving repeated, gradual increases in exposure to the adverse stimulus is an effective method of ridding the dog of its fear.

For dogs that fear the sound of thunder, fireworks, etc., owners must avoid direct attempts at comforting the pet, since by doing so would be indirectly rewarding the undesirable behavior. If your dog is the type that comes unglued in these situations, consider letting it "ride out the storm" in a travel kennel. In addition, playing a radio or television loudly in the vicinity of your pet might help muffle some of the fearful sounds, as well as make your canine feel more at ease.

Your veterinarian can prescribe anti-anxiety medications for your dog if it has an exceptional fear of loud noises. In any event, these should be used sparingly and only as needed.

Aggressiveness

Of all of the undesirable behaviors a dog can exhibit, this one is certainly the most disturbing and the most unacceptable. Aggressiveness can be directed toward other dogs or toward other species, including humans. Certainly dogs harboring an uncontrollable inherent aggressiveness towards the latter pose special problems to their owners in terms of liability as well.

Dominance   This certainly plays an important role in canine aggressiveness. Some dogs refuse to submit to authority and will lash out at anyone or anything that attempts to exert such. In many instances, these dogs were not properly socialized and/or trained when they were young. In others, sex hormones, namely testosterone, can exert a strong influence as well.

Treatment for such aggressiveness consists of a return to basic command and obedience training. In addition, exercises designed to re-establish dominance should be performed as well (see "Asserting Your Dominance" in this chapter). If the aggression is directed towards a particular person in general, he/she too should be included in these exercises. Remember: Extreme caution and a good, strong muzzle are both advised before any attempts at such dominance assertion are made! For domineering male dogs, neutering is recommended prior to any attempts at re-training.

Fear and pain   These are the two other common causes of aggressive showings in canines. If a dog feels threatened or overwhelmingly fearful, it naturally experiences a "fight or flight" syndrome—and might choose the former option over the latter, depending upon how it perceives its situation. In addition, dogs have been known to naturally lash out in fear at humans or other animals upon being startled, or more frequently, when they are experiencing pain. For this reason, sudden aggressive changes in personality with or without other signs of illness warrant a complete check-up by your veterinarian.

Treating fear-induced aggression is aimed at reducing the threat you or others pose to your pet. If fear aggression is induced by some outside stimulus, such as thunder, then proper restraint and isolation is recommended while the stimulus lasts. If a dog suffers from a vision or hearing deficit, attempts should be made to capture the dog's attention prior to approach. Also, remember that not only is physical punishment a useless tool for training, it can in itself lead to natural, aggressive backlashes due to pain (and fear). This is just one more reason why such punishment should be avoided. Finally, for those dogs suffering from injuries or illnesses, owners should remember to always approach and handle them with caution, for although they might not mean to, they could exhibit aggressive tendencies due to the pain associated with the disease.

Territorial defense   Dogs, male or female, will certainly defend that property they deem theirs, and they might not hesitate to fight for it. Territorial aggressiveness toward unwelcome animals or people is not uncommon, as any utility-meter reader would attest to! Such aggressive behavior can be just as easily sparked by a perceived encroachment while the dog is eating, or while it is playing with its favorite toy. Many bite wounds to humans have been inflicted because of such actions.

Again, a return to the basics of command training with or without neutering should help curb some of the territorial aggressiveness that might be exhibited by some canines. In those instances where dogs exhibit aggressiveness toward other dogs they deem a threat to their territory, neutering will usually help in the majority of the cases.

Certainly, showing some respect for a dog's "private property" (toys, bowls, etc.) and its eating privacy is a common-sense way to avoid this type of aggressive behavior. It is important to impress this concept upon children, too, because they are often the most frequent violators of this rule. If a dog seems particularly possessive over toys, bones, etc., then excessive sources of the problem should be reduced by eliminating all but one or two of the items. Also, consider feeding the dog in an isolated area of the house away from disturbances.

"Mean streaks"   Finally, certain breeds and canine family lines can have inherent "mean streaks" in them. For instance, chow chows are notorious among veterinary circles for their aggressiveness towards strangers. In addition, pit bull terriers, because of their ancestral breeding, pose a real threat to any other dog that might cross their paths.

In many instances, this inherent aggressiveness can be harnessed by way of proper socialization and by strict command training. Neutering can be of assistance as well in select cases.

The best treatment for most types of aggression is prevention. By adhering to the principles of proper socialization and by proper command training, most behavioral problems related to aggressiveness can be avoided altogether.

However, for any dog exhibiting aggressiveness, a thorough physical examination and consultation with a veterinarian is warranted. Ruling out underlying medical causes is certainly one reason for this; the other is that your veterinarian might choose to prescribe medications to assist in re-training efforts or as a direct attempt to curb the psychological aspects of your dog's aggressiveness. Human anti-anxiety medications such as ami-triptyline HCl and diazepam are being used more and more in veterinary medicine as effective replacements for progestin hormonal therapy (which can have many unpleasant side-effects) to help assist in the correc-tion of many behavioral problems, including aggressiveness. Ask your veterinarian for more details.

3

Preventative
Health Care

WHEN IT COMES TO HEALTH, dogs are just like people. Some
will go through their entire life without any health problems along the
way; others just seem to be prone to every illness that comes along. A
number of factors play a role in the susceptibility of dogs to illness,
including genetics, environment, nutrition, immune system competence,
and, very importantly, the extent of preventative health care provided to
them by their owners. In fact, for a dog that is genetically prone to illness,
this latter factor can do wonders to help counteract some of these inherent effects. Unfortunately, many pet owners fail to realize the importance
of preventative health care; as a result, their pet can ultimately pay the
price on down the line.

AT-HOME PHYSICAL EXAM

Do you worry about your dog's health even when it appears healthy?
Your veterinarian can ensure that your dog is thriving by performing a
thorough check-up, but what can you do between visits? Dogs cannot
verbalize their discomforts, and people often worry that they'll miss the
early signs of illness. If you learn to examine your dog at home, you can
have that all-important peace of mind between visits to the vet (FIG. 3-1).

During your next visit to the veterinarian, he or she will probably
begin with an examination of your dog. Watch how your veterinarian performs the exam and ask to participate in the process. Discuss your desire
to supplement the vet's exams with at-home checks that you will make.
Your veterinarian should be pleased with your desire to provide such
attention to your dog's health and should be happy to help develop your

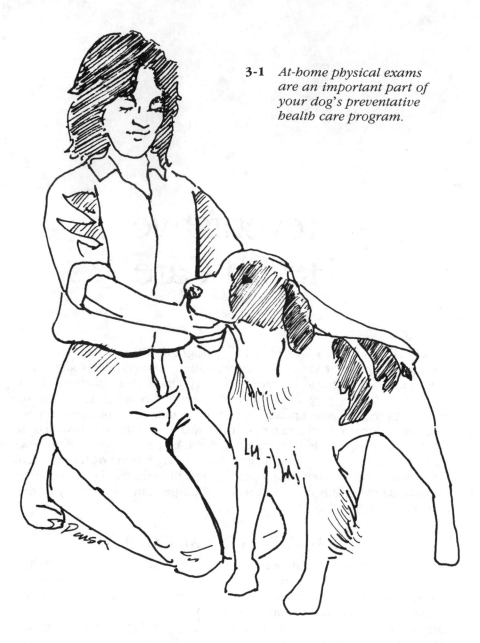

3-1 *At-home physical exams are an important part of your dog's preventative health care program.*

skills. Your teamwork will provide the consistent attention to details that could prevent a tragedy.

At-home examinations are no substitute for a veterinary checkup, but doing them might one day give you a jump on treating a minor or serious condition. For convenience, these exams can be combined with regular grooming sessions.

1. Observe your dog

Begin the exam by looking at your pet from a distance. Observe its general appearance. Watch it move back and forth. An abnormal gait with or without limping or lameness could indicate such things as nervous system problems or musculoskeletal disorders.

Does your dog stand erect and relaxed? Abnormal postures such as a wide stance with the neck extended could indicate breathing difficulties. An arching of the back could mean abdominal pain. Note the position of your dog's head. A tilted head is often characteristic of a dog with an irritated or infected ear canal. A droopy head can signify depression and overall malaise.

What is your pet's attitude? Is it alert, active, and friendly, or is it lethargic, depressed, or aggressive? Sick or injured animals, especially those in pain, often show aggressive behaviors; therefore, handle them with caution. Keep in mind that normal behavior will vary among individuals and in different situations.

2. Look for warning signs

Dog owners should be aware of certain clinical signs that could signify serious problems in their pets. Weakness, shortness of breath, coughing, labored breathing, and, as mentioned before, a wide-based stance could be the first signs of heart or lung problems. A pale blue or purple tongue (except in chow chows and Shar Peis) can signify poor tissue oxygenation, often the result of circulation problems.

If your dog shows any of these signs, obtain a pulse by gently pressing your fingers against the upper, inner portion of a back leg. Normal resting pulse for a dog ranges from 60 to 120 beats per minute. Abnormal pulse or any other signs of heart or lung problems should be reported to your veterinarian immediately.

A dog's normal temperature ranges from 99.5 to 102.2 degrees Fahrenheit. Excited or nervous animals might have elevated temperatures, but a temperature due to excitement should rarely exceed 103.5 degrees Fahrenheit (TABLE 3-1). To take your dog's temperature, lubricate the tip of a non-glass rectal thermometer. Insert the thermometer into the dog's rectum and hold it in place for at least two minutes (FIG. 3-2). If the reading is higher than 103.5, you should call your veterinarian for advice.

Get into the habit of weighing your dog every three months and record your readings. Unexplained weight loss or weight gain that is greater than 5 pounds or a pattern of continual loss or gain should prompt you to contact your veterinarian. Such fluctuations or patterns could signify some underlying medical disorder. Dogs that are 8 years old or older should be weighed monthly, and unexplained changes of 3 pounds in either direction should be reported to the veterinarian. Additionally, keep in mind that obesity poses the same health hazards in animals that it does in humans. An overweight dog should be put on a diet and an exercise program formulated and prescribed by its veterinarian.

**Table 3-1   Causes of Elevated
Body Temperature in Dogs**

Fear/excitement
High environmental temperature
Exercise
Infection
Tissue inflammation/trauma
Autoimmune disease
Cancer
Drug reactions
Endocrine disorders

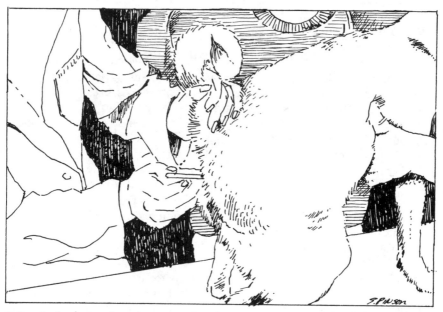

3-2 *A dog's temperature can be obtained using a rectal thermometer.*

3. Inspect the head region

You need a systematic approach to performing the examination. To prevent forgetting a checkpoint, I suggest beginning at the head and working toward the rear. As you go, check each body part for abnormalities. A check sheet might be helpful to remind you of each stop, and it will be an excellent record for future reference.

Eyes   Any abnormalities you detect involving the eyes should be brought to the attention of your veterinarian. Redness, cloudiness, discharge (or drainage), squinting, or unequal pupil sizes could signify trouble.

The whites of the eyes, called *scleras,* should be just that—white. If inflammation is present, the scleras are usually reddened. Yellow-tinged scleras or *jaundice* can indicate the presence of a serious condition, such as liver failure. A thorough exam by a veterinarian is the only way to determine the cause of the jaundice.

Check the dog's eyelids. Be sure that no foreign objects are irritating the surfaces of the eyes. Constant, untreated irritation can lead to corneal injuries, which are extremely painful. Eyelid abnormalities require immediate veterinary attention to prevent significant eye damage.

Ears   Inspect the ears and note any foul smell or discharge. A black or brown discharge could signify an ear mite infestation or a yeast infection. A yellowish, creamy discharge means a bacterial infection is present. Other signs of ear disease include constant scratching at the ears, head shaking, and head tilting.

Ear problems are very common in dogs; therefore, every dog owner should implement a program of ear cleaning to prevent problems from arising. Never insert anything directly into the ear canal. This would only push debris further into the canal and increase the chance of injury to the eardrum.

Excessive hair growth in or around the ear canal traps moisture and can lead to the development of infections. Breeds such as poodles, cocker spaniels, maltese, bearded collies, and other long-hairs should receive special attention. Hair should be plucked, not cut, from the ear canal. Cut hair can lodge in the ear and is very difficult to remove. A veterinarian or a qualified groomer can remove the accumulated hair, or he/she can instruct you in how to keep the area clean.

Nostrils   Discharges from the nostrils should alert you to a potential disease condition. Clear discharges usually indicate either allergies or viral infections. A green, mucoid discharge usually indicates bacterial infection, which can be caused by a variety of diseases or a lodged foreign object. Bleeding from the nose could result from trauma, tumors, foreign bodies, or a blood-clotting disorder. Look for tumors and ulcerations affecting the mucous membranes of the nose.

Mouth   Gently open your dog's mouth by grasping the head and upper jaw with one hand, tilting the head back and using your other hand to separate the jaws. The gums and mucous membranes should be moist and pink (except in animals with very dark pigmentation). Pale, dry mucous membranes might indicate anemia, dehydration, or shock.

If you suspect a problem, obtain a capillary refill time by pressing on the upper gum with your index finger. The gum region under your finger should turn white. Release the pressure and the gum should return to a pink color within two seconds. If it takes longer, consult your veterinarian.

Check the mouth for swollen gums, foreign objects, tumors, ulcerations and sores. A foul odor can be caused by excessive dental tartar or by tumors or infections in the mouth.

4. Inspect the body

Run your hands over your pet's entire body and feel for lumps or bumps. If you have any doubt that what you feel is normal, you should consult your veterinarian. Lumps can indicate abscesses, enlarged lymph nodes, cysts, foreign bodies, soft tissue swellings (such as hernias and bruises), or cancer. The earlier you detect and treat cancer, the better the chances are for complete recovery.

Be sure to check for lumps in the mammary region of female dogs (especially if they have not been spayed). The testicles of intact male dogs should be examined for abnormal swellings and masses. Intact males and females run higher risks of developing cancer than neutered animals. Why not have your pets neutered to prevent the development of these kinds of cancers?

Note any discharges from the reproductive tract. Not all discharges are abnormal, but some discharges indicate the presence of infections. For example, female dogs coming into heat can have a normal bloody discharge lasting up to two weeks.

Often an odor is the first noticeable sign of infection of the reproductive tract. If you have any doubt whether or not a discharge is normal, consult your veterinarian.

The stomach, intestines, liver, pancreas, spleen, and kidneys are all located in the abdomen. Gently press both sides of the abdomen just behind the ribcage (**Note:** some dogs immediately become tense when you do this). Slowly work your way to the hip region, gently pressing as you go. Unless you have training in *palpation* (the act of feeling with the hand to determine physical diagnosis), don't expect to know what you are feeling. The purpose of doing this is to detect any swelling, tenderness, pain, or obvious masses involving the abdomen. If you feel anything strange, seek the opinion of your veterinarian.

5. Inspect the skin and coat

Evaluate your dog's skin and coat carefully. Signs of skin problems include hair loss, itchiness, redness, oiliness, scaliness, crustiness, and infection. Look closely for parasites, such as fleas and ticks, which can cause a number of skin problems. Poor nutrition or a metabolic disorder (abnormal thyroid function, for example) can cause a dog's hair to become dull and lifeless. The potential causes of skin and coat disorders are so numerous that all such disorders should be diagnosed by a veterinarian. Your early-warning system will enable you to treat the problems before they become serious.

6. Other observations

If your dog scoots its rear across the floor, continually bites at its rear end, or has difficulty defecating, it could have impacted anal sacs. These sacs are located at the 4 o'clock and 8 o'clock positions beneath the dog's anus. Normally, the dog will empty the sacs when it defecates. Occasionally, fluid can accumulate in the sacs, and they will need to be manually expressed by you, your vet, or your dog's groomer. If left untreated, the sacs could become infected, and could eventually rupture.

If your dog struggles against your attempts to examine it, you might consider re-evaluating your obedience training. If you dislike struggling with your pet, so will your veterinarian. A dog that will not cooperate during the examination is difficult to diagnose and treat. This regular examination should teach your dog to stand still, which in itself is a very valuable lesson.

Remember: Your veterinarian wants to keep your dog in top condition, but he or she cannot do it alone. With a little practice, you should be able to complete your physical examination in a matter of minutes. This is time well spent when your dog's health is at stake (TABLE 3-2).

Table 3-2 Congential Disorders Detectable on a Veterinary Physical Examination

Eyes	Microphthalmia (small eyes)
	Juvenile cataracts
	Entropion/ectropion
	Glaucoma
	Prolapsed third eyelid
	Tear duct deformity
Ears	Congenital deafness
Nervous system	Epilepsy
	Brain underdevelopment
	Hydrocephalus
	Intervertebral disc disease
Integument	Umbilical hernia
	Inguinal hernia
	Demodectic mange
Digestive system	Cleft palate
	Abnormal dentition
	Overbite/underbite
Musculoskeletal system	Dwarfism
	Joint dislocations
	Patellar luxation
Cardiovascular system	Blood clotting disorders
	Heart murmurs
	Anemia
Respiratory system	Collapsed trachea
Reproductive system	Retained testicles

THE ABCs OF IMMUNITY

The theory behind vaccinating any pet is to provide artificial exposure to certain disease-causing organisms, thereby priming the body's immune system before actual exposure occurs. Doing so will allow for a rapid, effective immune response if this exposure does happen, without the lag time associated with a first exposure.

If their mother has been properly vaccinated prior to pregnancy, most puppies receive protective antibodies from their mother through nursing, primarily during the first 24 hours of life. These "passive" antibodies are important, since the immune system of a neonate under 6 weeks of age is incapable of mounting an effective response to any *antigen* (foreign organism or substance). Around 8 weeks of age, levels of these antibodies begin to taper off, leaving the puppy to fend for itself.

If a puppy who still has adequate levels of passive antibodies present in its system gets immunized, the vaccination will be rendered ineffective. For this reason, initial vaccinations for such puppies are usually given around 8 weeks of age, when levels of passive antibodies are low. Vaccination as early as 6 weeks of age is indicated in those instances where the mother was not current on her vaccinations, or if lack of passive antibody absorption is a possibility (i.e., inadequate nursing during the first hours of life).

Those diseases that are routinely vaccinated against in dogs include:

○ Distemper
○ Parvovirus
○ Coronavirus
○ Canine infectious hepatitis
○ Leptospirosis
○ Parainfluenza
○ Canine cough complex
○ Rabies

The first six vaccinations above are normally given as one injection; the rabies vaccine as a separate injection; and the canine cough complex vaccine administered via *intranasal* drops (through the nose). In addition to these vaccines, a new, injectible vaccine against Lyme disease has become available and could come into routine use if the prevalence of this *zoonotic* disease (a disease that can be secondarily transmitted to humans) continues to increase.

Depending on the type of vaccination that is being given, booster immunizations are normally given every three weeks until the puppy reaches 16 weeks of age. The purpose of this schedule is to successively prime the immune response to a higher level with each booster given to ensure that, if the puppy ever meets up with one of the diseases in question, a maximum immune response will be achieved.

Certain vaccines, such as rabies vaccines and some canine cough vaccines, do not require these three-week boosters to be given since they purportedly prime the immune system to its maximum with a single dose. However, a booster is a good idea if contact with the disease is suspected or confirmed.

Canines should receive boosters on all vaccines on a yearly basis. This is to ensure that the immune system stays alert and ready at all times. There are some exceptions, such as three-year rabies vaccines, but as a general rule, an annual protocol should be followed. Timely booster vaccinations are exceptionally important as dogs get older, since an aging immune system needs constant priming for maximum effectiveness.

Don't be lulled into a false sense of security simply because your pet is "never around other dogs" or "never goes outside." If its immune system is caught loafing by some disease you track in on your shoe, the results could be disastrous.

For more information regarding immune system function, see chapter 8.

STAYING AHEAD OF INTERNAL PARASITES

Left undetected, intestinal parasites can rob your dog of much-needed nutrients, can cause severe gastrointestinal upset, and can predispose it to secondary disease, such as parvovirus (see chapter 6). Internal parasites are widespread throughout the canine population. In fact, it is estimated that over 90% of puppies are born with some form of intestinal parasitism. To make matters worse, many internal parasites of dogs are also classified as zoonotic diseases; that is, they can be directly communicable to

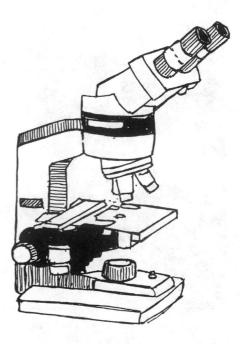

3-3   *Detection is the first line of defense against internal parasites.*

humans, especially children. As a result, controlling canine intestinal parasites is a vital part of any preventative health care program.

Management of canine intestinal worms should begin when a puppy is as young as 3 weeks of age. At this age, these puppies can harbor immature hookworms and roundworms without any evidence of eggs shed in the stool. Puppies should receive medications for these parasites at 3, 6, and 9 weeks of age, regardless of whether or not eggs are detected in the pup's stool.

Stool examinations

More treatments might be necessary for those puppies found to be actually harboring worms. Stool examinations on these pups should be performed by a veterinarian at 6, 9, and 12 weeks of age to ensure that your pet is indeed free of these parasites and is not shedding their eggs into the environment.

Frequent stool checks such as these will also assist in the detection of two other common intestinal parasites, tapeworms and coccidia. The latter parasite can especially cause severe gastroenteritis and sometimes even neurological problems in puppies if left undetected and untreated.

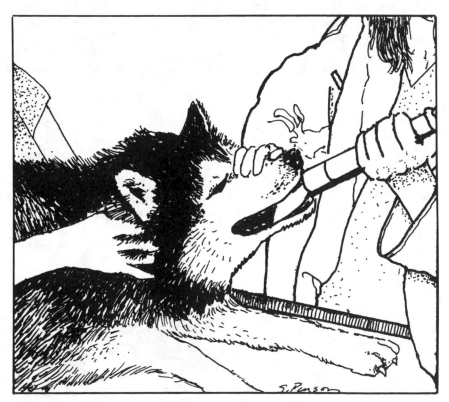

3-4 *Administering a dewormer.*

Although dogs over 1 year of age do not necessarily need routine dewormings, their stools should be examined for parasite eggs on at least an annual basis. Stool exams should also be conducted on any ill animal, regardless of clinical signs. Even when the illness is not directly caused by the worms, their mere presence and effect on the host's immune system can exacerbate any disease, regardless of cause.

Sanitary environment

Aside from routine stool checks, good environmental sanitation is another way to lessen the impact of canine intestinal parasites. Many parasite eggs that are shed into the environment via feces take days of sitting in the sunlight or in other favorable environmental conditions before becoming infective to other dogs. As a result, keeping all fecal matter, be it your dog's or an unwelcome visitor's, cleaned up out of your dog's environment on a daily basis is very effective way of protecting your pet (and yourself) from these worms.

For more detailed information on control of internal parasites in dogs, refer to the specific sections in chapter 6.

STAYING AHEAD OF EXTERNAL PARASITES

Much confusion exists in the proper approaches to external parasite control and prevention in dogs. Many different approved product types are available for external parasite control. The key to successful control is choosing and properly using the products that provide the best possible results for the specific external parasite and environment involved.

External parasites such as fleas and ticks require both environmental and pet treatment to eliminate them. Consultation with your veterinarian and exterminator is advised in choosing insecticidal products that are safe and effective for your specific needs (FIG. 3-5).

PRECAUTION: Young animals are ultra-sensitive to insecticides. Use only products recommended by your veterinarian on any pet under four months of age.

Control measures for the individual parasites include the following:

Insecticidal sprays

Flea and tick sprays are available in both liquid and aerosol forms. Sprays containing natural chemicals called *pyrethrins,* derived from chrysanthemums, are the preferred products over others for flea control due to their safety and efficacy if used properly. The big advantage of natural pyrethrins is that they are relatively safe for use on pets of all ages. The disadvantage is that they have poor residual flea-fighting activity, lasting only a day or so. Newer, synthetic pyrethrin products available on the market today have improved this residual activity while still maintaining a good safety margin.

If pyrethrin products are used, frequent spray application, both on

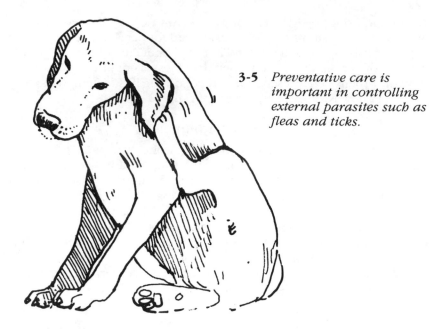

3-5   *Preventative care is important in controlling external parasites such as fleas and ticks.*

the dog and in its environment (bedding, carpet, etc.), is imperative for effective flea control (FIG. 3-6). In some instances, this means on a daily basis. Just be sure before doing so to check the label on the particular product you are using to confirm the safety of this practice. If you are in doubt, always follow label directions!

Remember to always wear hand protection anytime you are using any type of insecticidal product. Application of the spray should begin at the head with progression toward the rear and tail of the dog. The hair should be pulled forward with rubber-glove-protected fingers to ensure good penetration down to the skin. A light yet thorough application is desired.

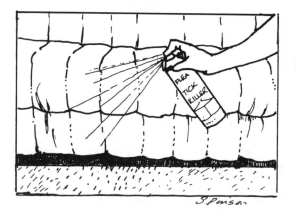

3-6   *Environmental control is a must in any flea-control program.*

Insecticidal powders

As with the sprays, pyrethrin-containing powders are preferred over others due to their low-toxicity potentials. Powders do not evaporate like liquid products and, therefore, under dry conditions, powders stay active on the hair and skin somewhat longer than sprays. Again, frequent application is required for best results, and three to seven weekly applications are advised. Exposure to water inactivates most insecticidal powders.

As with sprays, application should begin at the head with progression toward the rear and tail of the pet, and should provide good penetration down to the skin. The amount of powder applied to one specific area should be similar to that applied when salting a steak.

Powders should always be applied to a dry pet. Pyrethrin powders, like sprays, can also be applied to your dog's sleeping quarters to aid in essential environmental control.

Some powders contain another chemical called *carbaryl,* which belongs to the class of insecticides known as carbamates. Carbaryl is much stronger than pyrethrins and affords a better residual activity. It is also relatively safe when used according to label directions. It tends to have better activity against ticks than just pyrethrins alone.

Insecticidal shampoos

Insecticidal shampoos are common items in both retail stores and in most veterinary clinics. Many different insecticides in many different forms can be found in the various shampoos. Flea shampoos, like flea dips (see below), are best utilized as quick-kill measures for pet flea-infestation episodes. Shampoos with relatively safe insecticides, such as pyrethrins and/or carbaryl, offer flea- and tick-killing activity with low pet toxicity potential. Since shampooing too frequently can lead to excessively dry skin, alternate application of flea sprays or powders are advised over shampooing for routine flea control on your pet.

Insecticidal Dips

Dips are nothing more than highly concentrated preparations of insecticides. Chemicals such as pyrethrins, carbaryl, dl-limonene, and rotenone are all generally available in a dip formulation for use against external parasites.

However, for severe flea and tick infestations, or for sarcoptic mange infections, a more potent dip formulation containing one or more members of a class of insecticides known as *organophosphates* is desired. Since misuse of organophosphates can be harmful both to your pet and yourself, extreme caution should be exercised in both their preparation and their application.

As a flea-control technique, dipping is generally advised only as a quick-kill measure in cases of severe infestation. For routine control and/or prevention, milder products (sprays or powders) are safer and allow for more frequent usage. Always confer with your veterinarian in choosing a dip to suit your pet's particular problem, and always check on the label of the dip you are using for precautions concerning safe ages for use, frequency of application, and other pertinent facts.

When applying the dip, always wear rubber gloves. After shampooing or wetting the dog thoroughly with water, apply the dip by sponging the properly mixed product into the animal's hair coat, making sure that it penetrates down to the skin. Re-apply eye protection before dipping, and try to keep the dip off abraded areas of skin. Again, follow all product directions carefully!

Insecticidal collars

Insecticidal collars act via time release of insecticide vapors or powders. In general, the effectiveness of such collars is inversely proportional to pet size, environmental area involved, and amount of flea exposure. Quality insecticidal collars can help reduce the overall flea and tick load on the pet, but they seldom produce adequate control of these pests if employed as the sole control measure. The best results with flea and tick collars have been seen with small pets that experience relatively low environmental exposure to external parasites. Water reduces collar efficiency on powder-type collars.

The chemicals contained within the collar belong to any number of the classes of insecticides discussed so far. As a result, be sure to consult with your veterinarian before putting such a collar on your pet to be sure that it is safely compatible with the other products you are using for parasite control.

Internal insecticides

Insecticidal tablets and liquids designed to be taken internally are also available, through veterinarians, for flea control. Depending on which products are involved, the medications are administered either orally or topically. Regardless of the route, both methods of administration results in circulating blood levels of insecticide with its residual deposition in the pet's skin. The flea, in turn, is exposed to the insecticide when it feeds.

Such products can produce an overall reduction in pet flea load if environmental measures are also employed. However, since the flea bite must occur before the flea dies, the relief from flea-related problems such as itching, infections, and flea allergies is generally poor.

Obviously, potential toxicity problems, especially involving the liver, do exist with any internal type insecticides. Always follow all label instructions when utilizing such products.

Finally, when using internal flea control, the use of insecticidal shampoos, dips, collars, sprays, and powders should be discontinued to prevent inadvertent toxicity. You will find that there are a few select products, most of which contain pyrethrins, that are labeled safe for use with these internal products, but these should be employed only under direct supervision of your veterinarian.

Natural remedies

Throughout the years, countless natural remedies for parasite control have been touted as effective alternatives to insecticides. Some of these substances or devices are worn or applied externally; some are designed to be taken internally.

Products such as brewer's yeast, garlic, and B-vitamins have all been implicated at one time or another as flea-control remedies. Unfortunately, controlled scientific studies indicate little to no benefit in flea control with these products.

Certain products containing abrasive-type ingredients (e.g., silica gel, diatomaceous earth) are available for external flea control. These noninsecticidal products act by damaging the chitin exoskeleton of the flea. *Desiccation* (drying up) and death of the flea can result.

Moderate success has been reported with abrasive-type products. Drying and/or mild irritation of the pet's skin may occur with these products. Frequent application (four to seven times weekly) is required if these are to be used.

Electronic flea collars

Such flea collars have become quite popular in recent years as well. Although many manufacturers and pet owners will stand by their efficacy, scientific studies have shown that their worth in controlling external parasites is minimal. The idea behind them is that the device emits a high-pitched sound that can't be heard by humans or dogs, yet it drives fleas away. Unfortunately, aside from their relative ineffectiveness, some models might indeed deliver an audible pitch that can be heard by—and might be quite discomforting to—the dog wearing the collar.

Summary for controlling fleas and ticks

Start your control program by fogging your house or having it professionally exterminated to kill the existing flea population. Thoroughly vacuum the carpet, draperies, furniture, and your pet's bedding to help remove any adult and immature fleas from these areas. After treating the house, spray or dust the yard with an appropriate insecticide to kill the fleas there. Then, in two to three weeks, repeat both the house and yard treatment to eliminate any newly-hatched fleas.

As far as your dog is concerned, there are a number of flea shampoos, dips, and sprays available that are effective at fighting fleas. Flea baths and dips should be given at least every two weeks during peak flea season. In most areas, this runs from May to September. Between baths, pyrethrin sprays or powders can and should be used daily if needed.

Before using any flea-control product on your pet, be sure to always read and follow the label directions closely, and, to be on the safe side, consult your veterinarian before using any combinations of flea-control products directly on your pet.

Note: Ticks tend to be more resistant to the milder type insecticides than fleas, and can remain temporarily attached to the skin after dying. Dipping or spraying with appropriate products is advised as the best measure in killing ticks on your pet. Veterinary advice is imperative in choosing both a safe and effective product for tick infestations. Ideally, dead ticks should be allowed to fall off the pet without manipulation, since pulling and tugging could cause detachment of the mouth parts resulting in abscess formation at the attachment site. In addition, manual manipulation can increase the chances of exposure to Lyme disease and other zoonotic diseases.

Environmental measures are essential if pet infestation occurred in the home environment. Professional exterminators are recommended for environmental infestation problems.

PREVENTING CANINE HEARTWORM DISEASE

Heartworm disease is a devastating disease of dogs, responsible for tens of thousands of deaths each year. Most of these occur due to the destruction that these worms do to not just the heart, but the lungs, liver, and kidneys as well. In some cases, the worm burden within the heart and blood vessels can become so great that circulation of blood is actually compromised, resulting in sudden death. Other infected dogs can go years without showing any signs of heartworm disease, seemingly forming a symbiotic relationship with the parasites. Regardless of its presentation, the presence of heartworm disease puts a tremendous burden on the body's organs and immune system. (For more information regarding canine heartworm disease, see chapter 7.)

The good news is that this destructive disease is completely preventable!

Heartworm preventatives

Heartworm preventatives come in all sorts of sizes, shapes, and formulations. Depending upon the type of drug used, it should be given either on a daily or monthly basis during mosquito season. In cooler climates, this might mean only four to six months out of the year. In warmer climates, preventative should be given year-round. Your veterinarian will instruct you as to the proper medicating regimen for your particular area.

Diethylcarbamazine has been the traditional medication used to prevent heartworm infections. Due to its rapid metabolism within the dog's body, it must be given on a daily basis at a dose of 3 mg per pound of body weight. If administered to puppies, it is important to adjust the dosage accordingly as the puppy's body weight increases to ensure contin-

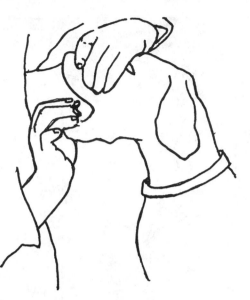

3-7 *Heartworm disease is easy to prevent.*

ued protection. Diethylcarbamazine comes in chewable and nonchewable tablet forms, as well as in a liquid (FIG. 3-7).

Once-a-month preventatives are becoming more popular among dog owners, owing to the ease and infrequency of administration. Preventatives containing the drug *ivermectin* provide this type of monthly protection. Available in chewable and nonchewable tablets, ivermectin performs its job quite effectively. It should be noted, however, that if ivermectin is to be used, only the commercially available canine formulation of the drug should be employed. Other formulations can prove to be toxic to dogs, especially to collies and collie-crosses.

Milbemycin, an antibiotic compound, represents the newest type of once-a-month heartworm preventative available to dog owners. It has a high margin of safety and should prove to be an effective addition to the anti-heartworm arsenal.

Before starting a dog on heartworm preventative medication for the first time, it must always be tested and deemed free from circulating *microfilaria*, or heartworm larvae (FIG. 3-8). (Exceptions to this rule are puppies under 5 months of age, who are too young to be harboring sexually mature adult heartworms.) If a dog has microfilaria in its blood and is given a heartworm preventative, a severe and often fatal allergic reaction could result.

For this reason, regardless of the type of preventative you choose, be sure to give it on a regular basis (daily for diethylcarbamazine; monthly for ivermectin and milbemycin). To be safe, if a treatment is accidentally missed, dogs should be re-tested before the medication is resumed. Similarly, dogs receiving preventative medication on a seasonal basis should always be tested before the first preventative of the season is given.

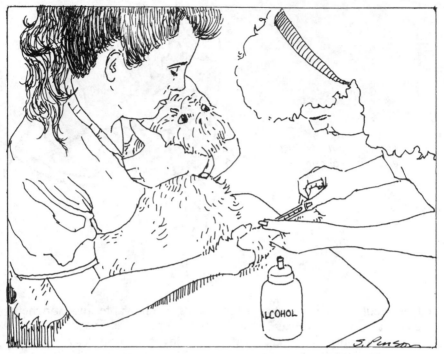

3-8   *Drawing blood for a heartworm test.*

HEALTHY TEETH MEAN HEALTHY DOGS

Periodontal disease, or tooth and gum disease, is one of the most common diseases affecting dogs today. In fact, most canines show some signs of this disease by the time they're 3 years of age. These signs can include tender, swollen gums, excessive drooling, loss of appetite, and—most commonly—bad breath. More importantly though, plaque and calculus build up on the teeth can lead to heart and kidney disease if left untreated.

A complete dental exam should be performed on all dogs at least once a year. For smaller breeds more prone to periodontal disease, these exams should be done every six months. If dental calculus is present at the gum line, the teeth should be professionally cleaned by your veterinarian (FIGS. 3-9 and 3-10). Because this cleaning can be a painful procedure, especially if periodontal disease already exists, a short-acting sedative or anesthetic is essential for your dog's comfort and safety. An ultrasonic dental scaler, combined with manual scaling instruments, is used to break apart and remove the hard calculus and deposits from the tooth surfaces. Afterwards, the teeth are polished with a special paste to restore their natural smooth surfaces.

Your pet's dental care doesn't stop there, though! At-home after care is a vital part of your dog's dental health. Toothpastes formulated for use

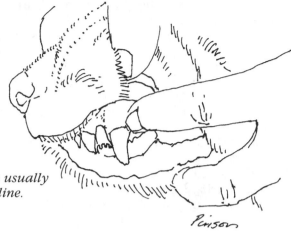

3-9 *Calculus build-up usually starts at the gum line.*

3-10 *Professional dental scaling can remove calculus from your pet's teeth.*

in canines are readily available from pet stores or from veterinary offices. Human toothpastes should not be used, as these can cause stomach upset if swallowed by your pet. The much-advocated home formula mixing baking soda and salt in water can be effective as a toothpaste alternative, yet due to the high sodium content of this mixture, it should not be used in older dogs or in those dogs suffering from heart ailments.

A regular, soft-bristled, human toothbrush can be used to apply the dental paste. For smaller dogs, a children's toothbrush can be substituted. Brush as you would your own teeth, concentrating on outsides of the large premolars and canine teeth. No rinsing is necessary.

As an alternative or supplement to pastes, specially formulated canine mouth rinses are also available. These can help slow the build-up of dental plaque and calculus. Choose one that contains *chlorhexidine;* this antibacterial compound can remain effective for up to 12 hours after application.

What about flossing? Yes, you can floss your dog's teeth, but not in the conventional way. Flossing devices in the form of chew toys have been developed to assist in dental hygiene (FIG. 3-11). Don't laugh; such devices can have a significant impact on dental health—assuming, of course, that your pet will play with them.

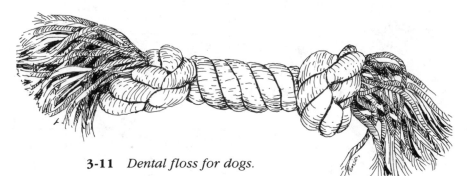

3-11   *Dental floss for dogs.*

Rawhides, nylon chew bones, and urethane chewing devices can also prove helpful in mechanically removing plaque from dental surfaces. Contrary to popular belief, feeding hard chew biscuits does little by itself to prevent periodontal disease; in fact, the starchy nature of such food items can promote plaque formation. The same holds true for the hard dog foods, although most contain substantially less plaque-promoting sugar than do their moist counterparts.

Remember: Good dental hygiene is important to the health of your pet. In fact, it can help it live a longer, happier life. If you have any questions concerning your pet's dental health, don't hesitate to confer with your veterinarian.

FEEDING YOUR DOG

There can be little doubt that proper nutrition is the cornerstone of a long, healthy life for all pets. As our understanding of the link between diet and health increases each day, so does the quality of foods which are available to feed your pet.

Not long ago, the diet of most dogs consisted primarily of table scraps, supplemented by whatever other foods they could find while roaming freely on ranches, farms, and the like. Today, our pets more often live indoors with us, and it is much more practical to feed them commercially prepared food which is complete and balanced for the particular stage of life of each pet.

While the quality of nutrition for dogs has improved considerably with the increasing use of prepared pet foods, there remains a great deal you should know about choosing the proper diet for your pet from among the many thousands of brands available in this country alone. Because dogs move through several "life stages" as they age, it is easiest to discuss the nutritional needs of these different life stages separately and in the order in which the dog experiences them.

Nutrition for puppies

For most dogs, puppyhood lasts for about the first year of life, although very large breed dogs (Great Danes, Newfoundlands, St. Bernards, etc.) may continue to grow rapidly until they are 18—24 months of age. During this time, the puppy requires higher levels of minerals like calcium and phosphorus, protein, vitamins, and energy (calories) than it will as an adult. Therefore, foods fed to young, growing dogs should contain these higher levels in balance with each other and with all other dietary nutrients. Such a pet food will carry a designation such as "canine growth," "puppy food," etc. to distinguish it from diets that contain levels of nutrients that are right for some other life stage, like adult maintenance.

Please note that the commonly held belief that if "a little is good, more must be better" is not true when it comes to feeding pets. Diets that contain very high levels of minerals, protein, and some vitamins are not superior to those that contain only the amounts required for growth. Excesses can actually be harmful to the growing pup as can the practice of supplementing a good growth diet with various human foods or vitamin/mineral preparations. Scientific studies have shown that high calcium and phosphorus intakes by young dogs can lead to a variety of bone problems, especially in large, rapidly growing dogs.

In addition, research has also shown that allowing your puppy to overeat even a high-quality, well-balanced growth diet can lead to some of these same problems because the pup grows too rapidly as a result of the high food intake.

To be sure your puppy gets all the good nutrition it needs for good growth and development, but never too much, follow these simple guidelines:

1. Feed a high-quality, balanced commercial dog food that specifically states on the label that it is intended for growth in dogs. Your veterinarian—who should examine, vaccinate, and deworm your pup—can recommend an appropriate brand. Remember that your puppy's start in life will influence its lifelong health and happiness.

It is very important that you invest in good nutrition at this crucial life stage.

2. Do not supplement a quality, balanced food; you will almost certainly unbalance your pet's diet if you do. Avoid giving table food, table scraps, or treats and snacks to your puppy for the same reason.

3. Do not leave unlimited amounts of food out at all times unless your puppy is very small or a very finicky eater. Most pups are very eager eaters and will tend to overeat a high quality, highly *palatable* (good-tasting) diet. It is much better to put down a large amount of food for a limited time—usually 15–20 minutes—allow your pet to eat all it wishes to eat in that time, and then remove the food entirely until the next meal. Most puppies can get by on 2 of these meal feedings per day. If your pet starts to become overweight, reduce the total amount fed or the time the food is available per feeding. Remember, overweight puppies tend to become permanently overweight adult dogs, with all the serious health risks that come with excessive body fat.

4. Keep fresh, clean water available at all times (FIG. 3-12).

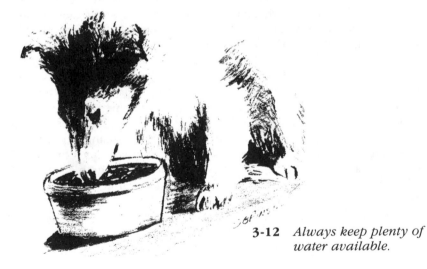

3-12 *Always keep plenty of water available.*

Nutrition for adult dogs

At about 12 months of age (about 18 months for larger breeds) you should switch your pet, now a full-grown dog, to a maintenance-type diet for adults. Once your puppy is grown, its needs for nutrition are considerably reduced from those during the rapid development of that first year. Continuing to feed your adult dog high levels of minerals—particularly calcium and phosphorus—protein, and energy (calories) could lead to problems later in life.

Just as we are finding that excess intake of certain dietary nutrients (like phosphorus, sodium, and fat) are harmful for humans over long periods, certain excesses might also contribute to diseases like kidney failure, heart failure, obesity, and diabetes in adult and older dogs. Also, we know that reducing the level of key nutrients in the adult's diet to meet but not greatly exceed its needs is never harmful. Good-quality, scientifically designed, adult-maintenance diets always contain these reduced and balanced nutrient levels.

Guidelines for feeding adult dogs include:

1. Feed a high-quality, complete, and balanced diet specifically designed for adult dog maintenance. Be aware that foods that say they are "complete and balanced for all life stages" are actually puppy foods, since they have been formulated to meet the needs of the most demanding life stage, growth. They contain excesses of most nutrients for the adult or older dog.

2. It is best not to give supplements or treats to your adult dog. If you must give an occasional food snack, either use a small amount of the regular food, or fresh, unsalted vegetables cut up in bite size pieces. Most dogs like vegetables, and eating them provides good chewing exercise for the teeth and gums (FIG. 3-13).

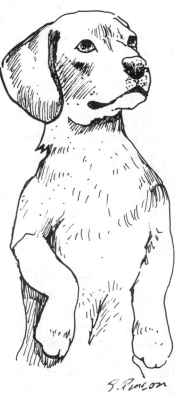

3-13 *Feeding dogs table scraps can lead to begging behavior.*

3. Most dogs should be fed their food in two or more equal meals per day. Use the manufacturer's recommended feeding amounts as a starting point only. If your pet gains weight, reduce the portion per meal. If your pet starts to lose weight, increase the amount you feed. Your veterinarian can help you decide what your pet's optimum weight is. Once you decide this, weigh your pet periodically to prevent weight loss or gain from becoming a problem.

4. Some dogs show a pronounced tendency to gain weight as they grow older, despite eating only moderate amounts of an adult-maintenance diet. Follow the instructions for overweight dogs in this chapter.

5. Dogs that are very active, do regular work, have nervous dispositions, or simply are not eager eaters will usually maintain condition best if they eat foods that contain extra calories. Such foods have levels of nutrients balanced to the increased energy of the diet, and they should not be supplemented with other foods.

6. The pregnant female dog will need extra nutrition in the last few weeks of her pregnancy and throughout the time she nurses her pups. Actually, she requires a good "growth" diet again, the same one she needed when she was young (FIG 3-14). Feed such a food starting in the last trimester of pregnancy and continue it until all puppies are weaned. Feed her free-choice, as much as she will eat, and do not add vitamin/mineral supplements unless your veterinarian recommends it.

7. Keep fresh, clean water available at all times.

A word about bones...

To get to the point, natural bones should not be fed to dogs. Now some might scoff at this, saying that dogs have been surviving on bones for centuries. While this is true, we still don't know how many of those dogs succumbed to impactions and to intestinal perforations. Why take a chance?

Bones, regardless of type, can splinter, causing penetrating wounds within the gastrointestinal tract. They can also add unwanted amounts of minerals to the diet. Nylon or rawhide substitutes more than adequately satisfy that bone-chewing urge and are much safer (FIG. 3-15).

Nutrition for the older dog

Once your pet is about 7 years old (5 years old for larger breed dogs), another dietary change becomes necessary. As people and animals age, many organ systems begin to show the effects of wear and tear. The kidneys especially begin to lose the ability to handle waste materials that must be removed from the bloodstream and excreted in the urine. Even older dogs that appear to be in perfect health could have kidneys which are much less effective than they used to be.

3-14 *Pregnant and lactating dogs need to be on a high plane of nutrition.*

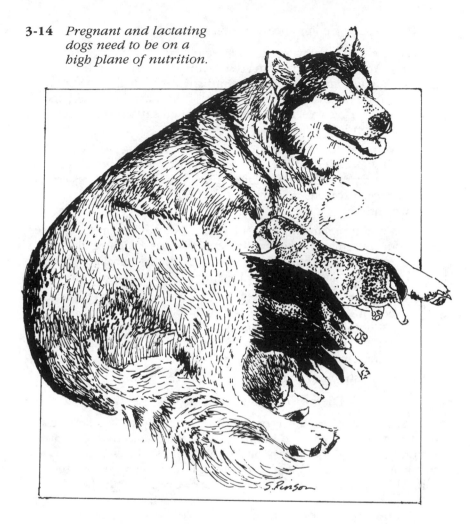

S. Pinson

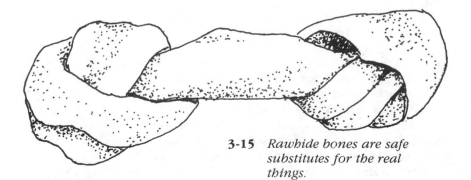

3-15 *Rawhide bones are safe substitutes for the real things.*

Guidelines for feeding the older dog include:

1. Feed a high-quality pet food specifically designed for the older dog. Your veterinarian can advise you of any special health problems that your pet already has and any other dietary changes that might be necessary. In many cases of "old age" diseases, special foods can be prescribed along with medication to help manage these conditions.

2. If you notice your older dog gaining or losing weight, consult with your veterinarian about any changes in diet which can correct the problem. At the same time, your vet will check for any medical problem that might be contributing to the change in weight.

3. Do not supplement your older dog's diet with anything unless your veterinarian specifically recommends it. The older dog is even more sensitive than the young dog to the unbalancing effects of frequent snacks, treats, and table food added to the diet.

4. Take your "senior" for regular (at least once a year) medical check-ups to catch problems early or prevent them altogether. The right diet throughout life is an important part of a sound preventative medicine program to safeguard the health and long life of your treasured pet.

5. Keep fresh, clean water available at all times.

Dietary management of disease

For years, medical research has been telling us about the benefits of eating a well-balanced diet for good health. In addition, we also know that special modification of the dietary intake in the presence of a disease state can be helpful in the treatment and/or long-term management of the condition. This same nutritional health concept can be applied to dogs, as well.

Many disease conditions in dogs, such as obesity (yes, obesity is a disease!), heart disease, kidney disease, and gastrointestinal disease, can be effectively controlled, and sometimes even cured, just through diet modulation alone.

For example, obesity, constipation, certain types of colitis, and diabetes mellitus all warrant an increase in the amount of fiber present in the ration. Dogs suffering from diarrhea, excessive gas production, and/or pancreatic problems can benefit from diets that are more easily digestible than standard maintenance rations. Finally, recommended management of dogs suffering from heart and/or kidney disease includes diets low in sodium and restricted in protein.

These special diets or rations aimed at fighting or counteracting canine diseases can be purchased through your veterinarian, or can be prepared at home via veterinary-supplied recipes. In general, the commercially available products, such as Hill's Prescription Diets, are preferred over the homemade rations. The cost of these diets is negligible when compared to continuing veterinary bills and the poor quality of life that would result by not feeding them. Just remember to follow your veterinarian's directions closely as to amounts and frequency of feeding of these diets if they are indeed used.

BATTLING OBESITY IN DOGS

Obesity is certainly one of the most prevalent diseases affecting the dog population today. For years, the frequency of this health disorder was skyrocketing at an alarming pace, owing primarily to improper feeding practices and inadequate time spent exercising due to owners' perceived lack of time. Sounds a lot like the cause of most obesity in humans, doesn't it? In fact, dogs are not much different than us in this respect. The problem, however, is that most overweight dogs were made that way not by themselves, but by their owners! Unfortunately, few owners realize that by encouraging their pet to get fat, they are at the same time endangering its health and unfairly reducing its quality of life.

The health-related ramifications in dogs are the same as they are in people. Although dogs don't suffer from atherosclerosis and "heart attacks" like we do, obesity does place a great strain on their cardiovascular systems. Other internal organs suffer the consequences as well. For instance, obesity promotes pancreatitis in dogs, among other gastrointestinal disturbances. Obese canines seem to suffer from more skin ailments and coat disorders than do their slim and trim counterparts. Musculoskeletal disorders, including intervertebral disc disease, occur with greater frequency in dogs carrying around excessive weight. In summary, it is safe to say that the overall quality of and length of life for these dogs is reduced, owing to these side effects of obesity.

Causes of obesity

The causes of obesity in dogs are numerous, but the first and foremost of them is plain, old dietary indiscretion: Too many table scraps! Realize that when you feed 10-pound Ginger that tiny piece of hot dog, that is equivalent to you eating two to three! In other words, it won't take many of these tiny pieces to make Ginger fat. Feeding one innocent cheese curl to a dog might be the same as eating half a bag ourselves, depending on the dog's size! I think you get the message. Table scraps do nothing but promote obesity and create an annoying beggar out of your dog.

Feeding dogs table scraps is no doubt the biggest culprit causing obesity in pets, but simply feeding the wrong type of dog food can do the same. Most dog food manufacturers produce products geared for different stages of a dog's life. For instance, on the market today you have growth formulas, high-protein rations, "light" formulas, adult-maintenance formulas, rations designed for senior dogs, and so on. The choices are so numerous that pet owners often become confused as to which type their particular pooch should be on, and this could lead to improper feeding practices and obesity.

The only type of dogs that need to be on a growth formula of dog food are puppies under 1 year of age, pregnant and lactating dogs, and, in certain instances, dogs that are recovering from or fighting off illness. Because energy requirements drop considerably as a dog matures, feeding high-energy, high-calorie growth formulas to an otherwise healthy adult dog can inadvertently cause obesity. The same holds true for geriatric pets over 8 years of age. These dogs should be fed "less active" or senior-type diets containing higher fiber and fewer calories instead of the regular adult maintenance rations.

Failure to adjust dietary requirements to specific individual needs is another predisposing cause of obesity. As a veterinarian, I am always being asked "Doc, How much should I feed my dog of this particular food?"

The first place to start is to consult a breed book or your veterinarian and find out what the ideal weight should be for your dog. Then look at the recommendations printed on the label of the dog food you are using. Even these printed guidelines should be considered averages, since the needs of each individual will vary, depending on individual metabolic rates, exercise levels, and eating habits.

For adult and senior dogs, the best approach is to feed the recommended amount of food over a 3 week period, monitoring your dog's weight each week. If weight gain is noted, cut back on the rations fed. If the opposite is true, then increase the rations slightly.

For puppies, follow the manufacturer's recommendations as to how much to feed. When your dog is still a pup, instilling solid feeding habits is more important than worrying about how much to feed.

Weight reduction

If your dog is overweight, simply cutting back on the amount you feed will not do the trick. In fact, doing so could conceivably lead to a mild state of malnutrition and will cause your dog to be constantly hungry (and begging!). Many dogs who are not receiving adequate nutrition will try to eat anything, which in itself can lead to a serious case of gastroenteritis.

Proper diet Instead of cutting back on its ration, switch your dog's feed to one that is specially formulated for weight loss. These diets are readily available from your veterinarian. They might cost a bit more than what you are accustomed to paying for dog food, but the switch is only temporary and the benefits to your pet are immense. These special foods have a high fiber content, which allows for calorie reduction while still giving your dog that feeling of fullness after eating.

Your veterinarian can assist you as far as how much to feed and how often to feed. Spreading out the total daily food amount over two to three feedings during the day might help satisfy your pet even more. Be patient with the results. You might not realize it, but even one pound of weight loss is significant in a dog.

It is vital that during the weight reduction period that you remain consistent with the feedings and avoid giving any snacks (a few kibbles of the special diet now and then can make for an excellent snack substitute). Rawhide bones are OK to give your dog to chew on during this time, but keep in mind that dogs that gulp down rawhides in a ravenous fashion can be susceptible to gastritis and intestinal blockages.

Exercise   As with people, lack of exercise does its part to promote obesity. House dogs kept indoors most of the time are the ones at greatest risk. Many are lucky if they just get acknowledged when their owner steps in the door from a hard day's work. When they do get to go outside, many times it is just to go to the bathroom, then back inside.

Regardless of whether or not your dog is kept indoors or out, make it a habit to devote a specific amount of time each day to social activity and exercise with your dog. It is not only important for its peace of mind, but it will keep its body fit and will keep the fat away.

A brisk, 15-minute aerobic walk twice a day is all that should be needed. Jogging with your dog is not required; in fact, in dogs that are already overweight, a jogging pace can place undue stress on the heart and musculoskeletal system and should be discouraged at least until your pet is physically conditioned for such a workout and is at its ideal weight.

When exercising your dog, just be sure not to overdue it. Stride for stride, most dogs need to work twice as hard to keep up with the pace you set. Avoid exercising during those times of the day when the heat and humidity is at their worst. And remember to keep plenty of water available for your dog's consumption. Dogs can't sweat like we can, and they rely heavily upon heat loss through panting and through dissipation from the oral cavity and tongue. Drinking water prevents these dogs from becoming dehydrated, and provides a cooling mechanism for their body.

Rule out medical reasons for obesity   Finally, just to be fair, the pet owner can't be saddled with the blame for his dog's obesity in all cases. There can be medical reasons behind a dog's weight problem. Hypothyroidism is not an uncommon condition in dogs, and it can lead to weight gain and lethargy by lowering the body's metabolic rate. One unique finding in hypothyroid dogs is that these dogs will gain weight despite a poor appetite.

The signs associated with this condition can be quite subtle and might lead you to believe that improper diet is the cause of your dog's weight problem. Because of this, all dogs that have a problem with their weight should have their thyroid function tested. Most veterinarians now offer a simple, inexpensive in-house thyroid screen that can detect problems if they exist. In these cases, supplementing thyroid hormone by mouth not only makes the pet feel better, but helps conquer the weight disorder at the same time.

In summary, follow these guidelines to protect your dog from the health risks caused by obesity:

1. Be strict when it comes to your dog's diet. Keep it regular and feed a formulation suited for its stage of life and physical activity. Avoid feeding table scraps! If your dog needs to lose weight, don't just cut back on your dog's ration. Switching to a specially-formulated high fiber diet is a must. Eliminate all treats and special snacks during the weight reduction period, and never use an automatic feeder (FIG. 3-16).

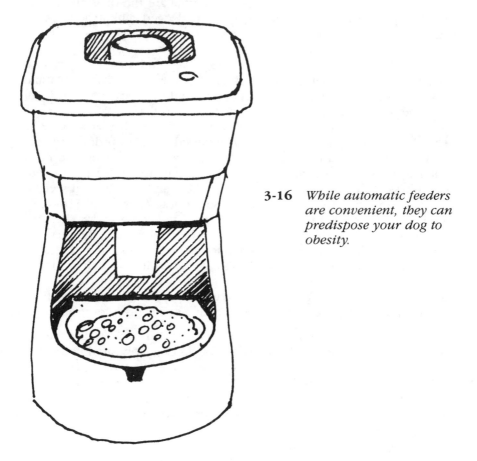

3-16 *While automatic feeders are convenient, they can predispose your dog to obesity.*

2. If you haven't already done so, implement an exercise program for your dog. Not only will you be helping control your dog's weight, you'll also be preventing potential behavioral problems as well. Don't overdo the exercise, and always keep plenty of water available at all times.

3. Always have a medical checkup performed annually on your pet,

or before embarking on any weight-loss program. Your veterinarian can tell you if your dog is actually overweight, and he or she can give you specific guidelines for weight reduction in your pet if needed.

CARING FOR THE CANINE EAR

Because of the unique anatomy of the canine ear, routine preventative ear care, involving cleaning, drying, and, when applicable, plucking, is recommended.

Cleaning

Many different types of ear cleansers and drying agents are available from pet stores, pet supply houses, and veterinary offices. Liquid cleansers are preferred over powders; powders can become quickly saturated with moisture, trapping it within the ear canal. Most liquid ear cleansers contain wax solvents as well as built-in astringents (drying agents) that help promote a healthy environment within the ear.

Isopropyl alcohol and hydrogen peroxide are two favorite home remedies that have been employed by some as ear cleansers, yet their efficacy in this role is questionable to say the least.

Cotton balls, cotton tip applicators, and tissues are also helpful accessories to have available. These are used to clean around the outer portions of the ear canal and surrounding structures. In no instances should a cotton-tipped applicator be placed down into an ear canal; you'll only serve to pack wax and debris down deep next to the eardrum or actually rupture the ear drum itself.

Be sure to consult your veterinarian before putting any medications or solutions into your pet's ears. This is especially important if those ears are inflamed or infected, since many solutions designed for use in healthy ears can cause serious problems if used in ears with unhealthy or ruptured cardrums.

Restraint during cleaning or treatment

The most important part of any preventative or treatment program for the ears is proper restraint of the patient. This is essential for effective application of medications, as well for the safety of both owner and dog. If necessary, don't hesitate to use a muzzle. Unfortunately, it is not uncommon for some dogs to object to having their ears medicated, especially if the ears are already sore from inflammation.

If at all possible, obtain assistance from a friend or family member for that extra set of hands. Smaller dogs can be placed atop tables or washing machines for a better working angle. This unfamiliar ground usually serves to pacify a fidgety protester.

Use good judgement: If it looks like all-out war is likely, abandon your efforts and seek the assistance of your veterinarian. Having to make repeated weekly trips back and forth from the veterinary office might be inconvenient, but try to keep the benefits afforded to your pooch's ears in mind. If your dog is suffering from an ear infection, consider leaving it at the hospital or clinic for a few days to make sure those ears are treated properly.

Proper procedure

The procedure for cleaning and/or applying medication to the ears is easy. To begin, the *pinna* (ear flap) should be pulled gently towards the handler in an outward, not upward direction. By extending it in this fashion, the external ear canal will be straightened, allowing easy access of the cleanser to the deep portions of the canal. On the other hand, if the pinna is pulled upwards, the ear canal will become flattened against the skull, rendering cleansing efforts ineffective.

Now carefully place the cleanser or medication into the external ear opening and squeeze a liberal amount of solution into the ear. The next step is to feel for the cartilage supporting the ear canal and, keeping the pinna extended outwards, gently massage the ear canal for a good 15 to 20 seconds. Once this time is up, the dog should be allowed to shake its head before proceeding to the next ear (FIG. 3-17).

After both ears have been treated, cotton balls, cotton applicators, or tissue can be used to wipe up excess cleanser, medication, or waxy debris stuck to the inside folds of the pinnae and the very outer portions of the ear canal. Again, never stick anything down into the ear canal itself. Seri-

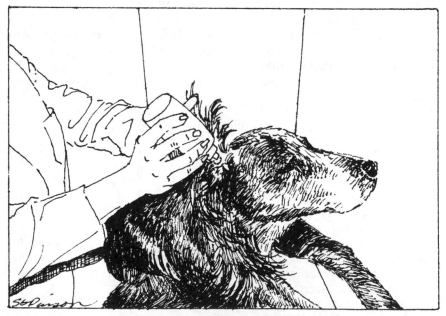

3-17 *Routine cleansings will help keep your dog's ears healthy.*

ous injury could result! Most commercial ear cleaners contain or come with drying agents, which makes manual drying of the ear canals unnecessary.

Hair in the ear canal

In some breeds, hair can occlude the ear canal, predisposing to inflammation and infection (FIG. 3-18). Poodles, terriers, and schnauzers are notorious for this. In a cases where excessive hair is visualized in the ear canal, an ear pluck should be performed by your veterinarian.

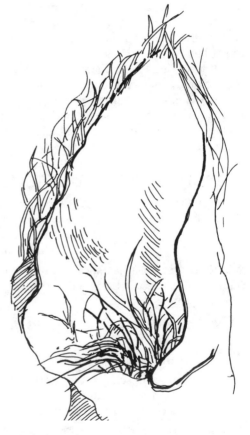

3-18 *Excess hair in the ear canals can predispose your dog to infection.*

Why not do it yourself? Well, there are three good reasons not to. First, ear plucking is a painful procedure, especially if inflammation is already a factor. As such, it requires effective restraint. In some instances, sedation might even be required to do the job.

Secondly, if done properly, an ear pluck should be focused not just on the hair visibly occluding the outside of the ear canal, but on the hair down deep within the canal as well. Special instruments are needed for this; the kind used by your veterinarian.

Finally, if done improperly, ear plucking can lead to infection within an ear canal. Since the act of forcibly removing hair from their follicles causes inflammation, the entire length of the plucked canal needs to be medicated afterwards to reduce this inflammation and prevent a secondary infection from occurring.

The bottom line is this: Ear plucks done improperly and without proper medicating afterwards can actually do more harm than good!

Routine weekly application of an ear solution can help keep ear canals healthy. In addition, using a drying agent in the ears after a pet goes swimming or receives a bath is also a good idea. Daily or every-other-day preventative treatment is not needed unless prescribed by a veterinarian; in fact, such frequent application could conceivably alter the normal flora and environment within the ear enough to allow disease-causing bacteria to proliferate.

Routine ear plucks should be performed on an as-needed basis. In most cases, this means every four to six weeks.

If the ears are being treated for an infection, follow the dosage and frequency guidelines prescribed by your veterinarian for the particular medications you are using. See chapter 15 for more information regarding diseases and disorders that can affect the canine ear.

MAINTAINING A HEALTHY SKIN AND COAT

Routine skin care for dogs with normal, healthy hair coats and skin should include good hygiene practices, including brushing and bathing.

Brushing

Whether your dog has short hair or long hair, brushing the coat thoroughly on a regular basis will aid in its appearance as well as promote healthy skin. It does this by:

○ Removing *telogen* (dead) hairs from the coat, making way for new ones to grow in

○ Preventing tangles and mats

○ Stimulating sebaceous gland activity, which keeps the skin moisturized and the hair coat shiny. Brushing also helps to spread these oils across the entire skin and coat.

○ Removing scale (excess keratin), which could lead to itching.

○ Increasing owner awareness of the presence of external parasites or other skin-related problems.

Long- and/or thick-coated breeds require more diligent brushing than shorter coated dogs due to high shedding and matting tendencies (FIGS. 3-19 and 3-20). Minor shedding is normal year-round in all breeds. However, because the shedding cycle in dogs is stimulated by changes in

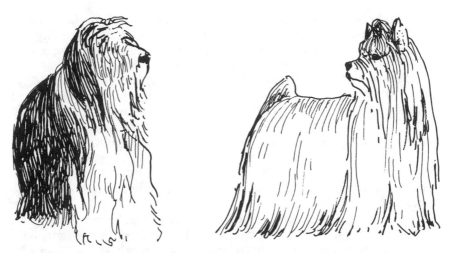

3-19 & 3-20   *Hair coats such as these require daily attention.*

day length, most will occur during the spring and fall months, when the days are getting longer and shorter, respectively.

During maximum shedding times, brush your long- and thick-coated breeds four to seven times weekly using a wire-pin brush. For dogs with short- to medium-length coats, one to four weekly brushings with a bristle-type brush should be adequate during maximum shedding periods.

Be sure to choose the right type of brush for your pet. In general, the wider the bristles or pins are placed on the brush, the longer the coat it is designed to be used on (FIG. 3-21).

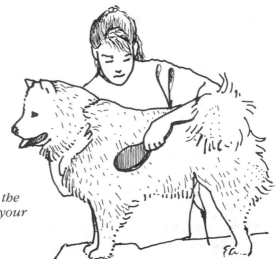

3-21   *Be sure to choose the proper brush for your pet's hair coat.*

In addition to wire-pin brushes, slicker brushes are another type of very popular brush. Most of these consist of a square head containing lots of tiny wire projections, and they can be used on almost any type of hair coat for removing shed hair and tangles.

Purchase of a comb is optional, unless you own one of the silky-coated breeds whose coat might be too delicate for many standard brushes. Combs can also come in quite handy for removing tangles and mats when used in conjunction with scissors. Like brushes, the teeth of combs are set at different widths apart for different types of coats; wide-spaced for thicker coats and closely spaced for longer, silkier hair. Just keep in mind that using the wrong type of brush or comb can be painful to your pet and actually damage the hair coat. For this reason, choose grooming tools with care.

Always use firm, short strokes when brushing, never forcing the brush through the coat. For dogs with short- to medium-length hair, brush with the grain of the hair. To help in the removal of shed hair, use towels or latex gloves to buff the coat after brushing. For those canines with thick undercoats, the initial direction of brushing should be against the grain of the hair. Once the undercoat has been groomed, then you can brush the outer coat with the grain.

If you encounter a mat, don't try to forcefully remove it with the brush. Instead, try to work it free with your fingers, using one hand to free the tangle and the other to stabilize the tuft of hair to keep it from pulling the skin. If the mat or tangle still can't be freed, insert a comb between the mat and the skin surface, then take a pair of blunt-nosed scissors and snip as much of the mat off as you can between the comb and the free end of the hair. Don't worry about cosmetic appearances. It will grow back! Mats that are left in place can promote infection involving the skin beneath. And always remember: If you brush your dog as often as you should, you won't have a problem with matting!

Bathing

Dogs with normal healthy skin and hair coats really do not require routine bathing. In fact, indiscriminate bathing can dry out the skin and predispose an otherwise healthy skin to disease. So when is bathing indicated? Our canine friends do need the suds when the following circumstances develop:

○ Accumulation of excessive dirt, grease, or other foreign substances on the skin and coat.
○ Build-up of waxy *sebum* (seborrhea), which often leads to body odor.
○ Accumulation of skin scale (dandruff).
○ Infestation with external parasites, such as fleas and ticks.
○ Skin infection.

Hypoallergenic or other mild dog shampoos are ideal for bathing dogs with otherwise healthy skin and coats. Shampoos containing insecticides are warranted if external parasites are a problem.

For medical conditions involving skin infections and seborrhea, use only those shampoos prescribed by your veterinarian. Using the wrong type of shampoo on such skin disorders will yield poor results and might even exacerbate the disorder in some instances. Even if your dog appears to have perfectly healthy skin, it is still prudent to consult your veterinarian in choosing a specific shampoo for your canine friend. He or she will be able to recommend products and give you valuable tips on how to keep your dog's *integument* (skin) in the top shape that it's already in.

Before you put your pooch into the tub, brush it out thoroughly and remove any mats and tangles. In addition, always apply some type of protection to both eyes to prevent accidental soap burns. Mineral oil has been used for this purpose; however, a sterile ophthalmic ointment is preferred. Such ointment is readily available from your veterinarian or favorite pet store, and provides greater eye protection than does plain mineral oil.

After you've treated the eyes, stick some cotton balls into the outer portion of each ear canal to keep bath water out. If the nails need trimming or the anal sacs need emptying, do this before the bath as well. Once these preparatory measures have been taken, you can now proceed with the shampoo and rinse (FIG. 3-22).

If you are using a medicated shampoo, allow it to lather and remain in contact with the skin for a good 10 minutes prior to rinsing. After rins-

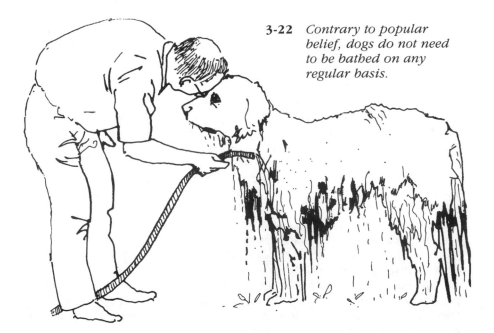

3-22 *Contrary to popular belief, dogs do not need to be bathed on any regular basis.*

ing, a towel, chamois cloth, or brush and blow dryer (on the low heat setting only) can be used for drying.

NAIL TRIMMING

As part of a routine grooming program, you should perform a nail trim on your dog every four to six weeks. The procedure itself is easy, assuming you have the right equipment and that your dog agrees to cooperate. If your pooch refuses to stand still for its manicure, let your veterinarian perform the deed. It will be less stressful on both you and your dog (FIG. 3-23).

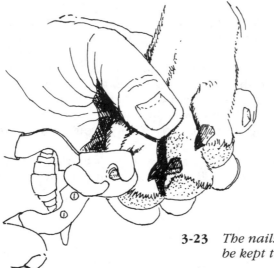

3-23 *The nails of dogs should be kept trimmed.*

There are many types and style of nail trimmers on the market today. The preferred choice is the guillotine-type nail trimmers with replaceable blades. These are available at pet stores everywhere.

The procedure itself is simple on clear nails: Observe the nail to be clipped and identify the endpoint of the blood supply, or the *quick.* Then, staying just in front of the quick, snip off the end portion of the nail.

On dark nails that don't have readily identifiable quicks, start snipping back the end of the nail in small portions at a time. Stop when the nail is short enough as to not contact the ground when weight is placed on the corresponding paw.

Invariably, the time might come when you accidently "quick" your pet's nail, causing it to bleed. If this occurs, there is no cause for panic. Using a clean cloth or gauze pad, apply direct pressure to the bleeding nail for five minutes to stop the bleeding. Alternatively, you can apply clotting powder or clotting sticks, both of which can be purchased at pet stores, to the end of the affected nail to quickly stop the bleeding.

Occasionally, a dog's nails might have grown so long that the quick has extended far down the nail, making it virtually impossible to clip the nail without making it bleed. In these instances, you might wish to employ the help of your veterinarian, who can perform a short nail trim with your pet sedated.

ANAL SAC EXPRESSION

The *anal sacs* are structures located on either side of the anal opening in dogs. Filled with a foul-smelling fluid that dogs use for intraspecies identification, these sacs normally empty with each bowel movement. Contrary to popular belief, these do not have to be manually emptied on a routine basis whenever a dog is bathed. In fact, by manually expressing healthy anal sacs, you could inadvertently cause inflammation and predispose to secondary impaction. Anal sacs only require attention if a dog is showing signs of impaction or anal sac irritation. These signs usually appear in the form of scooting the rear end across the floor or excessive licking of that region.

Mildly impacted anal sacs can be expressed by applying gentle, inwards and upwards pressure at the 4 o'clock and 8 o'clock positions surrounding the anal opening, using your thumb and forefinger respectively. If this fails to empty the sacs, or if the sacs are especially tender, stop what you are doing and call your veterinarian. In these instances the procedure is better performed at his/her office (See chapter 11 for more information regarding anal sacs.)

Note: If you happen to get anal sac secretion on your skin or clothes, you might lose your friends quickly unless you take appropriate action to neutralize the odor. Isopropyl alcohol can be employed to get rid of the smell. Better yet, many commercial odor neutralizers that are available at your favorite pet stores do the job even better.

GERIATRICS: CARING FOR YOUR OLDER DOG

It is estimated that in the United States alone, over 30% of all pets owned can be considered "geriatric status." Dogs are considered geriatric when they reach 7 years of age (5 years of age for larger breeds). Understand, though, that breed, genetics, nutrition, and environmental influences will all ultimately affect the aging process in a particular dog.

Smaller dogs tend to age more slowly and live longer than larger dogs. However, different breeds of large dogs can vary vastly in their life spans and the age at which they are considered geriatric. For instance, German shepherd dogs commonly reach 13 to 15 years, while an 8-year-old Great Dane would be considered ancient. Likewise, many bulldogs and boxers tend to age at an accelerated rate.

The overall care that a dog receives throughout its life will also have a great impact upon the rate of aging. Dogs that are well cared for throughout puppyhood and adult life tend to suffer fewer infirmities as they grow old. Furthermore, through diligent preventative health-care measures, age-related health problems can be detected early, greatly diminishing their impact. In contrast, neglecting a pet in husbandry or in preventative health care will greatly accelerate the aging process.

The canine species tends to age most rapidly in their first years, which allows for early maturity and ability to breed. This might be a holdover from primitive times when wild dogs were subject to early death from fights, disease, and the harshness of pack life. An early puberty allowed young dogs to raise litters and ensure speedy propagation of the species (TABLE 3-3).

Table 3-3
Chronological vs Biological
Age of Dogs as Compared to Man

Age of Dog (years)	Age of Man (years)
1	12
2	22
3	30
4	35
5	40
6	45
7	50
8	55
9	60
10	65
11	70
12	75
13	80
14	85
15	90

Physical changes noted as dogs age are related to wear and tear on all body systems. Again, these are variable between individuals and breeds, and can be greatly influenced by an owner who provides good environment, proper nutrition, and routine veterinary care throughout the dog's life.

Physical problems in older dogs

As with people, the overall metabolism of a pet has a tendency to slow as the years advance. This, combined with a decrease in the amount of exercise, can easily predispose a geriatric pet to obesity and all of its dangerous ramifications.

As dogs age, they don't suffer from many of the cardiovascular problems that humans do, such as hardening of the arteries and atherosclerosis. Yet as the canine matures, the heart does become less efficient at pumping blood during exercise or stressful situations that can arise. In addition, heart valve disease caused by wear and tear from years of normal use is not uncommon in older pets as well. This type of heart disease can sometimes be related back to untreated periodontal disease during the pet's younger years.

Bone and joint problems Arthritis is one of the more common ailments affecting dogs as they grow old. In addition, many of the larger breeds can suffer from the painful condition of the back known as vertebral spondylosis (see chapter 16). Furthermore, as intervertebral discs mature and become less resilient, the risk of disc rupture in these older pets increases at the same time.

Muscular problems The muscles of older dogs tend to atrophy due to a decrease in muscle activity and due to age-related protein loss from the body. A loss in flexibility can also occur, causing upwardly mobile canines to slow down somewhat.

Disorders of the skin and hair These can increase in prevalence in the geriatric dog due to aging effects upon the hair cycle and due to metabolic and endocrine upsets.

Aging kidneys It is a well-known fact that as a dog matures, its kidneys become less and less efficient at filtering the blood and ridding the body of waste products. Incredibly enough, however, it would take a loss of over 75% of the functioning capacity of both kidneys to lead to signs of kidney failure in dogs. As a result, care taken early to help ease the burden placed on the aging kidneys and keep them out of this percentage range will greatly enhance the longevity of a dog.

Reproductive problems Female dogs that were not spayed at an early age are more prone to uterine problems and mammary cancer as they enter into their geriatric years. At the same time, most older male dogs are afflicted with some degree of prostate enlargement. Furthermore, as one might expect, fertility and reproductive performance tend to decrease with advancing age.

Intestinal problems The aging gastrointestinal tract might begin to show signs of reduced efficiency and intolerance to excesses. For this reason, flare-ups of gastritis, colitis, and constipation can become more prevalent as a pet enters into the geriatric years. At the same time, liver function can decrease, making it more difficult to metabolize nutrients and detoxify wastes than it was during the younger years.

Weakened immune systems It is well documented that the efficiency and activity of the immune system is compromised with age. As a result, geriatric pets are more susceptible to disease, especially viruses and can-

cer. For this reason, preventative health care takes on even more importance in these pets.

Endocrine problems   As dogs mature, the activity of the glands within
the body may start to wear out, leaving the pet with hormone-related
problems. For example, hypothyroidism is not an uncommon condition
seen in maturing dogs. Diabetes mellitus can occur secondarily to aging
of the insulin-producing cells within the pancreas, or to repeated bouts of
pancreatitis over the years. In contrast, age-related tumors affecting
glands within the body can lead to over-secretion of hormones, resulting
in illness. Canine Cushing's disease is a prime example of this (see chapter
18).

Vision problems   Most older dogs will likely develop a slight grayish
white or bluish haze to the lenses of both eyes. This change, termed
nuclear sclerosis, is brought on by a complex deposition of body metabo-
lites into the eye lenses. It is a normal change and should not be confused
with a cataract. Unlike cataracts, nuclear sclerosis only mildly affects
vision.

Dogs with decreased visual ability might not be able to focus on an
object rapidly, so they might react suddenly if approached. Don't confuse
this with crankiness or irritability. A slow approach with a gentle hand
accompanied by a calm voice will allow a dog with failing vision to hear
and smell the familiar person approaching.

Hearing loss   Partial or total hearing loss is common in geriatric dogs. It
is often related to long-term, irreversible nervous changes in the inner ear.
Further hearing loss occurs with senile changes or damage to the eardrum
or ossicles (the bones of vibration conduction) housed within the middle
ear. Also, wax accumulation within the ears can play a role in deafness as
well.

Dependence on sense of smell   The sense of smell is usually the last
sense to fail in a dog. For this reason, the geriatric dog depends more and
more on its sense of smell to identify people, objects, and food. Also, the
senses of taste and smell are highly dependent on one another. As a result,
the appetite of older dogs will taper off as the sense of smell becomes
compromised.

The changes that occur with aging warrant special consideration
when it comes to husbandry practices and preventative health care for
geriatric pets. The following are five steps you can take to be sure your
pet's geriatric years are filled with health and happiness:

1. Adjust your dog's diet to match its health needs. Your veterinarian
   can assist you with this switch. If your pet suffers from a specific
   ailment, such as heart disease, special diets can be prescribed to
   reduce the wear and tear on the affected organ systems. For the otherwise healthy dog, feed a diet that is higher in fiber and reduced in

calories. Don't forget to weigh your dog on a monthly basis. Obesity is an enemy, and can significantly shorten your dog's life.

2. Maintain a moderate exercise program to keep the bones, joints, heart, and lungs conditioned. Always consult your veterinarian first as to the type and amount of exercise appropriate for your particular pet.

3. Be sure to groom and brush your pet daily. Skin and coat changes secondary to metabolic slow-down or adjustments within the body can often be managed with a stepped-up home-grooming program. In addition, keep those toenails trimmed short. Older dogs suffering from arthritis don't need the added challenge and pain of having to ambulate with nails growing to the floor.

4. Along with grooming and brushing, be sure to give your geriatric pet plenty of attention each day. As the senses start to fail, pets can become frightened by the gradual loss of sensory contact with their owners. As a result, you need to reinforce the care and companionship you are offering.

5. Semiannual veterinary check-ups and periodic at-home physical examinations for aging pets are a must. Remember: Early detection of a disease condition is the key to curing or managing the disorder. Also, because of the effects aging has on the immune system, be sure to keep your pet current on its vaccinations.

4

Breeding Your Dog

SINCE THE DAYS OF EARLY domestication, man has tried to understand and be able to assist in the propagation of this most helpful and
delightful of species, the dog. From acquired knowledge gathered
throughout the ages, new breeds and favorable characteristics were created, designed to meet the needs of each civilization. As creatures of status and show, dogs became the compatriots of kings and queens, who
appointed royal breeders to oversee the task of maintaining the formed
and functional purity of their favored breeds (FIG. 4-1).

Today, a sound knowledge of canine reproductive principles constitutes the livelihood of the professional dog breeder. But professional
breeders are not the only ones who need to know about these matters; all
dog owners desiring to breed their pet should do their homework first
prior to proceeding with such plans. For this purpose, this chapter will
come in quite handy. For an overview of canine reproductive anatomy,
see chapter 13.

PUBERTY AND THE REPRODUCTIVE CYCLE

Puberty is defined as the age in which female dogs first come into heat,
and when the male testicle first begins to produce spermatozoa. The time
at which this event occurs is not sex-dependent, but is governed by other
factors, including age, size, and breed. In general, the smaller the breed,
the earlier puberty is reached. For toy breeds, this can mean at 6 to 7
months of age; for giant breeds, it can take up to two years! On the average though, most dogs reach puberty around 8 to 10 months of age. However, just because puberty is reached does not mean that they have
reached breeding age.

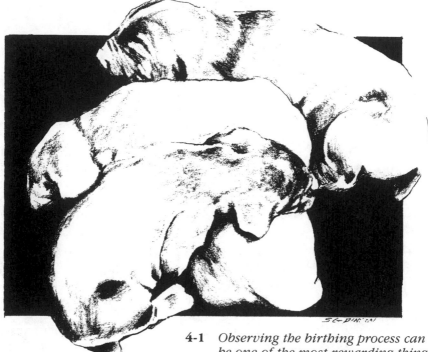

4-1   *Observing the birthing process can be one of the most rewarding things about being a dog owner.*

As a general rule, owners should wait until a male dog (*sire*) reaches at least 12 to 14 months before using it for breeding purposes; for females, breeding attempts should not be made until the second or third heat cycle. Even these guidelines can vary, depending on the dog's level of maturity, both mentally and physically.

The optimum breeding age for female dogs is between 3 to 6 years. Puppies born to females in these age groups tend to be healthier at birth, faster growers, and wean much easier when compared to others. After 6 years, reproductive performance in the female begins a steady decline.

Male dogs, on the other hand, have greater sexual longevity than do females, yet this too begins to decline as the dog advances in years.

The female estrous cycle

Estrous cycle is the term used to describe a series of events that occurs within the female reproductive tract between actual heat periods. On the average, this cycle lasts from 6 to 8 months in the female dog (*bitch*). Contrary to popular belief, smaller breeds do not have shorter, more frequent estrous cycles than do larger ones. The basenji, who averages only one heat period per year, is a prime example. As with breed size, seasonal changes also have no significant effect on the length of the estrous cycle.

There are four phases to the canine estrous cycle:

1. Anestrus
2. Proestrus
3. Estrus
4. Metestrus.

Anestrus   This is the period of time in which there is no reproductive activity going on in the ovaries at all. The duration of anestrus is typically four to five months in the average dog.

Proestrus   From anestrus, the reproductive cycle enters the period of proestrus. Signs seen during proestrus are related to the ovaries' increased production of the hormone estrogen, and they include vaginal bleeding and a gradual swelling of the vulva. Proestrus can last anywhere from 7 to 14 days. Normally, females will not stand to be mated until the waning days of this phase.

Estrus   As vaginal bleeding subsides and proestrus ends, estrus, or true heat, begins. (The term *estrus* should not be confused with *estrous cycle*.) As with proestrus, this heat period can last 1 to 2 weeks and is character-ized by sexual receptivity of the bitch to the sire and by ovulation of unfertilized eggs from the ovaries.

A common misconception among novice dog owners is that once a dog begins to bleed, they are "in heat." In actuality, they are just begin-ning proestrus and have yet to reach this stage. Unfortunately, many pet owners guarding against accidental pregnancies learn this fact two months later when an unexpected litter arrives!

Some breeds of dogs, particularly husky-type breeds and basenjis, can undergo a phenomenon known as *wolf heat*. Thought to be a carry-over from their wilder ancestors, dogs exhibiting such a pattern might not enter directly into heat after the proestrual period. Instead, the estrous cycle actually comes to a halt for two to three weeks before starting up again in estrus.

Another interesting fact about the heat period in the dog is that eggs that are ovulated from the ovaries can mature and become fertilizable at different rates. As a result, it is possible for mixed litters to occur if the female dog happens to be bred by more than one male.

Metestrus   The last stage in the estrous cycle is metestrus, which can last from 2 to 3 months. It is said to begin when the female refuses to accept the sire for breeding any more. It is the period of uterine repair, or—if fer-tilization is achieved—the period of pregnancy. False pregnancies appear during this phase as well.

When to breed

There are some guidelines dog owners can follow as to when the best time is to attempt breeding. Females entering into heat can be identified by the following:

○ The vaginal discharge changes from a red color to a brown or tan color as estrus arrives.

○ The vulva will turn flaccid in its appearance.

○ Females entering into estrus will often flag their tails; that is, they move the tail to the side of the body when touched around the rear end.

Another parameter used by some breeders is to start counting the days from when the first signs of proestrual bleeding appeared. Usually by day 10 after this bleeding starts, the female becomes willing to accept a male dog and attempts should be made to breed. If the female refuses to mate at this time, wait 2 days and try again. After the first mating occurs, a second mating should be performed 3 to 4 days later.

Your veterinarian can help you decide the best time to breed your female about to enter into heat. By microscopically examining slides containing smears of vaginal cells, your vet can pinpoint the exact dates when proestrus and estrus begin. This information is especially helpful for those female dogs who tend to exhibit subtle proestrual and estrual signs. In these, and in others, this vaginal cytology in an invaluable aid towards ensuring correct timing when it comes to matings.

Where and how to breed

When deciding where exactly the breeding should take place, it is better to take the female dog to the male's own environment, rather than vice-versa. Males tend to feel more comfortable in their own territory, and will perform their duties with less problems and distractions.

The male and female should be introduced to each restrained by leashes and with owners present. That way, if personality conflicts arise, they can be quelled quickly, before a fight breaks out. (Such conflicts may arise if the female is not yet ready to accept a male.)

If the two seem compatible, then breeding can be allowed to take place. Some experts recommend muzzling both dogs prior to breeding to prevent accidental injuries or personality surges. Whether you actually stick around for the mating is up to you; some of the more inexperienced dogs might need assistance. Most dogs don't mind the presence of a third party, but some might become uncomfortable.

A key point to remember is that once mounting takes place, it's best to leave the two alone from then on. After mounting, the two will "lock" together, forming what is termed a *tie*. While intercourse is maintained via the tie, the male might manipulate itself around so that both dogs' posteriors are facing each other, with their heads pointed in opposite directions. This is a normal mating position, and dogs so locked together should not be disturbed until the mating process has been voluntarily completed.

Normal ties will last from 10 to 30 minutes, although longer ones are not uncommon. After the tie is released by the male, the two will separate, and breeding is complete.

Breeding problems

Occasionally, you'll find that some dogs cannot breed properly due to personality problems or physical defects. In these cases, artificial insemination offers a viable way to obtain a litter from the impotent canine.

GESTATION

The gestation period for dogs ranges from 59 to 65 days, with the average being 63 days. Unfortunately, there are no simple blood tests that can confirm whether or not a dog is pregnant, and this problem is certainly compounded by the fact that canines can undergo *false pregnancies* that can mimic the real thing. As a result, alternate means of pregnancy diagnosis must be utilized.

Ultrasonography provides a reliable way to confirm pregnancy status as early as 28 days. If an ultrasound is not available, abdominal palpation by trained hands can often achieve similar results. However, there is much room for error with this method, especially if the female dog is tense during the examination. Abdominal enlargement and mammary development usually becomes noticeable after the first month of pregnancy. If an uncertainty still exists, radiographic X-rays can be used to confirm pregnancies as early as 42 days.

Care of the pregnant dog

Care of the pregnant dog consists of nothing more than maintaining a good plane of nutrition and reducing stress as much as possible. Pregnant bitches should be placed on a growth-type ration, similar to those used for puppies, during the gestation and lactation periods. Vitamin and mineral supplements are generally not required; however, if your dog is at risk of developing eclampsia (see chapter 13), your veterinarian might elect to start her on a calcium supplement a few weeks before parturition and continuing as such through the lactation period.

Stressful situations should be avoided if at all possible. Moderate exercise (two 15-minute walks daily) is certainly acceptable and encouraged during your dog's pregnancy. However, intense exercise and/or play sessions should be avoided.

While your dog is pregnant, administer all medications only upon your veterinarian's direct consent or under his/her direct supervision. Many drugs can harm both mother and unborn pups if given during pregnancy.

Always check the labels on insecticidal products used for flea and tick control before applying these products to pregnant pets. The label should state whether or not that product is safe to use on pregnant pets. If it doesn't say anything about it at all, play it safe: Don't use it.

Most heartworm prevention medications on the market are safe for use during pregnancy and can be used without interruption. Again, check the label.

THE BIRTHING PROCESS

One of the most fascinating and rewarding experiences associated with pet ownership occurs when a female pet undergoes *parturition*, the birthing process. In most instances, you need only to sit back and let nature take her course. While *dystocia*, or difficult parturition, is not especially common in dogs, it is important to be able to recognize problem situations that might arise in order to protect the health of both mother and offspring.

Dystocia can occur in any type of dog, yet smaller breeds and those that become pregnant during their first heat cycle might be more prone to these birthing difficulties.

It is important to record the actual breeding date of your dog in order to accurately predict when parturition will occur. If your dog is not already acquainted with the surroundings, be sure to allow her three weeks prior to the due date to become familiar and comfortable with her new environment. In addition, in order to satisfy her "nesting" instinct, provide her with plenty of clean towels and some sort of enclosure (a covered box or travel kennel) in which she can retire to if she so desires.

Interestingly enough, the season of the year can affect what time during the day that your dog will whelp. For instance, during the spring and summer months, whelping tends to occur during the early-morning hours. Whelpings during the fall and winter months commonly occur in the late afternoon or evening hours.

A yellow, gelatinous vaginal discharge might appear up to two days prior to whelping. In addition, 12 to 24 hours prior to parturition, the rectal temperature of your dog will drop to as low as 97 degrees Fahrenheit. This sign alone should alert you of impending parturition.

Stages of parturition

Stage one: prelabor This stage might last anywhere from 2 to 36 hours. Signs associated with this stage include pacing, anxiety, nest-building, loss of appetite, vomiting, and/or shivering.

Stage two: true labor Signs seen when a dog enters into true labor include straining, abdominal contractions, the appearance of the placental sac, and the actual birth of the puppy. Be aware that up to 40 percent of pups might be delivered "feet-first."

Stage three: expulsion The placenta might be passed with the puppy or soon after its birth. A greenish fluid should accompany a normal delivery.

The following guidelines are written in a quick reference, logarithmic format to help you through your dog's special time. If you ever have any questions or doubts concerning the health of your dog or one of its pups, don't hesitate to contact your veterinarian for advice.

Guidelines for parturition in dogs

Has your dog started to show ────► NO ────► Review and watch for signs.
signs of Stage 1 labor?   Contact your veterinarian if
                                               pregnancy lasts more than 63
↓   days.
YES

↓

Is there any evidence of a ────► YES ────► Contact your vet.
greenish, black, or red
foul-smelling discharge from
the vulva?

↓

NO

↓

Don't intervene prematurely.
Leave your dog alone in a
quiet environment with
minimal interruptions. Many
dogs have the ability to delay
parturition if interrupted by
the unnecessary presence of
the owner.

↓

Has your dog started to show ────► NO ────► Contact your veterinarian if
signs of Stage 2 labor?   Stage 1 lasts more than 36
                                               hours.
↓
YES

↓

Has a puppy been born ────► NO ────► Contact your veterinarian.
within 2 hours after the onset
of Stage 2 labor?

↓
YES

↓

Immediately after giving ────► NO ────► Remove the membranes.
birth, has the bitch removed
the placental membranes
surrounding the newborn?

↓
YES

↓

Has the puppy started ────► YES
breathing within one minute
after birth?

↓

No

Hold the puppy upside-down
to allow the fluid to drain
from its lungs, and
vigorously massage the skin.
A bulb syringe can be used to
suction excess fluid out of
the mouth and nose. If this
approach is not working
within two to three minutes,
institute artificial respiration
(see CPR pg. 646), and gently
expand the lungs, taking care
not to blow too hard into the
nostril. Avoid over-inflating
the lungs.

Has the bitch severed the ────────►YES
umbilical cord?

No

Tie off the cord with thin
gauze or thread by making a
knot about 1/2 inch from the
body wall of the newborn,
then sever the cord between
the tie and the membranes.
Discard the membranes.
Treat the end of the umbilical
stump with tamed iodine.

Has greater than three hours ────────►YES ────────►Contact your veterinarian.
elapsed between births?

After the birth

Following delivery and clean-up by the mother, newborn puppies will
usually find their way to their mother's milk supply. You should, however,
keep an eye out for puppies that might be rejected and ignored by the
mother for one reason or another. For instance, this rejection might occur
if the newborn's body temperature is lower than normal, if it is the runt of
the litter, or if it has any physical abnormalities.

Do you suspect a rejection of ────────► No
a newborn?

YES

Try warming the puppy with
a blanket or covered heating
pad (use the low setting!),
then place it back with
mother and the rest of the
litter. If this does not work,
you might need to hand-feed
the pup yourself.

It is wise to have your dog examined by your veterinarian as soon as
you think that it has delivered all of the puppies.

A dark, red discharge might be seen from the vulva following the last
birth. On the average, an entire litter is usually born within twelve hours
after the onset of parturition.

CARE OF NEONATAL PUPPIES

This section is included to alert you to potential health problems that
might arise in neonatal puppies (FIG. 4-2). If you suspect something is

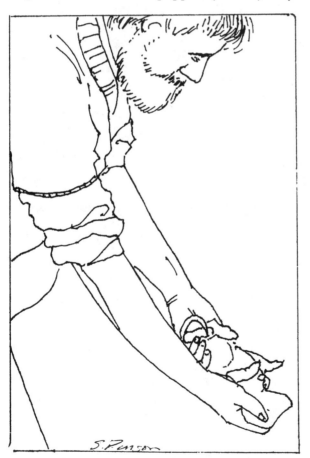

4-2 *Attempting to*
stimulate
breathing in a
newborn pup.

wrong, consult your veterinarian immediately. Normally, healthy puppies should be doing one of three things: eating, playing, or sleeping. Crying usually indicates hunger, and should cease when the puppy is allowed to nurse. If it doesn't, something might be wrong (FIGS. 4-3 and 4-4).

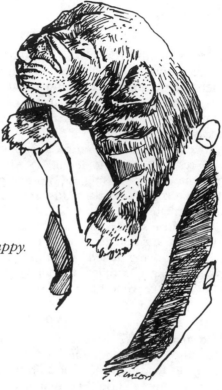

4-3 *A healthy newborn puppy.*

Hypoglycemia

Hypoglycemia, or low blood sugar, can result from lack of adequate intake of the mother's milk. It is often seen in orphaned puppies too weak to nurse. This condition requires immediate attention, for it can lead to profound weakness, convulsions, and death.

Commercial formulas available at your veterinarian or pet store are ideal milk substitutes. The amounts needed by the puppy are printed on the label. However, in emergency situations, you can prepare a homemade formula from 1 large egg yolk and enough homogenized milk to make 4 to 6 ounces of formula. The mixture might be sweetened by adding 1 teaspoon of honey to 8 ounces of formula.

Feed this homemade formula according to the willingness of the puppy to accept it. A general rule of thumb is 1 tablespoon of formula for each 2 ounces of the animal's body weight per 24 hours. For example, a 6-ounce puppy would get 3 tablespoons of formula in 24 hours.

Feedings should be performed every two hours. You can obtain a feeding syringe or pet nurser from your veterinarian or local pet store. If the neonate simply refuses to eat, tube feeding might be required. Ask your veterinarian for details. It should be emphasized this formula is only for emergencies, and the commercial formula should be started as soon as possible.

Diarrhea

Diarrhea is another dangerous condition in newborn puppies. Sometimes, the only sign of diarrhea you'll notice is an inflamed rectum, since mothers are so good at cleaning up after their young. *Toxic-milk syndrome* is one of the diseases that can cause diarrhea in neonates. "Bad" milk might result if *mastitis* (mammary gland infection) or uterine infection exists in the mother.

Affected neonates often bloat suddenly, cry frequently, run a fever, and are restless. When toxic-milk syndrome is suspected, puppies must be prevented from nursing the mother, and your veterinarian should be contacted. Oxygen, special fluids, and antibiotic injections might be necessary for treatment.

A newborn's hydration status might be easily evaluated by testing the elasticity of the skin over its back. If the skin fails to fall back to its natural position after being pulled up with your fingers, the puppy is most likely dehydrated. Since puppies can dehydrate 7 times faster than adults, this condition can prove to be rapidly fatal if not managed immediately.

Hypothermia

Another major cause of death in neonates is *hypothermia* (loss of body temperature). This condition is often seen in puppies rejected by their mothers. To help prevent hypothermia, the air temperature in the puppies' environment should be maintained at or above 75 degrees at all times, and care should be taken to prevent the young from being exposed to drafts and to cold floors.

Retained urine and feces

Finally, orphaned or neglected puppies less than 3 to 4 weeks of age can suffer from retained urine and feces, since they normally need to be stimulated by their mother to eliminate. To stimulate these necessary functions, puppies should be gently massaged in the genital area with a cotton ball soaked with warm water. This should be done after each feeding and at least once between feedings.

5

Elective Surgeries in Dogs

SOME OF THE MORE COMMON *elective* surgeries (surgeries not resulting from disease or illness) performed in dogs include neutering (ovariohysterectomy, castration), ear crops, and tail dock/dewclaw removals. Interestingly enough, where there is sound medical and sociological reasoning behind neutering dogs, many other elective surgical procedures commonly requested by dog owners have absolutely none. As a result, many of these procedures, such as ear cropping, have been coming under increasing public scrutiny as to their necessity and humaneness.

Whether or not you decide to have such procedures performed on your pet is up to you (and current laws governing such practices), but you are encouraged to communicate with your veterinarian before making a final decision. He/she will be able to answer your questions regarding benefits, risks, and controversy surrounding any particular elective surgery.

THE FACTS CONCERNING ANESTHESIA

Anesthesia is a word that tends to inspire uneasiness and fear in many people. In actuality, though, anesthesia is an indispensable tool in veterinary medicine (and human medicine, as well!). It is required for the painless performance of many important procedures, including surgery, dentistry, diagnostics, and restraint.

There are basically two types of anesthetics that are used alone or in combination in elective and nonelective surgeries. *Injectable anesthetics* are used quite often for procedures lasting for only a short period of time. For longer procedures, *inhalation* (gas) *anesthesia* is used for maintenance.

Isoflurane is the name of the newest, safest anesthetic gas available for use in pets. Because of its safety, most veterinary hospitals now employ this agent in their anesthetic routines. Regardless of the type of anesthetic agent used, it is important to remember that none, even isoflurane, are risk-free. It is difficult to predict how each pet will react while under anesthesia, yet with strict monitoring and adherence to basic anesthetic principles, many problems can be avoided.

Ideally, animals should be as healthy as possible prior to undergoing anesthesia. For this reason, laboratory work is often required to confirm the health status of your pet. Of course, certain situations will require the use of anesthesia in sick animals. It is easy to see how the risks of anesthesia tend to be greater in these patients. Older animals also tend to be at greater risk. Yet, again, with the proper laboratory work-up and a good physical exam performed by your veterinarian prior to anesthesia, the risks associated with the anesthesia can be greatly minimized.

Owners, too, have a responsibility to help ensure the safety of a pet undergoing anesthesia. Be sure to inform your veterinarian of any medications your pet is currently taking, as well as any changes you have noted regarding your pet's behavior (such as more frequent urinations, exercise intolerance, etc.). Don't hesitate to review your pet's past medical history with your veterinarian and to ask questions concerning the anesthesia to be used.

If the pet is to stay at home the night before the surgery, it is imperative that all food be taken away at least 12–18 hours prior to the scheduled procedure. Water, on the other hand, may usually be offered up to 4 hours before the scheduled anesthesia. Be sure to check with your veterinarian regarding this subject. If for some reason your pet does eat food or drink water when it's not supposed to, it is important that you relate this information to your veterinarian.

OVARIOHYSTERECTOMY

Ovariohysterectomy (OHE) involves the surgical removal of the ovaries and uterus from an intact female dog. The common term assigned to this procedure is *spaying*. OHE is a preferred method of birth control in dogs, since it is easy to do and ensures 100% sterility. Most veterinarians require a dog to be at least 6 months of age before undergoing such an operation.

Aside from birth control, there are many other reasons for performing an OHE on your female dog. For instance, it can be lifesaving as treatment for or prevention of *pyometra* (accumulation of pus within the uterus) as an animal matures. In addition, it has been used as a behavioral modification tool to calm excited or overly aggressive dogs.

Finally, and very importantly, research has actually shown that spaying a dog at an early age can reduce the risks of that individual developing mammary cancer in the future. In fact, the most protection is afforded if the procedure is performed prior to the first heat cycle. With each consecutive cycle a dog undergoes, this protective nature of an OHE becomes less and less until by two and one-half years of age, this potential benefit is lost altogether.

The operation

The operation involves making a small incision just under the navel. The abdomen is entered, and the uterus is retrieved with the help of a special spay hook. The veterinary surgeon must then manually break down a strong, fibrous ligament that attaches each ovary to the inner abdominal wall. Once this ligament is broken, the ovaries can be easily exteriorized. The blood vessels leading to the ovaries are then tied off (ligated) using suture material, and the ovaries are detached from their blood supply.

Next, suture material is again used to ligate the blood vessels supplying the uterus and the actual body of the uterus itself. Once accomplished, the uterus is excised just above the ligatures, and uterus, along with the ovaries, are removed. The abdomen and skin are then sutured closed (FIG. 5-1).

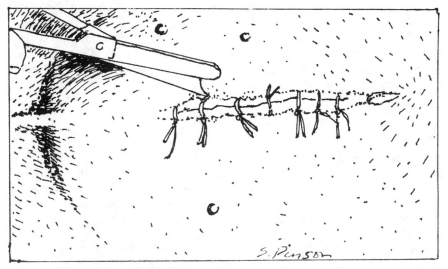

5-1 *Sutures are normally removed 8 to 10 days following surgery.*

The entire process takes anywhere from 10 to 20 minutes, depending upon the skill of the surgeon and upon certain patient factors. For instance, the procedure normally takes longer if the dog is in heat at the time of surgery, owing to an increased blood supply to the reproductive tract, requiring additional care and ligatures. The same holds true for pregnant dogs. Dogs that are excessively overweight are more difficult to spay because increased fatty tissue within the abdomen obstructs the surgeon's view. Finally, in the case of an OHE because of pyometra, the operation can take two to three times as long as it normally would, as the surgeon must use delicate care not to rupture the pus-filled uterus.

For whatever reasons, veterinarians often get asked if they can just remove the ovaries and leave the uterus (or vice-versa). While the intentions of such a request may be good, the medical reasoning that condones such a move is not. Dogs that have their ovaries removed without the uterus are still at risk of developing pyometra in the future. Similarly, dogs that have had their ovaries left intact, but have had their uterus removed, can still develop a pyometra in the stump of the uterus left behind. In addition, such an operation does little to reduce the risk of mammary cancer in that particular individual.

Common misconceptions about OHEs

One common misconception about spaying a dog is the belief that a dog needs to go through at least one heat cycle or have at least one litter of puppies before the deed is performed. Many incorrectly feel that this is necessary for the proper emotional development of their dog; it isn't. In fact, spaying before the first heat cycle can afford proven medical benefits to the dog, as mentioned.

Another false notion is that dogs that are spayed will get fat. Research has basically disproved this theory; most conclude that the obesity is due to poor feeding practices, lack of exercise, or certain medical conditions, such as hypothyroidism. Since most puppies are spayed at an early age, there is no sure way to tell whether or not these puppies would have been obese as adults regardless of the surgery.

CASTRATION

The technical term for *neutering* a male canine is *castration,* which involves the surgical removal of the testicles. This procedure is commonly employed for birth control, and for reducing territoriality and aggressiveness in male dogs. Castration is also employed as treatment for medical disorders that are directly influenced by testosterone, namely prostatic disease, perineal hernias, and certain tumors. Retained testicles (testicles that have failed to descend into the scrotum) are also candidates for removal, since they have high incidence of becoming cancerous. In general, castrations can be safely performed on a dog as early as six months of age.

The operation

The surgeon makes a small incision just in front of the scrotum, and each testicle is pushed forward and out through the incision. Once exteriorized, the blood vessels and associated structures leading to the testicles are tied off with suture material and incised, allowing the testicle to be completely removed. After both testicles have been removed, the skin incision is closed with suture.

Currently, studies are being performed on a new, nonsurgical method of castration. This method involves an injection of a sterilizing substance directly into the testicles, effectively rendering the dog sterile. If approved, it could make surgical castration obsolete.

Common misconceptions

The same misconceptions about ovariohysterectomies in female dogs exist for castrations in male. Yet, as with the former, these claims are without foundation.

TAIL DOCK/DEWCLAW REMOVAL

Established conformational standards dictate that select breeds of dogs have artificially shortened tails and be free of dewclaws.

Tail docking originated in centuries past as a way to prevent hunting and sporting dogs from traumatizing their tails while working in thick woods or underbrush (FIGS. 5-2 and 5-3). Even as certain sporting dogs have evolved into lap dogs, tail docking still remains in vogue as a cosmetic standard for many of these breeds.

Medical necessities might also warrant amputation of the tail. Trauma, infections, and tumors involving the tail may best be resolved by partial or complete amputation.

Dewclaws are actually functionless remnants of the first digit on each paw. Many puppies are born without any dewclaws at all; others are born with them on the front paws, but not the back, or vice versa.

Understand that, to conform with AKC standards, dewclaw removal is prohibited in some breeds. For instance, the Great Pyrenees is required to have double dewclaws on its hind feet and single dewclaws on the front ones to meet breed specifications.

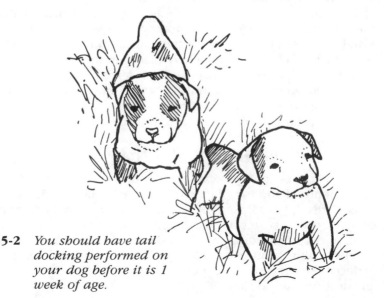

5-2 *You should have tail docking performed on your dog before it is 1 week of age.*

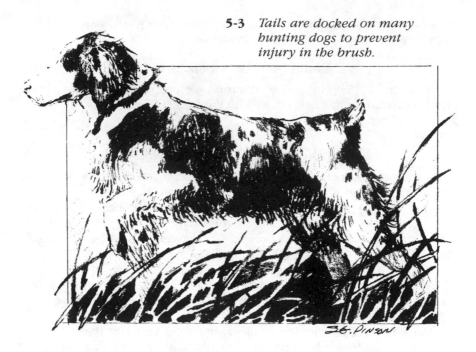

5-3 *Tails are docked on many hunting dogs to prevent injury in the brush.*

Cosmetics is not the only reason for removing these structures when a puppy is young. Dewclaws have a nasty habit of getting snagged and torn on carpet, furniture, and—in sporting dogs—underbrush. Secondary infections can develop if this trauma is repeated. For this reason, removal of dewclaws is a good idea if this is the case.

Tail docking and/or dewclaw removal are best performed within the first week of life. The operations simply involve snipping off the dewclaws and the desired length of tail (per breed standards) with surgical scissors. One to two sutures are usually placed in the tail; the site of the dewclaw removal is often cauterized and left open.

If tail docking/dewclaw removal is not performed within 7 days after birth, anesthesia will be required for the surgery. As a result, the procedures must be postponed until the pet is five to six months of age.

COSMETIC EAR TRIMMING

Cosmetic ear trimming, or ear cropping, is the surgical alteration of the normal anatomy of the ear pinnae in dogs to conform with accepted breed standards. It has sparked off a wave of controversy in recent years regarding its necessity and its humaneness. Many people feel that ear trimming puts a dog through needless pain and suffering. Veterinarians are even joining the bandwagon and are refusing to perform cosmetic ear trims, since they serve no useful purpose.

In Great Britain and Canada, cropped ears are no longer considered an acceptable breed standard, and cosmetic ear trimming has been officially banned by their respective kennel clubs.

The choice of whether to have it done or not is strictly up to you. If it is part of your dog's particular breed standard, and you plan on competing in the United States show circuit, then ear cropping will need to be done. In these instances, the surgery is best performed between 12 and 14 weeks of age. If, on the other hand, your dog is strictly for companionship, you should consider bypassing this procedure entirely.

POST-SURGICAL CARE FOR DOGS

Following any type of surgery, you should receive specific instructions from your veterinarian as to the type of post-surgical care your pet requires. It is important to follow these instructions closely to ensure an uneventful recovery for your pet. Post-surgical instructions should include the following:

○ Do not give your dog food or water for 30 minutes after arriving at home. To do so can cause nausea and subsequent vomiting.

○ Restrict your pet's activity for 8 to 10 days, or until the sutures, if present, are removed. Protect your pet from stressors, such as extreme exertion, excitement, temperature fluctuations, and drafts. Traveling should be kept to a minimum.

○ Check the incision site twice daily for any swelling and/or discharge. Keep the incision site clean and dry at all times. Avoid bathing your pet until all sutures have been removed.

○ Unless otherwise instructed, return to your veterinarian in 8 to 10 days for suture removal.

○ If medications are dispensed, follow all label directions closely. (See also instructions regarding oral medications, below.)

○ Don't hesitate to call your veterinarian if any problems arise or if you have any questions regarding your pet's recovery.

If you are required to give your pet oral medications, here's how:

Oral tablets Open your pet's mouth by placing your hand over the muzzle and your thumb and fingers behind the canine teeth. Now tilt the head back, and press inward and upwards with your thumb and fingers (FIG. 5-4). With your other hand, separate the jaws and place the pill far back on the center of the tongue, using your fingers or a commercially available pet-piller. Now close your pet's mouth and lower the head. It might be helpful to stroke its throat to encourage swallowing.

Oral liquids Simply "tent" the skin of the cheek out away from the gum line, and insert the syringe or spoon in the pocket formed. Now point your pet's muzzle upwards and deliver the medication (FIG. 5-5). Keep the head pointed up until the medication has been swallowed. Do not deliver liquid medications directly onto the tongue or into the back of the throat. To do so could cause choking.

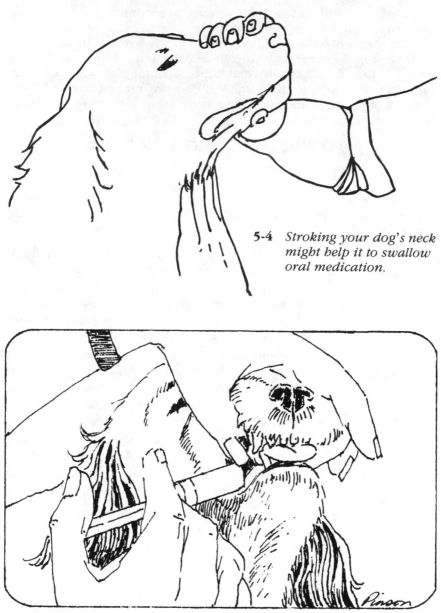

5-4 *Stroking your dog's neck might help it to swallow oral medication.*

5-5 *Injection of liquid oral medication.*

6

Infectious Diseases

INFECTIOUS DISEASES are those diseases directly communicable between pets. They are certainly among the most common canine illnesses seen by veterinarians. Infectious organisms responsible for diseases in dogs include a multitude of viruses, bacteria and bacteria-like organisms, and fungi. Multiple organ systems can be affected when an infectious disease is involved, resulting in a potpourri of clinical signs (FIG. 6-1).

VIRAL DISEASES

Viruses account for the majority of infectious disease seen in the canine population. Treatment for these agents is usually supportive in nature, owing to a lack of specific antiviral medications. Fortunately, most can be prevented through vaccination.

Distemper

This infamous viral disease of dogs used to be one of the leading causes of death in unvaccinated puppies throughout the world. Although the incidence of this disease has decreased dramatically over the years due to vaccination programs, the distemper virus is still out there and can strike without warning.

Symptoms
The virus itself is related to the human measles virus and can produce a number of different disease patterns in canines. Infected dogs shed the disease in all body excretions, and transmission usually occurs via air-

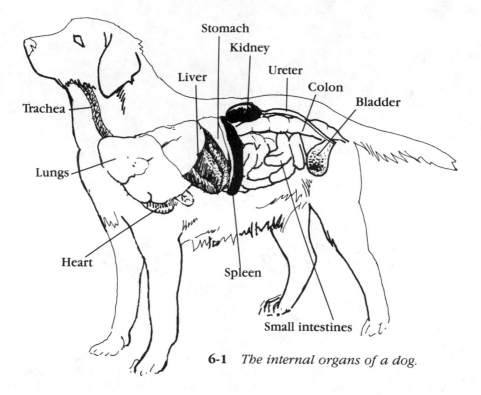

6-1   *The internal organs of a dog.*

borne means. As a result, like canine cough, it is highly contagious and can travel some distance on an air current.

Distemper is considered a multi-faceted disease; that, is it can affect a number of different body systems, including the respiratory, gastrointestinal, and nervous systems.

Early signs of the disease include fever, loss of appetite, and a mild conjunctivitis (eye inflammation). These signs can come and go, lasting only a few days. As a result, pet owners often miss or ignore this early phase of the disease.

As the disease progresses, signs become more serious and extensive. They can include coughing, breathing difficulties, eye and nose discharges, vomiting and diarrhea, blindness, paralysis, and seizures. The seizures associated with this disease often have their own unique presentation, called *chewing gum fits*. As the name implies, pets stricken as such will look as if they are chewing gum during the attack. In fact, many owners, when they see this, immediately think of rabies.

The final outcome of an infection with the canine distemper depends on the extent of exposure, the strain of the virus involved, and on the ability of the dog's immune system to mount a defense against the virus (with the help of supportive treatment). Depending upon these factors, the outcome of such an infection can present itself in one of four ways:

1. Death
2. Recovery with no lasting side effects
3. Recovery, with non-life-threatening side effects
4. Recovery, with life-threatening sequela.

The first and second outcomes are fairly self-explanatory. Non-life-threatening side effects that can result from distemper can include such conditions as *hard pad* and *enamel hypoplasia*. The former is characterized by a prominent thickening and proliferation of the pads of the feet, hence the name.

Enamel hypoplasia is a term used to describe the lack of normal enamel covering the tooth surfaces (see chapter 11). This occurs in puppies stricken with distemper at an early age, before their permanent teeth have erupted. What happens is the virus attacks and kills off those cells responsible for manufacturing the tooth enamel, hence the new teeth grow in lacking this vital component. Needless to say, teeth lacking enamel are not very strong and tend to erode quickly, becoming brownish in color.

These innocuous side effects might be all that linger, or they might be coupled with more serious sequela. One such side effect that could become life-threatening to some recovered cases is a degeneration of the nervous system, which can occur slowly or very rapidly. Dogs so affected sometimes show a progressive deterioration of both their motor skills and their mental abilities. Rhythmic muscle twitching can become so bad that it totally disables the unfortunate pet. Seizures, paralysis, and incoordination can also become factors as progression proceeds.

Diagnosis

A diagnosis of canine distemper is based upon a history of exposure, on the absence of proper vaccination, and on classical clinical signs associated with the disease (such as eye and nasal discharges, chewing gum fits, enamel hypoplasia, hard pad, etc.).

In addition, direct microscopic evidence of the virus within blood cells, or within scrapings of the conjunctiva of the eye or tonsils, can help out the veterinarian in his/her diagnosis.

Treatment

There is no specific treatment for the canine distemper virus; as a result, supportive care with antibiotics, fluids, and anticonvulsants is indicated. Unfortunately, the overall prognosis is poor, with over 50% of dogs that exhibit severe signs dying in spite of good supportive care. Of those dogs that do recover, about 50% of them can be expected to develop some form of nervous system complication down the line.

With recent advancements in veterinary dentistry, enamel restoration with artificial compounds has become available for those cases suffering from hypoplasia, and it is a viable way to prevent further tooth deterioration from happening.

Immunization at an early age with a canine distemper vaccine is the cornerstone for preventing this disease. Owners need to have their pets vaccinated starting at 6 to 8 weeks of age, then booster every three weeks until 16 weeks of age. Annual vaccination should also be performed. Breeding bitches should be boostered prior to pregnancy to ensure adequate amounts of maternal antibodies.

Any puppy or dog suspected of having the disease should be immediately isolated from its pack members. Disinfection of the contaminated premises with a dilution of 1:30 bleach will also help reduce spread.

Parvovirus

First identified in 1977, this virus, which is related to the feline panleukopenia virus, usually strikes young, unvaccinated puppies under the age of 6 weeks, although all ages can be susceptible to infection. It is highly contagious, spreading from host to host via oral contamination with infected feces. Parvovirus affects the intestines, the immune system, and/or the heart of infected canines and can quickly be fatal if neglected.

The parvovirus is attracted to those areas of the body wherein normal cells are actively dividing and multiplying. In dogs, the lining of the intestines, lymph nodes, and bone marrow are targeted areas. In addition, in puppies less than 6 weeks of age, the virus can infect heart cells, causing irreparable damage to this organ.

Symptoms

The intestinal form of the disease is by far the most common. Signs seen include loss of appetite, persistent vomiting, and profuse, odiferous diarrhea, often streaked with blood (FIG. 6-2). In severe cases, the actual lining of the intestines may be shed in the stool. As these signs develop, dehy-

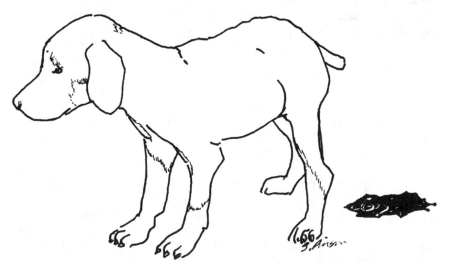

6-2   *Bloody diarrhea is one sign of parvovirus infection.*

dration and secondary bacterial infection can rapidly occur, especially in the young pup. If not treated immediately, both conditions can lead to organ failure and death.

The cardiac, or heart form of the disease is usually characterized by sudden death for no apparent reason, and oftentimes with no outward signs to indicate the virus's involvement. In a few cases, severe breathing problems may arise as the heart is attacked, which may then be followed up by vomiting and diarrhea as the disease progresses into its intestinal stage.

Diagnosis

Diagnosis of parvovirus infection is based on clinical signs, the absence of a vaccination history, and laboratory tests. Thanks to new technology, veterinary practitioners can now directly test for the presence of parvovirus right in their own clinics. Before this type of testing became available, a declining white blood cell count, which reflects the virus's invasion into the bone marrow, was the most consistent sign seen which alerted the veterinarian to the presence of parvovirus.

In fact, this parameter is still used as a prognostic indicator by veterinary clinicians for determining the severity of a particular infection. In general, if this white cell count continues to fall even after three days from the onset of clinical signs, the prognosis for recovery is poor. On the other hand, if the count rebounds, and starts its way back up by day 3, recovery is often imminent—provided, of course, that supportive treatment is continued.

Treatment

Because there are no specific antiviral agents available for this disease, treatment for parvovirus infection involves supportive care and the prevention of secondary complications. Success of treatment depends upon many factors, including how quickly it is instituted after the onset of signs, how aggressively treatment is applied, and which strain of the virus is involved.

Intravenous fluids are a must to treat existing dehydration and to prevent further from occurring. Supplementation with potassium, a substance vital to the normal motility of the intestinal tract, is also used to replace the amount that was lost due to vomiting and diarrhea.

Since an infected puppy or dog cannot keep any food down, a dextrose or sugar supplement and vitamins may be given intravenously as well. Antibiotics and drugs designed to control vomiting are also part of the support plan. Good nursing care to maintain an adequate body temperature and to reduce stress is also a must.

Starting immunizations at a young age is the most effective way to prevent serious complications associated with parvovirus exposure and infection. Puppies should be vaccinated starting at 6 to 8 weeks of age, and then every three weeks until they reach 16 weeks. Afterwards, yearly boosters are recommended.

Many experts feel that for dogs living in high-risk areas, or for those highly susceptible breeds—such as German shepherds and Doberman pinschers—booster vaccinations should be given every six months. To help reduce the chances of puppies coming down with the heart form of this disease, bitches should be fully vaccinated prior to breeding in order to ensure that optimum amounts of protective maternal antibodies will be passed on to the offspring.

Minimizing exposure is also an important control measure for parvovirus. This virus survives relatively well in the environment outside its host, so its contagiousness can last for days. All puppies and dogs, even those vaccinated, should be kept well away from dogs infected with the virus. Owners should also realize that some of these infected dogs can even shed the virus in their stools for weeks after clinical recovery. Puppies should be restricted in their contact with other dogs and with stressful situations until their vaccination program is complete. Contaminated environments can be cleaned with a 1:30 dilution of bleach to help inactivate the virus.

Coronavirus

Coronavirus infection in dogs is a highly contagious, gastrointestinal disease that causes vomiting, diarrhea, and dehydration. Because of similarity in signs, coronavirus infection is often mistaken for a parvovirus gastroenteritis. All ages are susceptible; however, young puppies under 4 months of age tend to contract the more serious disease (FIG 6-3).

The virus is transmitted via contact with shed fecal material containing the virus. This can present a problem when large groups of dogs are housed together, since viral shedding from one infected animal can continue for several weeks even after clinical signs have abated.

Symptoms

Coronavirus does not cause the same deadly destruction to the intestinal tract as does the parvovirus. Because of this, the true importance of this intestinal virus as a disease entity in dogs had been underplayed for years. In fact, the coronavirus had even been isolated in the feces of clinically normal dogs, causing no disease whatsoever.

Well, all of this changed when researchers discovered a surprising link between this virus and its nasty parvo counterpart. It seems that parvo-infected dogs who had a concurrent coronavirus infection had much severer clinical signs than those infected with parvovirus alone. In other words, the coronavirus was shown to potentiate or increase the severity of parvovirus infections. As a result, preventative vaccinations against this seemingly low-grade virus, even in older dogs, took on a whole new meaning.

Generalized depression and loss of appetite usually precede other signs. Once vomiting begins, it usually lasts two to three days. During this time, large amounts of diarrhea appear, which, when combined with the vomiting, often lead to rapid dehydration. Unlike parvovirus, blood is

6-3 *Coronavirus can be a serious disease in puppies.*

rarely seen in this stool. Fever is usually not a feature of this disease, although it can become a factor if secondary infections take hold.

Diagnosis

Diagnosis is afforded by a good history, clinical signs seen, and laboratory tests. One way clinicians differentiate an infection with this disease from one with parvo is by looking at the dog's white blood cell count. A reduction in the total number of white blood cells circulating throughout the body is usually NOT found with coronavirus infection, whereas, in a parvovirus attack, such a reduction is detected.

Treatment

There is no specific treatment for coronavirus. Supportive therapy consisting of intravenous fluids to correct or prevent dehydration, and antibiotics to prevent secondary infections, is indicated. Depending upon the severity, medications might also be given to help control the vomiting and diarrhea. If good supportive care is provided, the prognosis for a complete recovery is excellent. Be aware that once a pet has gotten over the initial stages of this disease, soft stools may persist for weeks. As a result, a bland diet should be fed during this time.

Vaccinations against coronavirus should be started at 6 to 8 weeks of age, and boostered every three weeks until 16 weeks of age. Again, owing to its unique relationship with the parvovirus, it is recommended that dogs of all ages be vaccinated.

Environmental control measures that can be taken include avoiding stressful situations and overcrowding of animals. If the environment is known to be contaminated with coronavirus, it should be treated with a 1:30 dilution of bleach to kill the existing virus.

Infectious canine hepatitis (ICH)

This disease is caused by the *canine adenovirus 1,* an organism found worldwide and known for its stability outside its host environment (it can survive up to two weeks!). The virus is shed in all body excretions, and can be found in the urine of a recovered dog for up to 6 months. Direct contact with such secretions by an unsuspecting dog, usually under 1 year of age and unvaccinated, is the method of disease transmission.

As the name implies, once the organism enters the body, it can set up a severe inflammation of the liver, or hepatitis. ICH does not, however, stop here. Other organ systems, including the eyes and kidneys, can be affected as well.

Symptoms

Loss of appetite, depression, and fever, sometimes reaching 106 degrees Fahrenheit, are initial symptoms seen. Enlargement of the tonsils and other lymph nodes occurs as the virus multiplies in these regions. As the liver is attacked, abdominal pain and jaundice become evident. In addition, inflammation of the blood vessels within the body can lead to clotting problems and internal bleeding.

One characteristic lesion of infectious canine hepatitis that can develop later as the disease progresses is called *blue eye*. In this condition, one or both eyes can take on a blue appearance due to fluid build-up and inflammation within the eye(s).

Diagnosis

Diagnosis of infectious canine hepatitis is based upon the age of the animal involved, vaccination history, and laboratory data. Such data will reveal elevated liver enzyme levels, a lowered white blood cell count, and increased clotting time. Biopsy samples might reveal the actual presence of the virus within the tissue itself.

Treatment

Treatment aims are preventing secondary complications, such as bacterial infections, and giving intravenous fluids to combat dehydration. In severe cases, blood transfusions could be required. Even when vigorous therapy is instituted, prognosis for recovery remains very guarded in the majority of cases.

Vaccination is the best way to prevent this disease from striking a pet. Interestingly enough, the organism used in the protective vaccine is not the canine adenovirus type 1; it's actually a cousin of the virus, the canine adenovirus type 2. This is the same virus that complicates canine cough (see discussion later in this chapter).

Researchers found that vaccination with a preparation of the type 1 virus could cause some undesirable side effects—including the "blue eye" previously mentioned and kidney disease. As a result, the type 2 virus is used in the vaccine. The immunity it stimulates provides protection against both viruses, without the side effects.

Vaccination programs should start at 6 to 8 weeks of age, and boosters should be given every three to four weeks until 16 weeks of age. After that, an annual booster is recommended.

Canine cough (kennel cough)

In the past, most pet owners regarded this respiratory disease as unimportant unless their pet was to be boarded or kept in a kennel environment (hence its nickname). True, it occurs more frequently in such surroundings, and in other areas where dogs are congregated (such as grooming salons and dog shows), but it is by no means restricted to these.

The disease is highly contagious, transmitted by air and wind currents contaminated with cough and sneeze droplets from infected canines. For this reason, all dogs, young and old, kenneled and unkenneled, can be threatened.

There is no one organism on which to solely place the blame for this disease; in fact, over six different causative agents have been isolated, causing disease by themselves or in combination with the others. The two most important of these agents include the parainfluenza virus and a bacterium called *Bordetella bronchiseptica*.

Symptoms

The classical clinical sign associated with an uncomplicated case of canine cough includes a relentless dry, hacking cough, usually nonproductive (FIG. 6-4). Occasionally, a clear discharge from the nose might appear. Gagging or retching might be noted at the end of a coughing spell and is often mistaken for vomiting. Affected dogs usually don't run a fever or seem to "feel bad," nor is it common for them to lose their appetite—that is, if the case doesn't become complicated with secondary infections.

Complicated cases of canine cough are characterized by a greenish eye and nasal discharge, and by obvious breathing difficulties as pneumonia rears its ugly head. In these instances, affected animals do run fevers, do lose their appetites, and do appear sick.

Diagnosis

Diagnosis of canine cough is based upon the presence of the classical clinical signs, plus a recent history of exposure to other dogs. Radiographs might be required to evaluate the extent of the lung and airway involve-

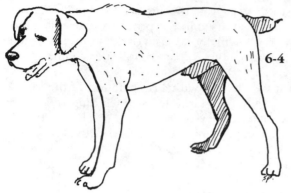

6-4 *A hacking cough is characteristic of canine cough.*

ment in complicated cases. Bacterial cultures are also indicated in these latter instances.

Treatment

Treatment of the disease consists of antibiotic therapy, and, in the case of nonproductive coughs, cough suppressants. Owners need to realize that coughing can persist for up to three weeks, even after treatment.

If complications exist, more specific therapy will be needed to battle the pneumonia and fever and to prevent dehydration. Vaporizers are often used to liquify secretions in the airway, allowing for greater ease of passage. A similar effect can be obtained by placing the affected pet in a steam-filled bathroom for 10 to 15 minutes. Just be sure the temperature within the room doesn't get too hot; drinking water should be provided to the dog to help prevent overheating.

An intranasal vaccine is available which has shown promise in protecting against agents that cause canine cough. It should be administered to dogs at least annually; every six months if the dog is kenneled a lot or is on the show circuit.

Protection against the canine adenovirus type 2, which can also play a role in canine cough, can be afforded by the regular combination vaccines normally given each year. Realize, however, that because there are so many different organisms involved in this disease complex, vaccinated dogs still might come down with this disease. Yet in most cases where this occurs, the clinical disease that results is normally much less in severity than that which would strike a totally unprotected individual. As a result, even though it might not afford 100% protection, regular vaccination is completely warranted.

Herpes virus

This virus poses no real threat to adult dogs; in fact, it is thought to be a natural inhabitant of the respiratory tract and sometimes the reproductive tracts of these adults. Its main importance rests in the disease it causes in puppies under 2 weeks of age.

As it turns out, this herpes virus does not multiply well in the higher body temperatures normally found in adult dogs. However, neonatal puppies, whose ability to maintain this body temperature is poor, are prime targets for the virus. They can become infected with it directly inside the mother's uterus, or they can become exposed after birth. Unfortunately, once clinical signs appear in these young puppies, there is not much that can be done to save them.

Symptoms

The time from exposure to the appearance of clinical signs is about 7 to 10 days. Afflicted puppies will cry constantly, become depressed, and stop nursing. Death usually occurs within 24 hours after the signs begin.

Because of its age specificity, herpes virus infection should be suspected anytime puppies under 2 weeks of age become ill and exhibit a constant crying. Further diagnostics performed on tissue samples after death can help confirm the diagnosis and shift focus on saving the remaining members of the litter.

Treatment

As mentioned before, once signs appear in an individual, death is inevitable. However, there are steps owners can take to try and spare the other puppies in the litter from the same fate. Be sure to provide a source of heat (remember: never allow a heating pad to come in direct contact with the body surface, and always keep heating pads on their low setting!) to the puppies to maintain their body temperatures above 100 degrees. This will help slow the multiplication of the virus. If indicated, supportive fluids and force-fed nutrition can also be helpful as well.

There is no vaccine available to help combat this disease.

Rabies

If there was ever a disease to strike fear into the hearts and minds of pet owners everywhere, this is it! Rabies is a deadly viral disease that can infect any warm-blooded mammal, including domesticated animals such as dogs, cats, horses, and cattle. As a disease to be avoided, rabies is one of the earliest to ever be recorded, dating back to almost 2000 B.C. It is found worldwide, except in a few countries, such as Great Britain and Japan, which have strict laws designed to keep the countries rabies-free.

The incidence of rabies within the United States varies with each state, depending upon the normal fauna found in that state and on existing vaccination laws. On the average, the United States experiences over 300 cases of rabies each just in dogs and cats alone.

It is estimated that 86% of all rabies cases occur in wildlife species of animals, with about 14% spilling over into the domestic pet and livestock population. It is certainly these latter groups that pose the greatest threat to public health.

Species that are commonly culprits of spreading wildlife rabies include skunks, raccoons, foxes, and bats. Opossums are noted for their resistance to this virus, and they rarely become infected. Rodents, such as rats and mice, are not significant carriers of the disease either, since most don't survive encounters with rabid animals in the first place.

Skunk rabies is most prevalent in the Midwest, Southwest, and California; raccoon rabies in the Mid-Atlantic and Southeastern United States; fox rabies in the Eastern states; and bat rabies—well, it's found in all states. Most cases seem to occur during the spring and fall months of the year.

The rabies virus is transmitted via the infected saliva of affected animals, usually through a bite wound or contamination therewith of an open wound or mucous membranes. Contrary to popular belief, however, this isn't the only way. Aerosol transmission has been known to occur as well, though certainly the incidence of this is very low. In addition, in skunks, oral ingestion of the virus leading to an active infection has been demonstrated. Regardless of the route of its transmission, the disease is almost uniformly fatal once contracted.

Dogs are a leading domesticated host for this killer, and are a major vector for transmission of the disease to humans. Studies have shown that rabies occurs in higher incidence in younger dogs, the median age being about 1 year. In addition, due to hormonally related roaming and territorial instincts, male dogs are at greater risk of exposure than are females.

Symptoms

Traditionally, when rabies is spoken of, most people visualize a snarling, frothing, dog snapping at anything in sight. While this is true in some instances, pet owners should understand that this represents only one of three stages that are part of the overall disease process. Depending upon each individual case, viciousness might take on a prominent role, or might not occur at all. These three stages of rabies include the *prodromal* stage, the *furious* stage, and the *dumb* or *paralytic* stage.

The first stage, which might last from one to three days, is characterized by a change in the overall behavior of the animal. Normally friendly dogs might suddenly exhibit aggressive tendencies towards their owners or towards other pets in the household. Affected individuals might also hide a lot, preferring to be left alone, and becoming upset when disturbed. Loss of appetite might become apparent, and owners might notice an increased sexual arousal and/or frequency of urinations.

Once the prodromal stage is complete, the victim then enters into the furious stage. This is the stage most persons equate with a traditional rabies presentation. Dogs in this stage often become quite restless, excitatory, and aggressive, losing fear of natural enemies. They might wander about aimlessly, snapping and biting at anything that moves. The character of the animal's vocalizations might noticeably change. In dogs especially, *pica,* or an abnormal desire to eat anything within reach (i.e., rocks, wire, dirt, feces, etc.), might become apparent.

As the disease enters the third stage, the swallowing reflex becomes paralyzed, making it impossible to eat, drink, or swallow saliva. This is what accounts for the excessive drooling seen in rabid animals.

The furious stage might last for up to a week before progressing into stage 3, the paralytic stage. Pet owners should be aware of the fact that some animals, especially dogs, might skip the furious stage entirely, going directly from the prodromal stage into the paralytic stage. When this happens, the disease can be easily mistaken for other nervous system disorders if the diagnostician is not careful. Because this quick transition can occur, the risk of human exposure is greatly increased. The paralytic stage presents itself as a general loss of coordination and paralysis. A droopy lower jaw with the mouth just hanging open is often characteristic. A general paralysis and death usually overtakes the unfortunate animal in a matter of hours.

Diagnosis

Rabies should be suspected anytime a dog exhibits behavioral changes with unexplained, abnormal nervous system signs. Unfortunately, the only way to definitively diagnose a case of rabies is to have a laboratory analysis performed on the animal's brain tissue, which means of course, euthanasia of the animal in question.

Treatment

There is no known treatment for this fatal disease; as a result, stringent control and vaccination measures are a must.

All puppies should receive a rabies immunization between 3 and 4 months of age. In most states, this vaccine must be administered by a licensed veterinarian. Depending on the vaccine used and on the state in which you live, a booster immunization is required every one to three years. Owing to the public health implications of this disease, dog owners who fail to keep their pets current on this immunization are putting their own health at risk!

Other preventative control measures that can be taken include discouraging night roaming and keeping all pets restrained on a leash when walking outside. Repairing or constructing fences and enclosures to help keep wild animals out of a pet's play area will also help reduce chances of exposure.

If a dog is bitten by a stray or wild animal, the wound needs to be seen immediately by a veterinarian, and, depending on when the last one was given, a booster rabies immunization should be administered. The animal should also be placed in quarantine for a minimum of 90 days, unless the particular animal that did the biting can be found and its rabies status confirmed as negative.

If the dog that was bitten by a known carrier of rabies has never been vaccinated before, immediate euthanasia is warranted. If an owner of such a pet refuses to do so, then, for safety sake, the pet should be quarantined for at least six months before it is declared uninfected.

Laws in most states spell out regulations concerning vaccinations, bites involving humans, and the ownership of wildlife in order to curb the impact of this disease. Any vaccinated dog that bites a human being needs to be placed in quarantine for a minimum of ten days to observe for signs of rabies. If suspicious signs appear, the animal is then euthanized, and samples are sent to the laboratory. If there is no history of the dog ever having a rabies vaccine in the past, or if a wild animal is involved, euthanasia and prompt laboratory examination of the brain tissue is warranted to expedite the diagnostic process.

Euthanasia should be carried out only by veterinarians or other public health and/or wildlife officials to ensure that the sample that reaches the lab has been properly handled and stored. Certainly any person bitten by an animal should contact his/her physician immediately. If the situation warrants it, prophylactic rabies treatment will be started on the bitten individual until the quarantine period is over or until the specific laboratory tests are in.

It is interesting to note that because the concentration of the rabies virus in the infected dog's saliva might be low or even absent in some cases, less than 50% of all bites from rabies-positive animals will result in the transmission of the disease. Yet because there is no way of knowing which fall into this category, prophylactic treatment is a must, just to be on the safe side!

Finally, ownership of wild animals, especially skunks (descented or not) and raccoons, should be avoided for a number of reasons. First, there are no licensed vaccines available for these wild pets. Secondly, because the incubation period of rabies can last for months, owners might be exposing themselves to rabies right from the start without knowing it. Finally, in many states, it is outright against the law to own such pets without a permit.

Parents should always discourage children from interacting with stray animals or wildlife. Their natural curiosity could lead to a serious bite wound and much anxiety, especially if the offender is not found.

BACTERIAL DISEASES

Primary infections caused by bacterial organisms are uncommon in dogs. In most instances, bacterial infections occur secondarily to other disease conditions, such as stress, viral infections, and parasites. As a result, whenever a bacterial disease is present, treatments should be directed against any underlying problems as well.

Bacterial skin disease

Bacteria can play an important role in diseases and disorders of the skin in dogs. For more information on bacterial skin diseases and their treatment, see chapter 14.

Leptospirosis

Canine leptospirosis is a bacterial disease of dogs characterized by jaundice, vomiting, and kidney failure. At least four different groups of leptospirosis organisms, all belonging to the genus and species *Leptospira interrogans*, have been implicated in this disease in dogs. Remarkably enough, most infections are subclinical; that is, few show clinical signs of disease. When clinical signs do arise, however, the results can be serious, even life-threatening. Leptospirosis becomes more of a problem in kennels where animals are kept together under poor sanitary conditions. Animals become infected with the organisms through contact with infected urine.

Symptoms

Leptospirosis is found primarily in young animals between the ages of 1 to 4 years. In addition, males seem to be more commonly affected than do females. Signs associated with the disease reflect the damage done by the organisms to the body's blood, liver, and kidneys. Fever, depression, vomiting, and diarrhea might be early signs that become noticeable. Anemia might set in as red blood cells are destroyed by the invading organisms, and distinct bruising on the skin surface might become evident as the body's blood clotting mechanisms are impaired. In severe cases, liver failure and/or kidney failure might appear, leading to rapid dehydration and to a urine with an orange-brown color, a feature characteristic of this disease. Left untreated, death will usually result.

Diagnosis

For diagnosis of this disease, veterinarians rely upon a thorough history (including a vaccination history and the type of quarters a dog is kept in), clinical signs, and laboratory work. The white blood cell count is usually elevated, in contrast to those seen with viral-type diseases. Blood and urine cultures might be called upon to confirm a diagnosis. Antibody levels measured at two week intervals have been used as well for this purpose.

Treatment

Treatment of leptospirosis consists of high levels of penicillin and aminoglycoside antibiotics, combined with fluid therapy to combat dehydration and medications to stimulate kidney function. Unfortunately, unless treated early enough, the kidneys could suffer irreparable damage, leading to unavoidable failure.

Because of the serious nature of this disease, dog owners need to focus their attention on prevention. Protection against this disease is usually provided in the standard DA2LPP vaccine used in puppies and annually in adults. Most of these vaccines protect against not just one, but several different groups of leptospira organisms that might infect dogs. In areas prone to the disease, dogs should receive a booster vaccination every six months or so, just to be safe.

Canine cough (kennel cough)

The bacterium *Bordetella bronchiseptica* is but one of the many organisms that can cause canine cough in dogs. Related to the same bacteria that causes whooping cough in humans, this bacteria can cause permanent damage to the airways of affected dogs if not detected and treated soon enough.

Higher bacteria

A special group of bacteria, called "higher bacteria," which share characteristics of both standard bacteria and fungi, can cause significant disease in exposed dogs.

Two of the more prevalent organisms in this class include *Nocardia* and *Actinomyces*. These agents, found in soil, are transmitted primarily via traumatic wounds. Draining, painful skin lesions and severe pneumonia are consequences of higher bacterial infections in dogs. Diagnosis and treatment for these diseases is similar to that of standard bacterial infections; however, surgical removal of infected tissue is often required to afford a complete cure.

FUNGI AND YEAST

Along with viruses and bacteria, fungal organisms can produce infectious disease (mycoses) in dogs. Probably the most common one pet owners are familiar with and have heard about is dermatophytosis, or ringworm. In addition, yeast infections can be a common problem in the ears of dogs. These types of yeast and fungi that affect mainly the outer skin surfaces are termed superficial mycoses.

Ringworm

The most prevalent fungal disease that afflicts dogs is ringworm. Ringworm can actually be caused by three different organisms, *Microsporum canis*, *Trichophyton mentagrophytes*, and *Microsporum gypseum*. The first two are contracted from infected animals, the third from contaminated soil.

Symptoms

In dogs, ringworm causes patchy hair loss with or without an accompanying lesion on the skin beneath. Since humans can be susceptible to the same type of ringworm, a diagnosis might be supported by reddened, circular lesions occurring on the owner as well.

Diagnosis and Treatment

Diagnosis of ringworm is confirmed by a fungal culture. Treatment can consist of iodine or chlorhexidine shampoos, topical anti-fungal medications (i.e., miconazole), and/or oral medications, such as griseofulvin. It

6-5   *Ringworm fungal spores.*

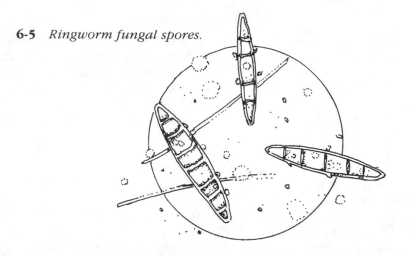

should be strongly emphasized that griseofulvin can cause birth defects and should not be given to pregnant dogs.

SUBCUTANEOUS OR DEEP MYCOSES

In contrast to ringworm, fungal and yeast infections involving the deeper tissues of the body are termed *subcutaneous* or *deep mycoses,* depending upon the level of tissue involvement. These organisms—including sporotrichosis, aspergillosis, blastomycosis, histoplasmosis, coccidioidomycosis, and cryptococcosis, can be quite severe, and even life-threatening at times.

Inhalation of fungal spores from infected soil through the respiratory tract is the primary mode of transmission for the majority of these deeper fungi and yeast (with the exception of sporotrichosis). As a result, often the first clinical signs seen relate to some type of respiratory problem. Many of these dogs just seem to do poorly, and often suffer from chronic weight loss. Others are presented to the veterinarian for a skin disorder or abscess, when in fact the skin problem is actually being caused by underlying drainage from the deeper fungal involvement.

Sporotrichosis

The fungus that causes sporotrichosis in dogs, *Sporothrix schenckii,* can gain entrance into the body via a direct injury to the skin or by inhalation, and then spread throughout the body by way of the lymphatic system.

Dogs afflicted with this soil-borne organism can exhibit numerous and tender lumps, nodules, and/or ulcerations anywhere on the body surface, but particularly on the extremities. Some of these lumps might actually resemble warts. In severe instances, liver, lungs, and other body organs can become involved as well. Inorganic iodide compounds, such as sodium or potassium iodide, are the treatments of choice for sporotrichosis.

Blastomycosis

Blastomyces dermatitidis is the organism responsible for this disease in dogs. Eighty percent of dogs affected will show some type of respiratory signs, such as a nonproductive cough. Skin involvement can occur with numerous draining lesions and abscesses, along with lymph node enlargement. Other organ systems can be affected as well. Blindness can result if the organisms spread to the eyes, and lameness, especially in the hind legs, occurs secondary to bone involvement.

Histoplasmosis

Histoplasmosis is caused by the organism *Histoplasma capsulatum*. Soil contaminated with the droppings of starlings and other birds appear to be an important source of this disease in dogs. Like blastomycosis, histoplasmosis can strike the respiratory system of affected dogs, leading to coughing and breathing difficulties. The gastrointestinal tract is often involved as well, resulting in chronic diarrhea. Bone, eye, and skin lesions can also result from a histoplasmosis infection.

Coccidioidomycosis

Infections with the fungus *Coccidioides immitis* are associated more with the dry, desert regions of North America. Hunting dogs and other canines allowed access to rodent burrows are most susceptible to exposure, since the soil in these areas might have a high concentration of fungal spores. As with other deep fungi, these spores are inhaled into the lungs, where the organisms set up housekeeping.

If the disease remains localized in the lungs, the clinical signs usually reflect this respiratory involvement. Coughing and breathing difficulties result from invasion of the lung tissue and from enlargement of lymph nodes within the chest cavity. If the coccidioidomycosis disseminates throughout the body via the blood and lymphatics, bone infection is common. Lameness, pain, and joint swelling usually occur as a result. Oftentimes, one or more draining tracts originating from the bone infection break through the skin and create unsightly lesions.

Cryptococcosis

Unlike the three conditions just mentioned, this disease is caused by a yeast organism, *Cryptococcus neoformans*, rather than a fungus. Soil contaminated with pigeon and bat feces is a main source of these yeast organisms.

Cryptococcosis in dogs is mainly an upper respiratory and nasal problem. A thick, copious, continuous nasal discharge usually results, and sneezing can be a clinical sign. From the nasal passages, cryptococcosis can spread throughout the body and cause lameness, enlarged lymph nodes, nervous system impairment, blindness, and skin infections.

Diagnosis and treatment for fungal infections

History, physical exam findings, and laboratory tests, including radiographic X-rays, and biopsies of affected regions can lead the veterinary practitioner to a tentative diagnosis of a fungal infection within the body. Microscopic examination of body fluids or drainages for fungal spores or yeast can also be helpful. In most cases, a definitive diagnosis is made by testing a blood serum sample for antibodies against the fungal organisms in question, or, less commonly, by culturing for growth.

Medications commonly used to treat fungal infections in dogs include amphotericin B, ketoconazole, 5-flucytosine, and iodide compounds. Depending upon which agents are used (many are used in combination with one another), duration of treatment required is often one to three months to afford a complete cure for these infections.

Radiographs and special immunologic tests can be used to monitor the response to treatment. In many cases, surgical excision of those regions infected with the fungus can afford faster recovery. The prognosis for dogs is good when fungal infections are detected and treated in their early stages; guarded to poor if dissemination throughout the body has occurred.

7

Parasitic Diseases

ALONG WITH INFECTIOUS diseases, internal and external parasites are responsible for the vast majority of illnesses and disorders seen in dogs. As a result, timely diagnosis and treatment for these pests is vital to the health of the dog.

FLEAS

Ctenocephalides canis (common dog flea) is by far the most common external parasite seen on dogs (FIG. 7-1). As every pet owner will attest to, these pests are the number-one health problem facing these pets. However, aside from causing relentless chewing and scratching, fleas are also disease carriers, and can threaten the dog owner's health as well. For these reasons, the development of a good control program to combat these irritating pests is a must.

It is important to understand that fleas spend the vast majority of their time off of the pet, reproducing and maturing in the pet's environment. As a result, environmental control measures are essential for successful flea control.

The flea life cycle includes four major stages: egg, larva, pupa, and adult stages. Both the egg and pupa stages are very resistant to insecticides, which can make complete flea control difficult. During summer months, the entire flea cycle (egg to adult) might be completed in 16-21 days. Heat and humidity tend to shorten this cycle period. In addition, fleas are most prolific during hot humid weather.

A complete approach to flea control should always involve three steps:

1. Treating the home
2. Treating the yard
3. Treating the pet.

Because fleas, on the average, will only spend about 10% of their time on dogs, treating the surrounding environment is probably more important than treating the actual pet. Remember: For every one flea seen on a dog, there's nine more in the house or yard.

For more information regarding flea control, see chapter 3.

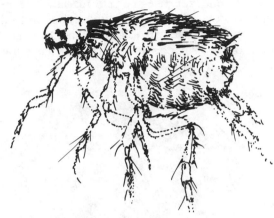

7-1 *The flea.*

TICKS

Ticks, unlike fleas, attach themselves to the pet's skin via their mouthparts. Ticks generally remain attached in one spot for long periods (FIG. 7-2). The head, neck, and interdigital (between toes) areas of the pet

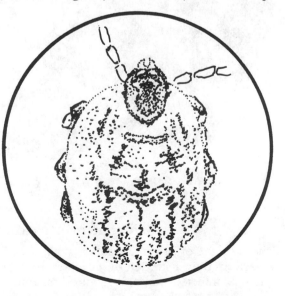

7-2 *The female tick.*

are the most common sites of severe infestation. Ticks produce local irritation and even anemia in heavy infestations. Ticks might serve as intermediate hosts for disease-producing microorganisms and might transmit these "germs" (such as Lyme disease) to the infested pet.

For more information on tick control, see chapter 3.

MITES

Mite infestation is commonly known as *mange* and requires the diagnostic and treatment expertise of a veterinarian. The common mites infecting dogs are microscopic requiring skin scrapes and subsequent microscopic examination by the veterinarian for diagnosis (FIG. 7-3). The three most common forms of mange and pertinent facts concerning each are listed below.

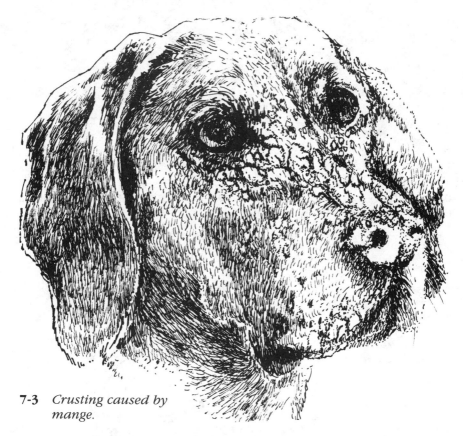

7-3 *Crusting caused by mange.*

Sarcoptic mange (scabies)

Caused by the organism *Sarcoptes scabiei* var. *canis*, sarcoptic mange is characterized by a sudden onset of severe itching (FIG. 7-4). Direct exposure to an infected animal is required for transmission.

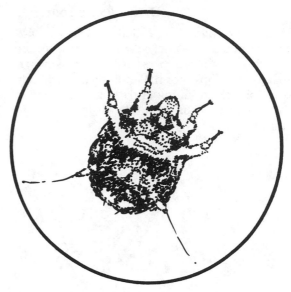

7-4 *Sarcoptes.*

Symptoms

The mite burrows into the host's epidermis and tunnels. Severe itching results, particularly on the abdomen, chest, legs, and ears. Thickening and scaling of elbows, hocks, and ear tips might be noted. Hair loss and skin irritation often results from the almost constant scratching and biting.

Scabies is highly contagious to other dogs. In addition, it might temporarily produce chigger-like bites and itching on exposed human family members.

Treatment

Pet treatment consists of proper diagnosis and miticidal dipping. Total cure can generally be achieved with one to three proper dippings. All dogs in the household should be treated due to the highly contagious nature of the scabies mite. Consult a veterinarian in cases of puppy exposure since milder type products are required for the young. If pet to human transmission occurs, contact your physician.

Cheyletiella mange

The mange mite *Cheyletiella* can cause skin scaling, intense itching, and hair loss in affected dogs. The common name for this parasitism is "walking dandruff," since the flakes and scales produced by the disease, when observed closely, appear to be in motion. Like sarcoptic mange, this mite can temporarily infest people who become exposed.

Diagnosis and treatment of *Cheyletiella* is the same as that for sarcoptic mange.

Demodectic mange

Demodectic mange is also called *follicular* or *red mange*. The demodectic mange mite, *Demodex canis*, might be found in the hair follicles of normal dogs in low numbers (FIG. 7-5). However, in cases where demodectic mange develops, normal immunity to the mite either fails to develop or is suppressed resulting in pathogenic proliferation of the mite within the hair follicles. Thus, demodicosis is not considered to be a contagious disease.

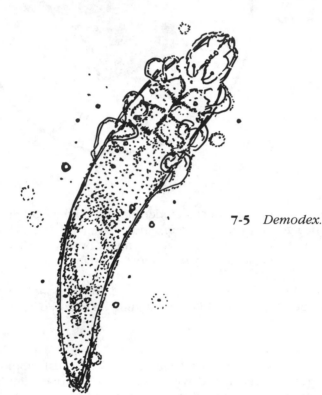

7-5   *Demodex.*

Symptoms

The majority of demodectic mange cases occurs in dogs less than 2 years of age whose immune systems are immature or temporarily suppressed. The first symptom observable is usually small areas of hair loss. The lesions might occur anywhere on the body but often begin in the head area. Diagnosis requires a skin scraping and microscopic exam by a veterinarian.

The lesions (areas of hair loss) might be localized to one area or generalized over the body. Secondary bacterial hair follicle infections (*folliculitis*) is a common sequel to some localized and most generalized cases. The inflammatory skin reaction which ensues might result in the reddened skin referred to by the term "red mange."

Treatment

With correct diagnosis and appropriate treatment, 80-90 percent of young dogs with demodicosis will recover. Maturation of the immune response plays a vital role in cases of complete recovery. Relapse might occur but is infrequent. However, unlike sarcoptic mange, demodicosis often requires long term therapy.

Demodectic mange in older dogs might reflect immunologic suppression elicited by an underlying disease. Liver disorders, viral infections, malnutrition, heat cycle changes, neoplasia, hypothyroidism, diabetes, and other problems might lead to impaired immune responses and demodicosis. A thorough physical examination is important in such cases. The success of the treatment varies being dependent upon the cause of immunoincompetence.

Special insecticidal dips are available for demodectic mange through a veterinarian.

Factors concerning a dog's immunologic ability to protect itself from developing demodectic mange are considered hereditary. However, since most cases of demodicosis resolve upon patient maturity, the significance of heritability is questionable.

LICE

Lice infection, or *pediculosis*, in dogs is usually seen in young animals kept in unclean breeding or kennel environments (FIG. 7-6).

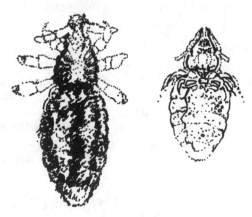

7-6 *Left: sucking louse; right: biting louse.*

Symptoms

Signs of such an infestation can include itching and reddened skin, with or without secondary bacterial infection. As with mites, lice can be identified by performing a skin scraping on an affected area and looking for the organisms under the microscope. In addition, the eggs of the lice can often be visualized attached to hair shafts near its attachment to the hair follicle.

Treatment

Lice are treated the same way that sarcoptic mange mites are treated: with insecticidal dippings. These dippings should be performed on a weekly basis for three or four treatments. In addition, the pet's environment should be treated as well to prevent reinfestation.

ESOPHAGEAL WORMS

The esophageal worm of dogs, *Spirocerca lupi*, is found primarily in the southeastern and southwestern portions of the United States. These worms, which are red and coiled in appearance, burrow into and inhabit the wall of the esophagus, and sometimes the stomach, of their host.

Direct transmission from dog to dog does not occur; rather, beetles, chickens, amphibians, and rodents all can act as intermediary hosts for this worm. When dogs come in oral contact with one of these hosts, infection can result. Once ingested, the worms migrate through blood vessels within the body, eventually ending up in the esophageal wall. From here, they produce more eggs, which are coughed up and swallowed, and then passed out in the feces.

Symptoms

Because the nodules formed by the worms interfere with swallowing, vomiting after meals is the most prevalent clinical sign seen with *Spirocerca* infections. To make matters worse, these nodules can have a propensity for becoming cancerous in a small percentage of cases. In addition, bony lesions along the vertebral column and in the bones of the arms and legs can result from the migratory habits of these parasites.

Treatment

Diagnosis of esophageal worms involves a fecal exam, radiographs, and direct examination of the esophagus and stomach using an endoscope. Unfortunately, once clinical signs are noticed by the owner, the majority of the damage has already been done, and treatment attempts are futile. Surgery can sometimes be used to actually remove the nodules and provide relief, yet it rarely affords a total cure. And considering the number of possible transport hosts for this parasite, environmental control is difficult at best.

TAPEWORMS

Tapeworms are considered segmented flatworms, belonging to a class of organisms called *Cestoda* (FIG. 7-7). One important characteristic of this class is that all utilize intermediate hosts in their transmission cycle. Intermediate hosts can include rodents, fleas and other insects, rabbits, sheep, swine, cattle, and in some instances, even humans!

Tapeworm segments containing eggs are shed in fecal material. When these eggs are accidentally or voluntarily consumed by an intermediate host, they hatch and the resulting larvae migrate into the body tissues and

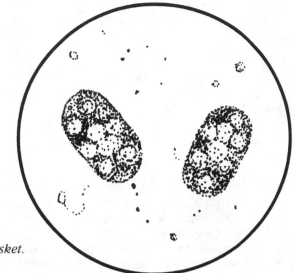

7-7 *Tapeworm egg basket.*

begin their development. Yet they won't reach their adult stage inside the tissues of this intermediate host. Instead, the life cycle is completed when this host or portions thereof is consumed by another, called the definitive host. Inside this new host environment, the larvae then proceed to develop into an adult tapeworm, which attaches to the intestinal wall, eats, and makes ready to repeat the cycle all over again.

The extent of disease caused by tapeworms depends on the type of worm involved, and if the affected individual is an intermediate host or a final host. As a rule, adult tapeworms living within the intestines of a definitive host are not usually life-threatening, causing varying degrees of gastroenteritis and malnutrition. Larval forms, on the other hand, tend to do more damage, simply because they migrate through the body tissues. Furthermore, if these larvae gain entrance into the tissues of an animal (or human) that is not a normal intermediate host for that tapeworm, the results can sometimes be deadly (see Zoonotic Diseases).

By far the most prevalent species of tapeworm seen in dogs is called *Dipylidium caninum*; the double-pored tapeworm. The reason it is so common is that it uses the flea as an intermediate host (the dog louse can also be a carrier).

Segments from the tapeworm are passed in the feces or actually "crawl" out onto the hair coat of an infested animal. Once outside, the segments dry out and release egg baskets into the environment. These eggs are then ingested by flea larvae looking for food, and a new tapeworm begins its development. If the flea happens to be ingested by a dog during chewing or self-grooming episodes, the tapeworm larvae will continue its development into an adult worm within the pet's small intestine.

Though less frequent, dogs can become infected with other types of tapeworms besides *Dipylidium*, depending on potential exposure to intermediate hosts. For instance, dogs fed raw meat or garbage are at risk. *Echinococcus granulosus*, the tapeworm responsible for hydatid cyst disease, is often transmitted to dogs in this way.

Symptoms

Dogs infested with adult tapeworms might or might not exhibit the typical signs associated with gastroenteritis, such as vomiting and diarrhea. Weight loss certainly can occur as the worms absorb nutrients from within the gut. Oftentimes, scooting and other signs related to anal sac discomfort might also tip an owner off as to the presence of these pesky parasites.

Diagnosis of a tapeworm infestation can be confirmed by actually seeing the white, moving, worm-like segments in fresh fecal material or on the hair coat around the hind region. Segments might also be seen upon anal sac expression. If dried, the segments will take on a brownish, "rice-like" appearance.

Microscopic examination of the stool might be helpful as well; however, because the shedding of the segments is sporadic, a negative finding cannot totally rule out an infestation.

Treatment

Tapeworms can be difficult pests to treat and totally eliminate. Praziquantel and epsiprantel are two effective medications used by veterinarians to eliminate tapeworms from the intestines. Other drugs, such as niclosamide and bunamidine, have also been used as well. Repeating the treatment in 2 to 3 weeks helps ensure thorough elimination. For tough infestations, administering an injectable form of the medication might be more effective than through oral means.

Flea control is the best way to prevent *Dipylidium caninum*. Other tapeworms, including *Echinococcus*, can be prevented by not allowing dogs access to garbage and/or raw meat.

ROUNDWORMS

Roundworms, known as ascarids or spool worms, are thick-bodied, whitish-to-cream-colored worms that can inhabit the small intestine of dogs (FIG. 7-8). This is one of the most common intestinal parasites affecting dogs and young puppies. In fact, research has demonstrated that over 95% percent of all puppies are born with some form of roundworms.

Adult worms exist unattached within the intestinal lumen and can grow up to eight inches in length. If present in large enough numbers, adult roundworms can cause prominent malnutrition and gastroenteritis. In some severe instances, rupture of an intestine jam-packed with roundworms has been known to happen. Immature roundworms can cause problems too, since they might migrate throughout the lungs, liver, and other tissues of the body before settling down as adults within the intestines.

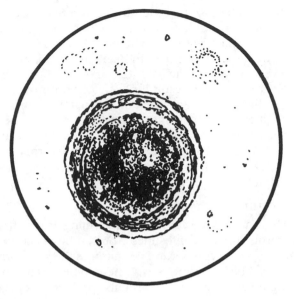

7-8 *Roundworm egg.*

Unlike tapeworms, roundworms do not require an intermediate host for their transmission. Each female worm sheds thousands of eggs into the environment by the way of feces. These eggs, which are covered by a thick shell, are very resistant and might remain viable in an environment for years prior to being consumed by an unsuspecting dog.

After consumption of a roundworm egg, it is possible for the hatched larvae to develop into adults without ever leaving the intestine. However, this is the exception rather than the rule. What usually happens is the larvae penetrate the bowel wall and migrate to the liver and the lungs, maturing and growing along the way. Once inside the lungs, they can enter the airways, be coughed up and swallowed again, allowing them to finish their development into adults within the intestines.

Alternatively, from the lungs, these larvae can enter the bloodstream and circulate throughout the body. In female dogs, these larvae might settle down and become dormant within the mammary tissue until such time as lactation begins. In this way, newborn pups can ingest roundworm larvae through their mother's milk. But this isn't the only reason for the high incidence of roundworms in neonatal puppies. They can also be exposed to the circulating roundworm larvae via the umbilical cord while they are still in the womb, and actually be born with an active infestation!

Symptoms

The clinical signs seen with a roundworm infestation depend upon the age of the dog affected, the stage of maturity that the worms are in, and their location within the body.

As a general rule, the younger the dog, the more severe the signs tend to be. In fact, some older dogs can actually develop a resistance to these parasites. If adult worms are within the intestines, signs often include stomach pain with a prominent "bloated" appearance to the abdomen, vomiting, and diarrhea. In many instances, actual adult worms might be revealed within the vomitus or stool. Ruptured bowels and intestinal obstructions can result if not treated promptly.

Because of the migration through the lungs, coughing, breathing difficulties, and other signs of pneumonia might be present. In severe cases, seizures and other nervous system problems can occur.

Veterinarians can diagnose roundworms by using a microscope to look for eggs in a sample of stool. Clinical signs and the dog's history are helpful in those cases where eggs might be absent from such a sample.

Treatment

There are a wide variety of deworming drugs effective at removing roundworms from the intestines. You can buy relatively inexpensive dewormers at grocery stores and pet supplies. Be sure, however, to consult a veterinarian before using one of these to be certain that it contains the correct ingredients for a pet's particular problem. Repeat dewormings should be performed three weeks later to ensure that any migrating larvae that reached the intestines since the first deworming are killed.

Young puppies suffering from roundworm-induced pneumonia require intensive veterinary supportive care to prevent life-threatening complications from arising. Most will recover with such care.

Research findings and the lack of effective drugs available that will remove roundworm larvae from the tissues (such as the mammary glands of expectant mothers), dictate that all puppies should be dewormed for these parasites, even if parasite eggs are not seen on an initial stool exam. These dewormings should commence at 3 weeks of age, and should be repeated at 6 and 9 weeks of age. Periodic stool exams are warranted to confirm a puppy's negative status.

Good sanitation procedures will help prevent reinfections and spread to other dogs. Realize, however, that once roundworms enter an environment, they are almost impossible to totally eliminate due to the hearty nature of the eggs. As a result, semiannual stool checks by a veterinarian are indicated to ensure pets remain parasite-free.

Visceral larval migrans, a human disease syndrome caused by migrating roundworm larvae, does pose a serious public health threat. As a result, good personal hygiene after handling pets, plus routine stool exams and treatments are a must to minimize the threat from this disease.

HOOKWORMS

The hookworm (*Ancylostoma, Uncinaria*) is another type of parasite that inhabits the small intestine of dogs (FIG. 7-9). Unlike the roundworm—which floats unattached within the intestinal lumen, absorbing nutrients through its skin—the hookworm actually uses teeth to attach itself to the

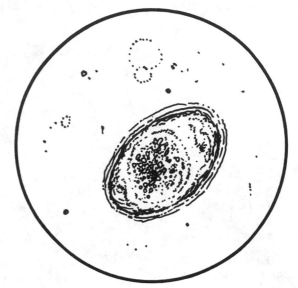

7-9 *Hookworm egg.*

wall of the intestine. Once attached, it begins to suck blood from vessels within the wall. In fact, it can become so severe that anemia and eventual death of the host animal could result if the hookworms are left untreated.

Compared to roundworms, hookworms are fairly small and thread-like, measuring up to one inch in length. Their life cycle (FIG. 7-10) begins with adult worms within the gut laying eggs, which are then passed out in the stool. If environmental conditions are warm and humid enough, the eggs hatch and give rise to larvae, which then search for a host canine.

Once a host comes along, the larvae can gain entrance into the body in a number of ways. They can be picked up by way of mouth, or they can actually penetrate the skin (usually the foot pads) and migrate through tissue before reaching the small intestine. Like roundworms, some of these migrating larvae might decide to stop and settle for a while within the tissues, making it possible for puppies of such females to become infected while still in the womb, or through nursing infected milk. As a result, puppies can be born with these blood-sucking parasites.

Symptoms

The severity of clinical signs depends largely upon the amount of worms present in the gut and the age of the dog infected. Generally speaking, young puppies suffer from more severe disease than do adults.

Lethargy, loss of appetite, and pale mucous membranes due to loss of blood are not uncommon in canines harboring a large worm burden. A dark, tarry diarrhea might or might not be present. If skin penetration has taken place, the foot pads or other areas might be reddened, bleeding, and/or infected due to the larvae. Intense itching is also be noted as a result of this penetration.

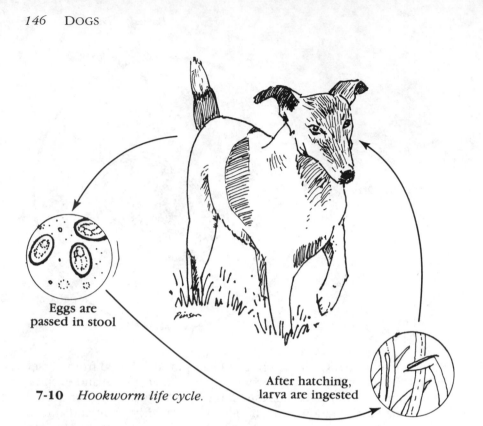

Eggs are
passed in stool

7-10 *Hookworm life cycle.*

After hatching,
larva are ingested

Treatment

Diagnosis of a hookworm infestation is based upon an examination of a
stool sample for the presence of hookworm eggs.

There are a number of safe dewormers available from veterinarians
that can help eliminate a hookworm infection. After the initial dose is
given, a follow-up deworming should be administered two to three weeks
later to kill any migrating larvae that have since reached the intestines.

In dogs suffering from anemia, supportive veterinary care is needed.
This might include blood transfusions if the loss of blood is bad enough.
Intravenous fluids and antibiotics might also be used to combat dehydration and secondary infections. Vitamin and iron supplements, combined
with a high-quality diet, are fed to provide building blocks within the
body for new blood to be produced.

It is known that some dogs can actually develop an immunity to
hookworms after an initial infection has taken place. However, this does
not preclude routine periodic stool checks by a veterinarian, since those
individuals that actually develop immunity can be difficult to identify.

Hookworm eggs are not as hearty as their roundworm counterparts;
hence, environmental control can be an effective way to prevent reinfec-
tion or spread to other dogs. Since the eggs require optimum environmental conditions before hatching will occur, keeping fecal material
picked up daily in and around the premises will reduce chances of expo-

sure. Studies have also shown that outdoor dogs kept on concrete stand less chance of infection than dogs housed in kennels with dirt or grassy floors. Again, this is assuming that daily removal of contaminating fecal material is performed.

Deworming female dogs prior to pregnancy will help reduce the chances of puppies being born with hookworm infections. However, because deworming will not eliminate larvae within the mother's tissues and mammary glands, all neonatal pups should be routinely dewormed for these parasites starting at three weeks of age.

Many heartworm preventative medications on the market today also help prevent or even eliminate hookworm infestations if given on a regular basis. In those instances where environmental contamination is difficult to control, administering such a preventative year-round might be the answer to keeping a dog hookworm-free.

As in dogs, some hookworm larvae have the ability to penetrate the skin of man, causing severe itching and dermatitis. This condition in man is known as *cutaneous larval migrans,* or "creeping eruption." It is seen most often in tropical climates and in the southeastern portions of the United States. Since hookworm larvae thrive in warm sandy soils, this disease is one major reason why in most areas, pets are denied access to public beaches.

WHIPWORMS

Trichuris vulpis, the dog whipworm, is a slender parasite that can reach four inches in length (FIG. 7-11). Unlike tapeworms, hookworms, and roundworms, which inhabit the small intestine, whipworms colonize the

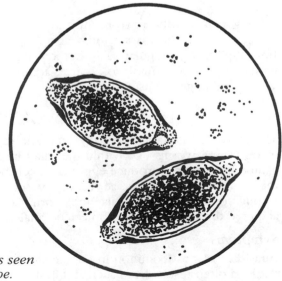

7-11 *Whipworm eggs as seen under a microscope.*

large intestine, particularly the cecum (this corresponds to the human appendix).

The life cycle of this parasite is fairly simple. Eggs are passed in fresh feces into the environment. These eggs are then swallowed by an unsuspecting dog, and hatch within the dog's gut. From there, they set up housekeeping within the large intestine and grow to maturity, sometimes taking up to three months to do so. Adult females then produce more eggs, and the cycle is repeated. Note that unlike hookworms and roundworms, whipworms are not known to undergo tissue migration.

Symptoms

Light to moderate infections with whipworms might not give any outward hints of their presence. Sometimes dogs so affected might develop rough, unkempt hair coats and lose weight. Diarrhea might or might not be a clinical sign. When it does occur, the stools are often blood-tinged.

Like other intestinal parasites, definitive diagnosis of a whipworm infection is made by identifying whipworm eggs in stool under a microscope. Whipworms don't seem to be as prolific as other gut parasites; as a result, multiple samples might need to be examined before any eggs are seen.

Treatment

Since whipworms are a common cause of chronic colitis in dogs, many practitioners might opt to deworm for these parasites in such cases, even if eggs are not seen on a fecal exam. In many instances, whipworms are indeed to blame, and the condition responds quite favorably to this empirical therapy.

Several different types of dewormers are effective at expelling whipworms. Some require only a single treatment; others need follow-ups.

As seen with hookworm infections, many heartworm preventative medications on the market today also help prevent whipworm infestations if given on a regular basis. In those instances where environmental contamination is difficult to control, administering such a preventative year-round might be useful.

THREADWORMS

Threadworm infestations usually limit themselves to tropical-type climates. These worms live within the small intestines as adults, and, like canine lungworms, produce eggs that hatch before being passed out in the stool. These active larvae that are passed can then enter a new host through oral ingestion, or, like hookworms, can penetrate the skin or be acquired through the milk of infected females.

Symptoms

Parasitism is most common in puppies under 4 months of age. Profuse diarrhea often results from such an infestation. In addition, if skin penetration occurred, intense itching at the sites of entry is seen. Following skin invasion, coughing might become a problem as the larvae migrate through the lungs on their way to the intestines. In severe cases, pneumonia can result.

Treatment

Diagnosis is made by direct microscopic examination of the live larvae in the feces. Treatment of threadworms can be difficult, requiring more potent compounds than those used to treat roundworms, hookworms, and the like. If diarrhea and/or coughing is severe, supportive veterinary care is also indicated.

Because threadworms thrive in warm, humid, unsanitary conditions, sound environmental management can help curb the spread of these parasites. This is especially important for public health reasons, since cross-infection between man and dogs has been known to happen.

LUNGWORMS

Lungworm infections in dogs are uncommon, yet worth mentioning. These delicate, transparent worms live within the respiratory tract of affected canines, burrowed within the wall of the trachea. Eggs are coughed up and swallowed. Hatching then takes place within the gut, and live larvae are passed out in the feces. As a result, contact with the latter is the mode of transmission from dog to dog.

Symptoms

Relentless coughing is the number one sign caused by this parasite. In severe infestations, actual suffocation resulting in death has been known to occur, especially in young pups. Because eggs are passed in the stool, fecal examinations can be used by veterinarians to diagnose an infection. Direct endoscopic examination of the airway nodules caused by the worms also provides definitive answers.

Treatment

Levamisole is the dewormer commonly used to tackle lungworm infestations in dogs.

HEARTWORMS

When we hear of parasites or worms our natural inclination is to think of those that inhabit the gastrointestinal tract. However, there is such parasite that, instead of residing within the gut, prefers the heart instead. That parasite is *Dirofilaria immitis*, the canine heartworm (FIG. 7-12).

Heartworm disease is a devastating disease of dogs, responsible for tens of thousands of deaths each year. Most of these occur due to the destruction that these worms do to not just the heart but the lungs, liver, and kidneys, as well. In some cases, the worm burden within the heart and blood vessels might become so great that circulation of blood is actu-

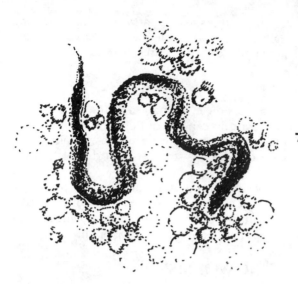

7-12   *Larval form of the heartworm.*

ally compromised, resulting in sudden death. Other infected dogs might go years without showing any signs of heartworm disease, seemingly forming a symbiotic relationship with the parasites.

Regardless of its presentation, the presence of heartworm disease puts a tremendous burden on the body's organs and immune system. The good news is that this destructive disease is completely preventable!

Heartworm disease is transmitted through the use of a vector, the mosquito. When a mosquito feeds upon a dog infected with heartworms, it picks up heartworm larvae (microfilaria) through its blood meal. Inside of the insect, the microfilaria begin to undergo primary development. Now when the mosquito gets hungry again, the larvae exit the feeding mouthpart of the mosquito and are deposited on the skin of the new host canine. From here, they gain access into the dog's tissue through the feeding port created by the mosquito, and begin a six-month migration to the heart, growing and developing along the way.

Once they reach the heart, they set up housekeeping and mature into adults (FIG. 7-13). Some of these can reach up to fourteen inches in length! Once mature, they start reproducing and the new larvae produced are deposited into the bloodstream, just waiting to be picked up by a hungry mosquito.

Heartworm disease is found worldwide, anywhere mosquitos are found. In North America, the Southeastern and Gulf Coast regions of the United States have a greater prevalence of the disease than other areas. However, infections have been documented as far north as Canada.

The incidence of this disease seems to be higher in dogs between the ages of 4 and 7 years. Males are more likely to contract the disease than are females. Larger breeds—who, as a general rule, spend more time outdoors—are also more susceptible to heartworms. Of course, this does not mean that small, indoor lap dogs are safe from exposure, since they can't

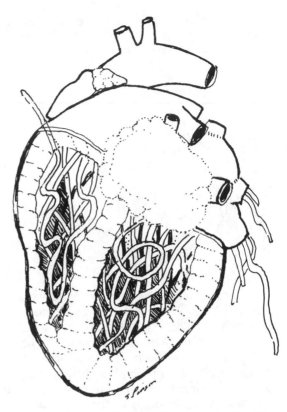

7-13 *Canine heartworm disease.*

be totally shielded from the wayward mosquito that happens to find its way indoors. Interestingly enough, the length of a dog's hair coat does not figure in when determining a dog's risk of contracting heartworm disease.

Canines are the primary host of *Dirofilaria immitis*; however, other mammals can become infected, including cats and foxes. Man has even been known to become an accidental host for this parasite. In these instances, the larvae will migrate into the lungs, where they are sealed off by the body and subsequently cause no clinical problems. The lung lesions created, however, might be easily confused with tuberculosis or cancer, causing some consternation in doctors and in the patients so affected.

Symptoms

Clinical signs of heartworm disease can include exercise intolerance, coughing and breathing difficulties, or sudden death. The worms primarily reside in the right portion of the heart and in the lungs. Heartworms cause thickening of the lung's blood vessels, causing an increase in blood pressure and the heart's workload. Congestive heart failure is not an uncommon sequela in these individuals as the heart eventually becomes unable to compensate for such an increased workload (see chapter 9).

This in itself has a "snowball" effect, causing fluid build-up within the lungs and a disruption of blood circulation to the vital organs. Damage to the liver and kidneys is an ultimate consequence (FIG. 7-14).

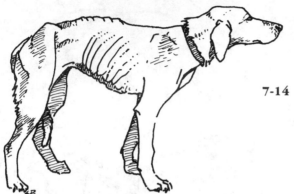

7-14   *The results of heartworms in a dog.*

Occasionally, the number of heartworms becomes so great that they can actually block the return flow of blood from other parts of the body to the heart. This condition and the resulting clinical signs are termed *caval syndrome.* Whereas the onset of clinical signs with a typical heartworm infection might be slow and gradual, the signs seen with caval syndrome occur abruptly and with fury. Dogs so affected might suddenly collapse, unable to breath, and in advanced organ failure. Actual surgical removal of the offending heartworms can be used to save the life of some of these dogs; in most, however, the disease is too far advanced to even attempt treatment.

Diagnosis

Diagnosis of heartworm disease is based upon a simple blood test and/or radiographic X-ray findings. Recent technological advancements have made heartworm detection much easier and testing much more accurate. Until recently, detecting microfilaria by passing a blood sample through a special filter was the standard test used to diagnose heartworms. However, through a new technology called *monoclonal-based enzyme immunoassays,* newer tests are now available which can actually detect the presence of adult worms within the heart and lungs, rather than relying on detection of larvae within the blood stream.

This is significant for a number of reasons. First, occult infections are readily identified by these tests. Secondly, newer tests readily differentiate between *Dirofilaria immitis* and another type of microfilaria that might be found in the dog's blood stream, *Dipetalonema reconditum*. Unlike the former, *Dipetalonema* is not considered dangerous to its canine host, yet its presence can easily confuse a diagnosis. Finally, since research has demonstrated that the time of day might have an effect on the number of larvae found in the bloodstream, the standard filter test might actually miss an active infection due to low numbers of larvae circulating in the blood. With the new technology, this margin of error has been eliminated.

Occult infections

Occult heartworm infections, or infections characterized by the absence of circulating microfilaria, can occur in 15-30 percent of all heartworm-infected dogs.

Occult infections might result from a number of factors:

1. Immature adult worms in the heart that are not yet reproducing
2. Infections involving worms of all the same sex
3. Destruction of larvae by the dog's immune system
4. Elimination of larvae as a result of giving heartworm preventative medication.

Until recent years, many occult infections went unnoticed, since the diagnosis of heartworms was generally based upon microscopic detection of larvae in a filtered blood sample. Unfortunately, many dogs (even those being given preventative heartworm medication) thought to be negative for heartworms based upon this type of testing actually harbored live adult heartworms within their hearts and lungs and suffered the consequences thereof.

Luckily for dogs and their owners, new tests have since been developed that do not rely upon this microfilaria detection; rather they detect the actual adult heartworms within the heart.

Treatment

Safe and successful treatment of a heartworm infection depends upon prompt diagnosis in the early stages of the disease, before secondary organ damage has occurred. The accepted drug of choice for treating heartworms in dogs is an arsenic compound called *thiacetarsamide*. Given intravenously, this medication kills the adult worms within the heart and lungs. Unfortunately, it can be highly toxic to the dog as well, causing damage to the liver and kidneys. In addition, some worms, especially females, might prove to be resistant to the effects of thiacetarsamide, resulting in an incomplete kill and necessitating the treatment series to be repeated.

Prior to treating a dog for heartworms, a complete laboratory workup, including radiographic X-rays, should be performed to determine the status of the internal organs, especially the heart, lungs, liver, and kidneys. If potential problems do exist, a "priming" dose of the thiacetarsamide might be administered to allow the body to adjust to this potent drug. Then in a month or so, if all looks well, a standard treatment is attempted.

The treatment involves a series of four thiacetarsamide injections; one injection given twice a day over a period of two days. Supportive medications such as antibiotics and vitamins are often concurrently administered during this time as well.

Complications from treatment

Complications from the thiacetarsamide therapy can arise, prompting immediate cessation of the treatment series. These can include loss of appetite, vomiting, and/or the development of icterus, indicating severe liver damage. As the adult worms die, pieces of them might lodge within the blood vessels of the lungs, and if extensive, protracted coughing and lung hemorrhaging can result. In addition to direct damage to the internal organs, intense inflammation and tissue sloughing can occur at the injection sites if any of the thiacetarsamide leaks from the vein after administration.

Recovery

If all goes well with the treatment series, patients are usually discharged from the hospital two to three days after the treatments are started to begin convalescence at home for the next four to six weeks. During this time, supportive treatments consisting of antibiotics, aspirin, and/or special diets might be prescribed.

It is of the utmost importance that a *strict limitation of exercise and stress be employed* during this convalescent period. In addition, preventative heartworm medication *is not* to be administered during this time.

Depression, loss of appetite, bleeding, and/or protracted coughing during this time should alert dog owners to potential post-treatment complications and warrant prompt veterinary attention.

Four to six weeks after treating the adult heartworms, special medication is administered to eliminate any circulating microfilaria that are present in non-occult cases. Once this is performed, preventative medication can then be given on a routine basis. At twelve weeks post-treatment, another heartworm test should be done to be certain that the infection was completely eliminated by the treatment. If not, the treatment series might need to be repeated, generally six to eight months after the first.

Because of the high toxicity of thiacetarsamide, veterinary researchers have been diligently at work trying to find an effective and less toxic alternative to it for treatment of heartworm disease. Newer, safer medications are being developed and tested for this purpose, and should become available in the very near future.

For information on preventing heartworm disease, see chapter 3.

FLUKES

Flukes are small, flat, tongue- or leaf-shaped parasites that inhabit the liver and/or lungs of parasitized dogs. Snails and fish can act as intermediate hosts for flukes, and dogs often become exposed by eating raw fish that is infected with the parasite. One such fluke, *Nanophyetus salmincola*, is also responsible for transmitting the organism that causes "salmon poisoning" in dogs. Seen primarily in canines living in or visiting California and other portions of the Pacific Northwest, the disease is contracted when these dogs consume raw or cold-smoked salmon or trout containing flukes. The disease syndrome seen somewhat resembles distemper and can cause a profuse, bloody diarrhea in affected individuals. Most dogs so affected will die unless treated promptly by a veterinarian.

KIDNEY WORMS

As with flukes, dogs can become infected with the canine kidney worm, *Dioctophyma renale* by eating raw fish. These worms are exceptionally large (some can grow up to three feet in length!) and cause damage to the tissues of the kidneys simply by their sheer size. Bloody urine is a common clinical sign seen, and eggs from the kidney worms can be visualized in the urine under a microscope. If parasites are found, surgical removal is warranted. Untreated dogs will eventually succumb to kidney failure.

COCCIDIA

Coccidia belong to a group of microscopic parasites called protozoans. These organisms primarily inhabit the small intestine of affected dogs. The disease caused by coccidia (coccidiosis) is rarely severe, yet the resulting diarrhea it causes can rapidly dehydrate a young puppy. Overcrowding and poor sanitation greatly contribute to the spread of these organisms within a group of canines. Eggs passed in fecal material can be directly ingested by another dog, leading to the development and maturation of the organisms within the gut of their new hosts.

If coccidia are ingested by animals other than their normal host (for example, if the feline *Toxoplasma* coccidia is ingested by a dog), tissue migration might occur, similar to that seen with roundworms. In most cases, this migration causes no problems, and the infection is quickly eliminated by the animal's immune system. However, if a young puppy is involved, or an animal with a compromised immune system, severe disease might result.

Symptoms

In younger dogs, diarrhea, abdominal pain, and weight loss are the most consistent clinical signs seen in an overwhelming case of coccidiosis. Older dogs might not show any signs at all.

If tissue migration has occurred (Toxoplasmosis), other signs might be seen, including fever, muscle soreness, and convulsions.

Treatment

A microscopic examination of a stool specimen will detect coccidia eggs if present. Treatment consists of administering an anti-coccidia drug in proper dosages. Sulfa drugs and nitrofurazone have been used by veterinarians to eliminate active coccidia infections in dogs. If dehydration is present, intravenous fluids are indicated to correct the disorder.

Good sanitation practices are the best ways to prevent exposure to coccidiosis. Routine stool checks performed by a veterinarian should also be utilized to ensure dogs remains parasite-free.

EHRLICHIOSIS

Ehrlichiosis, also known as canine typhus, is caused by the bacterial organism *Ehrlichia canis*. One of many tick-borne diseases, *Ehrlichia* is spread from dog to dog by the bite of the brown dog tick, *Rhipicephalus sanguineus*. First reported in the United States in 1963, this disease is most prevalent in the midwestern and southern states. Left undetected, ehrlichiosis can be quite devastating and ultimately fatal to its host (FIG. 7-15).

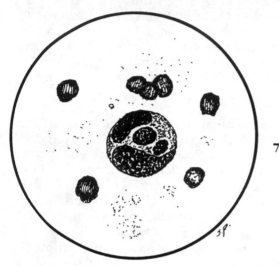

7-15   *Ehrlichia canis within a white blood cell.*

Symptoms

Once they gain entrance into the body, these parasitic bacteria set up housekeeping in various organ systems throughout the body within a week or two. As a result, clinical signs can be quite variable once they start to show.

Acute signs of infection include general depression, weakness, fever, weight loss, eye and nose discharges, and swollen lymph nodes. As the disease progresses over time and the organisms colonize the bone marrow, dogs will often become anemic and immunosuppressed. As a result, secondary pneumonia is not an infrequent finding in infected canines. Nosebleeds and bruising of the skin might also become apparent as the body's blood clotting mechanisms are interfered with.

Finally, in severe instances, the kidneys and brain might become affected, leading to kidney failure and nervous system disorders.

Diagnosis

A noticeable drop in the total number of white blood cells, red blood cells, and platelet (structures that play a vital role in the body's blood clotting mechanism) within an obtained blood sample are usually the first parameters that tip veterinarians off to a possible infection with ehrlichia (FIG. 7-15). In fact, in many cases, the ehrlichia organisms can be seen microscopically within the actual white blood cells themselves.

Clinical signs related to a bleeding disorder or involving a high fever also provide clues leading to such a diagnosis. Specific ehrlichia antibody detection tests are also available through veterinarians, and can help confirm what is already suspected.

Treatment

Current treatment of ehrlichiosis in dogs employs high doses of tetracycline antibiotics until clinical signs go into remission. Owing to the organism's ability to hide within blood cells and bone marrow, ehrlichiosis is difficult to treat. The sooner treatment is instituted after the appearance of clinical signs, the better the chances are for a complete recovery.

Chronic long-term infections, however, might never clear up totally with antibiotic therapy. A new experimental drug called *imidocarb diproprionate* has shown some promise in many of these cases, yet it is still in the testing stages. Until something new becomes available, continuous low-dose administration of tetracycline, combined with supportive therapy, including occasional blood transfusions, might be needed to keep these long-term infections controlled.

As of yet, there is no vaccine available to protect against ehrlichiosis; a good tick control program is still the best way to prevent this disease.

ROCKY MOUNTAIN SPOTTED FEVER

Rocky Mountain Spotted Fever is another tick-borne illness that can be transmitted to dogs. Many different tick species, including the brown dog tick can be carriers of the bacteria that can cause Rocky Mountain Spotted Fever. The incidence of this disease in the United States peaks during the late summer, then drops off as fall and winter arrive. As far as breed susceptibility to this disease is concerned, it is seen mostly in sporting breeds of dogs, simply because of their increased risk of tick exposure.

Symptoms

The clinical signs seen with Rocky Mountain Spotted Fever are very similar to those seen with ehrlichiosis. Bleeding, high fever, swollen lymph nodes, pneumonia, and seizures can all be seen with this disease. Yet unlike with ehrlichiosis, these clinical signs relate to an intense inflammation involving the blood vessels throughout the body. This can also result in marked abdominal pain, complete with vomiting and diarrhea.

Rocky Mountain Spotted Fever should be suspected whenever there is high fever, swollen lymph nodes, abdominal pain, and bruising of the skin and mucous membranes together with a history of tick infestation. Unlike ehrlichiosis, this disease is characterized in its later stages by an increase in the number of circulating white blood cells in the body; a clue that can help a veterinarian differentiate between the two diseases. Specific antibody tests can also be employed to obtain a definitive diagnosis.

Treatment

Treatment of this disease involves the use of high levels of tetracycline antibiotic for a minimum of 14 days. In many instances, response to treatment is slow, and favorable results might not be seen for some time.

Because there is no vaccine available, tick control is a must.

LYME DISEASE

In recent years, Lyme disease has come to the forefront in public awareness due to its ability to cause human illness. The disease, caused by the bacteria *Borrelia burgdorferi*, is primarily spread to dogs and to humans through the bite of an infected tick. Many different species of ticks can be involved, including the deer tick, the black-legged tick, and the Western black-legged tick.

Ticks, however, are not the only way the disease can be spread; fleas and other biting insects are capable of its spread as well. In addition, there have even been incidents in which Lyme disease has been transmitted via direct contact with infected body fluids. Because of this ease of transmission, Lyme disease is one of the most commonly reported tick-borne diseases, and it has been diagnosed in most states across the country.

Symptoms

Clinical signs of Lyme disease in dogs include loss of appetite, lethargy, high fever, swollen lymph nodes and joints, and/or a sudden onset of lameness. This lameness often resolves on its own accord, only to reoccur weeks to months later. In untreated dogs, kidney disease and heart disease can be unfortunate sequela.

Diagnosis

Diagnosis of Lyme disease is based upon a history of exposure to ticks and of recurring lameness. Veterinarians now have the ability to test for this disease in-house.

Treatment

Rapid treatment of a diagnosed case of Lyme disease is essential to prevent permanent damage to the joints or internal organs from resulting. Many different types of antibiotics can be used to treat this disease, and acute signs will usually disappear within 36 hours of instituting such therapy. Long-standing infections might not respond as well and require a more vigorous treatment approach.

A vaccine against Lyme disease is now available for use in dogs. After the initial immunization, a booster is recommended three weeks later, followed thereafter by annual re-vaccination.

Tick control is another important control measure to prevent Lyme disease. Since a tick must feed for about 24 hours before spread of the disease will take place, prompt removal of ticks will help break the transmission cycle.

The signs of this disease in humans are similar to those found in dogs. Vaccination of the family dog should help prevent it from becoming a source of human infection. In addition, prompt removal of ticks from the skin will help afford the same protection in people as it does in dogs.

8

The Immune System

WITHOUT A FUNCTIONING immune system, our pets (and ourselves) would fall easy prey to every hostile organism that came around. Immunity is designed to protect against such infectious invaders and eliminate any foreign matter or cells that somehow gain entrance into the body. Preventing the growth of cancer cells and tumors is also in its job description.

Although the immune system serves a rough and rugged function, a delicate balance does exist as far as its activity is concerned. Stress, poor nutrition, and hormone fluctuations are but some of the many factors which can deleteriously alter this activity, leading to a weakened defense system. As if this weren't enough, certain viruses, such as the canine parvovirus, have the ability to suppress the immune system. Such an overwhelming of the body's natural defense mechanisms can only lead to one outcome, and it isn't good.

This balance can be thrown the other way as well. There are certain disease conditions that might be caused by an overactive, overworking immune system. Allergies are a good example of this. Allergic reactions can even turn deadly if the response is exaggerated enough.

Other times the immune system, in carrying out its duties, will destroy or damage normal healthy tissue in the process. These *autoimmune* diseases usually result from the body's inability to turn off the immune response, with disastrous consequences.

ANATOMY AND PHYSIOLOGY

The immune system itself is a complex network of cells, organs, and special chemicals. No one division overshadows another; each team member relies on the others for support. In this way, they all work in unison towards a common goal.

Cells of the immune system

Special cells, called *stem cells*, located within the bone marrow give rise to all of the cells of the immune system. These cells that are produced are referred to as *white blood cells*. Within this general category there are numerous types, each serving distinct functions.

The *neutrophil* function to gobble up bacteria that gain entrance into the body. Also assisting in this function are white blood cells called *macrophages*. These cells usually come after the neutrophils are already in action. In addition to bacteria, macrophages also have the capability to eat viruses, fungal organisms, and foreign matter.

When a dog is vaccinated, special immune cells called *lymphocytes* are stimulated. *B-lymphocytes* are responsible for producing actual antibodies in response to the vaccine or foreign organism; *T-lymphocytes* don't produce antibodies per se, yet they assist the B-lymphocytes in doing so, and help modulate the immune response. They also have the ability to attack and kill cells within the body that are cancerous or infected with viruses (FIG. 8-1).

Both B and T lymphocytes are said to possess "memory"—that is, they remember the various organisms and invaders that they're fighting against. That way, if they show up again at a later date, they will be attacked without hesitation. Yet even with memory, this response can become slower and weaker over time if the immune system remains idle and unstimulated. This is why booster vaccinations are needed on a yearly basis in dogs—to keep their immune system in "code red."

Another important lymphocyte of the immune system is called the *natural killer cell*. These cells search out and destroy tumor cells and cells infected with viruses. Unlike their T-cell counterparts, natural killer

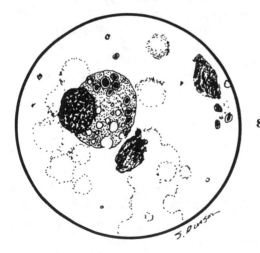

8-1   *White blood cell engulfing bacteria.*

cells do not possess memory, yet at the same time, most do not require a previous exposure to a foreign agent to respond effectively.

Organs of the immune system

The organs of the immune system include the bone marrow, the thymus, the spleen, and the various lymph nodes and aggregates of lymph tissue spread throughout the body.

Bone marrow   As mentioned before, all cells of the immune system originate within the bone marrow. Many stay put and undergo maturity right where they are; other cells are shuttled off to the thymus.

Thymus   The thymus is an organ located in the neck region of young animals. As that individual grows older and the immune system undergoes a mature development, the thymus gland gradually disappears. It is in this organ that most of the T-cells undergo their maturation.

Lymph nodes and tissue   From the thymus and the bone marrow, the cells of the immune system are then shipped to the front-line defenses, including the lymph nodes, tonsils, and other lymph tissue lining the gastrointestinal and respiratory tracts. This latter tissue, owing to its strategic location, comprises a first line of defense against organisms that try to gain entrance into the body. B-lymphocytes in this tissue produce special antibodies that coat the surface of the tract, and block such access.

Lymph nodes and tissue are responsible for filtering the body's blood and lymph for foreign agents and cells. *Lymph* is a special type of fluid that circulates throughout the body within its own separate channels or vessels, called *lymphatic vessels*. Fats that are absorbed via the intestinal tract enter into this lymphatic system, as do lymphocytes on their way to and from the front line defenses.

The spleen   The spleen is an organ most have heard about; its various functions include filtering blood like lymph tissue, and providing a storehouse for blood cells.

Chemicals of the immune system

Special chemicals produced by the cells of the immune system serve to assist them in their protective function. Among those chemicals generated are interferon, interleukins, and complement.

Interferon   is a protein that is produced and released by cells that have been invaded by or come in contact with a virus. Released within 2 hours after the cell is invaded, it acts as a messenger to surrounding healthy cells and stimulates the immune system to respond. It even has antitumor effects, preventing tumor cell replication in some instances.

Interleukins   are chemicals produced by macrophages that help control and modulate the activity of the T-cells during an immune response. Interference with the release of interleukins, which can occur with many viral diseases, can lead to immunosuppression.

Complement   is a special protein produced by the body that attaches itself to the surface of antibodies. When these antibodies bind to a bacteria or infected cell, the complement serves to "burn" a hole in the cell membrane, leading to the cell's destruction. In some instances, complement doesn't need the help of antibodies to fulfill this function.

Antigens

An *antigen* is defined as any substance capable of eliciting an immune response. Infectious organisms—such as bacteria, foreign matter, and even tumor cells—have antigens within their make-up and lining their outer surfaces. Since the body does not recognize such an antigen as one of its own, it mounts an immune response against it to try to eliminate it.

Upon initial exposure to an antigen, B-lymphocytes start to divide and differentiate into their antibody-producing form. It might take up to seven days before antibody production can be achieved. Even then, production is only moderate, and adequate levels generally only last about three weeks. In the meantime, however, other immune components, such as neutrophils, macrophages, and killer cells are called in to fight off the invader.

If the invader is a tumor cell, foreign body, or an organism that lives and multiplies within body cells (such as viruses do), then the T-lymphocytes start to multiply and prepare themselves for battle as well. As with the B-lymphocytes, they are specific for each antigen; that is, such a lymphocyte that responds to one type of antigen will not respond to any others. As a result, each different antigen that enters the body will stimulate its own group of antagonistic B and T-lymphocytes.

Following this first exposure, the lymphocytes that have been primed to the antigen retain "memory" of the experience. Sent to the front line defenses, they simply wait for the antigen to show up again. Now if it ever does, the lymphocytes are ready for it, without the seven day lag time. Antibodies are produced in high levels almost immediately, and the T-cells are primed and sent into action with minimal delay.

IMMUNOSUPPRESSION

As pointed out previously, the immune system is a complicated and delicately balanced system that performs a vital function within the body. If this balance is disrupted, serious trouble can develop.

A suppressed immune system leaves the body wide open to invasion by foreign organisms and cancer cells. This immunosuppression can occur secondarily to viral infections (such as parvovirus or canine distemper), drug therapy (including steroid treatments), severe stress, and disorders of the bone marrow. In addition, dogs can actually inherit poorly functioning immune systems. For instance, the incidence of an underactive immune system is higher in Doberman pinschers and rottweilers than it is in other breeds.

AUTOIMMUNE DISEASE

Autoimmune diseases are characterized by an overactive immune system that can irritate or damage its host's own tissues in response to an antigen invasion within the body. For example, atopic dermatitis in dogs results from an overactive immune response to inhaled pollens. Lupus erythmatosis and pemphigus are two more autoimmune disorders in dogs that, aside from causing significant skin lesions, can damage other organs of the body as well.

In autoimmune hemolytic anemia, the immune system actually destroys the body's own red blood cells, leading to anemia. Myasthenia gravis, a disease characterized by profound muscle weakness after only minimal exertion, is also classified as an autoimmune disease. Immune-mediated kidney disease and arthritis can also afflict dogs stricken with a genetic predisposition for these disorders. Finally, many cases of hypothyroidism are thought to be caused by an overactive immune system attacking and inactivating the thyroid hormone produced within the body.

Autoimmune reactions are controlled with high doses of corticosteroid medication, which has a suppressive effect on the immune system. However, because these steroids can have significant side effects at these high doses, such treatments should only be performed under the close, continual supervision of a veterinarian.

9

The Cardiovascular & Hemolymphatic Systems

THE SYSTEMS RESPONSIBLE for the effective transmission of oxygen and/or nutrition to all organs and tissues of the body are the cardiovascular/hemolymphatic systems. These systems are comprised of the heart and vessels, located within the chest or *thoracic cavity,* and the vessels that carry blood and lymph throughout the body.

ANATOMY AND PHYSIOLOGY

The heart is a hollow organ that serves as a double pump and is located approximately in the center of the thoracic cavity. Its walls consist of muscular tissue called *myocardium.* The pumping action of the heart causes blood to flow through the circulatory system, supplying oxygen and nutrients to the body tissue (FIG. 9-1). Inside the heart a wall of tissue separates the heart into two sections of pumps: the "right heart" and the "left heart."

Each side of the heart is made up of two hollow chambers: the upper chamber is the *atrium,* it receives blood; the lower chamber is the *ventricle,* it pumps blood from the heart. The cavities of the atrium and ventricle on each side of the heart communicate with each other, but the right chambers do not communicate directly with those on the left. Thus, right and left atria and right and left ventricles are distinct.

Blood flow is directed by a series of valves that have nothing to do with the initiation of flow. The driving force for blood comes from the active contraction of cardiac muscles. The valves only prevent the blood from flowing in the opposite direction. Heart murmurs are caused by the backflow of blood through defective or diseased heart valves.

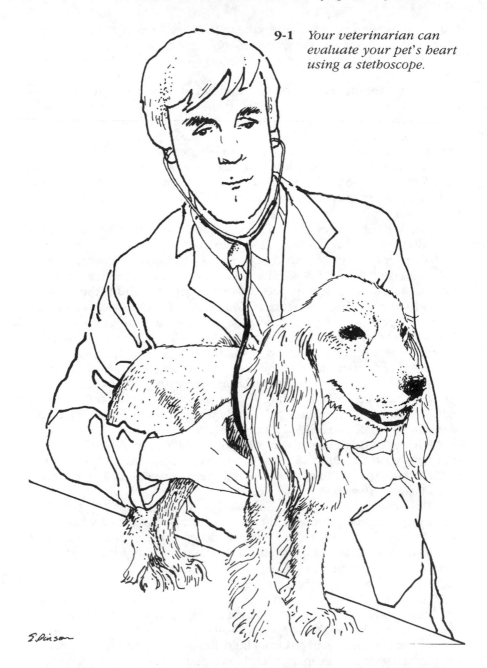

9-1 *Your veterinarian can evaluate your pet's heart using a stethoscope.*

A drop of blood that is in the right atrium is first pumped through a valve into the right ventricle. The ventricle then pumps the droplet to the pulmonary arteries and lungs. In the lungs, the blood takes on oxygen and releases the waste product carbon dioxide. The oxygen-rich droplet is now ready to nourish cells of the body, but first it must return to the heart. This time the droplet enters the pulmonary veins and goes into the left atrium. The atrium pumps it through a valve into the left ventricle. The left ventricle then pumps it out to the cells, tissue, and organs of the body.

Arteries are the name given to those blood vessels which carry oxygen-rich blood from the heart to the tissues. As these vessels approach their targets, they progressively branch out, creating smaller *arterioles*. Actual exchange of oxygen, nutrients, and waste products between the blood and the tissues occurs through microscopic, thin-walled vessels that originate from the arterioles called *capillaries*. Once this exchange has taken place, the capillary beds coalesce to form *venules*, which eventually empty into even larger *veins*. Blood is carried back to the heart via these veins.

The walls of arteries are much thicker and elastic than those of veins primarily to accommodate for the increased blood pressure within the arterial system caused by the pumping heart. Unlike in humans, *atherosclerosis,* characterized by a buildup of fat, calcium, and cellular debris, is not a significant problem in pets. However, pets can suffer the same ill effects from high blood pressure as do humans. Though stress can cause the blood pressure to rise, some type of impedance to normal blood flow—such heart failure, liver disease, and/or kidney disease—is the most common cause of its occurrence in animals.

Blood consists of a variety of cellular elements, including *erythrocytes* (red blood cells), which transport oxygen with the help of *hemoglobin* molecules contained within; *leukocytes* (white blood cells), which fight infections and foreign invaders; and tiny cell fragments called *platelets*, which initiate the blood clotting cascade.

Plasma is the noncellular portion of the blood. It consists of water, nutrients, waste products, and a wide variety of hormones, enzymes, and electrolytes. Plasma also contains special plasma proteins called *albumin, globulin,* and *fibrinogen.*

Albumin is a transport protein which escorts large molecules, including some hormones, through the bloodstream. Globulins include antibodies formed by the immune system and certain proteins needed for normal blood clotting. Fibrinogen is a plasma protein also involved in the body's blood clotting scheme. *Serum* is the term given to plasma that has had this clotting component removed.

The *lymphatic system* is an entirely different type of circulatory system found within the body. Lymphatic vessels that course throughout the body carry not blood, but a special substance called *lymph*. Lymph is a plasma-like substance derived from fluid and protein that normally leaves the blood stream at the capillary level to enter into tissues. Lymph components that are not used by the tissues enter into special lymphatic vessels, which carry them back into circulation. Lymph also contains fats absorbed from the small intestine.

Lymph nodes are special structures found all along the lymphatic chain that serve to filter bacteria and contaminates out of the lymph, while at the same time adding special immune cells called *lymphocytes* to the fluid for transport to the blood circulatory system. In dogs, *edema*, or fluid retention within the tissues, can be caused by parasites or tumors obstructing normal lymph flow through the lymphatic vessels.

HEART DISEASE & HEART FAILURE

Heart disease, with subsequent heart failure, is one of the most frequent problems in small-animal medicine. Because the heart functions to supply oxygen and nutrients to the rest of the body via the blood, serious ramifications result if this function is interfered with by disease. In addition, the decreased movement of blood through the circulatory system caused by a faulty heart leads to high blood pressure, and fluid buildup within the abdomen and/or the lungs (*congestive heart failure*), depending upon which side of the heart is involved. If the latter structures do become water-logged, oxygen exchange is reduced even further.

Mitral insufficiency

Different diseases involving the heart valves or heart muscle can lead to heart failure. By far the most common type of heart disease seen in dogs, aside from that caused by heartworms (see Heartworms, chapter 7), is called *mitral insufficiency*, which involves the heart valve separating the left atrium from the left ventricle. If this valve becomes diseased and fails to close properly when it is supposed to, blood is allowed to flow back into the left atrium when the left ventricle contracts.

This has two effects. First, the amount of blood pushed forward into circulation by each heart contraction is greatly reduced, which means that the heart (which, remember, is diseased) must work harder than it did when it was healthy to keep up with the body's demand for blood. Secondly, the back-up of blood that occurs as a result of the inefficient heart contraction leads to fluid build-up within the lungs, interfering with oxygen exchange between the blood and the lungs. As a result, a vicious cycle develops.

Mitral insufficiency can result from normal wear and tear associated with age, or—more importantly—it can appear secondary to other diseases, namely periodontal disease. Bacteria from the diseased teeth and gums can enter the blood stream and attach to the heart valve, setting up infection and inflammation. Over time, the heart valve becomes damaged and scarred, making it unable to function properly. The end result is often heart failure.

Other valve-related diseases

Though their frequency is much less, diseases involving the other valves in the heart can nevertheless occur. Disease of the triscupid valve, which separates the right chambers of the heart, can occur secondary to age or infection and can interfere with the normal return of blood to the heart from the body. Defects in the pulmonic or aortic valves, which separate the ventricles from the pulmonary vessels and aorta respectively, are usually *congenital* (present at birth) in nature and might not be detectable when the dog is young. However, as the dog matures and the requirements placed on the heart increase, signs of heart disease or failure could become apparent.

Cardiomyopathies

Diseases involving the actual heart muscle itself can also lead to heart failure. First, *cardiomyopathies* are diseases of the heart muscle that lead to enlargement of the heart. *Dilatative cardiomyopathy* is characterized by a thinning of the wall of the heart, whereas *hypertrophic cardiomyopathy* refers to an abnormal enlargement and thickening of the heart muscle.

In either case, normal contractility of the heart is disrupted, with end results similar to those caused by valvular diseases. Next, although dogs rarely suffer from overt heart attacks, *microinfarctions* (tiny regions of injury to heart muscle) resulting from diminished blood and oxygen flow to the heart muscle can be featured in any of the various forms of heart disease and can further interfere with heart's ability to contract. Infectious diseases such as parvovirus and Lyme disease, can also have a predilection for heart muscle and seriously damage cardiac function.

Birth defects

Birth defects involving the heart wall (*septal defects*), the heart valves (*valvular stenosis*), or the vessels leaving the heart (*patent ductus arteriosus*) can increase the workload placed on the heart and can lead to heart failure as the affected animal gets older. If detected early enough, many of these defects can be surgically corrected at a young age, before associated signs become severe. In those that cannot be repaired, treatment is similar to that of other forms of heart disease.

Symptoms of a failing heart

Regardless of the inciting cause, the clinical signs associated with a failing heart include coughing, especially at night and after exercise, breathing difficulties, distended abdomen, weight loss, and exercise intolerance. Suffering dogs might stand with their front legs spread wide apart and their neck lowered and extended to afford the passage of more air into the lungs. Affected dogs might collapse even after the slightest exertion or excitement.

If the right side of the heart is involved, owners might notice a bulging abdomen. This occurs secondarily to a back-up of blood within the abdominal vessels, leading to a fluid build-up within the abdominal cavity.

All of these signs might start off subtly, yet they usually become progressively worse as the disease progresses and failure begins.

Detection of heart disease

Diagnosis of heart disease or heart failure is made using clinical signs, radiographs, and electrocardiogram findings. In addition to the classical clinical signs listed above, many forms of heart disease are accompanied by *heart murmurs*, which can be detected by a veterinarian upon listening to the chest using a stethoscope.

A heart murmur is nothing more than an irregular sound caused by the disruption of normal blood flow within the heart. By far the majority of heart murmurs heard are caused by diseases of the heart valves and the abnormal blood flow through these valves that results. Still other murmurs can originate from the defects in the heart muscle or vessels which alter normal blood flow. Unusually forceful and rapid heart contractions, such as those seen within overly excited animals or in dogs suffering from anemia, can even lead to an irregular heart sound. Interestingly enough, murmurs are not commonly detected in dogs suffering from heartworm disease, even when their hearts are full of the parasites.

Heart murmurs are usually classified according to their intensity as heard through a stethoscope. A trained veterinarian can identify which portion of the heart is affected and arrive at a diagnosis just by pinpointing the area on the chest where the murmur is the loudest, and by determining when the murmur occurs, be it during the heart's contraction phase, relaxation phase, or both.

Other diagnostic tests

One parameter that cannot be determined from the intensity of a heart murmur is the stage of heart disease or failure the animal is in. For instance, severe mitral insufficiency might not be associated with any murmur whatsoever, whereas an early case might be accompanied by a loud one. This is because in the later stages, the valve might become so diseased and worn that if offers such little resistance to blood flow back through it that a murmur-causing disruption of blood flow might not arise.

Radiographs of the chest are essential for establishing a diagnosis of heart disease. Animals with primary lung disease, including pneumonia, can exhibit clinical signs very similar to those seen in patients with heart failure, and radiographs are needed to differentiate the two.

On radiographic X-ray film, most diseased hearts will appear abnormally enlarged. This enlargement can occur in compensation for the heart having to work harder to pump blood, or it could be due to a thinning and bulging of the heart wall resulting from constant bombardment with high-pressure streams of blood escaping through faulty heart valves. Regardless of the cause, an enlarged heart on radiographs, combined with clinical signs or murmurs, signifies heart disease. If such a combination exists, the next test most practitioners will perform is an electrocardiogram.

The *electrocardiogram* (ECG) is a test used widely to assess the condition of the heart. Remember that a heartbeat is produced when a wave of electrical energy moves through the tissues of the chambers, starting in the atria and moving down to the ventricles. This electrical wave then makes the muscle wall of these chambers contract, pumping out the blood contained within. The ECG helps evaluate the status of this electrical conduction system, and at the same time, can give the veterinarian useful information regarding the size of the heart itself, and indirectly, the condition of the heart as a pump (FIG. 9-2). In addition, with the information gained from an ECG, proper drug treatment dosages can be more easily established.

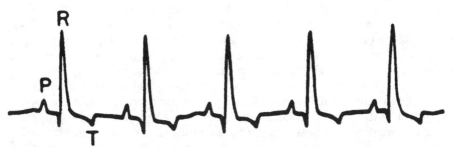

9-2   *An electrocardiogram measures electrical conduction throughout the heart.*

Treatment for heart disease

Because most cases of heart disease/failure are nonreversible, the treatment goal for any dog suffering from such is to create an environment that relieves some of the workload on the heart and slows the progression of the disease.

Canines with bad hearts need to be fed a special diet that is low in sodium to help reduce blood pressure and discourage the accumulation of fluid within the lungs and/or the abdomen. Diets formulated especially for this purpose are available from a veterinarian.

Diuretics, such as *furosemide,* are also used in heart failure patients to help mobilize and get rid of excessive fluid that might be accumulating within the body. In many instances, this diuretic therapy, combined with a low-sodium diet, might be all that it takes to relieve the coughing and discomfort seen in affected dogs. Be sure to remember that a dog on diuretic medication will drink water and urinate with greater frequency, so be sure to provide it with plenty of water to drink at all times, and be prepared to walk it outside more often.

Medications designed to dilate the blood vessels, making it easier for the diseased heart to pump blood through them, are usually the next in line if the special diet and diuretics don't seem to be enough to correct the problem. Two examples of such drugs that are frequently used in dogs include *hydralazine* and *captopril.*

If none of the above treatment regimens prove effective, the final medicating step often taken to manage the heart failure is to give the drug *digitalis* to help slow and strengthen the heart's contraction. Digitalis-type medications can have many undesirable and serious side effects if therapy is not carefully monitored by a veterinarian but, on the average, they will prolong the life of a dog in heart failure for 4 to 6 months.

ANEMIA

Anemia is defined as an overall reduction in the number of red blood cells within the bloodstream relative to normal levels within that pet. This reduction can occur from a number of processes, including an increased destruction or decreased production of red blood cells within the body. TABLE 9-1 lists some of the major causes of anemia. The overall consequence of anemia is the inability of the blood to supply desired levels of oxygen to the tissues.

Table 9-1
Potential Causes of Anemia in Dogs

Iron/B_{12} deficiency
Kidney disease
Addison's disease
Hypothyroidism
Liver disease
Toxins (e.g., lead poisoning)
Cancer
Ehrlichia canis
Trauma—blood loss
Hookworms
External parasites (fleas, ticks)
Blood clotting disorders
Gastric ulcers
Drug reactions
Autoimmune hemolytic anemia

Signs seen in an anemic dog include intense lethargy, weakness, increased respiratory and heart rates, and a pallor of the mucous membranes. Depending upon the cause of the anemia, signs related to a blood-clotting disorder might be seen as well. Finally, if red blood cells are being destroyed within the body, the skin and mucous membranes might become jaundiced.

A simple blood test performed by your veterinarian can tell you if your dog is anemic (FIG. 9-3). Treatment of anemia depends on the underlying cause. In severe cases, blood transfusions and oxygen therapy might be required to save the pet's life until the cause can be identified and treated.

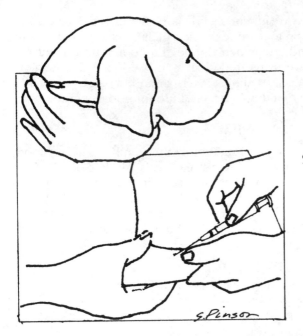

9-3 *A simple blood test can be performed to determine whether or not a pet is anemic.*

BLEEDING DISORDERS

Whenever an injury or illness compromises a blood vessel and leads to bleeding out of that vessel, a remarkable mechanism or chain reaction begins within the body in an effort to stop the leakage of blood from the damaged vessel and prevent the individual from bleeding to death. This mechanism is known as *hemostasis.*

When a blood vessel is compromised, the first reaction that occurs is constriction of the vessel to help slow blood loss. Following this, special blood cells called platelets begin to adhere to the injured vessel wall, forming a temporary plug. At the same time, a *coagulation* (clotting) pathway is activated within the body, involving a complex interaction of blood and tissue components, as well as calcium and vitamin K. The end result of this pathway is the formation of a more permanent clot at the site of injury.

Bleeding disorders can occur whenever any part of the clotting mechanism is interfered with. Platelet numbers or function can be interfered with by diseases or substances such as toxins, drugs, cancers, autoimmune hemolytic anemia, and infectious agents, such as *Ehrlichia canis.* In addition, kidney disease and certain congenital defects can also lead to poor platelet function and secondary bleeding.

Any disruptions of the coagulation pathway also spell trouble for hemostasis. For instance, most mouse and rat poisons contain substances which interfere with the vitamin K component of the coagulation pathway. If these are accidentally ingested by a dog, the dog's coagulation pathway will be effectively disrupted. Liver disease can lead to bleeding disorders because many of the components used in blood clotting are manufactured in that organ. Inherited defects in the coagulation pathway, leading to the bleeding disorders in dogs known as *hemophilia* and *Von Willebrand's disease* can occur as well.

Serious diseases or injuries such as heartworm disease, viral diseases, and massive trauma (such as that caused by a car) can lead to a secondary condition known as *disseminated intravascular coagulation (DIC)*. In DIC, tiny blood clots form all throughout the body. Not only are these clots detrimental to the health of the animal, but DIC also leads to a depletion of the body's clotting components. This, in turn, predisposes the pet to a bleeding disorder. DIC is invariably fatal to a pet unless rapid supportive treatment is instituted.

Clinical signs of a bleeding disorder usually include noticeable bruising of the skin and mucous membranes. Blood in the urine or feces, nosebleeds, joint pain, abdominal pain, and breathing difficulties might be seen as well. Because of the variety of potential causes, a veterinarian will need to run a series of tests to determine the exact cause and to formulate a proper treatment regimen (FIG. 9-4).

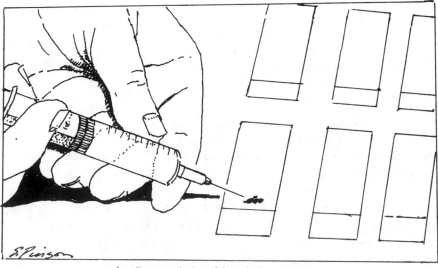

9-4   *Determining blood clotting times.*

Initial treatment for any bleeding disorder entails blood transfusions until the exact cause is discerned. If rodenticide poisoning is suspected, vitamin K injections, followed by oral vitamin K tablets, will help reverse the effects of the poison. These tablets should be given daily for a minimum of four weeks, since the ingested poison could linger within the body and exert its effects for this length of time.

Finally, for autoimmune clotting defects, steroid therapy can be used to help control the disease and subsequent bleeding.

10

The Respiratory System

THE RESPIRATORY SYSTEM works in conjunction with the circulatory system to provide oxygen to and to remove carbon dioxide from the body tissues. Oxygen is the driving force behind all chemical reactions that occur internally; obviously without it, life could not exist. As a result, the function of all body systems, including the respiratory system itself, depends first upon the ability of this system to deliver its product. In addition to this vital function, the respiratory system also serves as a means of *thermoregulation,* or body heat exchange, in the dog. Since dogs can't sweat in the conventional way, they rely upon heat transfer out of the body through exhaled air. Hence, dogs pant when they get hot.

ANATOMY AND PHYSIOLOGY

The respiratory system begins with the mouth and nose, which, under the influence of the breathing mechanism, facilitate the passage of air into the *trachea.* The wall of this cylindrical structure is lined with rings of tough cartilage which prevent it from collapsing during normal breathing activity. The trachea enters the thorax, or chest cavity, and eventually branches into *bronchi* and smaller *bronchioles* within the lungs themselves. The lungs and inner wall of the thorax are lined by thin membranes called *pleura. Pleuritis* is the term used to describe inflammation of these membranes, which can make normal respirations difficult and painful.

The smallest unit of the respiratory system is the *alveolus*, located at the terminus of the bronchioles. It is within these alveoli that gas exchange occurs between the lungs and the circulatory system. *Surfactant* is a special substance found lining the insides of normal alveoli. It is responsible for preventing alveolar collapse during the breathing cycle.

The major blood supply to the lungs and alveoli come from the pulmonary artery originating from the right ventricle of the heart. In dogs, heartworms reside in the right side of the heart and can effectively clog this artery and its branches supplying the lungs. The resulting disruption of blood flow and increase in pulmonary blood pressure can have devastating consequences as far as respiratory function is concerned.

The only air within the thorax, or chest cavity, is contained within the lungs. As a result, a negative pressure system exists which facilitates normal breathing. Intake or *inspiration* of air occurs as the *diaphragm*, the large muscular band separating the thorax from the abdominal cavity, flattens and lowers itself, and the ribcage expands. The resulting negative pressure caused by the increased thoracic size actively draws air through the trachea and into the lungs. Upon exhalation, or *expiration*, the diaphragm and ribcage are returned to their normal size, forcing air out of the lungs. *Pneumothorax* is a life-threatening condition in which air is allowed into the thoracic cavity, either through a penetrating wound through the skin and ribcage or through a tear in the lung tissue. Either way, the loss of negative pressure within the thorax quickly collapses the lungs, and renders the normal breathing mechanisms inoperable.

Defense Mechanisms

Because of its direct exposure to a hostile environment, the respiratory system contains several defense mechanisms to help keep foreign invader and particulate matter out of the lungs. The sticky substance called *mucus,* produced by cells lining the trachea and bronchi, serves to trap contaminants and foreign debris that might gain external access to the respiratory system.

In addition, tiny, movable, finger-like projections (called *cilia*) line the surface of airways and function to mechanically maneuver trapped contaminants in a direction away from the lungs. Any significant build-up of respiratory mucus or irritation to the respiratory lining results in a cough, and (hopefully) the forceful expulsion of any offending substance.

The airways are also lined with surface antibodies that provide a first line of defense against infectious organisms. In dogs, intranasal vaccines against the disease canine cough are designed to stimulate such antibody production. In an unprotected dog, infecting canine cough organisms can destroy the lining of the trachea, predisposing the unfortunate victim to all kinds of secondary infections and to a life of continual coughing (see chapter 6).

RHINITIS

Inflammation involving the nasal passages of dogs is termed *rhinitis*. The hallmark clinical signs seen with a case of rhinitis include sneezing and nasal discharge. Causes of rhinitis include bacterial infections, nasal tumors, trauma, and foreign bodies. In addition, the fungal organism *Aspergillus fumigatus* can invade the bones and tissues comprising the nasal passages, resulting in rhinitis. The nasal discharges associated with this fungal disease, which are usually green and thick in nature, might persist for months at a time. In addition, ulcerations involving the outer surface of the nose are sometimes seen. Aspergillosis can occur primarily on its own or secondarily to other conditions which might compromise the immune system.

TRACHEOBRONCHITIS

Inflammation occurring within the trachea and bronchi of the respiratory tree is properly termed *tracheobronchitis*. In dogs, the leading cause of tracheobronchitis is canine cough (see chapter 6). Other causes can include allergies, foreign bodies, and chemical or gaseous irritants.

Incessant coughing is the hallmark sign of tracheobronchitis. A dry, hacking cough is seen in cases of canine cough, whereas in other cases, such as chemical irritation, the cough might be moist and productive.

Treatment of tracheobronchitis depends on the underlying cause.

COLLAPSED TRACHEA

Collapsed trachea is a respiratory disease primarily seen in the smaller, toy breeds of dogs, such a toy poodles and Yorkshire terriers. It can occur in dogs of any age, but most cases are seen in dogs over 6 years of age.

The syndrome is caused by a weakening of the muscles that interconnect the band of cartilaginous rings which normally support the trachea. The end result of this malformation is that instead of the trachea maintaining its normal round shape during respiratory activity, it collapses or flattens out (FIG. 10-1). Depending upon which section of the trachea is involved, this collapse might occur on either inspiration or expiration. In some cases, it might be so severe as to become life-threatening.

Obviously, such a situation leads to noticeable respiratory distress in affected individuals. In addition, dogs suffering from a collapsing trachea can have a dry, harsh cough with a characteristic "goose-honk" sound to it.

Diagnosis is assisted by the type of breed involved and the type of cough heard. Radiographs taken of the trachea are usually diagnostic and will help differentiate this disorder from other diseases of the airways, including tracheitis, bronchitis, and pneumonia. Actual examination of the affected portion of the trachea with an endoscope can be used to help determine the extent and severity of the problem.

Mild cases of collapsing trachea can often be managed through medical means. If an affected dog is overweight, a weight-loss program is a good place to start. Cough suppressants and drugs designed to dilate the airways can help to relieve the symptoms. Overexertion and excitement should be discouraged, since the increased respiratory rate resulting from such activities can exacerbate the condition.

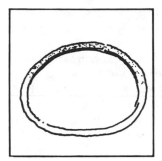

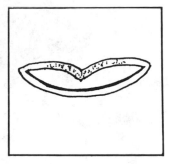

10-1 *Top left: Normal trachea; bottom right: collapsed trachea.*

Depending upon the location of the collapse, surgical correction might afford a more permanent solution to the problem. This involves the implantation of special polypropylene support rings around the circumference of the trachea for additional support. The postoperative complications associated with such a procedure are usually minimal.

PNEUMONIA

When inflammation strikes actual tissue within the lungs themselves, a condition of pneumonia is said to exist. Pneumonia doesn't necessarily mean that an infection is present; on the contrary, there are a number of non-infectious causes of pneumonia that need to be considered whenever a dog is showing signs of lung disease. For instance, *aspiration pneumonia* can result from the accidental inhalation of a substance originally destined for the stomach. Dogs suffering from seizures, persistent vomiting, or structural abnormalities, such as megaesophagus or cleft palate, are very susceptible to this type of pneumonia. Pneumonia can also result from inhalation of smoke and certain caustic chemicals. The damage caused by these noninfectious sources is often so severe that the unfortunate victims often develop secondary bacterial pneumonia as a secondary problem.

Dogs suffering from pneumonia will cough incessantly and often spit up mucus and phlegm. Obvious breathing difficulties are noticed in severe cases, with a reluctance by the pet to move or exert itself. Dogs so affected might stand with their front legs spread wide apart and their neck lowered and extended to afford the passage of more air into the lungs. Fever, lethargy, and loss of appetite are also seen in patients with pneumonia.

Clinical signs combined with abnormal lung sounds detected with a stethoscope can lead a veterinarian to suspect a case of pneumonia (FIG. 10-2). Chest radiographs are needed to confirm such suspicions. If a bacterial or fungal component is thought to exist, a culture of the fluid and mucus within the respiratory tree might be performed as well. Blood work will usually show an elevated white blood cell count.

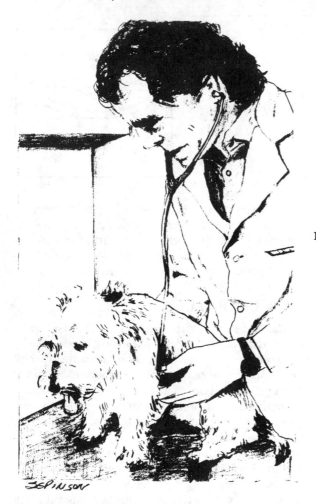

10-2 *Pneumonia is characterized by harsh lung sounds.*

With infectious pneumonia, high doses of an appropriate antibiotics and/or antifungal medications will be required to bring it under control. Drugs designed to expand the airways are helpful in improving air flow into and out of the lungs. Intravenous fluids are also useful to replace important body fluids lost in the increased respiratory secretions and to prevent existing secretions from becoming thickened as a result of dehydration. **Note:** In dogs, medication designed to suppress coughing should not be used, in most cases, since this only serves to prevent the removal of mucus and other respiratory secretions from the lungs.

Cases of aspiration or inhalation pneumonia are treated in a similar fashion, yet these carry a much poorer prognosis. Attempts can be made to suction the foreign material out of the lungs through the trachea are often unsuccessful. Dogs that survive are often afflicted with a residual cough for the rest of their lives.

METASTATIC LUNG DISEASE

One characteristic of most highly malignant tumors, regardless of their point of origin, is that they invariably spread to and end up in the lungs if not detected and treated soon enough. Some cancers spread, or *metastasize,* more readily to the lungs than others. For instance, malignant melanoma of the skin might be present in the lungs even before the actual skin tumor becomes noticeable.

The clinical signs exhibited by dogs afflicted with metastatic lung disease can be similar to those seen with pneumonia. Unfortunately, the prognosis for dogs harboring such tumors in their lungs is grave, even with specific cancer treatment.

11

The Digestive System

THE DIGESTIVE SYSTEM of the dog is made up of a collective network of organs designed to supply the body with the nutrition it needs
for growth, maintenance, and repair. It also functions to rid the body of
waste that it does not use. Because of this role in nutrition and waste management, diseases involving the digestive system can have a profound
effect not just on the region so afflicted, but on the entire body as well.

ANATOMY AND PHYSIOLOGY

Those organs or regions of the body categorized under the digestive system include the oral cavity (teeth, tongue, salivary glands, etc.), esophagus, stomach, small intestine, large intestine, rectum, anus, pancreas,
liver, and gall bladder. In order to better understand diseases and their
adverse effects, a brief overview of the digestive process is warranted.
Keep in mind, however, that the following description is an oversimplifi-
cation; the actual digestive process is so complex and involved that it warrants the devotion of an entire book in itself!

Once food enters the oral cavity, the process of digestion begins. The
teeth mechanically rip, crush, and grind down the food, while the saliva
secreted by the salivary glands into the mouth moistens and partially
digests carbohydrate portions of the food prior to it being swallowed. In
puppies, these teeth do not start their eruption patterns until around 2 to
4 weeks of age. By the time the puppy is 8 weeks of age, it should have a
full complement of *deciduous* (baby) teeth. By 7 months of age, all of the
permanent teeth should have fully erupted and replaced the deciduous
ones.

From the oral cavity, food, water, and saliva are passed back into the esophagus with the aid of the tongue and are swallowed. The walls of the esophagus consist of bands of muscle, which contract in a rhythmic fashion, pushing the food down towards the stomach. This unique muscle action is called *peristalsis.*

From the esophagus, the food passes through a muscular sphincter into the stomach. This sphincter is very important, for it keeps stomach acids and enzymes from entering into and burning the esophageal lining. If it is defective, ulcers and that feeling humans describe as "heartburn" can result.

The stomach is lined with cells that secrete acids and special digestive enzymes, designed to further break down ingested proteins and carbohydrates (FIG. 11-1). The muscular walls of the stomach help gently churn and mix the contents, until such time as they're ready for passage into the small intestine. Again, the food must pass through another sphincter to reach the small intestine. Once it passes through the sphincter, the stomach acids mixed in the digesta are neutralized and rendered harmless by secretions in the small intestine.

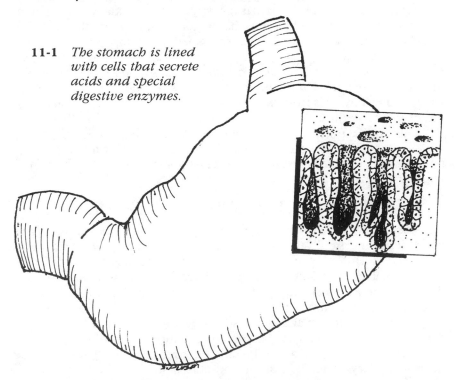

11-1 *The stomach is lined with cells that secrete acids and special digestive enzymes.*

The small intestine is the site where most digestion occurs, and where the resulting nutritional building blocks are absorbed into the body. Bile produced by the liver and stored in the gall bladder is added to the digesta here to break down fats. Enzymes from the pancreas further digest fats, proteins, and carbohydrates until finally, the nutrients can be absorbed through the intestinal lining and into the body.

The lining of the small intestine consists of millions of small, finger-like projections called *villi,* designed to increase the absorptive surface area within the intestine. And as if this weren't enough, each of these tiny villi are lined by even tinier projections, called *microvilli*—again, to further increase the surface area for nutrient absorption.

One reason that a parvovirus infection can be so deadly is that the virus can effectively destroy these villi lining the small intestine, blocking absorption of nutrients and "starving" the victim.

As digested nutrients are absorbed, they enter into either the circulatory system or into the lymphatic system. End products of protein and carbohydrate digestion travel by way of the blood to the liver, where any toxic by-products are promptly eliminated. Other functions of the liver include the production of serum proteins, the storage of vitamins and other nutrients, the destruction and removal of old red blood cells from the bloodstream, and the secretion and excretion of bile into the small intestine to aid in the digestive process.

Fatty acids, resulting from fat digestion, travel initially via the lymphatic vessels and later enter into the blood stream, where they are broken down and absorbed into the body tissues. The lymphatic system also plays an important role in immunity (see chapter 8).

Digesta and waste that is not absorbed from within the small intestine then passes into the large intestine, which is responsible for removing water and electrolytes from the material and lubricating it for its passage out of the body through the rectum and anus.

One special portion of the canine large intestine is called the *cecum,* which corresponds to our appendix. In dogs, whipworms inhabit this portion of the large intestine and exert their deleterious effects from within (see chapter 7).

GASTROINTESTINAL RESPONSE TO DISEASE

Considering what they have to go through each day, the stomach and intestines comprise a remarkable organ system. In the performance of their daily nutritional functions, they must be on constant guard to protect themselves from autodigestion by digestive acids and enzymes produced and must constantly battle foreign organisms and agents that are inadvertently taken in by mouth (FIG. 11-2).

When the stomach and/or intestines become acutely diseased, three major factors come into play that can quickly turn a sometimes seemingly harmless situation into a life-threatening predicament: These include pain, secondary bacterial invasion, and dehydration.

Pain

Any inflammation and/or excessive smooth muscle contractions occurring within the gastrointestinal system can be quite discomforting and

11-2 *Dogs with gastrointestinal upset invariably go off their feed.*

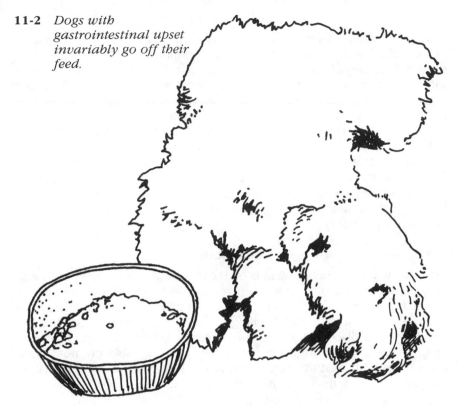

painful. In fact, in severe cases of viral enteritis, intestinal obstructions, and intussusceptions, this pain can be so great that the patient goes into life-threatening shock. As a result, the sooner therapeutic measures are undertaken to correct the problem and stifle the pain associated with it, the less the chances are of complications from occurring.

Secondary bacterial invasion

The second factor to contend with is secondary bacterial invasion. Normally, the intestines are inhabited by billions of bacteria that peacefully reside within without causing any problems whatsoever. In fact, the very presence of these non-disease-causing bacteria actually helps to prevent the growth of *pathogenic,* or disease-causing, bacteria within the intestinal setting. However, if disease strikes the small or large intestines, these "friendly" bacteria can be wiped out, allowing pathogenic ones to proliferate and cause disease themselves. If the inflammation persists, or if an intestinal perforation occurs, these and any other bacteria within the intestines can leak out of the gut and even gain entrance into the bloodstream, causing a life-threatening systemic infection and shock.

For these reasons, it is obvious that antibiotics become very important in the treatment of moderate to severe cases of gastroenteritis, even if the original cause is nonbacterial in origin.

Dehydration

The final threatening factor that arises when acute gastroenteritis strikes a pet is dehydration. Pets suffering from vomiting and/or diarrhea can quickly become dehydrated due to water loss through the bowels. Since inflamed bowels cannot regulate water absorption as they do when they are healthy, any fluid intake that indeed occurs will usually pass right out of the body via vomiting and/or diarrhea without being absorbed.

In fact, the disruption of normal motility and distension occurring within the affected bowel can actually attract and draw water right out of the body and into the intestinal lumen. As a result, dogs that have become dehydrated or are on the verge of dehydration due to gastroenteritis require intravenous fluids to correct the dehydration occurring within the body's cells, at least until the gut has healed sufficiently to resume these functions once again.

Treatment

Once the gastrointestinal system is on the mend, and all vomiting has been brought under control, a good plane of nutrition is required to counteract any malnutrition induced by the disease. Bland diets that are easily digested are prescribed until complete healing of the stomach and/or intestinal linings have taken place. Offering a convalescent dog some type of electrolyte replacement drinks during these first few days can also promote rapid recovery as well. Feeding plain yogurt is also helpful towards repopulating the gastrointestinal tract with nonpathogenic bacteria.

DISORDERS OF THE TEETH AND ORAL CAVITY

Diseases and disorders affecting the teeth or oral cavity interfere with a pet's ability to prehense and process food for digestion. In addition, other general signs associated with conditions involving these areas usually include increased salivation, swallowing difficulties, bad breath, gagging, and decreased appetite.

Malocclusion

Malocclusion occurs when the teeth lining the upper jaw fail to line up and fit properly with the teeth of the lower arcade. In the normal canine bite, the upper canine teeth should rest just behind the lower canines. Disruption of the normal bite pattern can be caused by trauma, by improper tooth eruption, and by genetics.

Brachygnathism refers to a condition in which an overbite, or overshot upper jaw, exists. Conversely, *prognathism* is the term given to the undershot jaw (underbite). Both conditions are inheritable traits, passed from one generation to another. In fact, prognathism is considered normal for certain breeds, such as Pekingese, Boxers, and bulldogs. Although not life threatening, these anatomic maladies can interfere with normal biting action and eating, and can predispose to dental and jaw problems in affected dogs. As a result, dogs suffering from distinct overbites or underbites (unless normal for the breed) should be surgically neutered to prevent the propagation of these undesirable traits.

Malocclusion can also result from improperly positioned deciduous teeth creating abnormal eruption pathways for the permanent ones. Dental examination of the deciduous teeth performed on puppies as early as 8 weeks of age can help identify potential problems. In many instances, simply removing the offending deciduous tooth clears the path for the proper eruption of its permanent successor.

Surgical repair or reconstruction of the jaw can be used to repair trauma-induced malocclusions. Orthodontic correction of brachygnathism and prognathism have been utilized in select cases, yet for ethical reasons, such procedures should only be performed for medical purposes, not for cosmetic gains.

Supernumerary teeth

Supernumerary teeth simply refers to extra teeth within the mouth. These can be retained deciduous teeth, or can actually be permanents (FIG. 11-3).

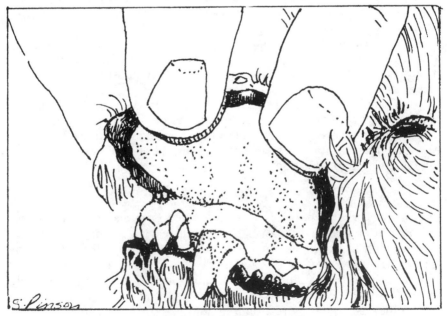

11-3 *Supernumerary teeth.*

Retained deciduous teeth are not uncommon in smaller breeds, including miniature poodles and Yorkshire terriers. In these dogs, the deciduous canine teeth have the greatest propensity for remaining behind. Such retained teeth can crowd the permanent ones, creating abnormal eruption pathways. In addition, due to their close proximity with their permanent counterparts, these extra teeth can serve as niduses for dental calculus build-up and infection. As long as the eruption pattern for the corresponding permanent tooth is not being interfered with, most veterinarians will postpone removal of the retained tooth (teeth) until another elective procedure, such as neutering or teeth cleaning is performed. However, if the permanent tooth is being interfered with in any way, immediate removal is recommended.

In rare instances, duplicated permanent teeth, consisting of one or two isolated ones, or an entire arcade, can erupt. Removal of these permanent supernumerary teeth is usually not necessary unless they interfere with the normal biting action of the dog. Because of the genetic preponderance of this condition, affected dogs should not be bred.

Enamel hypoplasia

This unfortunate condition involves the incomplete development of the hard, protective layer of enamel that normally surrounds the crown of the tooth. Enamel hypoplasia results when the enamel-producing cells within the dental arcade, called *ameloblasts,* are injured or destroyed prior to eruption of either the deciduous or permanent teeth. The canine distemper virus is the most notable culprit causing enamel hypoplasia to occur; other causes can include severe malnutrition and fluorine toxicity.

Teeth lacking in enamel have coarse textures (due to exposed dentin) and tend to stain brown. The absence of the protective enamel coating makes these teeth especially susceptible to decay and to traumatic fractures.

For puppies suffering from enamel hypoplasia on their permanent teeth, enamel restoration procedures (such as crowning) performed by a veterinary dental specialist can add a protective layer to exposed surfaces. Ask a veterinarian for more details regarding these new dentistry procedures now available for dogs.

Broken teeth

Occasionally, teeth will break or fracture due to trauma or due to disease (such as in enamel hypoplasia). If the pulp cavity of the tooth is not exposed by the break, treatment measures, aside from filing down any sharp edges, are usually not required. However, if the damage does extend down into the pulp cavity, inflammation, infection, and pain could result.

In the past, the only real option available to the veterinarian and to the pet owner was to remove the tooth in question. However, as the field of veterinary dentistry has blossomed in recent years, newer, more acceptable alternatives to extraction have arisen.

Endodontic therapy, or root canals, are being performed more and more to help save teeth with exposed or infected pulp cavities and dentin. The procedure involves the removal of the pulp tissue and infected dentin, thereby alleviating pain and the further progression of disease within the tooth. Cracks and fractures in the tooth can then be filled, completing the restoration procedure.

Discolored teeth

The administration of tetracycline antibiotics to a pregnant dog can result in yellow-stained dentin within the teeth of her offspring. The same holds true for adolescent puppies administered the drug prior to eruption of their permanent teeth. Though this staining has no effect on the health of the teeth, it can be unsightly, and detrimental in the show ring.

Calculus build-up can certainly discolor teeth so affected. If allowed to persist long-term, the tooth surface can often take on a yellow hue, even after the calculus has been removed. In these instances, the complete removal of the calculus is far more important than any discoloration left behind.

As mentioned previously, a brownish discoloration to the teeth could be the result of enamel hypoplasia. Enamel restoration procedures can be employed to deal with this problem.

Finally, a bluish-gray discoloration to a tooth is indicative of inflammation within the pulp cavity, warranting endodontic management if the tooth is to be saved.

Dental caries (cavities)

Due to a uniquely high pH of the saliva, cavities rarely form in the teeth of dogs. When they do, they are often secondary to some trauma that has disrupted the continuity of the dental enamel. Cavities in dogs are managed the same way as they are in people—through dental fillings.

Periodontal disease

Periodontal disease, or tooth and gum disease, is one of the most prevalent health disorders in dogs. Studies have shown that most canines show some signs of this disease by the time they are 3 years of age. Early signs can include tender, swollen gums, and, most commonly, bad breath. More importantly though, left untreated, periodontal disease can lead to secondary disease conditions that can seriously threaten the health of affected pets.

It all begins with the formation of plaque on tooth surfaces. This plaque is nothing more than a thin film of food particles and bacteria. Over time, however, plaque mineralizes and hardens to form calculus. Owners who lift up their dog's lip and glance at its teeth, especially near the gum line, might notice brownish to yellowish build-up of calculus on the outer surface of the teeth.

Calculus tends to accumulate worse on the outer surface of the large fourth upper premolars and on the inner surfaces of the lower incisors and premolars. This is because canine saliva is conducive to calculus formation, and the ducts from the salivary glands empty into the mouth at these particular sites. Build-up of this substance tends to be worse in smaller breeds of dogs, such as miniature poodles, Yorkshire terriers, Malteses, and schnauzers. In fact, it is not at all unusual for some of these dogs to start losing teeth by 4 to 5 years of age without at-home preventative dental care!

Along with these breed predispositions, diet can play an important role in the development of periodontal disease. For instances, moist foods high in sugar content promote plaque formation much more readily than do the dry varieties. In addition, diets containing too much phosphorus (such as all-meat rations) have been linked to periodontal disease.

Certain underlying disease conditions might also promote periodontal disease as a side effect. For example, hypothyroidism can lead to gingivitis and dental complications associated with it. Periodontal disease can also occur incidentally to tumors involving the gum tissue and/or teeth.

Symptoms

Dogs suffering from periodontal disease can exhibit a diverse selection of clinical signs. Early periodontal disease might be marked only by a decreased appetite due to swollen, painful gums. Dog owners often complain of bad breath in their pet, and might notice signs of gagging or retching as secondary tonsillitis sets in.

As the disease progresses, these signs might worsen, and other symptoms, such as gum recession, gum bleeding, and tooth loss, might arise (FIGS. 11-4 and 11-5). Infected teeth that do not fall out can form abscesses, marked by sinus infections, nasal discharges and/or draining tracts appearing on the face.

But the damage caused by periodontal disease doesn't stop there. Bacteria can gain entrance into the bloodstream by way of the teeth and gums, seeding the body with infectious organisms. In advanced cases,

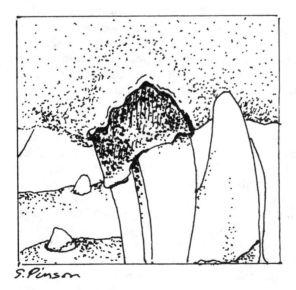

S. Pinson

11-4 *Receding gums are one consequence of periodontal disease.*

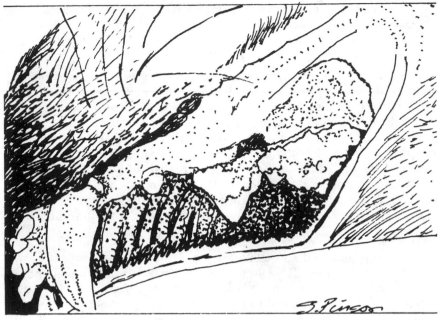

11-5   *Severe periodontal disease.*

these bacteria can overwhelm the host's immune system and set up housekeeping on the valves of the heart. The resulting valvular endocarditis in turn can lead to heart murmurs and eventual heart failure.

Besides the heart, the bacteria that gain access to the body because of periodontal disease can lodge in the kidney, causing infection, inflammation, and acute damage. Over time, signs related to kidney failure might develop in affected dogs.

Treatment

Early cases of periodontal disease can be treated by a thorough scaling and polishing of the teeth to remove the offending calculus. This scaling needs to be professionally performed under sedation or anesthesia to ensure complete removal of the calculus under the gum line.

Using special instruments to hand-scale a pet's teeth at home without anesthesia is not only dangerous, but highly ineffective at cleaning the teeth where it counts the most, up under the gum line. Furthermore, such scaling, if not followed by polishing, will leave etches in the enamel covering the teeth, which serve as foci for future plaque and calculus build-up.

Antibiotics will also be prescribed for dogs suffering from moderate to advanced periodontal disease to combat the associated bacterial infection. Teeth that are excessively loose within their sockets serve only to propagate infection, and should be extracted. For infected teeth that are still deemed viable, root canals can be performed as a salvage procedure.

See chapter 3 for prevention tips to help protect pets against the adverse effects of periodontal disease.

Tonsillitis

The tonsils are a pair of lymphoid tissue located in the back of the oral cavity near the esophagus. Since they are lymphatic tissues, tonsils have an immune function. *Tonsillitis* refers to the inflammation and/or swelling of these lymphoid structures in response to infections, foreign bodies, and sometimes even noninfectious diseases. For instance, long-term coughing, such as that seen in cases of canine cough, can result in a secondary tonsillar inflammation. Periodontal disease is another common cause of tonsillar swelling. Finally, certain tumors, such as lymphosarcoma and squamous cell carcinoma, can cause the tonsils to swell and should always be kept in mind anytime a dog develops a tonsillitis.

Symptoms

Signs of tonsillitis in dogs include gagging, retching, and difficulty swallowing. Affected animals might also go off feed and have a tendency to salivate excessively. Because tonsillitis is usually secondary in nature, other signs of illness related to the primary disease might be present as well.

Treatment

Diagnosis of tonsillitis is easy based on clinical signs and actually visualizing the swollen tonsils within the oral cavity. Treatment depends upon the underlying cause; for example, if the disease is infectious, appropriate anti-microbial therapy will clear up the tonsillitis. If a tumor is suspected, or if a seemingly simple case of tonsillitis is refractory to standard treatment, then the tonsils should be removed and biopsied.

Cleft palate

The palate is a fleshy structure located at the roof of the mouth that separates the oral cavity from the nasal passages. The firm portion located forward most in the mouth is termed the *hard palate,* whereas the softer, flexible portion towards the back of the mouth is called the *soft palate.* *Cleft palate* is a disease condition in which the palate fails to fully develop, leaving a communication gap between the mouth and the nasal passages (FIG. 11-6). This condition is inheritable in breeds such as English bulldogs, Boston terriers, and cocker spaniels. It can also be acquired secondary to foreign bodies puncturing the palate, or by burns caused by puppies chewing on electrical cords.

Neonatal puppies born with cleft palates often die because they are unable to suckle properly. Pups that do survive initially can develop nasal infections and aspiration pneumonia if the problem is not surgically corrected in time. The recommended time of surgery for these puppies is around 6 weeks of age. Until then, daily feedings using a tube passed directly into the esophagus is indicated to prevent these secondary complications.

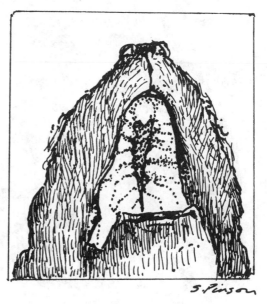

11-6 *Cleft palate.*

Oral tumors/epulis

Like other regions of the body, the oral cavity is not immune to its share of tumors and growths. A wide variety of tumors, including melanomas, sarcomas, papillomas, and carcinomas, can arise within the oral cavity of dogs. In contrast, *epulis,* or *gingival hyperplasia,* is the name given to a type of benign proliferation of the gum tissue within the mouth (FIG. 11-7).

Symptoms

Signs associated with oral tumors and epulis in dogs can include bad breath, oral bleeding, excessive salivation, and/or swallowing difficulties. In severe cases involving malignant tumors, actual facial deformities could occur secondary to the tumor growth.

Treatment

Rapid recognition of the presence of an oral tumor and concurrent treatment are essential, since malignant oral tumors in dogs will spread very rapidly to other areas of the body, including the lungs.

Epulis, on the other hand, requires no specific treatment unless the proliferation is so great as to interfere with normal function. In these instances, surgical removal of the overgrown gum tissue is indicated.

ESOPHAGEAL DISORDERS

Disorders involving the esophagus will manifest themselves as difficulty in swallowing. Effortless regurgitation of solid food, which must be differenti-

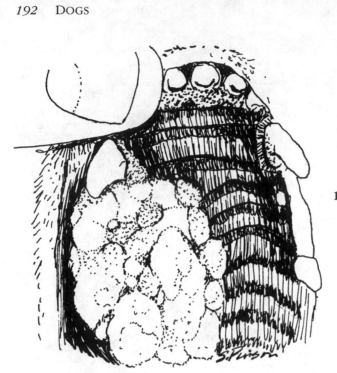

11-7 *Oral tumor.*

ated from vomiting and its associated abdominal spasms, often tips off the pet owner and veterinary practitioner to an existing problem with the esophagus. Due to the inability to properly swallow food, dogs afflicted with esophageal disease are at high risk of accidentally "breathing" or aspirating food into their lungs, causing serious, life-threatening pneumonia.

Megaesophagus

Megaesophagus is the term given to the condition in which a generalized enlargement of the esophagus occurs, making it unable to push food into the stomach. This condition might be inherited, or seen secondary esophageal obstructions or to neuromuscular diseases such as myasthenia gravis.

Diagnosis of megaesophagus is made by taking radiographs of the esophagus or actually visualizing the enlargement with an endoscope inserted into the esophagus via the mouth. Those dogs diagnosed with this disorder must be fed with their front end elevated on a chair or table to encourage gravity flow of food and water into the stomach. Feeding liquid or semisolid food will also help facilitate this passage into the stomach. Depending upon the cause, some individuals do improve with time. In select cases, surgery might be performed to help improve esophageal function.

Esophagitis

Inflammation occurring anywhere along the esophagus is termed *esophagitis*. Esophagitis can be instituted by foreign bodies which injure the organ's lining, by ingestion of caustic substances, and by reflux of stomach contents and acids up into the esophagus. In keeping with the latter cause, chronic, long-term vomiting can also lead to esophagitis.

Regurgitation, loss of appetite, and weight loss are the most frequent signs seen. If left untreated, damage to the lining of the esophagus could occur, causing strictures and secondary megaesophagus.

As with megaesophagus, diagnosis is made using clinical signs, physical exam findings, and endoscopic exam or radiographic X-rays of the esophagus using barium as a contrast media. Treatment of esophagitis consists of treating any primary problems that might be present, and, if stomach acid reflux is to blame, reducing the amount of stomach acid secretions and increasing the rate of stomach emptying.

Esophageal obstructions

Obstructions can occur secondary to tumors, infections, strictures, and the ingestion of foreign objects (especially bones). As with megaesophagus, obstructions can be diagnosed using radiographs and/or endoscopy. Treatment is aimed at the surgical removal of the offending obstructor (FIG. 11-8).

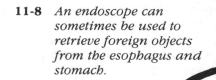

11-8   *An endoscope can sometimes be used to retrieve foreign objects from the esophagus and stomach.*

GASTRIC DILATATION-VOLVULUS COMPLEX (GDV)

Gastric dilatation-volvulus complex (GDV), or bloat, is a serious, life-threatening disorder that can strike the gastrointestinal system of dogs, particularly that of large, deep-chested breeds. Great Danes, St. Bernards, Irish setters, standard poodles, boxers, and English sheepdogs are but a few of the many breeds that can be suddenly afflicted with GDV.

Although they don't fit the anatomical mold of these other breeds, dachshunds and Pekineses also have a higher incidence of GDV than do other similar-sized breeds. Regardless of the size and age, death can quickly ensue in these dogs if the condition is not recognized and treated with speed.

Rapid ingestion of a large amount of food and water, followed by exercise, is an important predisposing cause to this disorder. As the stomach dilates due to the large food and water content within, and due to the gas formed within the stomach secondary to vigorous exercise, it can rotate or twist in such as way as to block off all entry into and exit from the stomach. The condition snowballs as the food, water, and gas within are not allowed to escape, and more and more gas and fluid are produced by the churning action and secretions of the distressed stomach. In addition, as the stomach dilates and/or rotates, it can effectively put pressure on the large blood vessels located within the abdomen and seriously reduce blood flow through them. This in turn places almost every major organ within the abdomen in serious jeopardy.

Symptoms

Dogs suffering from an acute case of GDV will exhibit signs such as a distended, bloated abdomen, vomiting, excessive salivation, and rapid breathing. In the early stages, the dog will be quite restless due to the pain; as the disease progresses, weakness, recumbency, and shock set in.

Treatment

A diagnosis of GDV is based upon history and clinical signs seen. As mentioned before, treatment must be instituted in earnest to save the life of the pet. The attending veterinarian will try to pass a tube into the stomach to relieve the stomach distension; however, if the stomach is twisted, this passage might be impossible. In these cases, immediate surgical intervention is required. Intravenous fluids, antibiotics, and steroids to combat shock are among the medications used in these patients. The prognosis is guarded with any dog presented with GDV, and reoccurrence is not uncommon.

If a dog likes to gulp down its food as soon as it is set down, protect it from the dangers of GDV by feeding smaller portions at more frequent intervals throughout the day. In addition, discourage exercise for at least one hour after mealtime. For dogs that have recurring bouts with GDV, surgical procedures can be performed as a preventative measure to "tack" the stomach down to the inner abdominal wall, thereby not allowing it to twist if bloating occurs.

GASTROINTESTINAL ULCERS

An ulceration within the stomach or intestines occurs when the protective mucus barrier covering the inner surfaces of the gastrointestinal tract is lost or destroyed, allowing stomach acids and bile acids to erode the gastrointestinal lining. The same type of heartburn humans can sometimes experience with this problem can affect dogs as well, leading to inappetence, vomiting, and lethargy.

Ulcers are actually a sign of disease rather than a distinct disease syndrome in themselves. Sharp foreign bodies or harsh chemicals that are swallowed can scrape, injure, and—in the case of the latter—burn the gastrointestinal lining as to cause a primary ulceration.

Ulcers occur secondary to stress, infectious diseases, intestinal parasites, and metabolic diseases such as Cushing's disease and kidney disease. Certain drugs, such as aspirin, can also have a deleterious effect upon the stomach lining when given orally.

Diagnosis of an ulcer relies heavily upon clinical signs seen and the history or evidence of an underlying disorder.

Radiographs taken after the oral administration of barium can be used to pinpoint the exact location of an ulcer. In addition, direct visualization of the actual stomach or intestinal lining using an endoscope is another means of diagnosing ulcers in a pet.

Obviously, when formulating any treatment regimen for ulcers, any underlying source for the ulcerations must be identified and treated. Specific ulcer treatment is aimed at reducing the amount of stomach acid secretion and providing a protective coating over the existing ulcer until it has time to heal.

As with humans, cimetidine and ranitidine are both very effective medications for reducing the amount of stomach acid secretion in dogs. Another drug often used to treat ulcers in dogs is sucralfate. This medication, when given orally, helps protect the gastrointestinal lining against the harmful effects of stomach acids.

INTUSSUSCEPTION

As with GDV, this is a life-threatening condition involving the gastrointestinal tract of dogs. An *intussusception* is abnormal invagination of a portion of small or large intestine into a dilated portion of bowel situated just ahead of it, causing obstruction to normal flow within the intestine. Peristalsis involving the affected gut segments further aggravate the intussusception, making it worse with time. In especially severe instances, the blood supply to the portion of the intestine involved will be cut off, resulting in the death of that tissue and serious health consequences. The site at which an intussusception is most likely to occur in dogs is where the small intestine links up with the large intestine (FIG. 11-9).

The causes of an intussusception can include any type of inflammation within the gut, viral infections, parasites, tumors, and swallowed foreign objects. Signs seen in dogs affected include lethargy, abdominal pain, fever, and vomiting.

Radiographs are the most useful tool in the diagnosis of an intussusception, since it has its own characteristic appearance on a radiograph. If intussusception is suspected or diagnosed, immediate surgery is neces-

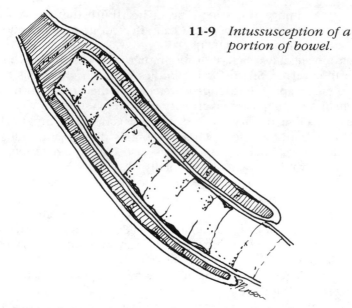

11-9   *Intussusception of a portion of bowel.*

sary to correct the invagination and to remove any dead portions of bowel that might be present. Obviously, the underlying problem that caused the intussusception in the first place must be corrected as well.

INTESTINAL OBSTRUCTIONS

In addition to intussusception, other items can obstruct normal flow through the gut and result in clinical signs, such as lethargy, vomiting, and black, tarry stools (FIG. 11-10). Swallowed foreign bodies (such as bones, rubber balls, stones), tumors, fungal infections, and herniations are all capable of causing either partial or complete obstructions if large or extensive enough. Unless the obstruction is relieved in a timely fashion, usually through surgical means, loss of blood supply to the affected portion can occur, resulting in the death of that portion of bowel, systemic infection, and shock.

COLITIS

Problems involving the large intestine of dogs are not uncommon in veterinary medicine. Colitis refers to the inflammation of the lining of the large intestine, resulting in diarrhea, with the feces often containing an abundance of blood and mucus. The blood seen with colitis is usually bright red, in contrast to small intestinal bleeding, which contributes a black tarry appearance to the feces. *Tenesmus,* or straining to defecate, is another prevalent sign that is often mistaken for constipation.

Symptoms
Acute colitis refers to a sudden onset of signs that usually lasts only a short

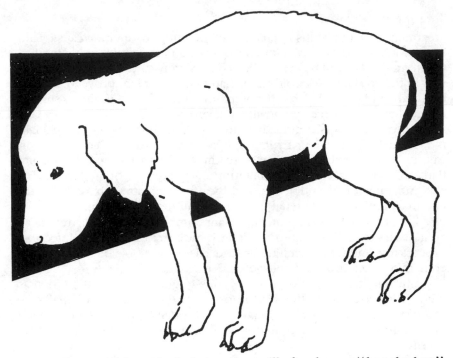

11-10 *Dogs with intestinal obstruction will often have a "hunched up" appearance.*

period of time with proper treatment. Chronic colitis is a long-term, recurring condition that might last an entire lifetime of the pet.

Parasites such as whipworms and coccidia are common causes of acute colitis in dogs; dietary indiscretions and stress-induced situations are two other prevalent sources. Less commonly, fungal infections, foreign bodies, intussusceptions, polyps, food allergies, immune system disorders, and tumors can all result in signs related to a chronic colitis.

Because of the variety of potential causes, colitis can strike a dog of any age. As far as breed dispositions to chronic colitis are concerned, boxers seem to have a higher prevalence than other breeds.

Diagnosis

Diagnosis of colitis is made from a predisposing history (such as dietary indiscretion), existing clinical signs, and physical examination. Stool examinations and other laboratory tests should be performed in an attempt to identify the underlying cause of the colitis. Radiographs, including barium contrast studies are indicated in non-responsive, recurring cases. Biopsies obtained using an endoscope or through exploratory surgery can also prove to be helpful for establishing a definitive diagnosis. In some cases, an exact cause of the inflammation can never be discerned, even with extensive laboratory tests.

Treatment

Treatment of acute colitis is aimed at eliminating the inciting cause. Parasites should be treated using proper dewormers and antiparasitic medications. Antibiotics can be used to help remove any disease-causing bacteria within the colon, and steroid anti-inflammatories might prove to be helpful in abating clinical signs. If polyps or tumors are presented, surgical removal might be necessary to afford a cure.

However, understand that in many cases of chronic colitis, especially those caused by stress or by immune system disorders, a complete cure cannot be achieved. In these pets, treatment goals are aimed at managing flare-ups as they occur and maintaining a good quality of life for the dog. Anti-inflammatories, antibiotics, and local protectants such as kaolin and pectin can help provide relief from these intermittent flare-ups.

Dietary management is an important component of colitis treatment. Acute cases of colitis caused by dietary indiscretion or some infectious process respond well to feeding a bland, easily digestible diet, such as one containing rice, eggs, and cottage cheese.

Chronic, recurring bouts with colitis might be managed by increasing the fiber content in the diet to normalize the gut motility. Finally, for those cases suspected of being caused by food allergies, a hypoallergenic diet composed of rice and mutton can help eliminate the effects of the allergy.

PLC

A special type of colitis, called *plasmacytic-lymphocytic colitis* (PLC), has been receiving special recognition in recent years as its diagnostic prevalence has been on the increase. Plasmacytic-lymphocytic colitis is a poorly understood disease that evokes much controversy among researchers. The hallmark characteristic of PLC is an infiltration of the gut wall with large numbers of lymphocytes, which suggests that this disease might have an immune component. An overactive immune response to certain dietary ingredients, parasites, and/or bacteria within the colon is believed to be underlying cause to this source of chronic diarrhea in dogs.

Symptoms

Clinical signs related to PLC are similar to those seen with other cases of colitis. Interestingly enough, most cases of PLC seem to strike young dogs under 3 years of age.

A diagnosis of PLC can only be made after obtaining a colonic biopsy. Before attempting this, however, other laboratory work, including stool exams and blood profiles, should be performed to rule out the other multitude of causes of colitis.

Treatment

Dogs that are diagnosed with PLC should be placed on hypoallergenic diets to rule out food allergies as a potential cause. If they respond favorably, then dietary management might be all that is needed to control the disease. Fiber supplementation has also been used with some effectiveness in the management of PLC, with the added fiber helping normalize the motility within the colon.

Drugs used to treat cases of PLC nonresponsive to dietary manipulation include sulfasalazine and/or corticosteroids. One potential side effect with long-term use of the former is decreased tear production, so that dogs on sulfasalazine should have their tear levels monitored on a regular basis.

Unfortunately, because of the apparent immune system component to this disease, a complete cure for plasmacytic-lymphocytic colitis is usually unobtainable. However, with the treatment measures just described, most cases can be managed enough as to allow the affected pet to live a relatively normal life otherwise.

ANAL SAC DISEASE

The anal sacs are special structures located at the 8 o'clock and the 4 o'clock positions just below the anus. These sacs are lined with special cells that secrete an odiferous liquid into the lumen of each sac, where it is stored. As feces pass out of the anus, these sacs are emptied of their stored material via small ducts located just below the anal opening. Some dogs even have the skunk-like ability to express these sacs free-will! No one knows quite for sure what the purpose of the anal sacs and their secretions are in dogs, but many suspect that they serve as a means of communication and identification between dogs.

Anal sac infections and irritation can occur if the material within the sacs isn't emptied on a regular basis (FIG. 11-11). Secretions that are allowed to remain for long periods of time within the sacs often become thick and gritty, making future emptying that much harder. Any inflammation of the skin, caused by allergies, fleas, etc., can lead to this problem. Changes in frequency or consistency of bowel movements caused by diarrhea, constipation, or dietary changes, can also result in improper emptying of the sacs and secondary anal sac disease. Tapeworm segments are notorious for finding their way into the sacs and causing marked irritation. Smaller breeds of dogs under 15 pounds seem to have more problems with their anal sacs than do larger breeds because the sac's emptying ducts are smaller as well.

Symptoms

Dogs suffering from anal sac irritation often show obvious signs of discomfort, including constant licking in that region, and "scooting" their hind end along the floor in an attempt to empty the sacs. In these instances, manual emptying of the sacs often leads to dramatic changes in the pet's overall disposition.

If one or more anal sacs become infected, actual pus or draining tracts might be observed around the affected region (FIG. 11-12). These

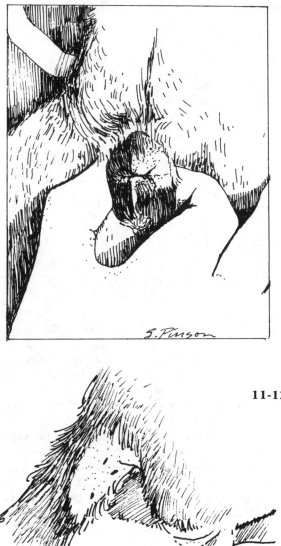

11-11   *Expressing anal sacs on a dog.*

11-12   *Irritated anal sacs can lead to dermatitis and hair loss.*

dogs are in a great deal of pain and will resist attempts at inspection. The amount of licking activity will also increase.

Treatment and prevention

Infected anal sacs need to be treated with topical antibiotics instilled directly into the affected sac(s) on a daily basis. In extensive cases, oral antibiotics might also be used to quicken the cure.

Anal sac problems can be prevented through a number of means. Increasing the fiber and bulk content in the diet, and hence the fecal material, will promote a more thorough emptying of the sacs with each bowel movement. If a dog is showing early signs of problems, such as scooting, prompt evacuation of the sacs by a veterinarian can help prevent further progression of the problem.

Routine expression of healthy anal sacs is not advised, since, if done improperly, it could actually inflame these sacs and lead to impaction. Surgical removal of the anal sacs is certainly an option for those dogs who suffer miserably from this affliction. If infection is present, it must be cleared up before this type of surgery is performed.

PANCREATITIS

Inflammation of the pancreas, or *pancreatitis,* is a painful condition characterized by an overproduction of digestive enzymes, which actually begin to damage the pancreatic tissue itself. This disorder tends to strike middle-aged, overweight dogs. In addition, female dogs seem to have a greater propensity for pancreatitis than do males. Dogs that are fed poor-quality, high-calorie diets with or without table scraps are also at high risk of developing pancreatitis. Finally, heredity can come into play as well, with certain breeds, such as schnauzers, being at greater risk than some of their canine counterparts.

Symptoms

Signs of a pancreatitis attack include loss of appetite, excessive salivation, vomiting, diarrhea, depression, and marked pain in the abdominal region on the right side just behind the rib cage (FIG. 11-13). Animals so afflicted

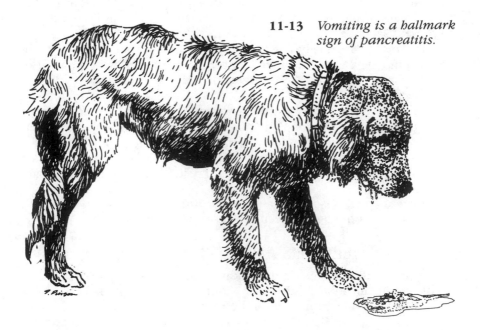

11-13 *Vomiting is a hallmark sign of pancreatitis.*

will sometimes assume a "praying" posture, with the front legs bent and the hind end stuck up in the air, in order to alleviate some of the pain.

In severe involvements, shock and death can result if the pain and inflammation isn't relieved promptly. Diabetes mellitus can also be an unfortunate consequence with repeated bouts of pancreatitis as the insulin-producing cells within the pancreas are destroyed by digestive enzymes. Because of the similarity of the clinical signs, acute bouts of pancreatitis must be differentiated from GDV and intestinal obstructions or intussusceptions.

Diagnosis

Dogs suffering from mild flare-ups of pancreatitis will often recover spontaneously when food and water is withheld. In fact, this is one method of diagnosing such a condition. Measuring the blood levels of the pancreatic enzymes amylase and lipase can also be a helpful diagnostic tool, since both tend to be elevated during an acute attack. Radiographs are useful for ruling out other potential causes of the clinical signs, such as GDV or obstructions.

Treatment

When treating pancreatitis, it is imperative that all food, water, and even oral medication is discontinued for a period of 48 to 72 hours. This will help lower the amounts of digestive enzymes being produced by the pancreas. Intravenous fluids are required to prevent dehydration during this time of fasting.

Pain relievers and medications designed to reduce pancreatic secretions are very important to prevent secondary complications from arising. Since the gastrointestinal tract is involved, antibiotics are indicated as well to prevent secondary bacterial infections.

Pancreatitis is usually a recurring problem that can never be eliminated completely. However, there are certain measures owners can institute at home to protect pets from acute flare-ups and the health problems associated with them.

Canines with a history of this disorder should be fed low calorie, easily digestible diets that don't require much pancreatic effort for their breakdown within the intestines. Such a diet, or a recipe for its formulation, is available from veterinarians. All table scraps should cease: Even sneaking a small treat from the table could result in a life-threatening pancreatitis attack.

Increasing exercise levels and promoting weight loss will also serve protective functions against recurrence of this disorder.

HEPATITIS AND LIVER DISEASE

While pancreatitis means inflammation involving the pancreas, *hepatitis* involves inflammation of the liver. Contrary to popular belief, not all cases of hepatitis are infectious and contagious in nature (i.e., infectious canine hepatitis, roundworms). There can be numerous noninfectious causes of liver inflammation as well. Some of these include diabetes mellitus, heart disease, accidental poisonings, starvation, and cancer.

As an organ responsible for metabolism of the multitude of nutrients absorbed from the intestines, and detoxification of poisons and drugs circulating in the blood, it is remarkable that the liver is normally very resistant to injury or breakdown resulting from its normal day-to-day functions. Unfortunately, because of this heartiness, clinical signs of liver inflammation usually won't appear until serious damage to liver function has already taken place.

Symptoms

Like so many other disease affecting the gastrointestinal tract, acute flare-ups of hepatitis can cause loss of appetite, vomiting, diarrhea, and fever in affected dogs. One unique sign often seen with hepatitis, both acute and chronic, is jaundice, or icterus. *Jaundice,* caused by elevated levels of bile pigments in the bloodstream, is characterized by a yellow discoloration of the skin, mucous membranes, and the liquid portion of the blood.

Other clinical signs that can result from chronic, long-term hepatitis and liver disease include a fluid buildup within the abdominal cavity (*ascites*) due to increased resistance to blood flow through the liver, bleeding tendencies, and anemia. Seizures and other neurologic disorders can also appear with advanced cases as blood levels of ammonia are allowed to build up.

Treatment

Diagnosis of hepatitis is made based upon clinical signs, elevated serum levels of liver enzymes, and/or the demonstration of an enlarged liver on radiographs. For those more subtle cases, special liver function tests and even biopsies might be required to confirm a diagnosis of hepatitis or discover its cause.

Treatment objectives for hepatitis and liver disease are aimed at eliminating the injurious agent and its harmful effect on the liver tissue and at promoting the healing of the affected tissue. The liver is one of the few organs within the body that can actually regenerate itself after injury—provided, of course, that the source of the injury is dealt with properly.

If vomiting is a problem, intravenous fluids might be needed until the stomach settles down enough for oral food and water (FIG. 11-14). An easily digestible diet with high biological value, such as Hill's Prescription Diet K/D, is ideal for patients suffering from a liver disorder. Oral antibiotics designed to eliminate ammonia-forming organisms are useful for those cases exhibiting neurological signs. Ascites can be treated with diuretic drugs such as furosemide and by reducing the amount of sodium in the dog's diet.

Finally, in chronic cases of hepatitis, steroids might be warranted to increase appetite and to counteract the loss of protein which can occur with liver disease.

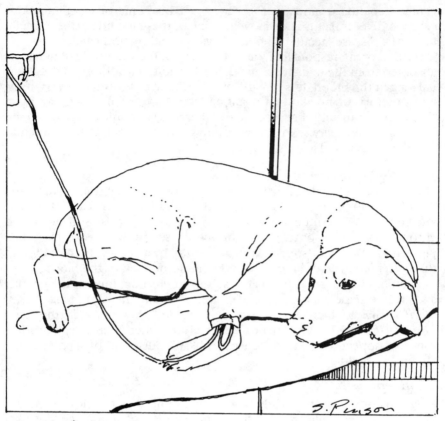

11-14   *Liver disease requires intense supportive treatment.*

12

The Urinary System

IN THE NORMAL, day-to-day functioning of the body, lots of waste material is formed as a result of metabolic activity. It is the function of the urinary system to handle and to rid the body of these waste products. In addition, through its ability to dilute or concentrate the urine, it serves to regulate fluid levels within the body.

ANATOMY AND PHYSIOLOGY

The urinary system of dogs is composed of two kidneys, the ureters, a bladder, and a urethra. The kidneys are composed of cells called *nephrons,* which are responsible for filtering the waste material out of the blood and returning vital fluids and nutrients that would otherwise be lost in the urine back into the bloodstream (FIG. 12-1). Those solids and fluids not put back into the blood by the nephrons will eventually make up the urine. All of the nephrons empty urine into a specific portion of the kidney, which then empties into the ureter for transport to and storage in the bladder.

The bladder wall is composed of smooth muscle and is capable of expanding to enormous sizes. Special muscular sphincters prevent the urine from passing out of the bladder prematurely. *Urinary incontinence,* characterized by an inability to voluntarily hold urine within the bladder, can result from malfunction of these sphincters. Once the bladder is ready to release its contents, the urine then passes out of the body by way of the urethra.

Because of its vital function, any interference or alteration of urinary system function can quickly have serious health consequences. For this

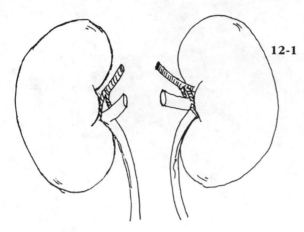

12-1 *The kidneys are responsible for filtering wastes out of the blood.*

reason, prompt and proper diagnosis of urinary tract disorders in dogs is essential. Periodic checkups by a veterinarian can help detect potential problems before they reach such a magnitude as to threaten the health of the pet.

KIDNEY DISEASE

The kidneys are responsible for eliminating waste products produced by the body's normal metabolism. If they fail to perform this function adequately, the body will literally poison itself. For this reason, special attention must be directed at keeping these organs healthy, or—if a disease state already exists—at treating to prevent further functional deterioration.

In dogs, kidney (*renal*) disease is the most common disorder associated with old age. In essence, through normal wear and tear, the kidneys become unable to perform their functions in the same way that they did when they were young. Worn-out kidney cells die and are replaced by scar tissue, which can't filter out toxins from the blood. When enough of these nephrons die and the buildup of toxins in the blood becomes great enough, then the pet begins to exhibit signs of kidney failure.

But don't get the idea that older dogs are the only ones that can suffer from kidney impairment. Young dogs might be born with inadequate kidney function, or they might suffer from other diseases or toxic agent which kill nephrons and impair renal performance.

For example, systemic infections, heat stroke, heart disease, and autoimmune diseases are but some of the acquired conditions that can lead to kidney disease and kidney failure. Many therapeutic drugs, such as aspirin and certain antibiotics, can be damaging to the kidneys if used indiscriminately. Antifreeze, or ethylene glycol, is deadly to dogs when ingested because of the profound damage to the kidneys it causes. Finally, periodontal disease, with its associated complications, can predispose dogs, both young and old, to kidney problems in the future.

Symptoms

The clinical signs associated with kidney disease can be quite variable depending on the extent of damage to the kidneys. Interestingly enough, dogs rarely show outward signs of kidney disease until at least 75 percent of the function in both kidneys is lost! As a result, when signs do finally become apparent, it is vital that therapeutic measures be taken quickly to prevent the loss of the remaining twenty-five percent.

Sudden, acute kidney failure, the type that can result from the ingestion of a poison such as antifreeze, can lead directly into intense dehydration, shock, unconsciousness, and death without showing any other signs.

Chronic, more long-term kidney disease and kidney failure rarely have such a dramatic presentation, yet such conditions can eventually turn into acute kidney failure if measures aren't instituted to prevent this progression. Dogs with chronic renal failure will exhibit an increased thirst and an increased desire to urinate. Depression and loss of appetite might also set in. In addition, since renal disease can cause stomach ulcers, vomiting might occur.

Diagnosis

Veterinarians can diagnose kidney disease through a series of laboratory tests performed on the blood and the urine. Two blood parameters, blood urea nitrogen (BUN) and serum creatinine will be elevated if the kidneys are failing.

The urine specific gravity is also an important parameter which helps the veterinary practitioner determine the extent of damage to the kidneys (FIG. 12-2). Under normal circumstances, the specific gravity of the urine, which measures how concentrated the urine is, should fluctuate depending upon the body's own needs for water. Diseased kidneys, however, are unable to conserve water for the body, hence, this specific gravity of the urine in a dog with advanced kidney disease will be diluted, even if the pet is clinically dehydrated.

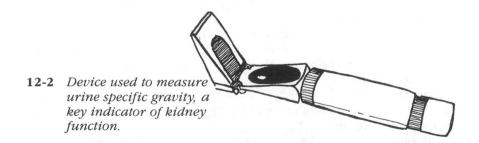

12-2 *Device used to measure urine specific gravity, a key indicator of kidney function.*

Treatment

Dogs suffering from acute renal failure must be hospitalized and placed on intravenous fluids to correct dehydration. Other medications designed to stimulate kidney function will be given as well. If the dog survives this acute attack, support measures for chronic kidney failure must then be implemented.

Stress reduction is vital in dogs with chronic renal disease and/or failure. Unlimited access to clean, fresh water should be provided at all times, since deprivation could lead into an acute kidney-failure crisis. Special diets that are low in protein should be fed to help reduce toxin build-up within the bloodstream. These are available from veterinarians. Vitamin supplementation should also be considered to replace those lost in the increased urine flow.

Since renal disease can alter, among other things, the blood levels of calcium and phosphorus, medications designed to keep levels of these electrolytes constant are used as well. If a pet is having trouble with vomiting, human antiulcer medications such as cimetidine can be employed to help settle the stomach.

Finally, since kidney disease places an incredible burden on the affected pet's immune system, all underlying disease processes and disorders (such as periodontal disease) need to be addressed and treated.

URINARY INCONTINENCE

Dogs that are unable to willfully control their urination habits are said to be suffering from incontinence. Pets with urinary incontinence might simply urinate spontaneously without warning, or might drip urine continuously throughout the day. Inappropriate urination during sleep is another common complaint. Dermatitis in the genital and hind leg regions can also be seen as a common sequella to incontinence and urine scalding in these areas.

The potential causes of urinary incontinence are numerous; as a result, a proper veterinary workup is essential to obtain a correct diagnosis. Spinal trauma, anatomical changes or irritation caused by congenital defects, infections, tumors, or urinary calculi, metabolic diseases such as diabetes mellitus or diabetes insipidus can all be underlying causes of incontinence. In these instances, treatment is geared towards correcting the underlying cause if possible.

It has been noted that a small number of female dogs that are spayed at an early age can suffer from incontinence when they enter their geriatric years. Although the exact cause of this incontinence is unknown, it can usually be controlled with medications designed to increase sphincter tone within the lower urinary tract. One such medication that has been used for years is the hormone diethylstilbesterol, which is usually given once to twice weekly.

Because of the unpleasant side effects that can sometimes accompany long-term usage of this drug, many veterinarians opt to avert such therapy in lieu of more advanced medications now available.

Puppies and even some adult dogs might urinate spontaneously when they become excited or frightened. Most puppies will "grow out" of this problem as they mature. For these and others, treatment for behavioral incontinence is geared towards minimizing the stimuli that cause the incontinence in the first place.

For instance, when dealing with dogs that urinate due to excitement, avoiding eye contact or exaggerated greetings when approaching the pet often help to curb excitement and prevent urination. For those dogs that urinate when frightened, easing their fear through behavioral modification is the key to a cure (see chapter 2).

BLADDER STONES (UROLITHIASIS)

Urinary tract infections that go unnoticed for a period of time can predispose a dog to urolithiasis. A urolith or stone results from the coalescing of crystals which form within the urine environment (FIG. 12-3). In dogs, these stones form more readily within the bladder than they do in other portions of the urinary system. Urolithiasis presents itself in dogs in two main forms: Cystic (bladder) calculi and urethral calculi.

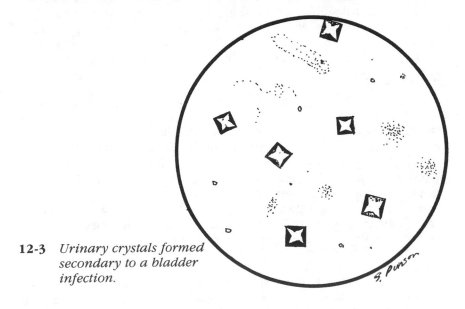

12-3 *Urinary crystals formed secondary to a bladder infection.*

The first of these, cystic calculi, are found mainly in females and usually result when infectious bacteria within the bladder cause an increase in the urine pH, which in turn causes the crystals to form. Most commonly, the particular crystals generated are termed *struvite crystals*. Stones formed by these crystals are often discoid in shape (FIG. 12-4).

Urethral calculi occur in male dogs and are typically composed of cystine or urate crystals instead of struvite. This type of urolithiasis is not generally caused by infections; rather, an inherent metabolic disorder is responsible for their formation. If these stones lodge in the male urethra,

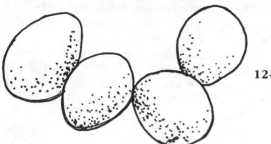

12-4 *Bladder stones.*

they can effectively prevent normal urination, and can seriously threaten the life of the pet.

Symptoms

Straining to urinate, bloody urine, constant licking at the urethral opening, and/or frequent unsuccessful attempts to urinate are all signs of a urinary problem. Stones might or might not be present in a dog exhibiting these signs, but it warrants a professional evaluation. Some dogs, especially females, might carry stones in their bladders for long periods of time without ever exhibiting any signs at all. This is one good reason for having a veterinarian perform a routine urinalysis on an annual basis.

Diagnosis

Diagnosis of urolithiasis is made based upon microscopic examination of the urine for crystal formation, abdominal palpation, and radiographs. Most stones will show up readily on regular radiographs (FIG. 12-5); however, those composed of urate or cystine might require special contrast radiographs in order to identify them. In addition, for male dogs suspected of having urethral calculi, impedance to the passage of a urinary catheter is a sure sign that stones are present.

In these cases and others, the attending veterinarian will often elect to run blood tests as well to be sure the kidneys and other organs are functioning properly in the presence of these uroliths.

Treatment

Treatment of urolithiasis depends upon the size and number of the stones present, and their location within the urinary tract. Obviously a male dog that is completely plugged by one or more of these stones requires emergency intervention at once. Catheterization is performed in an attempt to dislodge the stones, pushing them back into the bladder and freeing up the flow of urine. Most of the time, these stones must then be removed from the bladder surgically.

In those cases uncomplicated by obstruction, the size of the stones involved determines the treatment regimen. Large stones located within the bladder will undoubtedly require surgery for their removal. In contrast, cases marked by smaller stones or crystals only can often be effectively managed with special diets designed to dissolve the stones.

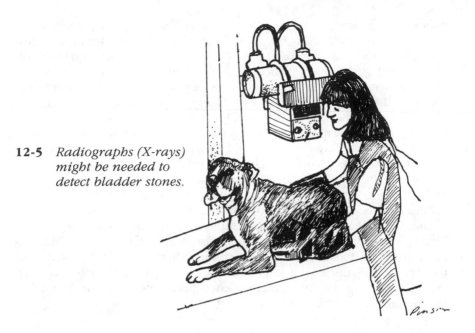

12-5 *Radiographs (X-rays) might be needed to detect bladder stones.*

Typically, this dietary approach to treatment might take anywhere from one to four months to accomplish the desired results. If a pet is placed on a urolith-dissolving diet, be sure to follow the veterinarian's instructions closely. These diets should not be fed for any term longer than that prescribed by the veterinarian. Once the stones have dissolved, the pet needs to be switched to a different diet.

Of course, whether a surgical or medical approach is used, concurrent antibiotic therapy is also necessary if an infection is underlying the bladder stones.

Prevention

Because the rate of recurrence of urolithiasis is relatively high even after successful treatment, preventative measures should be instituted to help lower the odds. For urethral calculi, special diets that can help promote a urine pH that is nonconducive to crystal formation are available from veterinarians. These diets are also low in those dietary components that might be incorporated into crystals.

Cystic calculi can be prevented in a similar fashion, using special diets designed for the prevention of struvite uroliths. In addition, prompt identification and treatment of urinary tract infections will help ensure that crystals and stones won't develop as a consequence.

URINARY TRACT INFECTIONS

Infections of the urinary tract can occur anywhere along the system pathway, including the kidneys, the ureters, the bladder, the urethra, and in males, the prostate gland. One particular site might be exclusively affected, or multiple sites could be involved at the same time. Most urinary tract infections are caused by bacteria gaining entrance into the body through external urinary orifices and traveling upwards into the system (termed *ascending infections*). Other routes of infection can include the blood or the lymphatic system, and through direct penetrating trauma.

Because of the shorter length of their urethras, female dogs are more prone to these type infections than are males. In all animals, regardless of sex, normal body defense mechanisms are constantly at work preventing the establishments of infections within the tract. Antibodies lining the surfaces of the bladder and urethra provide a first line of defense. Sphincter systems, controlled by contracting smooth muscle, help seal off the different portions of the tract from one another. An acidic pH to the urine is another safeguard against the multiplication of undesirable organisms. Finally, normal, frequent urination is also very effective at eliminating undesirable bacteria from the bladder and other parts of the system. For this reason, any disruption in the normal urination routine (for example, not taking a dog outside enough, dehydration, etc.) can predispose an individual to a bacterial infection.

Symptoms

Clinical signs of urinary tract infection will vary, depending upon the region or regions involved. Signs associated with infections of the bladder and urethra include straining when trying to urinate (often mistaken for constipation), passage of only small amounts of urine at a time, and/or bloody urine. In the latter case, blood noted at the beginning of urination often signifies a urethral infection, whereas blood noticed near the end of elimination might mean the bladder is involved. In many cases, dogs won't show any other signs of illness or fever.

If the kidneys or ureters are involved, similar clinical signs might be noticed, along with other obvious signs of illness, such as fever, depression, vomiting, abdominal pain, and/or back pain. In cases of upper urinary tract infections, it is vital that treatment be instituted at once to prevent permanent damage to the tissue of the kidney.

Urinary tract infections can be associated with other disease processes as well, so its presence can sometimes be overshadowed by clinical signs associated with another primary disease. For instance, diabetes mellitus can predispose to such an infection due to the high sugar content in the urine caused by the disease (sugar can provide an ideal growth medium for bacteria). Disorders of the nervous system can even lead to urinary infections if the nerve supply to the muscles and sphincters of the tract are disrupted, thereby eliminating some of the body's natural means of defense.

One unfortunate sequela that can result from any type of urinary tract infection that is not treated promptly is urolithiasis, or urinary stones. The reason for this is that these stones have a propensity to form when an increase in urine pH occurs, often as a result of bacteria acting within the urinary tract to break down urine. When this breakdown occurs, ammonia is released, increasing the pH of the bladder environment.

Diagnosis

Diagnosis of a urinary tract infection is based upon clinical signs, urinalysis, and urine cultures designed to identify the actual bacteria involved. In addition, a veterinarian might choose to order a blood workup done on a pet to rule out any disorders, such as diabetes mellitus, that might be underlying the infection. Furthermore, if crystals are noted upon microscopic examination of the urine, radiographs will be needed to make sure there are no bladder or kidney stones present.

Treatment

Treatment for urinary tract infections involves the use of an appropriate antibiotic for a minimum of 10 days. Since bacteria can become resistant to certain antibiotics over time, urine cultures to determine antibiotic sensitivity might need to be performed if a response to treatment with a particular antibiotic is poor.

Urinary stones, if present, might need to be removed surgically if their size is large enough. Smaller stones and crystals can often be dissolved by feeding a special type of diet designed to accomplish this task.

For those dogs that suffer from chronic, recurring flare-ups of urinary tract infections, long-term, low dose antibiotic therapy might be prescribed by a veterinarian. This usually involves the administration of a single dosage of antibiotic just before the pet's bedtime. Because of the long interval between bedtime and the next morning's first urine void, the antibiotic is allowed to reach high concentrations within the urine, effectively combating any bacteria that might be present. It is important to take a dog outside to eliminate just before bedtime, to assure that the new urine that is formed will contain undiluted high levels of the medication.

Prevention

Owners can help prevent the occurrence of a urinary tract infection in their dogs by providing plenty of fresh water to drink at all times, and by encouraging frequent urinations. Special diets that can help promote a healthy environment within the tract and help discourage infections are available from veterinarians.

For dogs with long hair, especially females, keep the hair trimmed up around the external urinary structures to reduce the chances of bacteria gaining entrance to the urinary system via contamination by this hair.

Finally, because uncomplicated urinary tract infections might not show any outwards signs, a routine urinalysis on a pet is encouraged on an annual basis along with its regular checkup and vaccinations.

13

The Reproductive System

DISEASES AND CONDITIONS involving the reproductive tract are not uncommon in nonneutered dogs. Most of the problems that arise tend to be either infectious or anatomical in nature. Prompt medical attention is warranted in any disorder involving the reproductive tract.

ANATOMY AND PHYSIOLOGY
The male reproductive system

Starting with the male, or sire, the major parts of the reproductive system include the testes (testicles) (with associated epididymis and ductus deferens), the scrotum (containing the testicles), the penis (containing the urethra), and the prostate gland.

The testes are the organs responsible for the production of spermatozoa. This production is directly influenced by the hormone testosterone, also produced by the testes. Aside from regulating sperm production, testosterone is also responsible for normal male sexual behavior, as well as the aggressive, territorial behavior exhibited by some male dogs.

Normally, the testicles should descend into the scrotum shortly after birth, usually no later than 8 weeks of age. If this event fails to occur, the dog is said to be *cryptorchid,* and surgical removal of the testicles is required to prevent medical problems in the future and to prevent the passage of that undesirable trait to offspring.

From the testicle, sperm is shunted into the epididymis, a structure closely attached to each testicle, where it finishes its maturation process. Upon copulation, the mature sperm is transported from the epididymis through the ductus deferens and to the tube-like urethra coursing within penis.

The canine penis, contained within a sheath of skin known as the *prepuce,* has the uncommon ability to swell near its origin during erection, effecting the unique interlocking "tie" with the female during reproduction. In addition, the latter half of the dog's penis contains a bony structure called the *os penis,* which is grooved underneath to allow for the passage of the urethra. If its support function seems somewhat sedentary, its medical significance is not. Because the penis and urethra are members of the urinary system as well as the reproductive, this os penis can exacerbate complications associated with certain urinary disorders, including urethral calculi.

The prostate gland, considered an accessory sex gland, is located surrounding the urethra near the neck of the bladder. It functions to produce prostatic fluid, which mixes with sperm to form semen, and helps to increase the survivability of the sperm within the female reproductive tract. Enlargement or inflammation of this gland is not uncommon as intact male dogs mature. Constipation, discharges from the penis, and painful urinations can be clinical signs of a prostatic disorder.

The female reproductive system

The major reproductive organs of the female dog, or bitch, include the ovaries, the oviducts, the uterus, the vagina, the vulva and the mammary glands. The ovaries are responsible for the production and release of eggs destined to be fertilized by the male sperm. In addition, several important reproductive hormones are produced by these structures.

Unfertilized eggs are released, or ovulated, by the ovaries, and pass into the small oviducts. It is within these oviducts that fertilization, if impending, takes place. After this is accomplished, the fertilized egg, or embryo, continues its passage down the oviducts on its way to the uterus.

When an embryo reaches the uterus, it attaches itself to the uterine wall and begins its development. If fertilization has not taken place, this attachment won't take place and the egg is eventually resorbed by the body.

The uterus is separated from the vagina by a ring of muscle known as the cervix. Most of the time, this cervix remains open. During pregnancy, however, the cervix will close, preventing outside access to the uterine environment. Then, at time of parturition, the cervix relaxes, allowing the birth to take place.

The external opening of the vagina is termed the vulva. As a female dog enters in to her heat cycle, the vulva will begin to noticeably swell, tipping owners off to the impending heat (FIG. 13-1).

Dogs typically have a total of 8 to 10 mammary glands (4 to 5 on each side), designed to supply newborn offspring with life-sustaining milk. The size of these glands will fluctuate, depending upon the stage of the estrous cycle and upon the pregnancy status of the bitch.

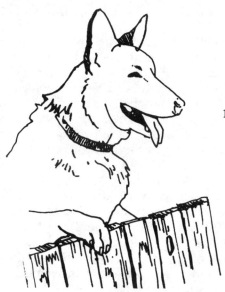

13-1

Male dogs will go to any lengths to be with a female in heat.

PREGNANCY-RELATED PROBLEMS
Accidental matings (mismatings)

The question about what to do with the female dog who is accidentally bred is not an easy one to answer. In the old days, all that dog owners needed to do was to take her in to the veterinarian for a "mismating shot or pill." What these treatments consisted of were formulations of the female hormone estrogen, which, if given within the first 36 hours after mating occurred, would effectively terminate a pregnancy.

This sounds all fine and dandy until you take into account recent research on the potential side effects of using such drugs in dogs to abort pregnancy. For starters, external sources of estrogens have been demonstrated to actually cause infertility in some female dogs, rendering them unable to conceive at later dates. On a more serious note, estrogens can also cause a life-threatening anemia in sensitive cases. And if that weren't enough, they can also predispose a dog to pyometra (see Pyometra, in this chapter) after administration.

To be on the safe side, use of such estrogen-containing drugs is not an acceptable method for dealing with mismatings in dogs. So what are the options open to pet owners? To begin, with valuable breeding females especially, it is best to just go ahead and let them have the litter of puppies instead of chancing it with mismating medications. If this is not acceptable, then either surgical removal of the puppies from the uterus at a later stage of development or an actual ovariohysterectomy is warranted.

Remember: All of this is assuming, of course, that a viable mating did indeed take place and that a pregnancy resulted from it! Many mismatings do not result in pregnancy, and grieve owners needlessly.

False pregnancy (pseudopregnancy)

When the ovaries of a female dog release eggs to be fertilized, they then start to produce a hormone called progesterone. Now the function of this progesterone is to maintain pregnancy if egg fertilization occurs. However, a unique feature about dogs is that even if fertilization does not occur, progesterone levels will remain high for up to 10 weeks after heat is over. It is precisely this behavior that is responsible for the condition dog owners know as *pseudopregnancy*, or false pregnancy.

All female dogs exhibit some form of pseudopregnancy after they come out of heat. In most, signs associated with it go unnoticed by the owner. However, some dogs do exhibit marked changes as a result of these high progesterone levels, including mammary gland enlargement with or without the production of milk, and behavioral changes which include restlessness, nesting, mothering of inanimate objects, and loss of appetite. In short, they might actually appear to be expectant mothers! Often, there is no way to be sure that they aren't, without the use of ultrasound or radiographic X-rays. Dogs that undergo marked false pregnancies are also prime candidates for mastitis, a common sequela.

Therapy to control signs associated with pseudopregnancies is generally not needed, unless mastitis becomes a recurring problem, or if marked behavioral changes occur as a result. Hormones prescribed by your veterinarian can provide relief in many cases, yet prolonged use of these can have undesirable side effects, especially in females used for breeding. Because of this, unless you have a valuable breeder on your hands, ovariohysterectomy is the safest and most effective way to deal with overt pseudopregnancies.

Eclampsia

Eclampsia is a serious, sometimes life-threatening disease that can occur in the bitch either just prior to giving birth or within three weeks after parturition has taken place. More common in the smaller, toy breeds, it is characterized by abnormally low levels of blood calcium in their systems (FIG. 13-2).

Early signs seen with eclampsia include nervousness, whining, pacing, and trembling. This might progress into uncoordination, muscle spasms, and seizure-like activity. Left untreated, death can result from respiratory difficulties and high fevers.

Diagnosis of eclampsia is based upon history, clinical signs and blood calcium levels. Luckily, treatment consisting of intravenous injections of calcium is highly effective and provides instant relief from the life-threatening signs seen.

After treatment is performed, and clinical signs have abated, owners need to take special precautions to ensure that a relapse does not occur. For starters, puppies should not be allowed to nurse for 24 hours after such an episode. Instead, a commercial milk replacement formula should be fed to them. In fact, periodic supplementation should continue even

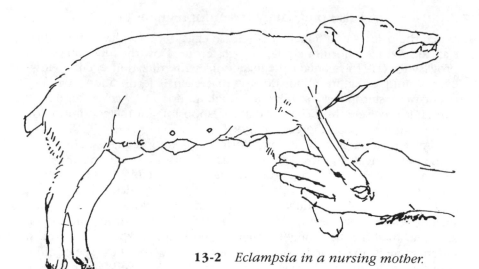

13-2   *Eclampsia in a nursing mother.*

after the puppies are placed back on their mother's milk to reduce the load on her. In some cases, putting the puppies back on their mother's milk will cause another episode of eclampsia, in which case, they should be permanently placed on supplements.

Bitches that are prone to eclampsia should be placed on oral calcium supplements throughout the nursing period. In fact, if there is a past history of such a problem, calcium supplementation started during the last two weeks of pregnancy and continued throughout lactation can be quite helpful at preventing a reoccurrence.

Placental subinvolution

Normally, after a bitch gives birth to a litter of pups, it might experience a thin blood-tinged discharge from the vulva for up to 6 weeks after whelping. If the discharge persists for longer than this, however, your dog could be suffering from a condition called *subinvolution* of placental sites. In layman terms, this means that the uterus fails to repair itself properly after the birthing process, resulting in a low grade blood loss. Over time, this blood loss could conceivably cause anemia if left unchecked. In addition, such a condition predisposes the female to uterine infections.

Most cases of placental subinvolution will resolve themselves within a few months, yet oral iron supplements should be given to the bitch to help prevent anemia. Antibiotics are required as well if infection is present. Finally, in recurring cases, or situations where the bleeding is severe, an ovariohysterectomy is recommended.

OTHER FEMALE REPRODUCTIVE PROBLEMS
Vaginitis/Metritis

Infections involving the uterus are termed *metritis;* those involving the vagina are properly termed *vaginitis*. Both vaginitis and metritis can occur independently of each other, or together. Causes of vaginitis/metritis can include such things as venereally-transmitted organisms, metabolic diseases like diabetes mellitus, retained fetuses or placentas, and, as mentioned earlier, treatment with estrogen-type drugs.

Female puppies under 1 year of age can suffer from a condition termed *juvenile vaginitis*, characterized by a thick, greenish vaginal discharge. Aside from the discharge, puppies so affected generally show no other ill effects, and the condition will in most instances spontaneously resolve on its own when the puppy enters into her first heat cycle.

Symptoms

Classic signs of vaginitis/metritis include a thick, yellow-to-green discharge seen coming from the vagina. Owners might notice their pets licking excessively around this area. In especially dour metritis cases, loss of appetite with an increased water intake, fever, and abdominal pain might become apparent. The discharge might also become discernibly blood-tinged. Because of the intimacy of the urinary tract with the reproductive tract in females, bladder infections that occur secondary to the vaginitis/metritis are also not uncommon.

Treatment

The type of treatment used for reproductive tract infections depends upon which portions are involved. For instance, in mild cases of vaginitis, including juvenile vaginitis, direct infusion of the vagina with antibiotics or povidone-iodine douches provides effective results. If the vaginitis is severe or if the uterus is involved, high doses of antibiotics given orally or by injection are required. To determine which antibiotics will work the best, a bacterial culture is indicated as well. Certainly, if there are any puppies nursing on the affected bitch, they should be removed and placed on formula.

In critical metritis cases, intravenous fluids might even be required for support. Unless the bitch is a valuable breeding animal, an ovariohysterectomy should be performed on these dogs to directly eliminate the source of the problem, and to prevent metritis from reoccurring at a later date. For those dogs who are considered too valuable to be spayed, special medications called prostaglandins can be utilized to help the uterus contract and empty. These, however, must be used with extreme care under the direct supervision of a veterinarian, and even then, only as a last resort.

Pyometra

In older dogs that have experienced numerous heat cycles, a special type of metritis, referred to as *pyometra,* can develop.

Because of repeated hormonal stimulation of the uterus year after year, glands lining the inside wall of the uterus become larger and more active with each heat cycle. Large amounts of fluid are secreted into the uterus by these glands, which can then accumulate, causing uterine swelling. Obvious problems can arise if this fluid is not allowed to drain out of the uterus. Unfortunately, this is precisely what happens in many instances. Because of high progesterone levels associated with metestrus, the cervix remains closed, prohibiting drainage from the uterus. At the same time, the trapped fluid provides an ideal medium for bacteria to grow in, leading to bacterial infections and pus formation. As a result, the uterus literally becomes a bag full of pus (FIG. 13-3). And because of the continued build-up of fluid and pus, an infected uterus can reach an enormous size within the dog's abdomen.

In advanced cases, actual rupture of the uterine wall might result, often with fatal consequences for the unfortunate dog.

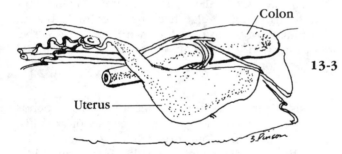

13-3   *Pus-filled uterus characteristic of pyometra.*

Symptoms

Bitches afflicted with pyometra usually exhibit the classic signs of metritis, including depression, loss of appetite with a markedly increased thirst, and abdominal pain. As mentioned earlier, a discharge might or might not be associated with pyometra, the lack thereof being associated with the more serious form of the disease.

Abdominal enlargement due to uterine filling might also become apparent, with radiographs revealing a huge uterine outline. Blood work performed on these patients will reveal an enormously elevated white blood cell count (sometimes over 30,000) and mild anemia (due to the long-term nature of the disease). Pyometra has also been shown to induce kidney disease in affected dogs; as a result, increased urinations, vomiting and dehydration might also be present.

Treatment

Complete ovariohysterectomy is the treatment of choice for pyometra. Those cases involving a grossly enlarged uterus filled with pus and fluid should be regarded as emergencies, and the surgery should be performed as soon as possible.

Pyometra and its associated complications can be prevented by spaying nonbreeding females at an early age (see chapter 10). For those bitches used for breeding purposes, spaying is recommended after their useful breeding life is finished (usually around 8 years of age).

Mammary tumors

Mammary tumors are among the most common type of tumor that afflicts dogs. These tumors are seen most often in unspayed female dogs over 6 years of age. Those glands closest to the hind legs are the ones most often affected.

Interestingly enough, the development of mammary tumors in dogs has a strong endocrine influence. That is, research has shown that dogs that receive an ovariohysterectomy before 18 months of age have a marked reduction in the incidence of future mammary tumors when compared to those dogs left intact. In essence, dogs that are allowed to go through more than two heat periods, even if they are spayed thereafter, have an increased risk of developing mammary tumors when they are older.

Mammary tumors can be detected upon physical examination via palpation. Biopsies can be taken as well to determine whether the mass is benign or malignant. Treatment of both benign and malignant mammary tumors involves surgical removal of the affected gland(s). If malignancy is suspected or confirmed, most surgeons will remove adjacent glands that communicate with the affected gland as well in case metastasis to these glands has occurred. Chemotherapy might also be employed if metastasis is suspected. Unfortunately, however, even with radical surgery and adjunct chemotherapy, the prognosis is poor for those dogs suffering from malignant mammary tumors.

For more information regarding the treatment of tumors in dogs, see chapter 54.

MALE REPRODUCTIVE PROBLEMS
Phimosis and paraphimosis

Phimosis and paraphimosis are two conditions that occur in male dogs resulting from a preputial opening that is too small.

The first, *phimosis,* refers to the inability to extrude the penis through the opening, effectively interfering with reproductive activity. The second, *paraphimosis,* is just the opposite: The inability to retract the penis back into the prepuce once extruded. The exposed organ is very susceptible to trauma and lacerations, which can exacerbate the problem even more (FIG. 13-4).

Phimosis can be treated by having the prepucial opening surgically enlarged. In cases of paraphimosis, reducing the penile swelling using

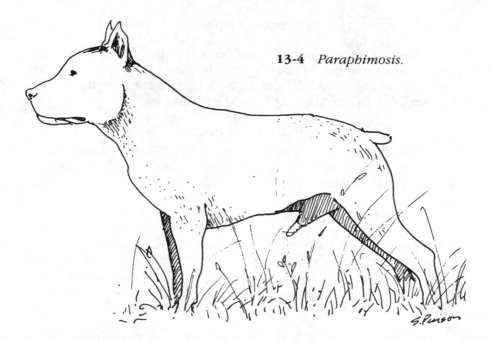

13-4 *Paraphimosis.*

epsom salts will usually allow the replacement of the penis back into the prepuce. Antibiotic ointment can then be instilled into the prepuce to speed healing.

Prostate disorders

The prostate gland in male dogs lies just at the base of the bladder at the origin of the urethra. Its normal function is to produce secretions that make up a portion of the semen. Disorders that can affect the prostate include bacterial infections, benign prostatic enlargement, cysts, and tumors. Signs of prostate disease include straining to urinate, painful urinations, blood in the urine, abdominal pain, and/or hind limb lameness.

Prostate pain or enlargement can be detected on a physical exam via rectal palpation and/or radiographs. If an infection is present, treatment consists of antibiotic therapy. If a tumor or cyst is suspected, surgical treatment is necessary. Neutering should be performed on all dogs that suffer from prostate problems to help prevent recurrences in the future.

14

The Skin and Hair Coat

THE SKIN, OR INTEGUMENT, functions to protect the body from outside foreign invaders and from loss of water. It provides a focus for the sense of touch and assists in the regulation of the temperature within the body. In addition, special modifications of the skin, such as claws and pads, provide a means of traction and defense, as well as shock absorbency.

ANATOMY AND PHYSIOLOGY

The skin of the dog is composed of three layers: the epidermis, the dermis, and the hypodermis. The *epidermis* comprises the outermost layer of the skin. Beneath the epidermis lies the *dermis* and *hypodermis,* which are composed of, among other things, an array of connective and fatty tissue. *Sebaceous glands,* embedded within these layers, secrete natural oils out onto the skin surface which lubricate and moisturize the skin.

The hair of canines consists of *guard hairs,* which make up the rougher outer coat, and the *wool hairs,* which constitute the fine dense undercoat of most breeds. In addition, special hairs called *tactile hairs* (more commonly known as whiskers!) can be found on the head region. These fulfill a sensory function.

A hair cycle exists in dogs which is responsible for the seasonal shedding of old hair with its replacement by new hair. This cycle is dependent on light, not on temperature, and it is triggered by increasing or decreasing amounts of daylight. As a result, peak shedding periods for the dog occur in the springtime, when the days begin to get longer, and in the fall, when the days get shorter. Of course, as more dogs spend more time indoors with artificial lighting, the hair cycle can be altered, with shedding occurring year-round.

Hair color is dependent upon the amount of pigment present within the hair shaft. Large amounts of pigment result in black hair; hairs which lack pigment are white. Different levels of pigmentation that fall between these two result in all other coat colors. Changes in the natural color of the hair can occur with inflammation, traumatization, or constant licking of a particular region or regions of the coat. Of course, as a dog enters its senior years, the appearance of gray hairs is not an uncommon sight as well.

THE ITCHY DOG

Many disease conditions can produce itching in the dog. However, only a few disorders result in severe and/or prolonged itching (FIG. 14-1). The primary symptoms of the "itchy dog" are scratching and biting of the involved skin. Early signs that might be noticed include wet hairs, reddened skin, and hair loss in the areas of biting and scratching. Prolonged itching results in further hair loss, excessive scaling, thickening, and discoloration of the involved skin. Secondary skin infection is not uncommon.

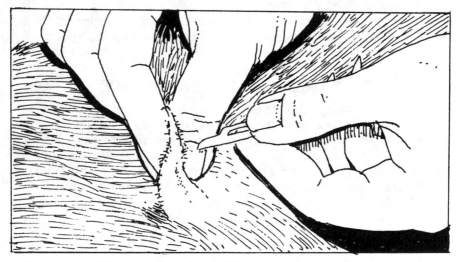

14-1 *Performing a skin scrape for mange.*

Severe and/or prolonged itching is most always a symptom of an underlying skin disorder. As a result, correction of the underlying problem is imperative if the symptom of itching is to be successfully controlled.

External parasites

Refer to specific discussions of external parasites found in this book (chapter 10).

Inhalant allergic dermatitis
(canine atopic dermatitis or atopy)

Inhalant allergic dermatitis represents one of the most common causes of itching in dogs across the United States, especially in the southern portions (TABLE 14-1). Atopy often produces severe itching and is frequently accompanied by skin infection (folliculitis), scaling, hair loss, and discoloration. Atopy parallels human hay fever with the exception of itching being the primary symptom in the dog rather than the respiratory symptoms exhibited by people. Licking and chewing of the feet and legs are commonly reported by owners along with generalized scratching.

Table 14-1 Wind-pollinated Plants & Trees That Can Lead to Atopy in Dogs

Common Name
Red-root pigweed
Meadow fescue
Bermuda grass
Johnson grass
Sweet vernalgrass
Quackgrass
Velvetgrass
Ryegrass
Russian thistle
Lamb's quarter
Western waterhemp
Box elder
Silver maple
Common sagebrush
Wild oat
Short ragweed
Kentucky bluegrass
Redtop
Smooth brome
Broncho grass
Prairie ragweed
Cocklebur
Sheep sorrel
Annual June grass
Oak
White elm

Atopy is hereditary and usually develops between the ages of 6 months to 4 years, following exposure to immune-system-stimulating substances called allergens. Being seasonal, sporadic, and relatively mild in its early stages, atopy often becomes perennial, and worsens in severity with time. Unfortunately, dogs do not outgrow these allergies. Dust (and dust mites), fungal spores, and pollens from trees, shrubs, and grasses can all initiate an allergy in dogs. Since these substances are present in the air and can be carried hundreds of miles by wind, trying to avoid them by restricting a dog's environment is not possible.

Diagnosis

Diagnosis of atopy in dogs is based upon clinical signs seen, seasonality of such signs, and allergy testing. There are currently two methods of allergy testing available: Intradermal skin testing and serum testing.

Intradermal skin testing involves injecting a number of different allergens into the skin of the patient and observing the injection sites for a corresponding allergic reaction. This type of testing has been used effectively for allergy diagnosis for years and provides the most definitive way to find out what a pet is actually allergic to.

Serum testing is a relatively new approach to allergy diagnosis. This test involves the evaluation of a serum sample from the allergic dog for antibodies to substances it might be allergic to. The advantage such testing affords over skin testing is that it is much easier to perform and causes little discomfort to the patient. However, since the accuracy of such tests is still being debated within the veterinary community, intradermal skin testing is still considered by some experts to be the most definitive way to diagnose atopy in dogs.

Treatment

There are three ways to approach treatment for atopy in dogs. These include:

Steroid anti-inflammatories (cortisone-type drugs) These medications temporarily suppress the itching sensations produced by the allergy. Steroid anti-inflammatories are never curative, yet they can offer effective relief from itching for days to weeks. Increases in water consumption, urination frequency, and appetite are sometimes seen in dogs placed on steroid therapy. Unfortunately, prolonged steroid usage over months might produce side effects much more unpleasant than these, including bloating (water retention), muscle atrophy, skin thinning, hair loss, and decreased resistance to infection. In addition, while these steroids are being administered to a dog, its body's ability to produce its own cortisone is suppressed, and might not return even when the steroid therapy is discontinued. If this happens, the dog could go into shock and die. As a result, long-term usage of these drugs for allergic dermatitis should be done only under the close scrutiny of a veterinarian.

Antihistamine/fatty acid therapy Scientific studies and experience has shown that antihistamine medications alone do little to suppress itching caused by atopic dermatitis. Because antihistamine drugs can cause drowsiness, they can be useful for helping calm down a frustrated dog who can't stop itching and chewing on itself.

In recent years, researchers have been looking with interest on the effects Omega-3 fatty acids have on the atopic dog. It seems that these fatty acids, which are derived from cold-water fish such as salmon, do have the ability in some cases to reduce inflammatory responses and stop itching. Some allergic dogs do fantastic just on these alone. Others require additional medications, such as antihistamines, in order to achieve an acceptable comfort level for the pet. Though the effectiveness of this therapy can vary between cases, it does provide a unique alternative to steroid therapy.

Allergy shots/hyposensitization An alternative approach to treating allergies aside from the ones just mentioned is an effort to hyposensitize the pet using allergen injections. This approach requires allergy testing to be performed, followed by a series of injections of the exact allergens or agents causing the reaction. Though not effective in all instances, some veterinary dermatology specialists do report upwards to an 85-90 percent success rate—this rate being based on greater than 50 percent overall improvement in the allergic pet's condition. However, since inhalant allergens are poor stimulators of immunity, this improvement takes some time. Owners should allow anywhere from one to six months before making a final judgment as to the effectiveness of the treatment. In most cases, maintenance injections given monthly will be required for the lifetime of the pet.

Flea bite hypersensitivity

Aside from the discomfort caused by the actual bite of a flea, dogs might develop an allergic response to the flea's saliva deposited in the skin during feeding. Moderate to severe itching and hair loss can result, especially along the back near the tail, hips, and rear leg areas (FIG. 14-2).

Some allergic dogs can harbor a staphylococcal bacteria not found on the skin of nonallergic dogs. Irritation resulting from flea bites can produce a skin infection (folliculitis) on the damaged skin surface and hair follicles. Toxins released from these bacteria might further intensify the itch-scratch cycle. As one might guess, successful treatment of a flea allergy is heavily dependent on the ability to control fleas on the pet and in the environment.

Food hypersensitivity (food allergies)

Food allergies are another potential cause of itching in dogs. Other dermatological symptoms might include hives and/or facial swelling as well. And besides these skin-related problems, food-related allergies have also been implicated in gastrointestinal disorders, such as diarrhea, vomiting,

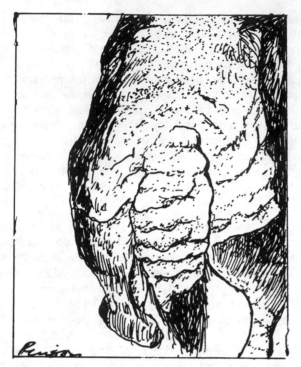

14-2   *Flea allergy.*

and/or excess gas. Fortunately, food allergies are relatively rare in occurrence.

Diagnosis of food hypersensitivity requires the exclusive feeding of a hypoallergenic (non-allergy-producing) diet for two to four weeks. A veterinarian can provide such a diet or suggest a homemade recipe that can be prepared if a food allergy is indeed suspected.

If a positive diagnosis is made, the dog will need to remain on the hypoallergenic diet indefinitely. Simply changing food brands or types seldom benefit food allergy cases since most commercial foods contain similar ingredients. Food items such as milk, animal proteins, and vegetable proteins are the most common culprits behind food induced allergies in dogs.

Contact hypersensitivity (contact allergy)

The hair coat of dogs offers an efficient protective barrier to many substances and agents that could produce an allergic reaction just by coming in contact with the skin. Therefore, those areas relatively devoid of hair such as the chest, abdomen, and feet are more susceptible to contact allergies.

The most common contact-allergy-producing agents are detergents, shampoos, pet sprays, insecticides, etc. which, in liquid form, can penetrate the normally protective hair coat. In addition, bedding that is moldy or has been chemically-treated can cause contact hypersensitivities.

Symptoms of such exposure include redness and swelling of the skin and intense itching. These signs will generally develop 24-72 hours post exposure.

Chemicals that can normally irritate the skin might produce similar symptoms immediately after contact. Such irritative reactions are not to be confused with slower developing hypersensitivity. Treatment of contact allergies requires the removal of the offending agent and administration of topical and/or systemic anti-inflammatory drugs. A thorough history of the pet's exposure to chemicals and exposure to any environment vegetation is imperative in the veterinarian's effort to identify the allergy-producing agent.

Bacterial infections

Bacterial infections involving the skin are itchy in themselves; as a result, when they occur secondarily to an allergy or parasitic infestation, it can mean sheer misery for a dog. It is for this reason that many treatments for other skin ailments are combined with antibiotic therapy.

HAIR LOSS (ALOPECIA)

Loss of hair either locally or generalized over the coat of a dog is another type of skin problem owners might be faced with. As with itching, the causes of hair loss can be quite numerous, and sometimes very complex. A proper diagnosis is essential for restoring the full-bodied hair coat that once was (TABLE 14-2). Here are some of the potential causes of *alopecia* in dogs:

Shedding

Though the normal shedding cycles for dogs tend to occur in the spring and fall, some pets, especially those kept indoors, might actually shed year-round. In fact, some of these dogs can fill a brush with hair every day! If the dog is otherwise healthy and is on a good nutritional program, this seemingly excessive shedding is of no real consequence. If normal shedding is truly the cause of the hair loss, rarely do raw spots or patches of exposed skin appear. If they do, another cause of the hair loss should be suspected. If the dog is of the type that sheds excessively, be sure to brush it daily to remove the dead hairs and make way for the new ones. Failure to do so can predispose the pet to skin infections.

Any event that is associated with abnormally high amounts of stress can cause increases in shedding activity and, in some cases, overt alopecia. A good example of this is a female dog undergoing pregnancy or lactation. The physiological stress and demands placed on such a dog's body might lead to an accelerated hair loss situation. Fortunately, in most instances, the hair will return once the stress abates.

Table 14-2 Diagnostic Aids for Dermatopathies in Dogs

Test	Purpose
Skin scraping	Detects mange mites, one of the most common causes of itching and hair loss in dogs.
DTM (Dermatophyte test medium)	Tests for the presence of the ringworm fungus, another common cause of hair loss and secondary skin infection.
Woods lamp (ultraviolet light)	A screening test for ringworm; may not detect up to 90% of actual cases; if negative, must be accompanied by a DTM
Thyroid testing and other hormonal assays	Detects hypothyroidism and hormonally-related dermatopathies; Hypothyroidism is a common cause of skin problems, ear problems, and obesity in dogs.
Blood and stool parasite checks	Detects internal parasitic organisms, some of which can cause itchy skin reactions
Cytology	This microscopic examination of fluid or cells from skin lesions is also used as a preliminary test for cancer
Biopsy	This microscopic examination of a tissue sample is the definitive test for cancer and autoimmune diseases
Bacterial culture/sensitivity	Used to identify which bacteria are causing the skin lesions and which antibiotics they are sensitive to
CBC/biochemical profile	Blood test used to identify internal diseases such as diabetes, which can outwardly manifest themselves as a skin and coat disorder
Allergy testing (skin test or blood test)	Helps identify which substances a pet is actually allergic to

Malnutrition

The hair cycle in dogs is dynamic and active, with new hairs constantly growing in to replace old, dead hairs that are naturally shed. These new hairs require a bounty of protein and other nutrients for their proper formation and development. If these are not supplied, the replacement hairs might not grow in at all, or they might be weak, brittle, and easily broken. As a result, dogs suffering from poor nutrition often have scanty, lackluster hair coats, not to mention unhealthy skin. Since the source of the problem is internal in nature, the distribution of this hair loss tends to be symmetrical over the entire body.

Feeding the wrong type of diet is not the only way to cause nutritionally related hair loss. Failure to have a pet checked routinely for internal parasites can also lead to malnutrition secondary to parasitism. Because intestinal parasites can steal vital nutrients, the hair coat can become deprived of essential nutrients and bear the brunt of the consequences.

Obviously, providing a good plane of nutrition and correcting any internal parasite problems that might exist are the two key means of restoring normal hair growth in these cases.

Itching

Virtually all of the disorders that cause itching can cause loss of hair as well. This hair loss might be due to self trauma from licking, chewing, and/or scratching, or it might be secondary to inflammation affecting the hair follicle (i.e., demodex, folliculitis). The distribution of the hair loss can be localized or diffused, symmetrical or asymmetrical, depending on the extent of the causative disorder. For instance, if allergies are to blame, the resulting hair loss is often symmetrical, affecting both sides equally. On the other hand, hair loss caused by mange or bacterial folliculitis usually appears localized to certain portions of the body at first, although this hair loss can spread to other parts if the disease is left unchecked.

Identifying and correcting the underlying problem is the most important step to take for restoring the scanty coat. Realize that in many conditions involving inflammation of the hair follicle, the coat might look worse with treatment before it gets better due to treatment-induced shedding of already dead or damaged hair. A good plane of nutrition, one that is adequate in protein and fatty acids, will also speed replacement of the lost hair in recovered pets.

Hormonal imbalances

Symmetrical, nonitchy hair loss in middle-aged to older dogs might be the result of hormonal disturbances within the body. Abnormally low amounts of thyroid hormone, deficiencies in insulin, and/or unusually high amounts of steroid hormones in circulation, can all cause this type of alopecia.

Although one would expect to see other signs associated with such disorders, this is not always the case. Imbalances in circulating amounts of sex hormones (estrogen and testosterone) have also been implicated in some cases of alopecia. Regardless of which hormone(s) are involved, stabilization and normalization of their circulating levels within the body is needed to correct the existing alopecia.

Ringworm

Fungal infections involving the skin and hair can cause hair loss without associated itching. Certainly the most prevalent fungal infection affecting the integument of dogs is ringworm. For more information on ringworm, see chapter 7.

Treatment of hair loss

As illustrated, canine itching and hair loss can be a complexing challenge to diagnose and treat. Owners should no longer ignore or simply blame external parasites in all cases of itchy or balding pets. A complete and thorough history provided to a veterinarian, combined with the vet's dermatologic examination, are important first steps in all cases of problem itching and/or alopecia.

SEBORRHEA

The term *seborrhea* refers to an abnormality in the normal turnover of skin cells, which can lead to excessive secretion of sebum by the sebaceous glands in the skin. Dogs afflicted with seborrhea might have dry, flaky skin (*seborrhea sicca*), or, if the sebaceous glands are active, greasy skin with a rancid odor to it (*seborrhea oleosa*). Itching and infections can also be unpleasant components of both types (FIG. 14-3).

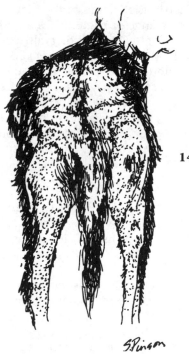

14-3 *Hair loss and seborrhea can occur secondary to endocrine diseases such as hypothyroidism.*

Seborrhea can be caused by a number of diseases, including allergies, fleas, and poor thyroid function. It can also be a primary disease entity, with no apparent underlying cause. Cocker spaniels and Doberman pinschers are two examples of breeds that can suffer from this primary seborrhea.

Diagnosis of a seborrheic condition is not difficult; what can be challenging is determining the underlying problems if they exist. Laboratory tests, including skin biopsies, might be needed to determine whether or not the seborrhea is primary or secondary. By knowing which it is, the better chance treatment stands of being successful.

Successful treatment of seborrhea depends upon correcting any underlying sources (secondary seborrhea), and then focusing attention upon normalizing the abnormal cell turnover occurring in the skin. Special medicated shampoos containing chlorhexidine, tar and sulfur, and/or selenium disulfide have all been used to clear up infections and remove dead epithelial cells and excessive oils associated with seborrhea.

In cases of dry seborrhea, moisturizing skin rinses and fatty acid supplements (available from veterinarians) can be helpful. In especially tough cases, prednisolone can be used to lessen the severity of signs and help stop the itching.

Due to its inherent nature, a complete cure will rarely be afforded in those cases of primary seborrhea. However, veterinary researchers are looking with interest at a new treatment for primary seborrhea utilizing vitamin A derivatives called retinoids. Although research is still ongoing, the results so far at least look promising.

Acanthosis nigricans

Acanthosis nigricans is a hormonal condition seen primarily in dachshunds and cocker spaniels, and characterized by hair loss, increased pigmentation, and thickening of the skin. This increased pigmentation usually begins in the armpit region and spreads to the chest and other regions of the body. As the skin thickens, it might become itchy and inflamed. Seborrhea and secondary bacterial skin infection could also result.

The exact cause of this disease is unknown, but a hormonal imbalance resulting in increases in the melanin pigment is suspected. Hyperthyroidism, although rare in dogs, must be ruled out as the cause of the increased pigmentation; so must allergic skin disorders. Skin biopsies can be used to help confirm or deny cases of acanthosis nigricans.

Treatment of acanthosis nigricans is nonspecific using corticosteroids to reduce pain and inflammation, and antibiotics to combat skin infection. Aloe vera gels applied topically can also be used to soothe and comfort irritated regions. Finally, if seborrhea is present, then antiseborrheic shampoos should be used as well on a weekly or twice-weekly basis.

BACTERIAL SKIN DISEASE

Bacterial skin disease in dogs usually does not occur unless there is some underlying disorder promoting it. Trauma, malnutrition, parasitism, hormonal abnormalities, and immune system malfunctions can all predispose to the proliferation of bacteria on the skin.

Healthy skin has several mechanisms by which it resists infectious organisms. A dry, outer layer of keratin, combined with periodic shedding of dead skin cells, helps to discourage population of the skin surface with harmful bacteria. Even sebum, produced by the sebaceous glands of the skin, is antibacterial at normal concentrations. Finally, a normal population of bacteria that resides on the skin surface and in the hair follicles competitively inhibit the growth of disease-causing bacteria.

Problems can start to occur when the integument becomes traumatized, or underlying disease alters the normal integrity of the skin. If the skin's defenses are penetrated in such a way, disease-causing bacteria found naturally in the environment can set up housekeeping.

Superficial bacterial skin disease can take on a number of appearances. These infections are limited to the outermost layers of the skin; although, if left untreated, they can spread to the inner layers, making treatment difficult and lengthy.

Acute moist dermatitis

Acute moist dermatitis or *hot spots*, are characterized by moist, weeping lesions with hair loss and noticeable redness and swelling of the skin. These lesions are quite itchy and painful to the touch, and can spread rapidly over the dog's body if not treated soon enough. Though any breed can be affected, thick-coated breeds such as golden retrievers and chow chows seem to suffer from these the most.

Impetigo

Impetigo, also known as *milk rash*, is a bacterial skin disease affecting puppies 6 weeks to 6 months of age. Characterized by small pustule formations especially in the abdominal region, impetigo is usually an after-effect of some debilitating disease that stresses the immune system, such as intestinal parasites or viruses. Most puppies seem unirritated by their presence, and with proper treatment, cases of impetigo clear up very rapidly.

Skin fold pyodermas

Skin fold pyodermas can strike those breeds with lots of extra skin. This type of infection occurs secondary to moisture, warmth, and friction occurring within prominent folds of skin. Many breeds and breed crosses can be affected by skin-fold pyoderma. For instance, cocker spaniels can have this problem in their lip region, Pekingese and similar flat-nosed breeds in their facial region, pugs in their tail region, and bulldogs and Shar Peis just about anywhere on their bodies! Keeping these areas clean and dry can help discourage this problem. In some cases, plastic surgery to remove the skin fold in question is truly the only way to afford a cure.

Folliculitis

Folliculitis is bacterial infection that affects the hair follicles. Because the hair within the follicle suffers from the infection, the coats of dogs with folliculitis often develop a moth-eaten appearance as the damaged hair falls out. In addition, as the inflammation progresses, pustules and small crusty lesions often form over the hair follicles. The amount of itching seen with folliculitis can range from mild to severe. One special type of folliculitis, called *bacterial hypersensitivity*, is a type of allergic reaction to the bacteria residing on the skin. Dogs affected with bacterial hypersensitivity exhibit severe itching and hair loss. In fact, because the hair loss is usually in a circular pattern, bacterial hypersensitivity is often mistaken for a case of ringworm.

Canine acne is another form of folliculitis which can affect the chin and lips of dogs. Seen primarily in young dogs, this condition will usually totally clear up once puberty is reached.

Deep pyodermas

Deep pyodermas extending into the depths of the skin layers warrant prompt attention. Unless hit hard with treatment, spread throughout the body is a possibility. As mentioned above, superficial pyodermas can easily become deep if neglected.

Juvenile pyoderma is a form of deep pyoderma that can strike young dogs under 6 months of age. Affected dogs have marked swelling, inflammation, and pain in the facial and ear regions. Lymph nodes in the neck region might be noticeably swollen as a result of such infections, and these dogs are noticeably depressed, sometimes running fevers of up to 104 degrees. Unless juvenile pyoderma is treated promptly and aggressively, permanent scarring and hair loss around the face and head can be unfortunate sequelae.

Cellulitis and *abscesses* are types of deep pyodermas that occur secondary to tissue injury. Cellulitis involves a poorly defined region of inflammation involving the deeper layers of the skin with no apparent rim or border, whereas abscesses do have a well-demarcated line of surrounding inflammatory cells that make them stand out. Both can be characterized by a painful build-up of pus, and usually cause fever and depression. Both can also lead to blood poisoning if not treated. Because of their isolated nature, veterinarians often lance and flush out abscesses to help speed the healing process.

Other types of deep pyoderma are named for the region of the body affected. These include, among others, *nasal pyoderma, interdigital* or *foot pyoderma,* and *elbow callus pyoderma. Generalized pyoderma* refers to a deep bacterial infection involving all areas of the body.

Treatment of bacterial skin disease

Prompt treatment of bacterial skin disease is a smart idea to prevent unnecessary complications. For all types, both superficial and deep, there are certain principles that should be followed when treating such diseases.

To begin, if there is an underlying cause for the infection, it MUST be identified and corrected first. For instance, if fleas seem to be the source, insecticidal treatment is warranted. If this problem is not controlled, chances are the infection will recur after other treatments are stopped.

Skin lesions should be kept clean and dry at all times. This is especially true for cases of acute moist dermatitis. Astringents (drying agents) should be applied daily to assist in healing and prevent further spread. Many of the ear cleansers available have excellent drying properties and can be used topically for such a purpose. Creams and ointments should not be used on moist skin lesions, since such vehicles are counterproductive to drying efforts. Ideally, bacterial skin lesions should be allowed direct access to surrounding air, which means that hair coat in the affected region(s) should be shaved and occlusive bandages avoided.

Antibiotics in high dosages and used for extended durations are the mainstay of treatment for bacterial skin infections. Mild, superficial infections might require only 10 to 14 days of medication to afford a cure; severe, deep infections might require antibiotic therapy that can last as long as eight weeks!

In recent years, bacterial resistance to the effects of certain antibiotics has become an unfortunate reality. As a result, do not be surprised if a veterinarian elects to perform a bacterial culture/sensitivity to determine the exact antibiotics that are effective against that particular infection. If a dog is placed on oral antibiotic therapy for a skin infection, it is imperative that owners complete the entire prescription as directed, even if the skin clears up after only a few days of medication.

Topical therapy for bacterial skin infections is an important adjunct to any treatment regimen. Many medicated shampoos that can be used to help speed healing are available. Those shampoos containing chlorhexidine are preferred, since this substance has excellent antibacterial properties. In some cases, these medicated shampoos should be used daily until the infection is brought under control. For best results, medicated shampoos should be allowed to remain in contact with skin in the affected area(s) for at least fifteen minutes before rinsing. Remember to follow all veterinarian's recommendations concerning the frequency and duration of this type of topical therapy.

Pets should be shampooed and rinsed thoroughly, then dried off well afterwards. This last step is vital because skin kept moist will only serve to promote the infection. If needed, a hand-held blow dryer set on low can assist in this task.

Medicated creams and ointments are also popular therapeutic additions for dogs with skin infections. Triple antibiotic formulations available over the counter or by prescription are preferred, and should be applied three to four times a day to the lesions. As mentioned before, use these products only on lesions that have been properly dried; do not use on moist lesions.

When using a medicated cream or ointment, avoid those preparations containing hydrocortisone or other steroid anti-inflammatories unless specifically prescribed or recommended by veterinarians. Indiscriminate use of such products could actually delay healing and allow the infection to worsen.

SKIN LUMPS AND MASSES

Whenever a lump or mass appears on/or beneath the skin of a dog, five possibilities exist as to its source:

1. An abscess
2. A hematoma/seroma
3. A cyst
4. A granuloma
5. A tumor

Obviously, because the cause can vary, owners will need to employ the help of a veterinarian for identification of the mass. A fine needle aspirate of the mass, or an actual biopsy sample will assist him/her in a diagnosis (FIG. 14-4).

Abscesses

Abscesses are usually painful to the touch and are often associated with other signs, such as fever, depression, and loss of appetite. They also tend to be fluctuant when direct pressure is applied to them.

Hematomas and Seromas

Hematomas and *seromas* result from leakage of blood or serum, respectively, from damaged blood vessels. Traumatic blows to the skin can result in hematoma or seroma formation beneath the affected area of skin. The swellings caused by these are also fluctuant, and due to the traumatic nature of their occurrence, they can be painful as well.

In most cases, the swellings caused by hematomas and seromas will resolve on their own with time, assuming infection does not set in in the meantime.

Cysts

A *cyst* is nothing more than a well-defined pocket filled with fluid, secretion, or inflammatory debris. Unlike abscesses, cysts are usually not painful to the touch.

Sebaceous cysts or *epidermoid cysts* develop within the skin of dogs when the sebum normally formed within sebaceous glands is not allowed

14-4   *Obtaining a cell sample from a skin mass.*

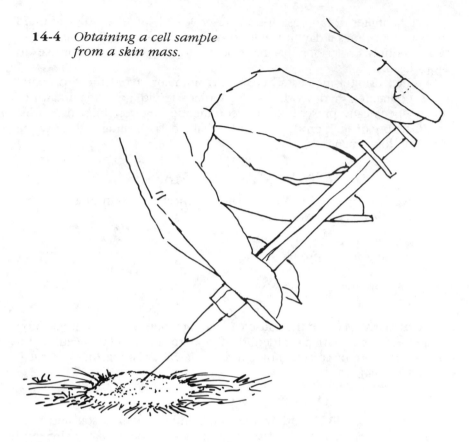

to escape. There does seem to be a breed predisposition for this problem, with cocker spaniels, springer spaniels, terriers, and shepherds most commonly affected.

Sebaceous cysts can arise in multiple locations over the body of these dogs, and can constantly reoccur throughout the life of the pet. Though they pose no specific danger to the health of a dog, especially large cysts should be surgically excised.

Granulomas

Granulomas are firm, raised masses consisting chiefly of inflammatory cells sent to the particular area by the body in response to skin penetration by a foreign substance or infectious agent. In essence, the body attempts to quickly surround and wall-off the foreign invader before it can spread to other parts of the body. Thorns, insect stingers, vaccines, fungal organisms, and certain bacteria are but a few of the things that can incite granuloma formation.

If a pet develops one of these growths, an attempt should be made to determine the cause of its appearance. If an infectious agent is suspected, appropriate antimicrobial therapy is warranted to prevent further development of the granuloma.

Granulomas might recede with time, depending upon the cause. In some cases, surgical removal of the mass gets rid of the unsightly lump and its inciting cause all at the same time.

Tumors

Skin tumors or *cancers* can appear in a variety of types, sizes, and shapes. Common tumors that might appear as a lump or mass on or beneath the skin of a dog include sebaceous adenomas, lipomas, carcinomas, sarcomas, and mast cell tumors. It is imperative that a biopsy is performed in all instances to determine whether or not the tumor is malignant.

Sebaceous gland tumors are among the most prevalent of all skin tumors. These wart-like growths are especially common in cocker spaniels and poodles. They can appear anywhere on the body, including the eyelids. The vast majority of these growths are benign and cause no problems whatsoever, unless they become traumatized due to sheer size. Excision of these tumors is curative locally, but others often appear elsewhere with time.

Lipomas are benign, soft, fatty tumors that often form beneath the skin of dogs and cause noticeable lumps. They occur with greater frequency in older dogs that have a weight problem. Although a diagnosis of lipoma might seem obvious, a fine needle aspirate should always be performed to rule out the presence of its less-common malignant counterpart, liposarcoma.

Lipomas can be surgically removed, yet because they can infiltrate into the muscle bundles and surrounding tissue, this removal might be unknowingly incomplete and the tumor reoccurs. As a result, many practitioners will choose to remove only those lipomas that are especially large or those diagnosed as malignant.

Histiocytomas are classified as a canine skin tumor, yet many researchers believe they represent instead an inflammatory reaction by the body to some foreign invader, similar to a granuloma. Although they can develop at any age, most histiocytomas occur in dogs less than 2 years of age. These tumors are disc-shaped and often reddened and ulcerated. The head, ears, and/or extremities are the prevalent sites of appearance.

For more information on tumors, refer to chapter 54.

15

The Eyes and Ears

THE EYES

THE VISUAL ACUITY of the average dog has been compared to that of a human at sunset. Most see only generalized forms rather than distinct images or features. Exceptions to this rule include the sight hounds (greyhounds, afghans), who indeed have a keen eyesight.

Contrary to popular belief, dogs might not be as colorblind as people think; in fact, the canine eye possesses all of those structures necessary to perceive their world in color. Now whether or not they take full advantage of this is still a matter of speculation. It seems, however, that since the sense of sight is not as vital to most dogs than, let's say, the sense of smell, there might be no real need for color perception.

Anatomy and physiology

Each eye is housed within a bony socket of the skull, and is surrounded by an upper and a lower eyelid. In addition, a *nictitating membrane,* or third eyelid, is located on the inside corner of each eye. Serving a protective function similar to the conventional lids, this third eyelid will passively extrude over the eye in the event of injury or illness (FIG. 15-1). Special glands lining the inside portion of this lid also bear significance in the disease condition known as *cherry eye*.

The *conjunctiva* is the delicate membrane seen lining the pink inner portion of the eyelid and a substantial portion of the eyeball itself. *Conjunctivitis* is the term applied to inflammation involving this membrane. It often results in red, weeping eyes.

The white portion of the eyeball is properly deemed the *sclera*.

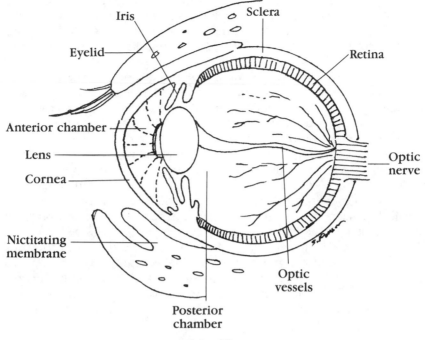

15-1   *The eye.*

Changes in the color of the sclera can be indicative of underlying disease. For instance, a sclera that is yellow-tinged could be reflecting jaundice, and a serious underlying liver or bleeding disorder.

The *cornea* is the clear, transparent structure at the front of the eye through which the colored iris and black pupil can be seen. When light passes through the cornea, it enters into the fluid-filled anterior chamber of the eye, which is located between the cornea and the iris.

Monitoring the pressure maintained within the eyes by this fluid is a valuable diagnostic tool for the veterinarian trying to diagnose eye disorders in pets. For instance, glaucoma, or increased pressure within the eye, is a serious disease that can lead to blindness if not treated promptly. It can originate as a result of increased amounts of this anterior chamber fluid. On the contrary, a decreased pressure reading signifies active inflammation within the eye itself (uveitis), prompting appropriate treatment measures.

The *iris* is the structure that contains the pigment that gives the eye its characteristic color. In dogs, brown is by far the dominant eye color seen, with a few blue eyes interspersed here and there.

The *pupil* is a hole formed by the iris. The size of the pupil is determined by the contraction and expansion of the iris in response to varying degrees of light. Thus, the iris serves to regulate the amount of light that is actually allowed into the eye.

Pupil size can be affected by injury or illness. For example, poisonings caused by organophosphate insecticides can cause the pupils to be pin-point in size. Furthermore, pupils that are unequal in size can be indica-tors of a primary neurological disease, including disorders of the middle ear.

Once through the pupil, light enters into the posterior chamber of the eye, containing the *lens* and the *retina*. The lens serves to gather incoming light and then focus it in upon the retina, which lines the back surface of the eye. Special fibers attaching to the lens allow it to change sizes to accommodate for distances.

The retina contains a multitude of nerve endings that, when stimu-lated by light, send nervous impulses which feed into the optic disk and then into the brain. The end result is a visualized, perceived image. The appearance of the retina can be altered by a variety of disease states, offer-ing valuable diagnostic insight to the veterinarian attempting to pinpoint the source of a canine illness.

The *tapetum* is a specially pigmented structure that lines the back surface of the eye along with the retina. The tapetum serves to act as a light gathering, reflective device which improves night vision in the dog. It is responsible for the characteristic green color seen when light from approaching automobile headlights or other sources catches the eyes of dogs in the dark.

Corneal ulcers and scratches

The transparent cornea enclosing the front portion of the eye is a remark-able organ in itself. Responsible for gathering light and directing it into the eye, healthy corneas are essential for proper vision. It stands to rea-son, then, that *ulcerations* (loss of surface epithelium) or scratches involving one or more corneal surfaces can seriously threaten eyesight if not managed promptly (FIG. 15-2).

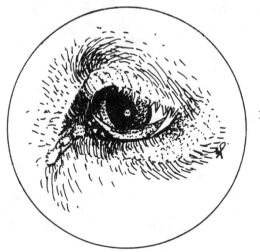

15-2 *Corneal ulcers can lead to red, weeping eyes.*

Corneal ulcerations in dogs can occur secondary to poor tear production, entropion/ectropion, dust and foreign debris in the eye(s), nail scratches and other direct trauma, and infections.

One of the most common sources of corneal ulceration seen by veterinarians is soap or shampoo burns caused by inadequate eye protection when bathing. Dog owners should always apply a sterile ophthalmic ointment to their pet's eyes prior to any procedure which involves potentially caustic substances around the eyes. Since canine corneas are so sensitive, even shampoos with touted "no tears" formulations should never be used without applying this protection first.

Symptoms

Clinical signs of a corneal ulcer include squinting and aversion to light, ocular discharge, and obvious discomfort, often signified by pawing at or rubbing the affected eye. A change in the normal color or transparency of the corneal surface is also an indicator that something is wrong.

Definitive diagnosis of a corneal ulcer is made by veterinarians using special fluorescein dyes to stain the corneal surfaces. Dead, diseased corneal tissue will readily take up such stain whereas healthy tissue will not.

Treatment

Luckily, the cornea is one organ that will heal quite rapidly if treatment is administered vigorously and in a timely fashion. For ulcers involving only the superficial layers of the cornea, topical antibiotic ointments or solutions designed for use in the eyes and applied three to six times daily will help speed healing.

Drops or solutions designed to dilate the pupils (such as atropine or tropicamide) are sometimes used to reduce pain and discomfort associated with the ulceration. These agents will also prevent adhesions from forming between the iris and the lens or cornea should any inflammation spread into the interior of the eye itself.

Of course, if an underlying cause, such as foreign debris, still exists in the eye, it must be removed before proper healing can take place. Superficial ulcers can heal in 36 to 48 hours with proper treatment applied.

Deep corneal ulcerations

Deep corneal ulcerations are treated the same way that superficial ulcerations are, yet these require close observation for progression or worsening of the ulcer. Bacterial cultures of such ulcers are necessary to be certain that the antibiotics being used are effective against the organisms involved, if any.

For deep ulcers that worsen, or even fail to respond to conventional treatment, additional procedures might be necessary to speed healing or to prevent the cornea from actually rupturing. A new, favorite procedure among veterinarians consists of surgically freeing and extending a portion of the thin conjunctiva over the ulcer and actually tacking it down against the ulcer using suture material (conjunctival flap). The flap of conjunctiva provides nutrition and speeds healing to the ulcer, and also allows any medications applied directly to the eye(s) to reach the ulcer without hindrance. Once healing has been accomplished, the flap is released, and excess conjunctival tissue is trimmed away from the healed surface.

Conjunctivitis

Inflammation of the thin, transparent mucous membrane lining the inner portion of the eyelids and front part of the sclera is termed conjunctivitis. Conjunctivitis is the most common cause of "red eyes" in dogs. Other signs seen with conjunctivitis include discharge, swelling, and, if other eye structures are involved, pain.

Symptoms

The type of discharge present can sometimes give a clue as to the underlying cause of the conjunctivitis. For instance, a watery discharge can indicate irritation from an allergy, virus (canine distemper), or contact with dirt or dust; a mucus-like discharge often links the problem to abnormal tear formation ("dry eye") or to a bacterial infection, either primary or secondary to any of the causes previously mentioned.

Because conjunctivitis can be secondary to other problems, diagnostic tests performed by veterinarians should be directed at identifying any underlying causes. Corneal staining using a fluorescent stain is usually performed to determine whether or not the cornea is concurrently affected. If a mucus-like discharge is present, a tear flow test should be performed to rule out "dry eye" as the cause of the conjunctivitis.

In cases of conjunctivitis that don't respond to conventional therapy, a bacterial culture/sensitivity should be performed as well to be sure treatment measures being used are correct.

Treatment

Treatment of conjunctivitis is aimed at treating or eliminating any inciting causes, and at controlling the localized inflammation. If dust or pollens are the source of the conjunctivitis, daily flushing of the eyes with a sterile saline solution designed for use in the eyes or daily application of a sterile ophthalmic lubricant can help reduce the irritation caused by these offenders.

Ophthalmic drops or ointments containing antibiotics are necessary if a bacterial infection is present (FIG. 15-3). In addition, ophthalmic preparations containing steroids can be used to reduce the inflammation present, provided that the surface of the cornea is intact. Preparations containing both antibiotics and steroid compounds for use in the eyes are readily available for pets through a prescription from a veterinarian.

Glaucoma

Glaucoma is a condition characterized by an increase in fluid pressure from the aqueous humor within the eye(s). In the normal eye, pressure

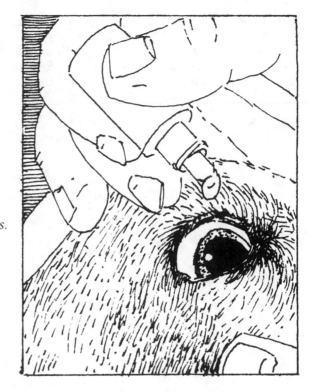

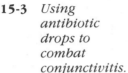

15-3 *Using antibiotic drops to combat conjunctivitis.*

and aqueous levels are maintained at a constant level by the continual drainage of excess aqueous humor out of the eye through tiny ports (drainage angles) located where the edge of the iris meets the cornea. If for any reason this drainage is obstructed or altered in any way, a rise in pressure within the eye can result. Unfortunately, even short-term rises in this pressure can lead to irreversible damage if not detected and treated in a timely fashion.

Conditions such as a buildup of inflammatory material within the eye, luxation of the lens due to trauma or cataracts, and synechia, where the iris "sticks" to the lens or cornea, can all effectively prevent the normal drainage of the aqueous humor from the eye.

Heredity is also thought to play a role in some cases of glaucoma, with basset hounds, beagles, and cocker spaniels having a higher incidence of the disease due to improper development of the drainage angles. In addition, a predisposition for lens luxation has been identified along family lines for many of the terrier breeds, predisposing them to glaucoma as well.

Finally, allergies and overactive immune system responses are currently being investigated as important precursors to glaucoma in dogs.

Symptoms

Clinical signs of a glaucomatous eye include a marked redness both affecting the conjunctival tissue and the sclera; a blue, hazy cornea; a dilated, unresponsive pupil; and apparent blindness due to the increased pressure the fluid is placing on the optic nerve. In instances where the glaucoma has been present for quite some time, enlargement of the affected eyeball might become noticeable, and actual rupture of the cornea could occur.

Treatment

Diagnosis of glaucoma can be easily confirmed by a veterinarian through the use of an instrument called a *tonometer* (FIG. 15-4).

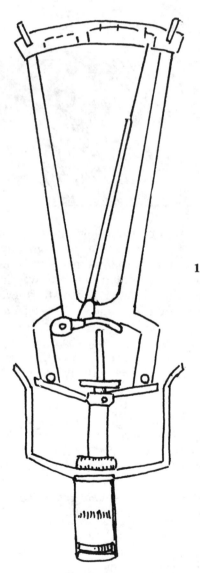

15-4 *A tonometer is used to test for glaucoma.*

This instrument, which is placed directly upon the surface of the cornea, measures the exact pressure occurring within that eye. If the pressure reading is indeed elevated, then treatment should be instituted immediately to prevent lasting damage to the eye.

Treatment for glaucoma is aimed at decreasing the pressure within the eye to an acceptable level as quickly as possible, and then stabilizing this pressure to prevent increases in the future.

Drugs designed to quickly draw fluid out of the eye and into the bloodstream will initially be used by a veterinarian to reduce the pressure within a pet's eye(s); other drugs which act by decreasing the production of aqucous humor and by increasing the size of the drainage angles are then prescribed and given for the long-term management and prevention of recurrence. At the same time, anti-inflammatory medications can be used topically on the eye to clear up any primary or secondary inflammation that might be aggravating the glaucoma.

In instances where a luxated lens is causing the increase in pressure, surgical removal of the offending lens should always be performed. In addition, a new type of surgical treatment and preventative measure involving *cryotherapy* (freezing), is being tested more and more in veterinary teaching hospitals across the country. Cryotherapy involves surgically inserting a special needle within the eye and freezing the cells within the eye responsible for the production of aqueous humor. With this technique, aqueous production has been reduced by up to 30% in some patients.

Cataracts

Any opacity involving the lens of the eye is termed a *cataract*. Cataracts can be inherited (juvenile cataracts) or might develop as sequella to eye trauma, infections, or metabolic disease, such as diabetes mellitus. As lens opacity increases, the amount of light allowed to reach the retina is diminished, and partial blindness ensues.

Cataracts can also predispose to rotation or luxation of the lens. Such lens movement can disrupt normal fluid flow within the eye and lead to secondary glaucoma.

True cataracts must be differentiated from lenticular sclerosis seen in older dogs. Lenticular sclerosis is a lens opacity caused by a normal hardening of the lens material due to age. It is a normal aging change seen in some dogs, and rarely leads to loss of sight as do cataracts. As a result, no specific treatment is required for most cases of lenticular sclerosis. Lenticular sclerosis and cataracts can be differentiated with an ophthalmologic examination performed by your veterinarian.

Treatment for cataracts usually involves surgical removal of the offending lens or lenses. A new, less invasive surgical technique for removal is called *phacofragmentation*. This procedure employs the use of ultrasound to break up the lens material into small pieces, which can then be drawn or sucked out of the eye using special instrumentation.

Once cataracts are removed, vision is effectively restored in the affected pet.

Dry eye (Keratoconjunctivitis sicca)

Keratoconjunctivitis sicca (KCS), or "dry eye," is a condition affecting the cornea and conjunctiva of the eye resulting from inadequate tear production. In actuality, only the water portion of the tear film is deficient; the mucus portion is still produced in adequate quantities. This leads to the characteristic green, mucoid buildup in and around eyes affected with KCS. The lack of adequate tear moisture also predisposes the cornea to damage and ulcers.

Symptoms

Long-term sequella include pigmentation of the corneal surface and blindness.

KCS can have a number of underlying causes. In many breeds—such as Yorkshire terriers, schnauzers, cocker spaniels, bulldogs, and beagles—KCS can be an inherited trait. Other potential causes include canine distemper, certain medications (such as sulfa drugs), hypothyroidism, diabetes mellitus, and autoimmune disease.

Treatment

Diagnosis of KCS is made using tear flow tests to determine the amount of tear production. Treatment of KCS involves the use of tear replacement drops, followed by an application of a tear replacement ointment to seal in the drops (FIG. 15-5). These replacements must be applied every three to four hours to be truly effective. If infection or inflammation is present, antibiotics and anti-inflammatory medications should be instilled into the eyes as well.

Medications designed to stimulate more tear production have been used for treatment in the past with varying success. Pilocarpine 2% is one such medication that can be added to the pet's food to help combat KCS. However, its use and the use of other similar medications might soon be superseded by a new experimental drug called *cyclosporine.*

Research has revealed that cyclosporine can be quite effective at stimulating renewed tear production in some dogs with KCS. For more information on cyclosporine, owners should contact their veterinarian.

In especially advanced cases of KCS, surgical intervention might become necessary. The standard surgical treatment used, called *parotid duct transposition,* involves repositioning a duct from a salivary gland to the corner of the affected eye(s), thereby providing a constant source of moisture (saliva) to the eye.

Prolapse of gland of third eyelid (cherry eye)

The third eyelid of dogs contains a gland that might occasionally become inflamed and protrude over the edge of the third eyelid, producing a clas-

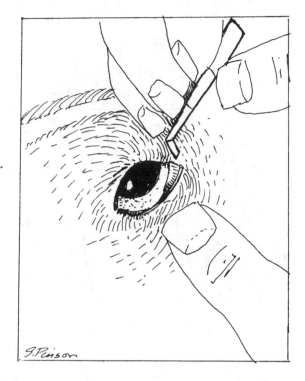

15-5   *Testing for tear production.*

sic "cherry eye" appearance. Certain breeds—such as the cocker spaniel, Lhasa apso, Pekingese, and beagle—seem to be more predisposed to this condition than others (FIG. 15-6).

In the past, treatment for a prolapsed gland of the third eyelid involved complete surgical removal of the gland. However, researchers now conclude that the gland might play an important role in tear production; hence, complete removal of the gland might predispose a pet to keratoconjunctivitis sicca. As a result, newer surgical procedures involve removal of only a portion of the gland, or actually tacking down the prolapsed portion of the gland to the inner surface of the third eyelid.

Entropion

Entropion is an ophthalmic condition in which the eyelids roll inwards, allowing lashes and hair to irritate the surface of the eyes. The condition is inheritable, or it can occur secondary to other types of eye irritation (spastic entropion) or eyelid injury. Congenital entropion has a high incidence in chow chows, shar peis, English bulldogs, poodles, and rottweilers.

Symptoms

Signs of entropion problems include excessive tearing, squinting, constant rubbing of the affected eye(s), excessive redness to the eye(s), and a noticeable inward roll to the eyelid, especially the lower lid.

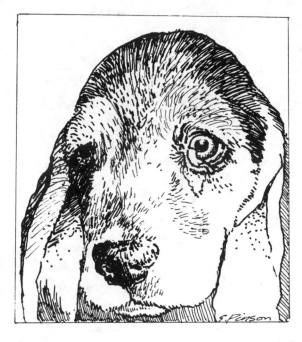

15-6 *Prolapsed gland of third eyelid in a puppy.*

Treatment

If a pet is suffering from entropion, surgical treatment might be essential to prevent lasting damage to the surface of the eye(s). Some puppies afflicted with this disorder might grow out of it as they mature, hence, surgery is usually delayed in these young animals until they are at least 6 months old unless the damage to the eye is severe.

In the meantime, topical lubricants designed to protect the corneas can be used on a daily basis in these patients. In some pups, especially Shar Peis, temporary eversion of the offending lids with sutures implanted in the skin of the lids can also help prevent complications until they grow out of the entropion or until they are old enough for the surgery.

Entropion surgery involves the removal of a flap of skin just beneath (lower lid) of above (upper lid) the inverted lid. Suturing close the resulting gap of skin will then provide enough tension to roll the lid back out. In many instances, more than one surgery is necessary to achieve just the right amount of eversion.

After surgery is performed, care must be taken to prevent the dog from irritating the incision line and causing swelling. Hospitalization for a few days after the procedure is performed will help reduce this occurrence.

Because of the inheritable nature of this disorder, all dogs affected with entropion should be neutered to prevent its passing to future generations. When selecting a new pet, especially one that falls into the high risk category, owners should examine the pup's parents closely for any signs of entropion or for evidence that surgical correction has been previously performed.

Ectropion

Ectropion is the exact opposite of entropion; it is the outward rolling of the eyelid(s), which exposes the pink conjunctival lining within. As with entropion, this condition is inheritable, with cocker spaniels, St. Bernards, and bloodhounds having a higher incidence. Facial nerve paralysis, such as that seen secondary to otitis media can also result in ectropic lids.

Symptoms

Mild cases of ectropion usually cause no problems whatsoever in affected individuals. Moderate to severe cases are often accompanied by conjunctivitis, excessive lacrimation, and eye discharges.

Treatment

Keeping the eye(s) clean and free of discharge on a daily basis using saline solution or medicated drops or ointments will help keep slight cases of ectropion under control. For more extensive involvements, surgical correction designed to release the tension placed upon the skin of the eyelid, allowing it to roll back to its correct position, might be required.

Masses involving the eyelids

The integrity of the eyelids is vital for the protection of the eyes from environmental hazards. Any disruption or alteration in the normal lid anatomy can place vision in jeopardy. And certain masses involving the lids can do just that if they become large enough.

Chalazion   are masses involving the eyelid that originate from the small meibomian glands which line the edge of the lid. They result from a buildup of secretion within the meibomian glands due to blockage of the duct leading from the gland. Chalazions appear as yellow to white swellings beneath the conjunctiva on the inner lid margin. Puncturing or incising these to remove the trapped contents will afford a cure.

Hordeolums   are pus-filled masses caused by infections within the meibomian glands or hair follicles lining the lid margin. As with chalazions, these can be punctured and expressed to help speed healing. Topical or systemic antibiotics are also used to eliminate the inciting infection.

Tumors   that affect the eyelid can be very serious due to the inability to remove surgically without disrupting the integrity of the lid. Sebaceous gland adenomas are common lid tumors, especially in older dogs. Others include adenocarcinomas, papillomas, and melanomas. As an alternative or adjunct to surgical removal, radiation therapy, chemotherapy, and cryotherapy (freezing) can all be used as well, depending upon which type of tumor is involved.

THE EARS

The sense of hearing in the average dog is much more fine-tuned than that in a human, allowing it to detect much higher sound pitches. The upper range of canine hearing is thought to be around 50,000 cycles per second; almost 30,000 cycles per second higher than that for people.

Silent dog whistles were invented based on this principle, with the pitch emitted being just above human hearing range but well within that of the dog being summoned. Unfortunately, contrary to popular rumor, the high pitch emitted by many of the new electronic flea collars available on the market might fall within the dog's hearing range, raising serious questions as to their safe use.

Anatomy and physiology

The canine hearing apparatus can be divided into three portions: the *inner ear, the middle ear,* and *the external ear canal* and associated structures (FIG. 15-7).

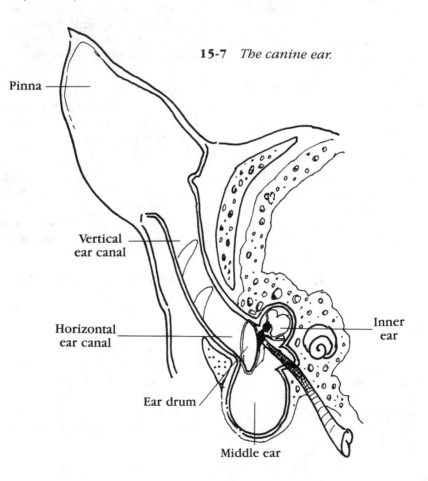

15-7 *The canine ear.*

Pinna

Vertical ear canal

Horizontal ear canal

Inner ear

Ear drum

Middle ear

The inner ear is that portion containing the nerve endings responsible for the hearing sensation. It also plays a leading role in maintaining balance and equilibrium in your pet (dogs can get car sick, too!). The inner ear apparatus lies protected within the bony confines of the skull. The nerves and associated structures within the inner ear are very sensitive and can be damaged through continued exposure to loud, high-pitched noises, infections, and/or toxic medications (see Deafness in this chapter).

The middle ear communicates directly with the inner ear and is contained within a pear-shaped bony cavity originating from the skull called the *tympanic bulla.* This middle ear cavity is normally filled with air and contains blood vessels and nerves which supply the head and face. Inflammation involving the middle ear can adversely affect these nerves, leading to paralysis of the muscles of the face.

The ear drum, or *tympanic membrane,* separates the middle ear from the external ear canal. This external canal directly communicates to the outside world, but not without first going through some significant anatomical changes along the way. A horizontal portion of the canal courses a short distance directly away from the eardrum before angling sharply upwards to form a long vertical portion. This distinct bend has medical significance in that it can lead to the entrapment of wax, hair, and debris deep within the ear, predisposing to inflammation and infection.

The vertical external ear canal—and to a lesser extent, the horizontal ear canal—are lined with special glands that produce ear wax, or *cerumen.* In the past, cerumen was thought to exert some beneficial antibacterial effects in the ear. Yet research has disproved this and has shown that too much of a waxy build-up can actually promote bacterial growth and infections. In the healthy ear with normal amounts of cerumen produced, this doesn't present much of a problem. Yet when an ear becomes inflamed, wax production increases, and can predispose to infectious complications.

Surrounding the opening of the external ear canals is the ear flap, or *pinna,* which come in all sorts of sizes and shapes, both natural and man-made (FIG. 15-8). Each pinna is supported by a sturdy band of cartilage that courses from the vertical ear canal to the tip of each flap. Long droopy ear flaps that hang down over the ear openings can effectively cut off proper air circulation within the ear canal. This can potentially lead to ear problems in these dogs unless preventative measures are instituted on a routine basis (FIG. 15-9).

Otitis externa

Inflammation involving the external ear canal is called *otitis externa.* It is estimated that up to 20% of the dog population in the United States alone suffers from some form of otitis externa. Anatomical features that predispose certain breeds to ear disorders include long, pendulous ears (cocker spaniels), long, narrow ear canals (poodles), and excessive hair within the

15-8 *Dogs with erect ear pinnae are less prone to ear problems than those with droopy ones.*

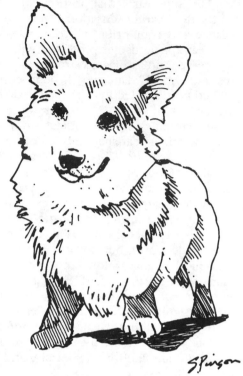

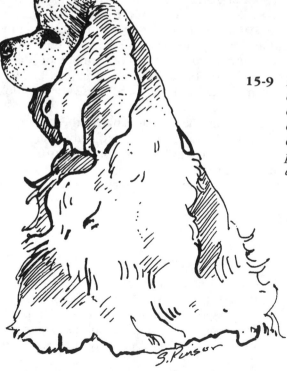

15-9 *Long, droopy ear flaps can cut off air circulation through the ear canal and lead to ear problems unless preventative measures are taken.*

ear canal which entraps wax and restricts air circulation (poodles). Dogs that spend a lot of time in the water, such as hunting retrievers and spaniels, are also prone to otitis externa.

Since the external canals are nothing more than inward extensions of the skin, conceivably anything that can cause skin inflammation can cause otitis externa. This can include allergies, metabolic diseases (hypothyroidism, seborrhea), trauma, foreign bodies such as grass awns and twigs, and parasites such as ticks and mites. Anal sac disease has even been implicated in cases of otitis externa, even though the exact mechanism of involvement is not completely understood.

Symptoms

Signs of otitis externa involving one or both ears include head shaking, itching, painful ears, personality changes, and/or odiferous discharges coming from the ear canal(s). Hair loss might be noticed around the pinnae due to scratching. Aural hematomas might also develop in the wake of such self-trauma.

Treatment

Diagnosis of otitis externa is based on clinical signs, physical exam, and selected laboratory tests if needed to determine the underlying cause of the inflammation. An *otoscopic* (ear) exam performed by a veterinarian will help rule out foreign bodies and parasites. This exam is also needed to assess the health of the eardrums. Since many medications cannot be used if the eardrum is torn or ruptured, never attempt to treat otitis externa at home without first having a veterinarian perform this otoscopic exam.

The type of medications prescribed by a veterinarian for the treatment of otitis externa will vary, depending upon the nature and extent of the causative agent or condition. See chapter 3 for proper techniques at instilling medications into the ears.

Yeast infections

Malassezia pachydermatis is the name of a yeast organism most commonly involved in otitis externa (FIG. 15-10). This is not surprising, since malassezia is normally found within the ear canals of healthy dogs, causing no problems whatsoever. However, if inflammation strikes for whatever reason, the yeast takes advantage of a good situation and begins to proliferate. When this growth reaches a certain level, it too can promote inflammation. A characteristic brownish discharge is seen with a buildup of yeast within the ears.

Ear ointments or solutions containing miconazole, thiabendazole, or nystatin can be used to effectively treat yeast infections in the ear. Treating the ears twice daily for ten to fourteen days will take care of most infections.

Because malassezia is considered an opportunist, it is important that the underlying source of the inflammation which led to the yeast infection be identified and treated concurrently.

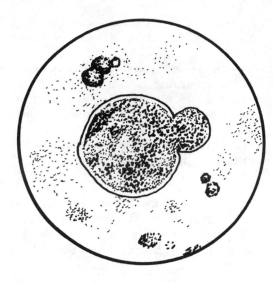

15-10   *A budding yeast.*

Bacterial infections

Failure to detect and treat inflammation within the external ear canal early enough can lead to the establishment of a bacterial infection within the ear. Oftentimes, these infections result when the harmless bacteria that normally inhabit the ear get killed off by the inflammation, allowing their not-so-peaceful counterparts to proliferate and take over.

Symptoms

A creamy brown to yellow discharge carrying a foul odor is characteristic of a bacterial disorder within the ear. Bacterial infections can even be found together with yeast infections within the same ear(s), leading to a discharge having characteristics of both types.

If not treated promptly and vigorously, bacterial infections can become firmly entrenched within the ear canal, making a complete cure difficult. For this reason, veterinary practitioners rely heavily upon bacterial cultures and sensitivity tests to tell them which bacteria are involved and which antibiotics will be most effective.

Treatment

Otic preparations containing appropriate antibiotics, often combined with anti-inflammatory medications, are used to combat cases of bacterial otitis externa. Five-percent vinegar (acetic acid) solutions have also been used with effectiveness against bacteria within the ear.

If a ruptured ear drum is suspected, selection of treatment agents must be made carefully. For example, antibiotics belonging to the class known as *aminoglycosides* (examples include gentamycin and neomycin) should not be used in the ear directly, since they can cause nerve deafness if exposed to the inner ear. The same holds true for astringent preparations and acetic acid solutions. In addition, if a ruptured eardrum is suspected, only water soluble treatment solutions should be used; ointments should be avoided, as they can become entrapped within the middle ear.

In especially severe cases of bacterial otitis, oral antibiotics might be given concurrently with topical ear medications to afford faster results. In chronic long-standing infections that can't be cleared up with antibiotics, a surgical procedure known as a *lateral ear resection* might be necessary to increase the treatment effectiveness. This involves the surgical reconstruction of the external ear canal to eliminate the vertical portion, allowing easy, direct access to the horizontal portion and the ear drum. Although the results might not be the most cosmetic, a lateral ear resection can mean the difference between a life of misery or comfort for a dog afflicted with chronic otitis externa.

Ear mites

Otodectes cynotis is the name of the most common mite that inhabits the canine ear canal.

Symptoms

These tiny parasites, which are transmitted by close contact with other infected animals, live on the skin surface within the ear and feed on body fluids. Their presence irritates the glands lining the ear canal, leading to an increased cerumen production. Secondary infections with the Malassezia yeast are not uncommon, leading to the brown, crusty discharge so often seen with ear mite infestations. In isolated cases, intense allergic reactions to ear mites can occur, causing severe inflammation and secondary infection.

Diagnosis of an ear mite infestation is confirmed by identification of the mites directly on otoscopic exam or through a microscopic examination of an ear swab.

Treatment

Treatment involves the use of medications containing antiparasitic compounds, such as pyrethrins, rotenone, and/or thiabendazole. Mineral oil has also been employed as a home remedy for killing mites by suffocation. Since secondary yeast infections are commonly found with ear mite infestations, an anti-yeast medication should be used concurrently with anti-mite preparations.

Ear mites can be difficult pests to eliminate. Daily treatment for three to four weeks might be needed to ensure a complete kill. All animals in the household, regardless of whether or not they are exhibiting signs of infestation, should be treated at the same time. In addition, to prevent reinfestation from the hair coat, an insecticidal spray or shampoo should be used at least twice during the treatment period.

Otitis media and interna

Otitis media, infection involving the middle ear, usually results from a chronic, untreated or recurring otitis externa. In such cases, the ear drum might become so diseased as to tear or rupture completely, allowing direct access of infectious organisms into the middle ear chamber.

Symptoms

The clinical signs of otitis media are essentially the same as those for otitis externa, with a few notable additions. Dogs so afflicted will usually exhibit a head tilt towards the side of the affected ear.

In severe cases, paralysis of the facial muscles on the side of the lesion might be seen as the nerves passing through the middle ear become involved. This can result in a characteristic drooping of the eyelids, cheeks, and lips. In addition, a decreased tear production, pinpoint pupil, and protrusion of the third eyelid might be noted in the eye on the affected side.

If the infection extends from the middle ear into the inner ear apparatus, the signs become even more pronounced. Since the inner ear functions in maintaining balance and equilibrium as well as hearing, dogs suffering from otitis interna tend to become very uncoordinated and might fall down frequently or move in circles to the affected side. A characteristic twitching of the eyeball, called nystagmus, also becomes more noticeable.

Treatment

Although the clinical signs seen are often diagnostic, radiographs of the skull are quite helpful at confirming a diagnosis of otitis media/interna and determining the extent of the disorder.

Therapy for otitis media/interna must be instituted promptly to prevent permanent damage to the hearing apparatus. Oral antibiotics should be started immediately. In cases of otitis interna, continued treatment with antibiotics might be required for up to thirty days to afford a complete cure. In select cases, anti-inflammatory medications have been used to reduce signs associated with inflammation. If not already ruptured, the ear drum on the affected side is usually punctured to allow for thorough drainage of the middle ear cavity and to allow for the direct infusion of medications. Of course, such treatment steps must be carried out in a veterinary hospital under heavy sedation or anesthesia. In tough, refractory cases, surgical placement of a drain in the bony tympanic bulla affords excellent exposure to the middle and inner ear spaces.

Ruptured ear drums

Ear drums can tear or rupture as the result of direct trauma from a foreign body (such as a twig, cotton-tip applicator, etc.), sudden pressure changes, or, most commonly, as a secondary complication due to otitis externa. Though a serious and painful condition, a torn ear drum will heal quite quickly provided the underlying cause of the perforation is eliminated.

Medications designed for use in the ears must be used with caution if a dog suffers from a ruptured eardrum. Not only can their application be painful, but, as mentioned previously, certain antibiotics and solutions, if allowed direct access into the middle and inner ear chambers, can cause damage to the auditory nerve endings, resulting in deafness. As a result, be certain to follow a veterinarian's recommendations closely.

Deafness

Veterinarians are often confronted by frustrated owners claiming that their dog is going deaf! Now whether this is a valid claim or rather an actual ploy conceived by a defiant Fido will not be known until a thorough ear examination is performed. A dog's apparent inability to perceive sounds can result for a number of reasons.

First, there might be impedance to the sound waves traveling through the ear. An external ear canal clogged with wax and debris can certainly be the culprit, as can constrictive swelling of the ear canal caused by otitis externa. The effective transmission of soundwaves to the middle and inner ears can also be diminished by torn or ruptured eardrums.

Interestingly enough, some researchers feel that a dog's ear drums are not altogether necessary for efficient conduction of soundwaves; rather, soundwaves permeating the bony, air-filled tympanic bullae directly fulfills a major portion of this conductive function. Regardless, researchers do know that sound waves must pass through the middle ear cavity before reaching the inner ear, and that fluid or inflammation secondary to otitis media can lead to diminished hearing.

Besides interference with the transmission of sound waves, deafness in dogs can also be caused by developmental defects of damage involving the actual nerve endings within the inner ear.

Congenital (inherited) nerve deafness has been reported in some breeds, including dalmatians, collies, and rottweilers. Certain drugs, such as the aminoglycoside antibiotics, are well-known for their adverse affects upon the hearing function in dogs. Chronic, untreated bacterial and fungal infections within the middle and inner ears can undoubtedly lead to nerve deafness, as can certain viral organisms, including canine distemper (see chapter 6).

Symptoms

How can an owner tell if their dog is deaf? Undoubtedly a sudden or progressive change in obedience or attentiveness on the part of the pet could tip you off that something is up. Dogs that once responded abruptly to spoken commands might suddenly appear insubordinate. Unfortunately, many owners resort to harsh discipline in such instances, leaving the pet quite confused and the problem unsolved.

One way you can test for hearing function in your dog is to stealthfully approach it in a manner that it is not immediately aware of your presence. Then, using a hand clap or a whistle, observe your dog for a response. Your dog should either turn to face you, or you should notice a twitching of the ears as the sound is evoked. Be sure to stand a good distance away from it when you do this to be sure that your actions or your scent won't inadvertently alert your pet to your presence.

If an owner is still not sure as to the status of their pet's hearing, have a veterinarian take a look. As mentioned before, a simple otoscopic examination might reveal a simple solution to the hearing problem. Special instruments are even available at universities and teaching hospitals across the country that can measure the amount of nerve activity taking place within the inner ear.

Treatment

Treatment for deafness obviously depends upon the inciting cause. Hearing loss caused by impedance of soundwaves through the ear is usually reversible once the underlying condition is addressed. Unfortunately, this optimism is lost when it comes to actual nerve deafness. In most cases, the injury sustained by infections or toxic medications is irreversible. Whether or not the damage done to the nerve endings is partial or complete can only be determined by special nerve testing. Believe it or not, hearing aids have been developed for dogs suffering from partial nerve deafness! Although their usefulness is limited by patient compliance, hearing aids can prove to be beneficial in some cases. If you feel that your dog might be one to benefit from such a device, don't hesitate to discuss it with your veterinarian.

Aural hematomas

Fractures or trauma to the cartilage supporting the pinna of the ear can lead to the accumulation of blood and serum within the affected flap. These aural hematomas cause the pinna to swell, sometimes to enormous sizes. In the majority of cases, the fluid accumulation occurs on the inside portion of the ear flap.

Researchers don't know what precipitates many cases of aural hematomas, but they do have a few suspicions. Since these hematomas are often accompanied by otitis externa, many feel that the trauma induced by scratching and shaking the head predisposes to aural hematomas, especially in those dogs with pendulous ears. Still others suspect that an overactive host immune system is the culprit behind this disorder. Regardless of the cause, aural hematomas are painful and irritating, and need to be drained as soon as possible after initial appearance.

Surgical drainage of the hematoma has been the standard treatment for years. This involves making an elliptical incision in the skin on the inner portion of the pinna, then tacking down the remaining skin tightly to the underlying cartilage. The procedure results in a portion of the cartilage remaining exposed to the outside, allowing for continued drainage to occur. In time, the wound heals over, hopefully with enough scarring to keep the skin and cartilage bound together.

A newer form of management involves draining the hematoma with a needle and syringe, then injecting anti-inflammatory medications directly into the affected part of the pinna. This noninvasive procedure has shown promise in the treatment of aural hematomas, prompting support for the "overactive immune system" theory.

16

The Musculoskeletal System

THE MUSCULOSKELETAL SYSTEM in mammals is responsible for locomotion, plus support and protection of vital internal organs. The components of this system include muscles, bones, and a variety of supportive structures, including ligaments, tendons, and cartilage. Disorders of the musculoskeletal system can be quite debilitating to a dog and be accompanied by a lot of pain.

ANATOMY AND PHYSIOLOGY

The type of muscle involved in skeletal locomotion is termed *striated* muscle. This type of muscle is in contrast to the cardiac muscle found in the heart, and the smooth muscle found in many of the internal organs, both of which are under involuntary control by the nervous system. Striated muscle consists of interlocking bands of cells capable of contracting with great force, thereby achieving movement. *Tendons* are those tough, fibrous bands that anchor the striated muscle to bone and allow this movement to occur. A *strain* is said to have occurred upon injury to a muscle or a tendon.

The *axial skeleton* of the dog consists of the skull, the vertebrae, and the rib cage. The *appendicular skeleton* consists of the bones making up the front and hind limbs, as well as the pelvis.

Each type is made up of a hard mineralized matrix with bone cells interspersed within. The centers of most bones are hollow and filled with soft *bone marrow*. This substance is an important component of the host immune system as the location for white blood cell production. Red blood cells and *platelets*, those structures involved in the blood-clotting scheme, are also produced exclusively within the bone marrow.

Bone is a dynamic tissue, constantly being reabsorbed and regenerated throughout the life of the individual. Long bones grow in length by means of a special structure called an *epiphyseal plate*, located at the ends of the bones. It is interesting to note that the overall health and growth patterns of bony tissue is very much dependent upon proper nutrition; malnutrition and vitamin/mineral deficiencies can wreak havoc upon the development and/or integrity of the skeletal system.

A *ligament* is different than a tendon in that it connects bone to bone, not muscle to bone. Injuries involving ligaments are properly termed *sprains*.

A *joint* is nothing more than a site at which two bones meet. Not all joints are movable, such as those making up the skull. However, for purposes of discussion, the types of joints referred to most are called *synovial joints*. These joints, found throughout the body, allow for free movement between bones and also serve in a shock-absorbing capacity. Each synovial joint consists of ligaments, cartilage on which the ends of the bones move or articulate, joint fluid designed to lubricate the joint and provide nutrition to the articular cartilage, and a tough, fibrous capsule surrounding it all. In addition, some synovial joints contain special pads of cartilage, called *menisci,* which act as super shock absorbers. The knee joint, or stifle, is a good example.

ARTHRITIS AND DEGENERATIVE JOINT DISEASE

Arthritis is the term used in both human and veterinary medicine to describe any type of joint inflammation. *Polyarthritis* describes inflammation involving multiple joints throughout the body. This inflammation might be accompanied by loss of cartilage or bony changes within the joint(s) in question. Causes of arthritis in dogs include infections, autoimmune diseases, and trauma. Even certain drugs, such as sulfa antibiotics, can promote joint inflammation if used indiscriminately.

Osteoarthrosis, or *degenerative joint disease*, describes the condition in which a cartilage defect or cartilage erosion occurs within a given joint. Though not considered a true inflammatory condition, many people use the term interchangeably with arthritis. Osteoarthrosis often occurs as a result of a hereditary defect that may show up at any age. For instance, hip dysplasia is one of the more infamous forms of inheritable degenerative joint disease, and it's one most dog owners have heard of.

But osteoarthrosis doesn't always have to be inherited; it can also occur secondary to joint injury, or it can even be a part of the normal aging process in older dogs.

Symptoms

Regardless of the cause, the clinical signs associated with joint disease are basically the same. Stiffness or lameness involving one or more limbs is often the most obvious sign of a joint problem. In many instances, this lameness is aggravated by colder weather and/or exercise.

Affected pets might be reluctant to play or jump, and they might become more irritable due to pain. If the hips are involved, inability to rise after lying down is a common clinical complaint. Joints can be swollen and painful to the touch, especially with infectious or autoimmune etiologies. Depression, fever, and loss of appetite could become apparent with the latter as well.

Treatment

Diagnosis of a joint disorder is based upon physical palpation of the joint(s) in question, observing the abnormal gait or movement associated with the disorder, and by obtaining radiographs.

Treatment approaches for arthritis and osteoarthrosis depend upon the cause and severity of the condition. In recent years, new medications and innovative surgical techniques have been introduced which show promise in the treatment of canine joint disease and alleviation of the pain associated with it. Where applicable, these new treatment approaches will be expanded upon in the following sections.

Infectious arthritis

As mentioned above, joint inflammation can be secondary to an infectious process. Bacteria that gain entrance into the body's blood stream can circulate to one or more joints of the body, setting up housekeeping within the joint fluid. Bacterial endocarditis caused by periodontal disease can be an important source of these organisms.

Arthritis can also be a prominent sign in ehrlichiosis, Rocky Mountain spotted fever, and Lyme disease. Left untreated, permanent damage to the cartilage and other joint structures can result.

Fever, depression, and painful, swollen joints are prominent clinical signs seen in most cases of infectious arthritis. Laboratory testing, including cultures of the fluid within the joint, may be needed to positively identify the offender. Once this I.D. is accomplished, specific treatment, usually involving high doses of antibiotics, can then be instituted.

Arthritis due to autoimmune disease

Sometimes, an overactive immune system can lead to an arthritic condition. In these instances, immune complexes consisting of antibodies coalesce within the joints of the body, causing inflammation. The resultant polyarthritis can be very painful and debilitating. Fever and a generalized depression are also features of these diseases.

Dogs can get rheumatoid arthritis just like people can. In dogs, this autoimmune-related disease is seen more frequently in the toy breeds than in any others. Another autoimmune disease in dogs that can cause arthritis is called *systemic lupus*. In contrast to rheumatoid arthritis, systemic lupus usually favors the larger breeds of dog, such as German shepherds and St. Bernards.

Special blood tests and/or tests on joint fluid are used to diagnose autoimmune disorders in canines. Treatment usually consists of high dosages of steroid anti-inflammatory medications designed to curb the body's overactive immune response.

Hip dysplasia

Hip dysplasia refers to a hereditary arthritic condition involving one or both hip joints of affected dogs. It presents itself as a partial dislocation, or in severe cases, a complete dislocation of the hip joints. With time, the cartilages lining the joint surfaces wear down due to the abnormal stress and strain placed on the joint, and arthritis results (FIG. 16-1).

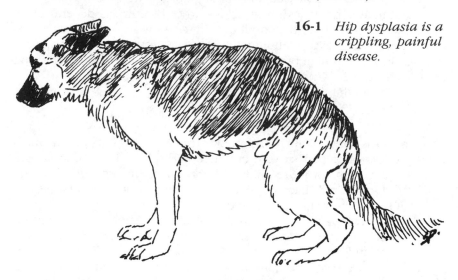

16-1 *Hip dysplasia is a crippling, painful disease.*

Although hip dysplasia can be a problem in any breed, it is seen most often in larger purebred dogs, such as German shepherds, golden retrievers, Labrador retrievers, and St. Bernards. In German shepherds alone, the incidence is thought to be as high as 80%!

Because of its inherited nature, signs associated with hip dysplasia may appear as early as 4 weeks of age, although as a rule, most cases show up around 8 to 12 months of age. These clinical signs consist of posterior pain, unsteadiness on the hind limbs, difficulty in rising from a prone position, and a reluctance to move or exercise. Manipulation of the hip joints will reveal obvious pain. In less severe cases, signs might only appear after intense activity and exercise.

Diagnosis of hip dysplasia in a dog is based upon the breed and age of animal involved, as well as clinical findings. A definitive diagnosis can only be made by having radiographs taken of the hip joints.

In older dogs who are poor surgical candidates, anti-inflammatory medications such as aspirin or prednisolone can be used to temporarily decrease pain and discomfort associated with hip dysplasia. A program of regular exercise and weight loss can also benefit these patients. In young dogs exhibiting marked lameness due to dysplasia, a number of different surgical techniques can be employed to help relieve pain and lameness caused by the disease, and/or to actually reconstruct the hip joint(s). Total hip joint replacement with prosthetic devices has also been employed in a number of select cases, with varying results. In general, the smaller the dog involved, the better the results achieved through surgical intervention.

In recent years, experimentation with a new type of drug called *polysulfated glycosaminoglycan* (PSGAG) has revealed promising results so far relieving pain associated with hip dysplasia and other arthritic conditions. PSGAG works within the affected joints to stimulate repair of damaged cartilage, thereby helping to eliminate the pain associated with arthritis. If your dog suffers from the ravages of hip dysplasia and arthritis, ask your veterinarian about this new nonsurgical treatment modality.

Because hip dysplasia can be inherited, affected dogs should be neutered to prevent the passage of the disease along family lines. Use care when selecting a new puppy, especially one of the high-risk breeds, to examine the pedigree closely and request proof of OFA certification. The OFA (Orthopedic Foundation for Animals, University of Missouri, Columbia, Missouri) is an organization that maintains a registry of dogs and pedigrees that have been determined to be free of hip dysplasia.

These determinations are based on hip radiographs taken when these dogs are at least 2 years of age. Veterinary experts at the Foundation review the radiographs and determine whether or not anatomical signs of hip dysplasia are present, regardless of whether or not the dog is showing any signs of the disease. The OFA will not certify dogs under 2 years of age because most cases of dysplasia in apparently healthy dogs can't be detected radiographically until this age is reached. For more information regarding OFA certification for dogs, contact your veterinarian.

Osteochondrosis

Osteochondrosis describes a condition characterized by abnormal development and growth of joint cartilage (FIG. 16-2). It is seen in young dogs and usually strikes larger breeds. Thought to be predisposed to by trauma and overfeeding, osteochondrosis can precipitate painful joint inflammation and lameness in these pets. The shoulder joint is the region most commonly affected.

Radiographic X-rays are used to definitively diagnose osteochondrosis in a dog. In many of these dogs, healing will occur spontaneously over four to six weeks with strict cage rest. If the cartilage defect is extensive, or if pieces of cartilage have broken off and are floating freely within the joint, surgical intervention might be necessary to remove any dead cartilage and to stimulate healing.

Recently, much attention has been focused towards the use of newer drugs such as PSGAG (see Hip Dysplasia in this chapter) in the conservative treatment of osteochondrosis in dogs. As in hip dysplasia, this drug

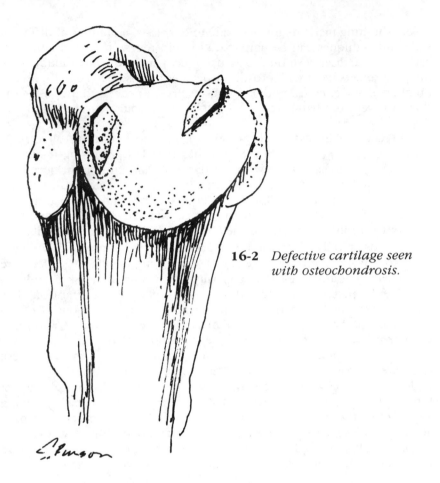

16-2   *Defective cartilage seen with osteochondrosis.*

appears to satisfactorily set the stage for healing to take place within the defective cartilage.

Legg-Perthes disease

Legg-Perthes disease, or *ischemic femoral head necrosis,* is an orthopedic condition involving the hips of smaller breeds of dogs, such as Yorkshire terriers and miniature poodles. This condition is characterized by a degeneration of the head of the femur bone—that portion which fits into the socket of the pelvis to form the hip joint (FIG. 16-3). Hereditary in nature, Legg-Perthes disease usually appears around 3 to 9 months of age. Clinical signs associated with this disease include lameness and painful hips.

Upon radiographic diagnosis, treatment for Legg-Perthes disease involves surgical removal of the head of the affected femur(s). Most dogs, because of their light weight, can return to normal locomotion and activity within a matter of days to weeks after such a surgery.

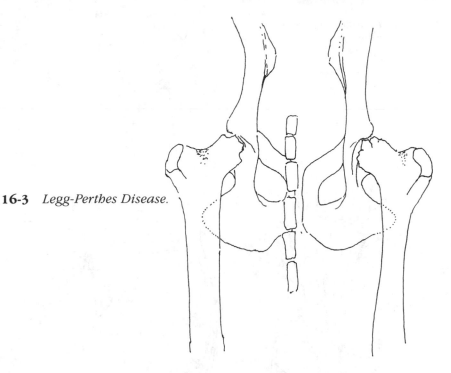

16-3   *Legg-Perthes Disease.*

PATELLAR LUXATION

Patellar luxation is an orthopedic condition in which the patella, or kneecap, "slips" to one side of the knee joint, causing pain and loss of the joint function (FIG. 16-4). *Medial patellar luxation,* in which the patella slips to the inside surface of the joint, is most often seen in the toy breeds, such as Yorkshire terriers, poodles, and Pomeranians. *Lateral patellar luxation,* where the knee cap migrates to the outer surface of the knee joint, shows no true breed disposition, with larger dogs sometimes affected. Luxations of the patella, regardless of the type, can occur secondary to direct trauma to the joint, or they can be caused by an abnormal anatomic development of the bones comprising the knee joint.

Symptoms

Signs of this problem can occur as early as 6 months of age in affected dogs. Milder cases often go unnoticed for years until arthritis of the affected knee sets in.

Symptoms associated with patellar luxation include intermittent lameness, with the dog often reluctant to put the affected back leg on the ground. Dogs affected with this problem might seem fine one minute, and then suddenly let out a yelp and come up overtly lame. Many times, the patella will slip back into place on its own and the dog will seem fine again. However, if this condition goes on for a long time, arthritis of the knee joint eventually occurs, and the lameness signs will fail to disappear.

16-4   *Left: Normal patellar
alignment at knee joint.
Right: Patellar luxation.*

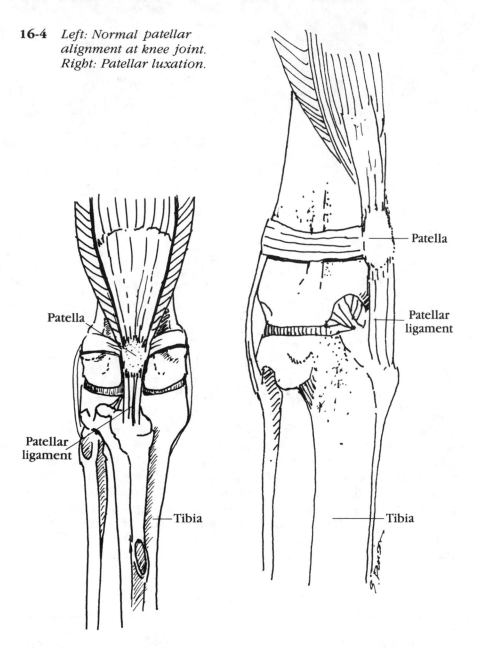

Patella

Patella

Patellar
ligament

Patellar
ligament

Tibia

Tibia

Treatment

An easily displaced patella found upon physical examination will confirm
a diagnosis of patellar luxation. Radiographs are helpful as well to determine the extent of arthritis involvement, if any at all.

Surgical correction of patellar luxation is the treatment of choice in
these pets. This involves altering the anatomy of tibia (the shin bone that

makes up the lower portion of the knee joint) in such a way as the patella is not allowed to slip to either side. The prognosis after surgery is good to excellent for complete remission of signs. In those dogs that have problems with both knee joints, surgical repair of both legs may be necessary.

TORN KNEE LIGAMENTS (CRUCIATE INJURIES)

The knee joints of dogs (and of people, for that matter!) are held together by a fibrous joint capsule and a number of ligaments, the most prominent of these being the *cruciate ligaments*. Because of their configuration, the range of motion allowed the knee joint is limited to simple flexion and extension. If an abnormal force is placed upon the joint from trauma or from planting the leg wrong on the ground, these ligaments could tear or rupture, leading to instability and pain within the affected knee joint. This instability, if not corrected in a timely fashion, will lead to arthritic changes and permanent pain within the joint.

As with humans, cruciate injuries seemingly affect active, athletic canines more than others, but older, obese dogs also have their fair share of this type of problem. Ruptured cruciates can also occur secondary to patellar luxation in toy breeds (FIG. 16-5).

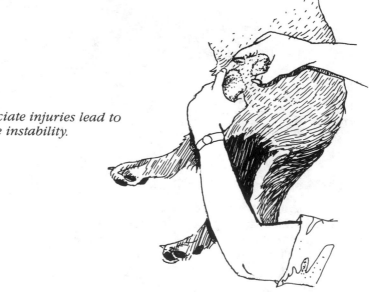

16-5   *Cruciate injuries lead to knee instability.*

Acute ruptures or tears involving the cruciate ligaments usually result in a sudden, non-weight-bearing lameness in dogs so affected. Over time, a gradual return to function can occur even if the condition is not treated, but the lameness will undoubtedly return as the activity level of the dog increases or as arthritis strikes the joint.

A diagnosis of torn knee ligaments is made if a veterinarian can demonstrate an obvious laxity within the affected knee joint. Due to the pain involved with such a diagnostic procedure, sedation might be necessary in order to obtain an accurate assessment. Radiographs might be helpful, depending upon the duration of the problem.

Treatment of this condition involves surgical repair and reconstruction of the torn ligaments in an effort to restore normal knee joint stability. Many techniques for such repair are available for use, depending upon the extent of the injury and other circumstances involved. In general, smaller dogs who do not have to carry as much weight around on their knee joints as do larger dogs have the most satisfactory post-surgical results.

HIP LUXATION

One common sequela to car accidents and other types of trauma involving dogs is dislocation, or *luxation,* of one or both hip joints. These dogs usually have a non-weight-bearing lameness on the affected leg, and it is quite painful (FIG. 16-6). Diagnosis can be made with a physical examination and radiographic X-rays of the hips and pelvis.

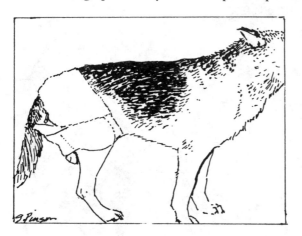

16-6 *Special sling used in dogs with a hip luxation.*

Treatment involves realigning the hip joints under sedation and strict cage confinement for a period of three to four weeks as healing takes place. If indicated, special slings designed to prevent re-luxation can be applied as well. In severe cases, orthopedic surgery is often needed to stabilize the joint.

FRACTURES

Most bone fractures in dogs are trauma-related. In isolated instances, metabolic diseases, such as nutritional osteodystrophy and bone cancers, can also be underlying causes as well. A fracture will present itself as a non-weight-bearing lameness, with noticeable swelling and pain in the region of the affected bone. *Crepitus,* or the grinding feel made by broken ends of bone rubbing together, and an anatomical distortion of the site, such as a shortening of an affected limb, might be seen as well.

Diagnosis of a fracture is based upon physical exam findings and radiographic X-rays. Treatment depends on the type of fracture and the region involved, and it consists of any combination of cage rest, bandaging/splinting, and surgery to reduce and stabilize the fracture.

Minor fractures involving the pelvis will often heal up nicely with cage rest alone; whereas malaligned fractures of one or more limbs might require surgical fixation using orthopedic pins, screws, and/or bone plates. In general, uncomplicated fractures usually heal quite readily in dogs.

OSTEOMYELITIS

Infections involving bony tissue within the body are termed *osteomyelitis*. Bacterial osteomyelitis in dogs can occur secondary to a deep bite wound or some other type of penetrating trauma. Open fractures can also predispose to bone infections. Furthermore, fungal organisms, such as histoplasmosis and blastomycosis, can also spread from other areas of the body via the blood and infect bony tissue in dogs.

Dogs with osteomyelitis are lame and feverish, and usually quite painful at the affected site. These signs, combined with the localized swelling that often occurs, can easily be mistaken for a fracture and must be differentiated from one. To do this, radiographic X-rays should be taken of the suspected skeletal region. In addition, bone biopsies might be necessary to differentiate some cases of osteomyelitis from bone tumors, and to collect samples for bacterial or fungal cultures.

Because infections that become embedded in bone can be difficult to clear up with antibiotics alone, surgery is usually needed to actually remove those portions of bone severely affected. Drain tubes are placed as well to allow for post-surgical drainage and flushing of the site with medicated solutions. Following surgery, antibiotic therapy might be required for one to two months; if a fungal organism is involved, medications might need to be given for four to six months.

SPONDYLOSIS DEFORMANS

Spondylosis deformans is a degenerative bone condition that seems to be related to the aging process in some dogs, especially the larger breeds (FIG. 16-7). It is characterized by the development of bony spurs that originate from intervertebral discs and grow to bridge the gap between adjacent vertebrae. These spurs are evident on radiographic X-rays. Most dogs afflicted with this disorder show no clinical signs whatsoever. However, in some dogs, pressure and pain originating from these bony growths can cause prominent hind-end weakness and reluctance to move (FIG. 16-8).

Unfortunately, there is no cure for spondylosis deformans. Discomfort associated with the condition can be temporarily relieved with aspirin or other anti-inflammatory medication.

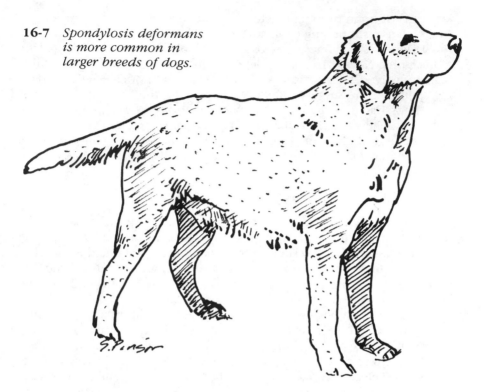

16-7 *Spondylosis deformans is more common in larger breeds of dogs.*

METABOLIC BONE DISEASE

Metabolic bone diseases are characterized by a thinning and loss of bony mass, predisposing the bone to fractures and to growth deformities. The most common metabolic bone disease seen in dogs is *hyperparathyroidism*. This condition is characterized by a calcium deficiency within the body that leads to abnormal bone growth and bone resorption as the body tries to correct the low calcium levels in the bloodstream. Hyperparathyroidism can result from feeding dogs all-meat diets (which are naturally low in calcium), or it can result secondary to kidney disease.

Puppies and dogs afflicted with metabolic bone diseases exhibit lameness, weakness, bone and joint deformities, and spontaneous fractures. Diagnosis is based on radiographic X-ray findings and on blood calcium measurements. Treatment for nutritionally related bone disease obviously involves changes in the diet and calcium supplementation. There is no effective treatment for kidney-related hyperparathyroidism.

MYOSITIS/MYOPATHIES

Myositis is inflammation of muscle tissue which results in pain, weakness, and muscle atrophy (shrinking). Dogs suffering from severe bouts of myositis are reluctant to move and can actually appear as if they are paralyzed due to the inflammatory effects on the muscles.

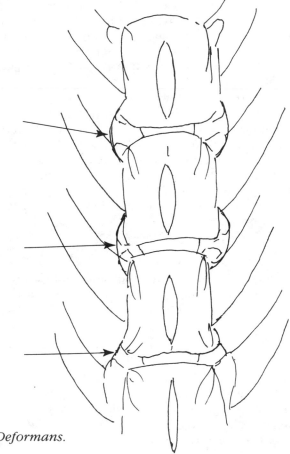

16-8 *Spondylosis Deformans.*

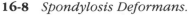

Myositis in dogs can be caused by a number of different disease entities, including toxoplasmosis, leptospirosis, bacterial infections (abscesses), and autoimmune disease. One special type of myositis, called *masticatory myositis,* affects the facial muscles of the affected dogs, causing atrophy and the inability to chew normally. This autoimmune disease is seen most frequently in German Shepherds.

Myositis is diagnosed using clinical signs and blood tests designed to detect increased levels in muscle enzymes within the blood. In especially elusive cases, biopsy samples taken from suspected muscle tissue can help veterinarians obtain a definitive diagnosis.

Treatment for myositis is aimed at the underlying cause. If infections are to blame, appropriate antimicrobial or antiparasitic therapy will help relieve the myositis. Antiinflammatory medications can also be used to relieve the pain and discomfort associated with the inflammation until the underlying cause is treated.

Autoimmune myositis, such as masticatory myositis, is treated with high levels of glucocorticosteroids (such as prednisolone) in an effort to suppress the immune response causing the inflammatory response in the first place. The prognosis for complete recovery in dogs with autoimmune myositis is poor, yet with medications, the signs associated with the disorder can be kept under control.

The term *myopathy* refers to abnormal anatomy and/or function of skeletal muscle tissue within the body. Most myopathies in dogs are inherited. Chow chows, golden retrievers, and Irish terriers are examples of breeds that can suffer from congenital myopathies. Dogs suffering from a myopathy exhibit abnormal postures, stiff gaits, and generalized shrinking or atrophy of the muscles. Because of the inherited nature of these diseases, the onset of clinical signs usually occurs within a year of age. Unfortunately, there is no effective treatment to stop the progression of these myopathies.

HERNIAS

A *hernia* results from a tear or defect in a muscular wall, allowing the contents contained behind the wall to protrude through the opening in the muscle. In dogs, the four most common types of hernias include umbilical hernias, inguinal hernias, perineal hernias, and diaphragmatic hernias.

Umbilical hernias   occur on the midline of the dog's stomach at the location of the *umbilicus,* or the belly button. These usually result from trauma to the muscle wall in this area that occurs as when the bitch severs the umbilical cord after birth. Umbilical hernias pose no real health problems, since fatty tissue is usually the only item that ever protrudes through the opening. These hernias can be sutured and repaired at the time of other elective surgeries.

Inguinal hernias   occur in the inguinal region of the abdomen, or that region where the abdominal musculature meets that of the hind legs. They are seen as birth defects or secondary to trauma. These hernias are more serious than umbilical hernias, since the herniated material often includes intestines. As a result, normal digestive processes can be disrupted. Treatment involves surgical replacement of the herniated material back inside the abdomen and suturing the defective muscle.

Perineal hernias   result from a weakening of the musculature in the region located beneath the tail on either side of the anus. Seen primarily in older male dogs that have not been neutered, perineal hernias can involve portions of the colon and cause impactions and elimination problems if not surgically corrected. Because the hormone testosterone seems to play a role in the development of these hernias, neutering these dogs is also recommended to prevent a recurrence.

Diaphragmatic hernia   By far the most serious type of hernia is the diaphragmatic hernia. The diaphragm is the thick wall of muscle which separates the thorax or chest cavity from the abdominal contents. Tears or ruptures occurring in this band of muscle, resulting either from congenital defects or from traumatic incidents, can allow liver, intestines, and/or other abdominal contents to herniate through into the chest cavity. When this happens, the pressure applied to the crowded lungs and heart results in, among other things, breathing difficulties, weakness, and/or gastrointestinal disturbances.

Definitive diagnosis of a diaphragmatic hernia can be made by coupling history, clinical signs, and a physical examination with radiographic X-ray findings. Surgical repair of the torn diaphragm will alleviate the signs and usually result in a complete recovery.

17

The Nervous System

THE NERVOUS SYSTEM involves a complex interaction between special elements designed to originate or to carry unique electrochemical charges to and from the various organs within the body. Like its endocrine counterpart, the nervous system initiates and regulates bodily functions and ensures its owner of an awareness to the surrounding environment.

ANATOMY AND PHYSIOLOGY

The smallest component of the nervous system is the *neuron*; there are over 10 billion of these dynamic cells in the body, and they have the ability to originate and propagate nerve impulses. These result from changes in electrolyte ratios, namely those of sodium and potassium, occurring across the cell membrane of the neuron (for this reason, abnormalities in the amounts of sodium and potassium within the body can have devastating effects on nervous system function).

Generated impulses are transmitted to their respective targets along special cellular projections, originating from the cell body, called *nerve fibers*. Speeds of transmission along these nerve fibers can reach over 110 meters per second. Groups or bundles of fibers coursing together are what are referred to as *nerves*.

Within the nervous system, neurons can link together to form a continuous chain to allow for the uninterrupted passage of a nerve impulse to its desired destination. A *synapse* is described as this connection between two nerve cells. Special chemical transmitters located at synapses (*neuro-transmitters*) transfer the impulses from end of one neuron to the receptive end of another, allowing the impulse to continue in its travels. Neurotransmitters are also found at the junctions between nerve fibers and their target muscles or organs. In dogs, organophosphate insecticidal poisoning exerts its deadly effects by interfering with the normal breakdown of *acetylcholine,* one of these neurotransmitters.

The *brain* is the control center for the entire nervous system. Internally, it is composed of *gray matter*, which is nothing more than a collection of neuron cell bodies and synapses between nerve cells, and *white matter,* made up of nerve fibers originating from the neuron cell bodies.

The mammalian brain is divided into three divisions, the *cerebrum,* the *cerebellum,* and the *brainstem.* The largest of the three, the cerebrum, is responsible for memory, sensory awareness, learning, and muscular movement. The cerebellum, located in back of and just beneath the cerebrum, functions to coordinate muscular activity and movement, and control body posture. The final division of the brain, the brainstem, serves a variety of functions. It acts as the important middleman by relaying messages between the cerebrum, cerebellum, and the spinal cord, and influencing activities such as heartbeat, breathing, vision, and hearing. A special portion of the brainstem, called the *hypothalamus*, provides an important link between the nervous system and the endocrine system.

The *spinal cord* is the major highway of activity for the transmission of nerve impulses between the brain and the rest of the body. It runs along the course of the back within the *spinal canal* formed by the *vertebral column*. Like the brain, the spinal cord also contains gray matter and white matter. Large spinal nerves containing numerous smaller nerve fibers branch off from the main cord along its course and travel to respective target muscles and organs. The spinal cord can also serve as coordinating center for certain reflex activities involving the muscles of the limbs without first requiring a nerve impulse to be sent to the brain. Clinicians can often assess the extent of damage to a spinal cord by evaluating these *spinal reflex arcs*.

Spinal nerves branching off from the spinal cord contain two main types of nerve fibers. *Somatic* nerve fibers carry information to and from skeletal muscle, skin, joints, and appendages. Effects, such as muscle contraction, produced by somatic fibers are said to be under conscious, or voluntary control from the brain. *Autonomic* nerve fibers innervate glands and internal organs throughout the body. Unlike somatic nerves, autonomic nerves act mainly on reflex, with little voluntary control. Blood pressure, cardiac output, breathing, gastrointestinal motility, body temperature, and hormone secretion are but some of the many vital life functions under the influence of this unique system.

Both the brain and the spinal cord are covered by three thin layers of tissue called *meninges*. Between these layers is found a special type of fluid, called *cerebrospinal fluid*. Meninges with their accompanying cerebrospinal fluid serve to protect, support, and nourish the underlying nervous tissue. Abnormal increases in the amount of cerebrospinal fluid can cause serious damage to spinal cord and brain. *Hydrocephalus* is the term used to describe such a condition affecting the brain.

SEIZURES

Those who own a dog that has suffered from seizures know first-hand how scary these episodes can be. A *seizure* is defined as uncontrollable behavior or muscle activity caused by an abnormal increase in the brain's nervous activities. *Epilepsy* is the term used to describe recurring seizures.

Seizural activity in dogs can be quite obvious or quite subtle. In essence, seizures should be suspected anytime a dog undergoes sporadic, unexplained behavioral changes.

Causes of seizures

What causes seizures? The following are some potential causes (FIG. 17-1).

○ Viral infections (e.g., distemper)
○ Toxoplasmosis
○ Fungal infections (e.g., cryptococcosis)
○ Epilepsy
○ Hydrocephalus
○ Brain tumor
○ Intestinal parasites
○ Low blood sugar
○ Low blood calcium
○ Insecticidal poisoning
○ Heat stroke
○ Idiopathic (unknown)

Because causes for seizures are so numerous, a thorough examination and blood workup by a veterinarian is warranted any time a dog exhibits seizures. In some cases, managing or eliminating an underlying cause will eliminate the seizures. In others, such as with *idiopathic epilepsy*, there is no known cause, yet by ruling out the other potential causes and establishing a pattern of occurrence, most cases can be effectively managed with anticonvulsant medications.

With idiopathic epilepsy, seizures can begin at any stage in life, yet, for the most part, they begin around 1 to 3 years of age. While the cause of idiopathic epilepsy is unknown, it has been shown to be inheritable in some breeds, including beagles and dachshunds.

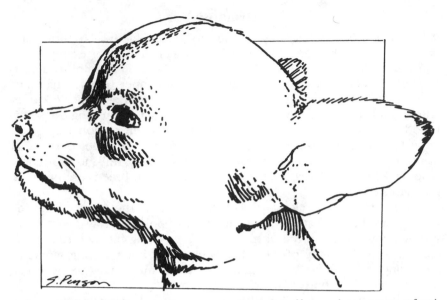

17-1   *Hydrocephalus, or "water on the brain," can be a cause of seizures.*

Characteristics of seizures

Most seizures themselves are rarely life threatening, unless some physical harm comes to the dog as a result of the fit. However, there is one seizural presentation called *status epilepticus* which can prove fatal to a dog unfortunate enough to be afflicted with such. This condition is characterized by continual seizures occurring one right after the other. Unless appropriate emergency medication is administered intravenously to stop the seizures, these dogs can lapse into a coma and die. As a result, prompt recognition and action on the part of the pet owner is essential.

The typical seizure or epileptic fit has three stages, or phases. The first of these, the *preictal phase*, is marked by anxiety and restlessness on the part of the pet. The actual period of the seizure activity, *ictus,* follows next. Its duration might be for only a few seconds or it might be minutes. Certainly the longer the seizure lasts, the more dangerous it is to the health of the pet.

The *postictal phase* following the seizure is characterized by an overall depression or confusion. Postictal dogs can appear to be blind, running into walls and objects, or they might just sleep a lot. This phase can last for a few hours or for days, with the dog returning to its normal state after its conclusion.

Diagnosis

When attempting to diagnose the cause of seizural activity, veterinarians will first look at the age and the type of dog involved. For example, seizures occurring in dogs under 1 year commonly result from birth defects or from infectious diseases, such as canine distemper or intestinal parasites, whereas seizures occurring in a very old dog often indicate kidney failure or cancer. In smaller, toy puppies and in active hunting dogs, low blood sugar brought on by illness, stress, or overexertion can be an important inciting cause. Seizures occurring in a pregnant dog or one that has just given birth are more than likely caused by milk fever, or low blood calcium. Finally, as mentioned above, certain breeds are prone to idiopathic epilepsy.

A good history is also vital to help determine the cause of the seizures. Does the dog have access to any type of poisons? Has the dog ever suffered any type of physical trauma, such as being hit by a car, in the past? Has the intensity of the seizures gradually been getting worse or increasing in frequency? The answers to these and other questions can help a veterinarian narrow the choices a bit.

A complete blood profile and urinalysis should be performed to help rule out the metabolic and infectious causes of seizures. Radiographs and ultrasound can prove to be helpful in certain instances as well. If no underlying cause can be found, and the history supports it, a diagnosis of idiopathic epilepsy is made and treatment is started on this premise.

Treatment

For cases other than idiopathic epilepsy, treatment is geared toward correcting or managing the underlying problem, be it kidney failure, poisoning, low blood sugar, etc. In instances in which idiopathic epilepsy is suspect, anticonvulsant medications can be used to control or even eliminate the seizural activity.

Dogs suffering from idiopathic epilepsy do not necessarily need to be on any medication unless the seizures last for more than two minutes at a time or occur more often than every two months. For those dogs that require medication, oral *phenobarbital* is usually the drug of choice to start with. For tougher cases, *primidone* or *phenytoin* are often prescribed.

Determining the exact dosages of any of these medications for a pet might require frequent adjustments at the start in order to accommodate its individual needs. Pets taking anticonvulsant medication should have liver-function tests performed at least annually, since some of these medications, such a primidone, can damage the liver over the long-term.

PARALYSIS

Paralysis can be defined as a disruption of the nervous system leading to an impairment of motor function and/or feeling to a particular region or regions of the body. This impairment can be in the form of a spasticity of the muscles in the involved region, or these muscles may become completely limp. In either case, the muscles involved are unable to function in the manner they were intended.

Paralysis involving the sensory portion of the nervous system can result in an increased sensitivity to pain or in a complete absence of it. Finally, paralysis resulting in the inefficient function of certain internal organs can occur as well if the nerves supplying these structures are disrupted in any way.

Any disease or disorder that traumatizes the brain, spinal cord, and nerves has the potential to cause paralysis. In dogs, some of the more common causes seen by veterinarians include infectious diseases and parasites, being hit by a car, ruptured discs, and in the case of facial muscle paralysis, ear infections.

Treatment of paralysis is geared towards identifying and treating the underlying cause. If it has been caused by trauma, anti-inflammatory agents combined with drugs designed to draw fluid out of the central nervous system might help reverse signs of paralysis, yet their usefulness is dependent on the extent of the nervous injury and how quickly therapy is instituted.

Dogs who have sensory paralysis in a limb might require limb amputation to prevent self-mutilation to the leg. In instances where an irreversible paralysis involves more than one limb, or involves the malfunction of internal organs, pet owners must seriously consider not only their dog's quality of life as a paralytic, but their own as well, before prolonged therapeutic or rehabilitative measures are undertaken.

DEGENERATIVE DISC DISEASE

Coursing along the length of the back, the spinal cord travels protected within the bony vertebral column. Separating each vertebra, and located beneath the spinal cord itself, are structures called *intervertebral discs*. These discs serve as cushions between each individual vertebra, absorbing shock and forming joints that allow the vertebral column to bend. Each circular disc is composed of an outer band of tough, fibrous tissue called the *annulus fibrosus* surrounding an inner gelatinous center called the *nucleus pulposus*. This latter structure is responsible for absorbing any shock placed upon the disc (FIG. 17-2).

Characteristics

Degenerative disc disease is characterized by the slow degeneration of the nucleus pulposus within one or more intervertebral discs. As these continue to degenerate, they become less resilient and can even calcify, leaving the intervertebral disc without its shock-absorbing unit. As a result, the discs so affected become very susceptible to compression dam-

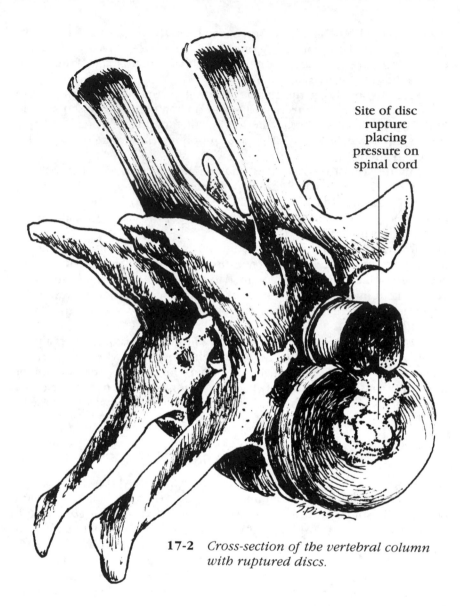

Site of disc
rupture
placing
pressure on
spinal cord

17-2   *Cross-section of the vertebral column*
with ruptured discs.

age, even from the normal day-to-day activity. In dogs so affected, continued stress or sudden trauma to the disc or vertebral column can lead to an
overt tearing or rupture of the annulus fibrosus, and extrusion of the
degenerating nucleus pulposus. Unfortunately, since the top portion of
the annulus is much narrower than the bottom portion, this extrusion
usually occurs upwards directly into the spinal canal, damaging the spinal
cord and associated nerves.

Overt disc ruptures may be classified as partial or complete. In partial
ruptures, the annulus can either be stretched and displaced into the spinal

canal, or it can partially rupture, allowing a small amount of the nucleus within to escape and pressure the spinal cord. With complete ruptures, the entire nucleus content is allowed to escape into the spinal canal. Obviously, the consequences of a such a rupture vs a partial one are much more severe.

The region of the vertebral column most susceptible to rupture is that portion extending from the last rib to the pelvis. The neck region is another area that can be affected. In a dog suffering from degenerative disc disease, even the slightest wrong move, such as jumping off the couch or running too fast can cause an affected disc to rupture (FIG. 17-3).

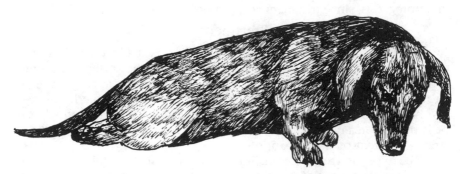

17-3 *Degenerative disc disease can lead to paralysis.*

Although any dog can suffer from degenerative disc disease, there do seem to be some breed dispositions. The dachshund breed certainly leads the list in the number of cases reported. Other breeds commonly afflicted with degenerative disc disease include poodles, pekingeses, and Lhasa apsos. Beagles and cocker spaniels also have a notable incidence of degenerative disc disease in their neck region.

Problems with degenerative disc disease can show up in smaller breeds as early as 3 years of age. In larger dogs, the onset of signs might not occur until they are six to seven years old. Overweight dogs are at an especially high risk of developing complications associated with intervertebral disc disease.

Symptoms

The clinical signs seen with degenerative disc disease and/or disc rupture depend on the location of the lesion and the amount, if any, of the rupture that has taken place. In fact, the extent of pressure or damage to the spinal cord can be estimated based upon the signs seen.

Dogs with early or mild cases of disc disease causing slight pressure upon the cord will be quite painful and reluctant to move. Many will cry or yelp when picked up. If the neck is involved, any manipulations attempted will be met with vigorous protests. These pets often prefer not to be bothered, and have the tendency to isolate themselves. Appetites are usually reduced as well. Since nerve fibers responsible for coordinated muscle movement run within the outer layers of the spinal cord, owners may also notice weakness and/or incoordination when their pet attempts to walk.

With more severe disc ruptures, damage to the deeper portions of the spinal cord can become a serious factor. When this occurs, partial or complete paralysis of one or more limbs might result, depending on the location of the rupture. If the entire depth of the spinal cord is involved, these animals will also lose all pain sensation to one or all four limbs, again depending upon the areas of the spinal cord involved. Such severe cases carry a very grave prognosis, since treatment at this stage is rarely successful.

Treatment

In most cases, confirmation of a ruptured disc is made via a thorough examination, clinical signs, and with radiographs of the vertebral column. If the exact location of the spinal lesion cannot be pinpointed with regular radiographs, a special test, called a *myelogram*, is performed. This test involves injecting a dye directly into the spinal canal. The dye, which can be identified on a radiograph, helps to outline the cord lesion and demonstrate the extent of the disc rupture.

The type of treatment instituted for disc disease and/or rupture depends on the extent of the damage done by the disc to the spinal cord.

For those dogs showing only pain with some mild incoordination, A STRICT TWO WEEK CONFINEMENT period either at home or in a hospital setting, is a must! Although anti-inflammatories are sometimes used to reduce the swelling and pain, many veterinarians prefer to forego them altogether since any pain experienced by the affected dog serves to discourage excessive movement and mobility, which, in turn, prevents further damage to the disk and cord until natural healing can take place. After a week or so, short 10- to 15-minute physical therapy sessions—involving controlled exercise, including swimming—can be performed twice daily to help speed recovery and return to normal function.

For cases in which the affected dog is having great difficulty walking, strict cage confinement combined with anti-inflammatory therapy and other specific treatment is indicated. If the disease is such that the dog is unable to support weight on the limbs at all, even after medical therapy, then surgery is required to reduce the pressure placed on the spinal cord by the ruptured disc.

This surgery, called a *laminectomy* or *hemilaminectomy*, works best if performed within the first 24 hours of the injury. It involves the removal of part of the vertebra over the affected cord segment. By eliminating the enclosed space through which the spinal cord runs, the pressure on the cord caused by the inflammation is allowed to dissipate. At the same time, surgeons often elect to perform *intervertebral disc fenestrations*, aimed at removing the offending nucleus pulposus from the disc in question and from adjacent discs as well.

The prognosis is poor for those pets who are unable to walk and have lost deep pain sensation in their legs as a result of a ruptured disc. The loss of deep pain indicates that the entire depth of the spinal cord is invariably involved, and surgical salvage procedures are rarely successful.

In those instances where surgery is unsuccessful, or in which paralysis is permanent, euthanasia is not always the only option left to the owner. Special "wheelchairs" for dogs have been developed for dogs paralyzed by a ruptured disc or other neurological accidents. Though not for every patient, these carts can help afford mobility to select patients willing to wear the apparatus and an alternative for those owners willing to devote much time and care to their paralyzed pet. If you think such a device could be applicable to your own pet's situation, ask your veterinarian for more details regarding this and other management options available.

Prevention

There are specific measures that pet owners can take to help protect their dog from a ruptured disc(s). The first and most important is to prevent obesity. Overweight dogs are prime candidates for such complications; hence, they should be placed on a strict diet to reduce this risk factor.

Jumping should be discouraged in dogs predisposed to intervertebral disc disease. Many ruptured discs result from pets jumping off and on furniture. Pets so inclined should be assisted up or down whenever possible. Even better, a small chair or ottoman ramp can be placed in front of its favorite piece of furniture to allow easier access.

Whenever lifting a dog with back problems, be sure to firmly support both the front and hind ends, keeping the back as straight as possible. This stabilizes the position of the spine and affords the handler with better and safer control should the pet struggle (FIG. 17-4).

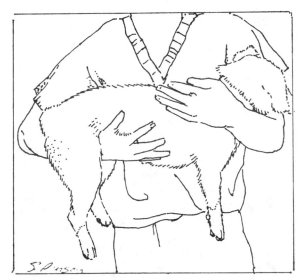

17-4 *Be very careful in how you handle a dog with vertebral or spinal problems.*

Surgical intervertebral disc fenestration is often used as a preventative measure in dogs that have previously suffered from bouts of intervertebral disc disease. As mentioned before, this involves the penetration and removal of the nucleus pulposus from one or more intervertebral discs suspected of causing current or future problems. By doing so, the danger associated with later disc rupture is removed with the nucleus.

VERTEBRAL INSTABILITY (WOBBLER'S DISEASE)

Seen primarily in Great Danes and Doberman pinschers, vertebral instability is characterized by instability and deformities in the vertebra of the neck region, leading to pressure on the spinal cord in that region. The condition in these breeds is hereditary in nature; however, trauma can predispose any dog to Wobbler's Disease.

Signs associated with vertebral instability include incoordination, weakness, and paralysis. Pain is not usually a feature of this disease.

Diagnosis of vertebral instability is made with radiographic X-rays. Treatment involves the use of anti-inflammatory medication to reduce the spinal cord inflammation. Surgical decompression of the spinal cord is also warranted in severe cases.

18

The Endocrine System

WITHIN THE BODIES of all mammals, a complex network of glands called the endocrine system is responsible for the production and secretion of special proteins and lipids (fats) called hormones. In turn, these hormones serve to regulate many vital functions within the body—from growth and development to digestion and utilization of nutrients. Like the nervous system, the endocrine system assumes a regulatory role within the body, and its proper function is essential to the overall health of the animal. Without the endocrine glands and their hormones, a state of chaos would quickly ensue within the body as the functional harmony existing between the various organ systems would cease to exist.

ANATOMY AND PHYSIOLOGY

Hormones can be protein in nature, or they can be fashioned from special fatty components, known as steroids. *Steroid* is one of the most misused and widely misunderstood terms in today's society (see The Use of Steroids in Veterinary Medicine, in this chapter).

Corticosteroids are a special group of steroids produced by the adrenal glands that are vital to many everyday functions within the body. Synthetic derivatives of this steroid group are commonly used, among other things, to reduce pain and inflammation resulting from musculoskeletal injuries.

Androgens (i.e., *testosterone)* and *estrogens,* the sex hormones that influence reproductive activity and secondary sexual characteristics, are also types of steroid hormones produced naturally within the body.

Anabolic steroids, probably the most notorious members of the steroid family, are actually man-made derivatives of the male androgenic steroid hormones. This is the group that has been largely exploited by athletes for increased muscular strength and size.

Although all of the different classes of steroids mentioned above, whether natural or synthetic, share a similar structural design, it is easy to see that their functions and effects differ greatly between each class.

Both protein and steroid-type hormones are secreted directly into the blood stream from the glands or organs that produce them, and circulate to their specific target cells or organs, where they exert their effect. The amount of hormone required to exert its particular effect is precise. If present in too great a quantity, or if supplies are deficient, abnormal function of its target cells or organs result. As a result, hormonal activities within the body are governed by complex negative feedback mechanisms, which ensure proper blood levels at all times. Unfortunately, certain disease conditions involving the endocrine glands and organs can disrupt this delicate balance, which can pose serious health problems.

The *hypothalamus*, located at the bottom portion of the brainstem, functions as an integration center between the nervous system and the endocrine system. Nervous system functions of the hypothalamus include regulation of body temperature, emotional behavior and sleep, and control of food and water intake. As an endocrine organ, the hypothalamus secretes the hormone *ADH* (anti-diuretic hormone), which controls the water balance within the body, *oxytocin*, which stimulates lactation and uterine contractions, and a variety of other hormones that exert control over the pituitary gland.

The *pituitary gland* produces hormones that have effects on other endocrine glands, such as the thyroid and adrenal glands. In addition, pituitary hormones also influence growth and reproductive patterns. In dogs, *Cushing's Disease*, a condition characterized by an oversecretion of adrenal gland hormones, is most commonly caused by a tumor of the pituitary gland.

Hormones produced by the *thyroid gland* control the rate of growth and metabolism within the body, as well as decrease calcium levels within the bloodstream. Closely associated with the thyroid gland are the *parathyroid glands*, which produce a hormone that counteracts the action of a certain thyroid hormone by increasing blood calcium levels. This balance between the thyroid and parathyroid glands helps to ensure proper blood levels of calcium at all times. Too much parathyroid hormone can result in excess resorption of bony tissue, resulting in metabolic bone disease (see chapter 16).

The *adrenal glands* produce a variety of hormones, each exerting unique effects within the body. Among other things, adrenal hormones influence carbohydrate and protein metabolism and storage (*cortisol, cortisone*), help the kidneys regulate sodium and potassium levels (*aldosterone*), and control blood pressure and heart rate (*epinephrine [adrenalin] and norepinephrine).*

Certain organs can double as endocrine glands. The pancreas is not just responsible for producing digestive enzymes; it secretes two hormones, *insulin* and *glucagon*, both involved in carbohydrate (sugar) metabolism within the body. Insulin functions to lower blood sugar by increasing its uptake and utilization by the body organs. Counteracting the effects of insulin, glucagon increases blood sugar levels by decreasing its uptake into the liver and fatty tissue. *Diabetes mellitus* is a disease in which not enough insulin is produced by the pancreas, prohibiting cells and organs from extracting carbohydrates out of the blood stream.

Other organs exhibiting endocrine functions include the stomach, which produces hormones that regulate digestion; the ovaries and testicles, which, together with the adrenal gland and placenta (in pregnant females), produce the sex hormones; the kidneys, which secrete hormones that influence blood flow and filtration within the kidneys themselves; and the thymus gland, whose hormonal activity influences the activity of cells of the immune system.

THE USE OF STEROIDS IN VETERINARY MEDICINE

If there ever was a group of drugs that revolutionized both human and veterinary medicine, it is steroids. These chemicals are produced naturally by the body and have been produced synthetically by man. Although they are vital to life and can be used therapeutically in a wide variety of useful ways, steroids are also, in the public's eye, one of the most misunderstood of all drug groups. When the word "steroid" is mentioned to the layperson, images of muscle-bound athletes or of unhealthy side effects are often conjured up. Yet what most of them fail to realize is that, used correctly, steroids can be safe and unsurpassed in effectiveness in treating a wide variety of diseases and conditions.

One point to keep in mind is that "steroid" is a catch-all phrase used to describe those compounds sharing a similar, yet not necessarily identical biochemical make-up. For instance, glucocorticosteroids, the types used most frequently in veterinary medicine, should not be confused with anabolic steroids, which are actually synthetic derivatives of the male sex hormone testosterone, (these are the steroids that have caused so much controversy within athletic circles). Although the chemical make-up of anabolic steroids may be similar to glucocorticosteroids, their functions and effects are not. The sex hormones, such as estrogen, progesterone, and testosterone, and the mineralocorticosteroids, probably the closest group in biochemical structure to glucocorticosteroids than any of the others, are also types of steroid hormones produced by the body.

Glucocorticosteroids

The glucocorticosteroids are by far the class of steroid used most in veterinary medicine. Some names from this group that you might be familiar with include *hydrocortisone, prednisone, prednisolone,* and *dexametha-*

sone. The first is a steroid produced naturally by the body; the latter ones are synthetic steroids created in the laboratory.

Glucocorticosteroids can be further classified into groups based upon the duration of their effects once they are administered for treatment purposes. For instance, hydrocortisone is considered a short-acting corticosteroid, with effects lasting anywhere from eight to 12 hours. Prednisone and prednisolone are termed intermediate-acting steroids, with durations of action up around 12 to 36 hours. Finally, corticosteroids such as dexamethasone are long-acting drugs, exerting their effects for up to 48 hours after administration.

Therapeutically, what are glucocorticosteroids used for? In veterinary medicine, their primary uses are to reduce inflammation associated with disease, to regulate immune responses, and to combat shock. They are the first line of defense against autoimmune diseases, or those diseases caused by an overactive immune system. Pet owners probably know them best for their ability to provide prompt relief from itching and skin irritation in those dogs suffering from allergies.

Although glucocorticosteroids can prove to be useful, and even lifesaving in many instances, they can't be employed with indiscretion. For example, because they do have the ability to suppress the immune system, especially at high doses, glucocorticosteroids need to be used with caution or avoided altogether in those instances in which severe parasitic, fungal, or bacterial disease is present. Also, if given to a pet during pregnancy, these steroids could cause premature labor and abortion. Even their use on the eyes should be avoided in those cases where an early ulceration has occurred on one or both corneas, since doing so could actually make the ulcers worse and lead to loss of the eye(s). Lastly, as with other anti- inflammatory medications, corticosteroids can also upset the gastrointestinal tract.

Long-term, indiscriminant use of glucocorticosteroids can eventually be detrimental to the health of a pet. Granted, the nature of some diseases do require extended and sometimes even lifetime use of these compounds. In such cases, these pets must be placed on a strict treatment regimen and be monitored closely by a veterinarian while they are on the medication.

The problem with the daily use of corticosteroids rests in the fact that whenever they are administered to a pet either through injection, orally, or even topically on the skin, the body's hypothalamus and pituitary gland signal to the adrenal glands to stop their natural production of glucocorticosteroids. In addition, if the adrenal glands remain dormant for any appreciable amount of time, they might actually *lose the ability* to make their own corticosteroids. If this happens, and if the corticosteroid therapy is abruptly stopped, the pet's life could be endangered because of a lack of corticosteroids within the body. Similarly, as high levels of glucocorticosteroids remain in the bloodstream, over time, signs of Cushing's disease could actually develop.

Because of these potential problems, pets that must be on daily glucocorticosteroid therapy for more than two weeks are placed thereafter on alternate-day dosing regimens using a short or intermediate-acting synthetic steroids, such as prednisolone, at the lowest possible dose. Giving the corticosteroid every other day instead of daily should prevent total suppression of the adrenal glands and allow the body to continue to produce its own steroids. In addition, by using the lowest dosage possible in this fashion, there is less chance of causing Cushing's-like disease. If the situation ever arises where the corticosteroid therapy is to be halted, then a gradual weaning off of the medication, usually in the form of a slow reduction in dosage over four to six weeks time is indicated.

HYPOTHYROIDISM

The thyroid gland, through production of thyroid hormones, functions to influence nutrient and oxygen utilization within the body, hence affecting overall metabolism. As a result, deficiencies in thyroid hormone or interference with its function can have profound effects on the body.

In dogs, immune system malfunctions, iodine deficiencies, incomplete thyroid gland development, and pituitary gland malfunctions can all lead to a condition of *hypothyroidism.* Predisposed breeds include cocker spaniels, dobermans, dachshunds, and golden retrievers (FIG. 18-1).

18-1   *A simple blood test can be used to assess the thyroid status of a dog.*

Symptoms

Clinical signs associated with this disorder are varied, owing to the tremendous scope of thyroid hormone function. Dogs with hypothyroidism tend to be lethargic—sleeping a lot and tiring easily after exercise. Some exhibit a profound intolerance to cold floors or cool environmental temperatures. Puppies so affected might seem to be slow learners when it comes to training. As the skin around the face of these dogs often thickens as a result of the disease, a dog's voice might change to a lower pitch, and facial features might appear droopy or sad.

In addition, hypothyroid dogs may also have poor appetites, yet still gain weight. Over 50% of dogs afflicted with hypothyroidism will exhibit changes to the skin and hair coat. A loss of the undercoat occurs, resulting in a thinned, poor-looking coat. Skin thickening occurs, and secondary seborrhea is not uncommon. Finally, eye problems, neurologic disorders, reproductive infertility, and arthritis could all have their roots in a thyroid disorder.

Treatment

A veterinarian can evaluate your pet's thyroid function right at the office. A simple blood test can be used to screen thyroid hormone levels within the body. If a problem is found, then more extensive thyroid function tests may be ordered to help determine the extent of the problem. If a dog is taking corticosteroid hormones for other problems at the time of the testing, the results could come back falsely low. As a rule, however, if clinical signs correlate with blood test results, then it is safe to assume that a condition of true hypothyroidism exists.

Regardless of the underlying cause, treatment of hypothyroidism in dogs involves daily supplementation with synthetic thyroid hormone tablets. The most commonly used type is called *sodium levothyroxine,* and it is given on a daily or twice-daily basis.

Thyroid hormone levels will need to be monitored during the initial stages of treatment to assure that the proper dosage is being met. For the most part, this is a medication that affected dogs will need to stay on the rest of their lives. Clinical response to medicating is usually seen within two weeks after initiation, with resolution of signs occurring soon after.

HYPERADRENOCORTICISM (CUSHING'S DISEASE)

Steroid hormones, specifically the class known as glucocorticosteroids produced by the adrenal glands, serve over 50 vital influences within the body. Some of the more important ones have to deal with carbohydrate, protein, and fat utilization and with maintaining water and electrolyte balance within the body. Veterinarians fighting allergic reactions or inflammation in dogs rely on glucocorticosteroids for their anti-inflammatory effects when given at low dosages. Similarly, since high doses of glucocorticosteroids can suppress the immune system, they are quite useful in treatments against autoimmune diseases in dogs, including *pemphigus*, a disease that causes severe skin lesions in affected dogs.

Unfortunately, since steroid hormones help maintain a delicate balance within the body, an overproduction of them within the body can upset this balance. This is precisely what happens in Cushing's disease. An overproduction of glucocorticosteroids from the adrenal glands occurs within the body, usually the result of a tumor affecting one or both glands, or, more commonly, a tumor affecting the pituitary gland. The disease is most common in dogs over 8 years of age. Furthermore, poodles, boxers, and dachshunds seem to be afflicted with a greater frequency than other breeds.

Symptoms

Some of the clinical signs seen in dogs with Cushing's disease include a marked increase in water and food consumption, an increase in elimination activity, lethargy and exercise intolerance, and a generalized reduction in muscle size and tone, which, when it affects the muscles of the abdominal wall, leads to a characteristic pot-bellied appearance (FIG. 18-2).

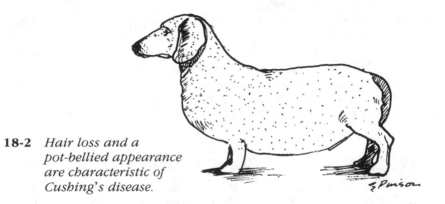

18-2   *Hair loss and a pot-bellied appearance are characteristic of Cushing's disease.*

The skin and coat changes that occur in a dog with Cushing's disease might be the first clues as to the existence of the problem. A generalized thinning of the hair coat and skin will be seen, with flakiness, pigmentation, and secondary infections. Eye problems are common in these dogs too, with reoccurring ulcers affecting the cornea. Because high levels of steroids have a suppressing influence on the immune system, secondary infections, especially bladder infections, are often seen in these dogs as well.

Finally, if a tumor is present in the pituitary gland at the base of the brain, neurological problems might occur as pressure is increased on the brain.

These signs can lead a clinician to suspect Cushing's disease, but it usually requires more extensive blood testing and radiographic X-rays to confirm a diagnosis. Measuring actual blood levels of steroids within the bloodstream is one way to test for Cushing's disease; other methods include injecting small amounts of special synthetic hormones, designed to alter the production of steroids within the body, into the dog and measuring the body's response to them. If the steroid production cannot be altered by these hormones, then a diagnosis can be made.

Treatment

Once a dog is diagnosed with Cushing's disease, therapy may be instituted in a number of ways. Surgical removal of the tumor in either the adrenal glands and/or pituitary gland can be attempted, yet this is a very difficult procedure associated with many post-operative complications.

Chemotherapy, using the drug o,p'-DDD can be employed to target the adrenal glands and reduce the amount of steroids being produced by them. Used correctly, this treatment can reduce or eliminate the clinical signs seen and greatly improve a dog's quality of life. Since it is a chemotherapeutic agent, a veterinarian will need to monitor an affected dog closely for side effects during the initial treatment stage. Therapy is usually required for life.

Because of the intense management required with these modes of therapy, some pet owners prefer to stick to conservative treatment when dealing with this disease in their dog. In these cases, dogs should be placed on high-protein diets to counteract protein loss caused by the disease. In addition, treating secondary problems as they arise—such as skin infections, bladder infections, and corneal ulceration—is necessary. Because the tumors responsible for Cushing's disease are usually slow-growing, most dogs can live up to two years with this treatment approach alone.

HYPOADRENOCORTICISM (ADDISON'S DISEASE)

While Cushing's disease is caused by too many corticosteroids circulating within the body, Addison's disease is caused by the exact opposite: inadequate amounts of circulating corticosteroids. This includes not only the glucocorticosteroids produced by the adrenal glands, but the mineralocorticoids as well. Because the latter are so vital at maintaining a fluid and electrolyte balance within the body, Addison's disease can be acutely life-threatening in the affected individual.

Causes of this disease in dogs can include tumors, infections, autoimmune diseases, and toxins. It can also occur secondarily to overtreatment with corticosteroids.

Symptoms

The clinical signs seen resemble those exhibited by pets afflicted with viral or parasitic gastroenteritis—namely vomiting, diarrhea, and dehydration. Loss of appetite and weight loss accompanies these signs as well, yet there might be an increase in water consumption.

Because the levels of sodium and potassium, two electrolytes vital to proper muscle contraction, are disrupted, profound muscle weakness, including a slowing of the rate at which the heart muscle contracts, are also observed. In severe cases, collapse of the entire circulatory system, with shock and then death, have been documented.

Diagnosis of Addison's disease can made based upon the history (i.e., long-term corticosteroid therapy), clinical signs seen and determining the ratio of sodium to potassium in the bloodstream. Marked increases in potassium and decreases in sodium is indicative of primary Addison's disease. Physical examination and electrocardiograms will reveal abnormal heart activity in these patients as well.

Treatment

If Addison's disease is diagnosed or suspected, treatment should be instituted immediately. Dehydration is combatted with intravenous fluids, and injections of mineralocorticoids are administered to stabilize fluid and electrolyte levels.

For cases of primary Addison's disease, periodic injections with mineralocorticoids will be required throughout the dog's life to prevent relapses from occurring. If the condition was caused by the sudden cessation of glucocorticosteroid therapy, such therapy is reinstituted and then gradually tapered off over weeks to months.

SEX HORMONE IMBALANCES

Although rare, imbalances involving testosterone, estrogen, and progesterone have been known to occur. For instance, in male dogs with too much circulating estrogens, skin disorders, hair loss, increased skin pigmentation, enlargement of the mammary glands, seborrhea, otitis externa, and behavioral changes can result. Estrogen-secreting tumors involving the testicles, called *Sertoli cell tumors,* are the main cause of increased estrogen levels in dogs. Cryptorchid canines, or those with one or both testicles retained within the abdomen, are at highest risk of developing such a tumor. Neutering those dogs so affected is the only effective way to treat this disorder. In some cases, giving testosterone supplements may be required as well for full abatement of clinical signs.

Similarly, if a female dog has too much circulating estrogens in her system, then she can suffer from the same clinical signs as her male counterpart. Hair loss, seborrhea, and increased pigmentation of the skin, especially in the areas of the flank, are common signs. Performing an ovariohysterectomy on these dogs will effectively reduce the amount of circulating estrogens and clinically effect a cure.

A condition known as *hypoestrogenism,* or inadequate amounts of the estrogen hormone, have been documented in older female dogs who were spayed at an early age. A gradual hair loss, especially around the hind end of these dogs, could be all that is seen in these pets. In addition, dribbling of the urine has been reported in older dogs suffering from this lack of estrogen. Fortunately, low-dose supplementation with an estrogen compound is usually all this is needed to clear up these clinical signs.

DIABETES MELLITUS

Diabetes mellitus is one of the more common endocrine diseases affecting dogs. The condition is caused by a deficiency in the hormone called insulin, which is normally created by the pancreas. Insulin is responsible for regulating the uptake of blood sugar, or glucose, into cells and tissues of the body for use as energy. Deficiencies in this hormone can be caused by any disease involving the pancreas, including chronic pancreatitis. In addition, autoimmune disease, in which the dog's body creates antibodies against its own insulin, has also been known to occur. Finally, there is evidence that, in dogs, the propensity for diabetes can be inherited. Middle-aged female dogs seem to be more at risk than others.

When a deficiency in insulin does occur, this transfer of glucose from the bloodstream to the tissues does not occur; hence, blood glucose levels become elevated. At the same time, the cells, tissues, and organs of the body don't receive the proper nutrition needed to maintain their function, and they start to look for other sources of energy in the body, namely proteins and fats. And this is where the problems start.

Symptoms

Dogs with this disease will exhibit an increase in water consumption and, consequently, urinations. As the body calls on these alternate sources of energy, pronounced weight loss results. In addition, as bodily fat stores are called upon and metabolized for energy, an excess of *ketone bodies,* by-products of fatty breakdown, accumulate within the body. In large amounts, these ketone bodies have the ability to damage the liver and to depress the nervous system, leading to depression and coma. Over time, the increased glucose levels within the blood can lead to cataracts and blindness.

Diabetic dogs have a decreased resistance to infection; as a result, they often suffer from chronic skin and bladder infections. Damage to small capillaries within the body caused by diabetes mellitus can lead to secondary kidney disease, blindness, and gangrene of the skin and extremities.

The clinical signs associated with diabetes mellitus are similar to diseases such as Cushing's disease, kidney disease, and diabetes insipidus; therefore, a thorough laboratory work-up is needed to ensure a correct diagnosis. Blood tests on dogs with diabetes mellitus will consistently reveal elevated glucose levels, and evaluation of urine samples will reveal the same. Such findings, along with the ruling-out of other potential causes of the clinical signs, can lead to a definitive diagnosis of diabetes mellitus.

Diabetes mellitus can be classified as uncomplicated or complicated. Uncomplicated cases might exhibit mild to moderate signs of the disease, yet none are truly life-threatening. In contrast, dogs diagnosed with the disease and exhibiting marked depression, vomiting, diarrhea, heavy breathing, and/or severe weight loss should all be considered complicated cases and should always be considered medical emergencies.

In most of these cases, the high levels of ketone acids produced as a result of increased fat metabolism lower the pH of the blood significantly enough to cause the harmful effects represented by the clinical signs. These dogs are usually become severely dehydrated at the same time.

Treatment

Treatment consists of immediate hospitalization with intravenous infusion of replacement fluids, medications designed to increase the pH of the blood (if indeed the pH is too low), and insulin (FIG. 18-3). The insulin is either given as a large bolus or as a continuous drip in the replacement fluids. Regardless of how it is administered, the levels of insulin given and corresponding blood glucose must be monitored closely, since too much insulin is even worse than not enough. If excess insulin is given, the pet could quickly become hypoglycemic and go into convulsions. Good monitoring and careful planning on the part of a veterinarian will help prevent this.

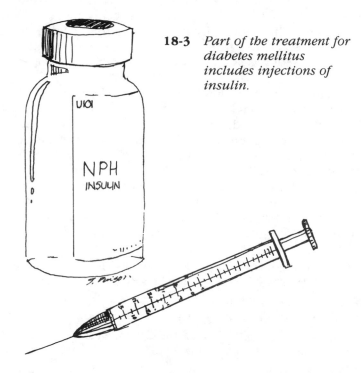

18-3 *Part of the treatment for diabetes mellitus includes injections of insulin.*

Often, dogs are presented with complicated cases of diabetes mellitus because of some underlying disorder adding to the problem. For instance, many of these dogs suffer from coexisting disorders such as obesity, pancreatitis, kidney disease, and heart disease. In order to increase the chances of recovery from a complicated case of diabetes mellitus, these disorders must be addressed at the same time.

For those cases of uncomplicated diabetes mellitus exhibiting no immediate life-threatening clinical signs, treatment is aimed at keeping blood glucose levels between 200 mg/dl just prior to insulin administration and 60 mg/dl at the peak of the insulin activity. Because of the danger of insulin shock (hypoglycemia) if too much insulin is given, the first few injections should be performed by a veterinarian in a hospital to help establish a proper starting dosage.

Pet owners should realize that there are different types of insulin. The type that should be used for maintaining blood glucose levels in dogs is called *NPH insulin,* and it, along with insulin syringes for administration, are available at pharmacies with a prescription. This type of insulin reaches its peak action after administration in six to 12 hours and lasts anywhere from 18 to 24 hours total. As a result, only one injection per day is required.

At-home care for diabetic dogs

When a pet finally comes home, it will be the owner's job to ensure that a proper dose is given each day and that adjustments are made in the dosage if necessary. This is done by monitoring urine glucose levels using special test strips available from pharmacies. These test strips will represent urine glucose levels as either a percentage or as a number followed by a +.

For example, each morning, a urine sample should be obtained and a urine glucose strip be run. Ideally, the strip should read 1 + (1/4%)to **trace** (1/10%) just prior to the administration of the day's insulin. If it indeed does read this, then the same dose of insulin that was given the day before should be administered again. If the urine glucose strip reads **negative**, then the dosage of insulin used must be cut back. Along the same lines, if the reading is greater than 1 + (1/4%) then the insulin dosage must be increased accordingly. The following is an insulin dosing schedule that should be used to help establish and maintain a proper insulin dose for a diabetic pet. All injections should be given under the skin in the neck or shoulder regions.

If the morning urine glucose levels are at **4 +** (2%) *increase* the previous day's insulin dosage by *2 units* and administer.

If the morning urine glucose levels are at **3 +** (1%), then *increase* the previous day's insulin dosage by *1 unit* and administer.

If the morning urine glucose levels are at **2 +** (1/2%), then *increase* the previous day's insulin dosage by 1/2 unit and administer.

If the morning urine glucose levels are at 1+ (¹/₄%) or **trace** (¹/₁₀%), then give the *same* dose of insulin as was given the previous day.

If the morning urine glucose level is **negative**, then *decrease* the previous day's insulin dosage by *2 units* and administer.

Keep in mind that it is better to give too little insulin than to give too much. Adjustments to insulin dosages need to be made slowly and carefully in these uncomplicated cases. Giving too much insulin can cause insulin shock (hypoglycemia), which can be fatal. Signs of this can include trembling, weakness, incoordination, and, if it is not rapidly corrected, seizures. Owners of diabetic pets should always keep a bottle of pancake syrup or honey around in case of insulin shock. Two tablespoons or more given orally should be used if such a reaction is suspected.

Owners must keep accurate records each day as to their pet's morning urine glucose levels, insulin dosage, overall attitude and/or clinical signs that day, and appetite. These will not only come in useful in regulating insulin levels, but such records can provide a veterinarian with valuable information should a question or problem ever arise.

Strict feeding schedules for dogs with diabetes mellitus must be followed. Rations high in fiber and protein with restricted fat and carbohydrates are ideal for maintaining the diabetic dog. One-third of the total daily ration should be fed at the time the insulin injection is given; the rest of the ration should be offered eight to ten hours later. A small portion of this latter feeding may even be set aside to feed just prior to bedtime. Just be sure to remain consistent in all feeding practices.

Diabetic dogs must also be kept on a consistent exercise program, since fluctuations in the amount of exercise performed from one day to the other can effect blood glucose levels and make proper insulin dosing difficult. If a dog is obese to start with, it will need to be placed on a weight reduction program.

Finally, if you own an intact female dog that is diabetic, your veterinarian will recommend that it be spayed. By eliminating female hormonal influences on glucose levels in the body, achieving and maintaining proper insulin levels will be greatly enhanced.

If you have any questions regarding dosage regulations, clinical signs seen, or any abnormalities you note in your records, don't hesitate to contact your veterinarian at once.

DIABETES INSIPIDUS

This type of diabetes should not be confused with diabetes mellitus, which involves abnormal glucose metabolism. *Diabetes insipidus* involves abnormal water metabolism, and it occurs when there is a lack of the hormone antidiuretic hormone (ADH). ADH is normally produced by the hypothalamus of the brain, yet it exerts its effects on the kidneys, causing water to be recaptured from the kidney tubules rather than being lost in the urine. As a result, the delicate water balance within the body is maintained with this hormones influence.

Too little ADH may be produced by the hypothalamus as the result of an inherited defect or due to head trauma that damages the hypothalamus. In addition, defects present in the kidneys at birth or acquired later in life can make the kidneys unresponsive or only partially responsive to the effects of ADH. If any of the above situations occur, then diabetes insipidus results.

Symptoms

Dogs with diabetes insipidus exhibit increased urinations, incontinence (especially at night), and an increased water consumption. Routine laboratory work usually reveals nothing too significant except for very low urine specific gravity (dilute urine). However, a laboratory work-up will help rule out other potential causes of the clinical signs seen, such as diabetes mellitus, Cushing's disease, and kidney disease. If these are ruled out, then a tentative diagnosis of diabetes insipidus becomes more likely. To obtain a definitive diagnosis, special laboratory tests, such as water deprivation tests, plasma ADH determinations, and ADH trials, are required.

Treatment

Diabetes insipidus caused by poor ADH production from the hypothalamus can be treated by administering a natural or synthetic ADH supplement. Injections of such supplements can be administered at home, or, more recently, synthetic ADH drops can be applied directly into the eyes, with subsequent absorption into the body. Such treatment will be required on a daily basis to control the clinical signs. Therapy is usually for life.

Diabetes insipidus caused by kidneys that are nonresponsive to ADH is more difficult to control. Special drugs called *thiazide diuretics* can be utilized to slow water loss and reduce thirst in dogs so affected.

Providing free access to water at all times is the most important therapeutic measure for all dogs suffering from diabetes insipidus. Doing so will help prevent dehydration and its undesirable effects from setting in as a result of the excess water loss through the kidneys.

The prognosis for most dogs with diabetes insipidus is good to excellent, assuming that medical therapy and free access to water is provided. Because these pets are prone to dehydration, any signs of illness such as loss of appetite, vomiting, diarrhea, etc. warrant prompt veterinary attention.

CATS

IF THERE EVER WAS a creature that stirred the fascination and admiration of mankind throughout the ages, it is the cat. Cat fanciers have existed for thousands of years, captivated by the personal, yet seemingly independent nature of these graceful animals.

The cat is a descendent of *Miacis*, a cat-like creature that lived over 40 million years ago and gave rise to not only the modern-day cat, but to the dog and the bear as well. The modern cat, *Felis catus*, is a direct descendent of *Felis libyca*, the African wildcat, and *Felis sylvestris*, a European wildcat with a tabby-like appearance.

Interestingly enough, over the years, the cat has not had much selective breeding brought on by domestication. As a result, it has the closest ties to its "wild" ancestors when compared to other domesticated animals. Evidence of this is the similar size and anatomic features of all cats. Save for certain muzzle and coat lengths, as well as color, different breeds of cats all look alike. Compare this, if you will, to the dog, which comes in so many sizes, shapes, and varieties, brought on by domestication and selective breeding.

Cats first associated with man back in the Stone Age, where they probably hung around the camp for food scraps and leftovers. It was not until ancient Egyptian times that man and feline became true companions. Cats were used to hunt birds and catch fish for the Egyptians, and to rid their granaries of rats and mice. So revered did the cat become in this society that goddesses were fashioned after its image, and separate burial grounds were set aside for the mummified remains of those felines that departed from this world.

As the world trade routes opened up and the high seas became an important means of interaction between countries and peoples, the cat spread throughout the civilized world. Longer-haired varieties soon developed, and became highly favored in the European community—favored, that is, until the Dark Ages, when superstition began to run rampant and cats became symbols of evil and witchcraft. They quickly lost their favored status, and the European cat population fell into decline. Unfortunately, when the Crusaders returned from the Holy Land carrying plague-laded brown rats with them on their ships, there were few cats around to meet this threat.

As the bubonic plague devastated Europe, the importance of the predatory nature of the cat increased, and numbers were soon back on the rise. As their status in society was regained, cats found their way back into the farmer's granaries and into the courts of royalty. To this day, in the eyes of millions of cat fanciers, they still command a royal status in our society!

19

Choosing the Right
Cat for You

WHEN IT COMES TIME to choose that perfect feline companion, what criteria should you follow to be certain your selection is a sound one? Some questions you should ask yourself include the following:

○ What type of cat do I want?
○ Will my cat be housed indoors or outdoors?
○ How will existing pets (if any) be affected?
○ How much time and money am I willing to devote to my new cat?

The manner in which you answer these questions will have great bearing on your selection process.

WHY DO YOU WANT A CAT?

Companionship is the most popular reason for choosing a cat as a pet. Although they can be somewhat independent at times, cats can be just as loving as a big, shaggy dog and can provide owners with hours of enjoyment at a time just watching their antics! Any breed, pedigreed or otherwise, can make a wonderful companion, so choose based on your own individual fancy (FIG. 19-1).

Cats and children

Cats can provide an excellent means for educating and teaching children about responsibility of pet ownership and about the cycle of life itself. Before obtaining one for your children, however, keep these following guidelines in mind.

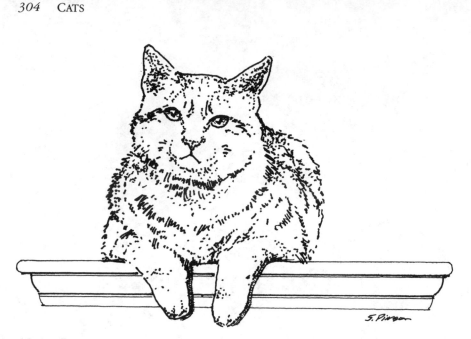

19-1   *Be sure to choose your cat based on your own personal fancies.*

First, for maximum benefit and enjoyment, consider waiting until your children are at least 5 years of age before acquiring a new kitten or cat. Younger children, some of whom might just be starting to crawl or walk, stand a greater chance of being accidentally hurt by a playful nip or scratch than do older ones. In addition, older children are better equipped to learn about and undertake responsibilities associated with cat ownership and can become active participants in the feeding, care, and—don't forget!—the litter box duties—of their new friend.

Choose a kitten with an outgoing personality; one that can stand up to the rigors of ownership by a child. Shy, introverted kittens rarely satisfy the energy requirements of children, and these cats might not think twice to scratch or bite when annoyed.

Along these lines, domestic short-hairs or long-hairs are preferred over pedigreed cats as pets for children, simply because they are considered less excitable than some of the more emotional purebreds.

Where children are concerned, it is best to limit your selection of a kitten to one that is between 8 and 12 weeks of age. Because socialization naturally occurs during this time, a greater bond will form between the cat and your child. One word of caution: Be certain that your child is not allowed to abuse or hurt his new kitten during this sensitive period. Such an adverse interaction could easily ruin their relationship for years to come. It is every parent's responsibility to teach their children that their new cuddly friend is not a toy, and that it needs to be handled with loving care.

Breeding

Some people look to cat ownership for money. For many, breeding pedigreed cats is looked upon as big business. Yet it is a financial responsibility and should never be taken lightly. Most novices find out the hard way that breeding operations, if done correctly and humanely (and they should always be), represent a considerable investment in time and in money. If you are a beginner to the cat-breeding business, be sure to become an expert on the business and on the breed or breeds you want to propagate before your first purchase.

It is wise, if you are a beginner, to confine your efforts to one of the more popular breeds, such as the Siamese or Himalayan, rather than starting with those more exotic, delicate strains, such as the Egyptian Mau and Havana Brown. Remember, the more popular the breed, the greater the demand will be for your kittens, resulting in greater financial rewards.

But beware: When selecting your initial breeding stock, closely scrutinize the pedigree of the parents. All that it takes is one genetic defect to appear in one or more of the offspring, and your reputation as a cat breeder could be ruined!

Competition

For cat lovers, the pleasure of ownership and/or breeding is compounded by the thrill of competition in the show ring. Competitive events involving cats have been around since the 1800s. Each year, events are sanctioned by a number of different cat fanciers' associations throughout the world. At such functions, serious breeders have the opportunity to earn the reputation of producing champion-quality felines—rewarding not only to the ego, but also the pocketbook!

But you don't need to own a purebred cat to enter the show ring. Most events have a special show class in which an average house cat can compete. If you are interested in showing cats, there are many good books available at the library or bookstore that can help you on your way. For a list of upcoming competitions, contact a local cat club or breeder listed in the phone book.

A word of warning . . .

Although your intentions might be pure and good-hearted, never, ever surprise someone with a new cat or kitten unless you are positively, absolutely sure that they want one in the first place. Think about it: Your gift to them not only includes that furry bundle of energy, but a hearty commitment to time, money, and responsibility.

Unfortunately, too many people do fail to think about this, and as a result, our nation's pounds and shelters are overflowing with unwanted cats turned in by disgruntled or disinterested gift recipients or picked up off of the street. Allow these people to come to a decision about pet ownership by themselves, and don't force it on them with your good intentions. Everyone will be happier in the long run!

WHAT TYPE OF CAT DO YOU WANT?

The choice of your cat's pedigree is entirely up to you. If you choose to go the purebred route, expect to pay more up front for your purchase. In addition, because of selective breeding, you might run a greater risk of facing congenital problems inherent to that particular breed or pedigree. However, such risks can be minimized by being very cautious and prudent in your selection process.

If you are like many cat fanciers, you may be less finicky about a lengthy pedigree and instead prefer your average domestic short-hair (DSH), medium-hair (DMH), or long-hair (DLH) cat. These certainly cost much less than their papered counterparts, and they might even exhibit a genetic phenomenon known as *hybrid vigor,* which has a positive impact on the health and longevity of these individuals (TABLE 19-1).

Table 19-1   The 10 Most Popular Cat Breeds

1	Persian
2	Siamese
3	Abbysinian
4	Maine Coon
5	Burmese
6	Oriental Short Hair
7	Exotic Short Hair
8	American Short Hair
9	Scottish Fold
10	Burman

Source: Cat Fanciers Association, 1990

DO YOU WANT AN INDOOR OR OUTDOOR CAT?

For some reason, many cat owners are under the false impression that a cat cannot be happy unless it is roaming free outdoors. Although this might have been the standard of thinking years back, it is time that cat owners change their attitudes towards this subject. Aside from the obvious health hazards afforded to outdoors cat—such as car fenders, hostile dogs, hostile humans, and feline leukemia— there is another important reason that has just come to the forefront in recent years: Feline AIDS. The epidemic is real, and unless cat owners shield their pets from contact with carriers of the disease roaming the neighborhood, there is a good chance their cats will also be exposed to the disease (see chapter 24).

In addition, cats allowed to roam freely outdoors stand a greater chance of transmitting a zoonotic disease, such as ringworm, toxoplasmosis, or larval migrans to their owners.

HOW WILL YOUR EXISTING PETS BE AFFECTED?

Are there other dogs or cats in your household already? Jealousies or incompatibilities could arise, and you need anticipate them before you bring home your new kitten or cat.

Any newcomer should be gradually introduced to the old-timer, a day at a time. Keep your new kitten or cat in a separate room or yard, allowing interactions to take place only under your direct supervision. These gradual encounters should eventually help break the ice between the two and help establish a social pecking order within your furry family.

ARE YOU WILLING TO BE A RESPONSIBLE PET OWNER?

Reduced time requirements is a big reason many people choose cats over dogs as pets. Cats are indeed fairly self-sufficient, seemingly needing only food, water, a clean litter box, and very little training. While this is true in many instances, all cats also need some type of daily attention and grooming given to them as well.

Although behavioral problems associated with attention deprivation aren't as common with cats as with their canine counterparts, keep in mind that many cats need just as much daily pampering as dogs do to keep them content. If you aren't able to devote much time to your new pet, consider substituting an additional feline companion in your place.

The financial aspect of pet ownership is a major consideration if you are in the market for any type of pet. The actual cost of owning a cat—food, supplies (including litterboxes, scratching posts, etc.), and veterinary care—can easily exceed $300 per year. Are you willing to accept financial responsibility for your cat's preventative health care, or for medical treatment in an event of an injury or illness? Sometimes this can run into the hundreds, maybe into the thousands of dollars. If you feel uneasy about such responsibility, you might not be ready for pet ownership.

FINDING THE RIGHT CAT

Once you've decided on a particular type or breed of cat, now is the time to start your search. Newspapers, pet stores, veterinary hospitals, and word of mouth are fruitful avenues to utilize for information.

If you're not interested in a pedigreed feline, check the local humane society or animal shelter in your area. These are excellent places to start, and they are often jam-packed with cats and kittens eager to be adopted into happy homes. Usually one can be yours to love for a nominal adoption fee. As an added benefit, you will feel good knowing that you've saved an unwanted pet from an uncertain future.

If a registered purebred fits your fancy, check pet stores, or contact cat breeders within your area. Local veterinarians and groomers can often provide specific recommendations. Magazines catering to cat owners can also be excellent reference sources. Finally, cat shows provide a means of giving you a first-hand glimpse of the cream of the crop and for meeting prominent breeders in person.

Before you go shopping, do your homework. Find out what the going rate is for the particular breed you want. Beware of the small-time operator who advertises or offers you a great deal on a "registered" kitten. These so called "great-deals" could end up costing you more in the long run in medical bills and emotional drain. Where quality counts, stick with reputable breeders who can provide you with the complete pedigrees of both parents, and with references of satisfied clients.

This rule holds true for pet-store purchases as well. Before buying from a pet store, ask where the kitten came from; who the breeder was. Ask to see the pedigrees of both parents. Reputable pet stores will have all this information readily available for your inspection. And ask for references from satisfied customers. If the store is unwilling or unable to divulge such information, look elsewhere.

Whatever you do, don't rush your decision. Remember: You are fixing to make a long-term commitment. Take your time, and pick out that special feline just right for you!

PRE-PURCHASE EXAM

Once you think you've found the perfect companion, now what? For starters, you want to be sure you are getting a healthy specimen. Be sure to inquire about the cat's vaccination/deworming history. You might be told that all of the "shots" and dewormings have been given. While this might be true, don't hesitate to ask for dates and names of products used in writing. This list can then be reviewed for completeness by your veterinarian during his/her pre-purchase exam. Inquire as to any prior feline leukemia or feline AIDS testing. Kittens can be born with these diseases, so be certain you know their status before you buy.

Even before your veterinarian becomes involved, perform your own pre-purchase exam on the prospective feline. Such an exam is easy to do on-site, and it will help illuminate many problems that might otherwise elude the untrained eye.

1. Environment For starters, take note of the surrounding environment the kitten or cat is being kept in. Does it look and smell clean, or is it filthy, with unkempt litter boxes or no litter boxes at all? You can bet that if it appears unclean, you should begin to question the integrity of the seller.

Observe all of the kittens in the litter. Do any appear sickly, depressed, or otherwise unhealthy? Infectious diseases such as feline upper respiratory infections can have free run through such a congregation of kittens, and it could be just beginning to rear its ugly head within the group.

2. Attitude   Now focus your attention on the actual candidate. Start with overall attitude. Does it appear active and healthy, or is it lethargic and depressed? Are breathing problems evident? Does it seem friendly and outgoing to people, and to the other kittens in the group, or does it seem shy and introverted? Cats and kittens destined to be good pets should take an instant fancy to people and should outwardly show this affection. At the same time, avoid those individuals with overbearing and domineering personalities. Observe how your favorite treats other members of its group. Domineering personalities are usually quite evident. As a general rule, choose one that is middle of the road: Not too domineering, yet not too shy.

3. Skin and Coat   Once attitude and personality have been evaluated, check out the skin and coat. Any fleas or ticks present? How about any hair loss, scabs, or signs of infection? These could be indicators of diseases, such as mange or ringworm, both of which have *zoonotic* (diseases passed from pets to people) potential. Also, since cats are such meticulous self-groomers, an unkempt hair coat could signify parasitism or some other underlying health disorder.

4. Abdomen   Does the kitten's belly seem distended? If so, it could be full of food, or it could be full of worms or coccidia. Check beneath the tail, looking for tapeworm segments (see chapter 25) and for evidence of diarrhea. Soiling on and around the hair in this area should tip you off to this.

5. Other Anatomical Considerations   Observe leg conformation, and the way the kitten walks and runs. Any obvious deformities and/or lameness should be noted. In males, check for descent of the testicles. Both should be down at birth; if they aren't, be prepared to neuter at a later date, not only for health reasons, but also to prevent the passage of this inheritable trait to future generations.

6. Head Region   Now focus in on the head region. Using your eyes and your nose, check the ears for discharges or strong odors (usually a sign of infection or ear mites). Both eyes should be free of matter, with no cloudiness or redness. Compare both eyes, making sure they are of the same size, and that the pupils are of the same diameter. Glance at the nose, noting any discharges or crustiness to it. Finally, look into the mouth. The gums should be nice and pink; if they are whitish, the kitten could be anemic. Notice any severe underbites/overbites, or any missing teeth. Also look at the roof of the mouth. In young kittens, a cleft palate is a serious birth defect, and unless it is surgically corrected, it will ultimately lead to secondary aspiration pneumonia and death.

Consulting your veterinarian

Let's say you've completed the above exam and have found some potential problem areas. What do you do next? Well, first of all, don't get discouraged. Many of these potential problem areas have quick, inexpensive solutions. This is where your veterinarian comes in handy.

Don't feel awkward asking the seller to pick up the tab for a professional pre-purchase exam by a veterinarian of your choice. Those sellers confident in the quality of their product should have no qualms about this. If they balk, a warning light should flash in your head. And don't get suckered into a "money-back guarantee" or a "lifetime guarantee" on a pet as an alternative to a professional pre-purchase screen. Such a guarantee doesn't protect you against the emotional distress caused by returning a pet you've already grown fond of.

Follow your veterinarian's recommendations as to the purchase quality of the cat or kitten in question. If the one you have your heart set on has medical problems that can be corrected easily, talk to the seller and see if he or she won't deduct these costs from the purchase price. They aren't obligated but by character to do so, so you must decide on your next move if they refuse or fail to compromise. The extra expense out of your own pocketbook might be worth it if you think you have truly found the feline of your dreams! You be the judge.

CAT-PROOFING YOUR HOME

Upon arrival home, you'll want to do everything in your power to make your new cat feel comfortable and secure in its new home (TABLE 19-2). Your new cat's first encounters with your family are important. Be sure initial introductions, be they with children or other adults in the family, turn out to be positive ones. Carefully supervise children-pet interactions, and stress to the former the importance of gentle play and handling.

Table 19-2 Supply Checklist for Your New Cat

☐ Food and water bowls	☐ Litter box
☐ Cat (kitten) food	☐ Cat litter
☐ Harness/collar	☐ Bed
☐ Leash	☐ Travel kennel
☐ Toys	☐ Nail trimmers
☐ Identification tag	☐ Ear cleanser
☐ City license (if required)	☐ Toothbrush/paste
☐ Proof of rabies vaccination	☐ Brush/comb
☐ Scratching post	☐ Flea control products

Instruct your children and other adults on the proper way to pick up and hold the new kitten. Cats should not be picked up solely by the front legs or by the midsection; instead, the entire body should be picked up as one unit, with the hind end supported, not left dangling in mid-air. Picking a cat up by grasping the skin over the back of the neck is acceptable as long as the hind end is supported as well.

If they had it their way, most children—and some adults, for that matter—would love to play with a new kitten 24 hours out of the day. You need to stress the importance of rest times for their new kitten after periods of play, and lay strict ground rules against disturbing it while it is in bed or in the litter box.

Although most cats kept indoors have the run of the house, yours should have one special area it can call its own. When you bring your new friend home for the first time, have a special area equipped with a cushioned bed or basket set aside. For kittens, cardboard boxes work just fine, assuming that easy access into them is provided. Be sure this sleeping quarter is in a part of the house away from noise and disturbances.

Your cat's litter box should also be placed in an area in the house where interruptions are not likely to occur. For very small kittens, an aluminum pan or shallow tray may be used; for larger kittens and adult cats, your standard plastic varieties available from a pet shop work just fine.

Avoid using boxes or other cardboard devices for a litter box. Not only do they have a tendency to leak, but their porous nature is most unsanitary to your cat. Covered litter boxes have the advantage of keeping the litter from being strewn across the floor—assuming, of course, that the cat will even enter such an enclosure!

You can use standard clay, a mixture of clay and potting soil, shredded newspaper, or most commercial cat litters in the litter box. Avoid those products containing chlorophyll to mask odors; this substance can irritate a cat's nose and prevent it from using the box. Regardless of the type of litter you use, fill the bottom tray with about one and 1/2 inches of litter. For sanitation purposes as well as esthetics within the house, make it a habit of changing your cat's litter box on a daily basis. **Note:** Pregnant women should pass this duty on to someone else, in order to reduce their risk of exposure to toxoplasmosis (see chapter 53). Litter boxes should also be emptied and cleaned with soap and water at least weekly to maintain sanitary conditions and to control odor.

Finally, here's a valuable tip regarding litter box duty: Feeding your cat a high-quality diet cannot only cut down on stool volume tremendously, making your job much easier, but many of those diets can also cut down on stool odor as well. Ask your veterinarian for more details.

Unless you plan to have your cat declawed at a young age, you will also need to invest in a good scratching post to hopefully spare your furniture and fixtures from the ravages of nature (FIG. 19-2). Clawing comes naturally to cats, who use such behavior to keep their nails in good working order and to mark their territory. The scratching post should be made of sturdy material and be heavy enough or braced so they don't fall over when the cat attempts to scratch. A sturdy piece of soft wood is ideal for this purpose; other types can be obtained from pet stores. Avoid those lined with thick, compliant carpet, as this might not satisfy your cat's needs, causing it to look elsewhere for a surface that will (see chapter 20).

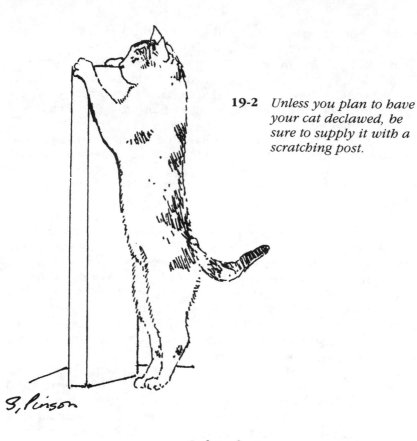

19-2 *Unless you plan to have your cat declawed, be sure to supply it with a scratching post.*

S. Pinson

Safety first

For your cat's sake be sure to take necessary steps to pet-proof your home. Because cats can be very inquisitive creatures, and because they have the ability to scale heights, you will need to take even more care when you are doing this than if a dog was involved.

Keep all plants out of reach. Cats and kittens love to chew on foliage, and they also enjoy using potting soil as litter. As a result, they have the ability to quickly dispose of precious house plants in either of these manners. Also, if they decide to nibble on a harmful ornamented variety of plant, they could poison themselves.

Next, keep electrical cords well out of reach. This might mean banishing your cat or kitten from certain areas of the house, but it's a minor inconvenience compared to a potentially fatal accident.

Pins, needles, knives, rubber bands, yarn, string, ribbons, aluminum foil, cellophane, and holiday tinsel are just a few items that could cause serious health problems in the cat accidentally or purposely allowed to play with them. Inquisitive cats have been known to get their heads lodged within open cans and jars, and because cats possess a strange attraction to bags of all types, plastic bags can become death traps if entered.

Finally, because of the cat's desire to explore its environment and to see how high it can climb, washers/dryers, drawers, high ledges or balconies, hot irons on ironing boards, and stovetop burners left on can all be insidious dangers to your cat's health.

When selecting toys for your new kitten or cat, be sure they cannot be torn apart easily and that they do not contain small parts that could be swallowed. Wrinkled paper and shoe boxes are intriguing to most cats. Rubber balls or mice too large to swallow, as well as catnip toys (again, constructed for safety), are also considered safe toys. If a string is attached to a toy in order to entice a cat to play, always remove it after the play session is over. Along the same lines, never use ribbon or laces as play items. If a cat swallows such things, they could damage the intestines and require surgical removal.

NAMING YOUR CAT

Naming your new pet should be fun and involve the entire family. You can even find at your favorite bookstore entire books that are dedicated to choosing the right name for your cat. Stick to names having two syllables; this will allow your cat to differentiate between its name and those one-syllable commands you might choose to teach it. You can further set its name apart from potential commands or reprimands by adding a vowel sound to the end of it.

TRAVELING WITH YOUR CAT

When transporting a cat by car, the comfort and safety of both driver and passenger must always be considered. Whether you are bringing it home for the first time, or simply taking it on a Sunday afternoon drive, keep three rules in mind which will make the ride easier and safer for the both of you.

For starters, when traveling by car, it is always recommended that your cat be confined to its travel carrier or kennel (FIG. 19-3). Not only will this help provide a secure feeling and ease travel anxieties , but it will also ensure a safe trip for you.

Regardless of trip length, keep the interior of your car well-ventilated and cool. Excited or nervous cats forced to travel in hot, stuffy environments, or ones filled with cigarette smoke, are prime candidates for car sickness. Cigarette smoke in itself can be quite irritating to the eyes, nose, and mucus membranes of cats, so if you have to smoke in the car, don't forget about your friend next to you. Crack the windows a bit, yet not enough to allow your cat to escape if it gets out of its carrier!

Car exhaust fumes can also be nauseating to traveling cats. For this reason, crack the windows about a third of the way open while you are traveling to ensure adequate ventilation.

Finally, if the car ride is going to be over three hours in length, be sure to take along litter box accommodations and plenty of water for your

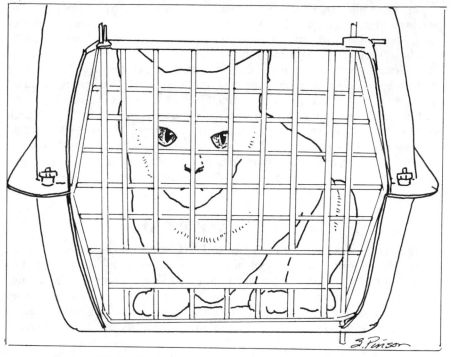

19-3 *Most cats prefer to travel in a carrier.*

cat to drink. Cats traveling via automobile have the potential to lose lots of body water through panting, and can develop quite a thirst in a very short period of time. Keep water in the carrier itself. Freeze some water prior to the trip in the water bowl intended for the carrier to provide a long-lasting source of water for those extra-long sojourns. Take rest stops every few hours to allow your pet to relieve itself in the litter box, and allow some time for exercise sessions (this is where harness-training a cat can come in handy!).

If motion sickness becomes a problem for your cat, there are a few measures that you can take. First, observe when your pet gets car sick: Is there normally food in the vomitus, or is it just liquid? If food is present, be sure to withhold food before further travels.

If, on the other hand, food is not present, try feeding your cat a small amount prior to the trip. For cats with sensitive stomachs, a little bit of food in the stomach is often all it takes to do the trick.

For those cats absolutely terrified of the car, actual tranquilization prescribed by your veterinarian might be necessary. Though this should be used only as a last resort, it can be an effective tool for taking the edge off of your feline friend and make the ride much less stressful for everyone concerned.

If your feline is traveling by air, you will need to obtain a health certificate from your veterinarian usually within 10 days of your trip. In addition, many airlines require their own flight certificates endorsed by the pet's veterinarian certifying that the pet is healthy enough to undergo the plane ride. Check with your flight carrier to see if such an authorization is required.

Try to take only nonstop flights with your pet; connecting flights and airplane changes only serve to increase your cat's stress and increase the chance of "lost baggage" (such as your cat!).

Carrying flight insurance on your cat might help to increase the gentleness and care with which it is handled. The night prior to the trip, freeze some water in the travel carrier water dish to ensure your cat continued access to water during the trip. Tranquilization should be reserved only for those cats that are absolutely terrified of travel.

20

Training Your Cat

ONCE YOUR NEW FAMILY member has settled into its new home, you are now ready for the next step: Training. Contrary to popular belief, many cats can be just as trainable as dogs. Keep in mind that the sometimes inherent independent nature of cats can make certain training procedures a bit tricky, but if you maintain an understanding attitude towards it, your frustrations will be minimal and your rewards plentiful.

BASIC TRAINING

All cats should be trained to walk on a leash at an early age. Why? By teaching your cat to accept a leash and harness, you will be able to institute a daily exercise program for it, keeping it fit and healthy. In addition, since allowing a cat to roam freely outdoors these days is becoming more and more dangerous because of the many life-threatening diseases cats are susceptible to, a leash-trained cat can enjoy the great outdoors, yet in a supervised manner. Finally, many travelers find that leash-training comes in quite handy at rest-stops during lengthy trips (FIG. 20-1).

Before you attach a leash to your kitten or cat, it must become accustomed to a halter. Because halters provide more control and security than do collars, the latter should not be used to walk a cat on a leash. Place the new halter on your cat and allow it to wear it around the house for 10 to 15 minutes at a time. Then take it off, and repeat the process at three-hour intervals throughout the day. Eventually lengthen the time you leave the halter on until your cat will wear it all day without a fuss.

At this point, attach a leash to the halter and allow your cat to drag the leash around for 10 to 15 minutes at a time before removing it. Repeat this

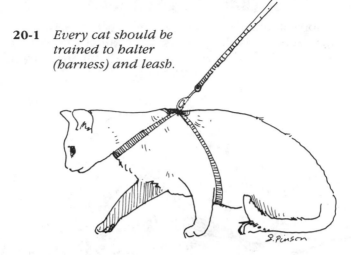

20-1 *Every cat should be trained to halter (harness) and leash.*

procedure throughout the day for a week or so. Keep in mind never to let your cat walk around unsupervised with the leash dangling free. If it gets snagged on something, your cat could seriously injure itself.

Once you feel your cat has become accustomed to the leash, then practice lead walking with it indoors for a week or two. Only after your cat gives you total compliance should you attempt the same maneuver outdoors. If everything goes as planned, be sure to reward your cat for a job well done. A scratch behind the ears or under the chin, or a favorite food treat, does wonders to help solidify and promote such favorable behavior.

Other commands

If you so desire, teach your cat commands as you would a dog (see chapter 2). Remember: Because of the very nature of the feline, you can't always expect 100% compliance; simply take all successes and run with them! One helpful tip to apply is to hold your training sessions when your cat is hungry. In that way, food rewards become powerful motivators for good behavior.

LITTER TRAINING YOUR KITTEN

Kittens will be instinctively drawn to litter or dirt in which to eliminate as early as 4 to 6 weeks of age. As a result, housebreaking a kitten usually involves minimal effort on the owner's part. Introducing new kittens to the litter box after eating, playing, waking up, or just before bedtime will help accustom your new addition to its litter box and encourage repeat use. If your cat doesn't seem to catch on, there might be some reason for its reluctance to use the litter box. If so, it is your job to find out why (see House Soiling).

SOCIALIZING YOUR CAT

As with a puppy, a kitten's socialization period falls between 3 and 12 weeks of age. During this short time span, a kitten will learn who it is, who you are, and who and what all of those other living, moving beings in its surroundings are as well (FIG. 20-2).

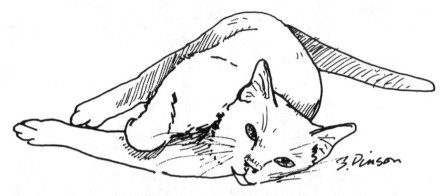

20-2   *Socialization is just as important for cats as it is for dogs.*

If for some reason a kitten fails to be properly introduced to members of its own species, or to other species as well (including children) during this time, then there is a good chance that it will not "recognize" these individuals for who they are, and your cat might even show aggressiveness or excessive timidity towards them. An excellent example of the socialization principle is the relationship between cats and mice. Cats and mice can become the best of buddies if they grow up together and a strong socialization takes place; if such socialization is missed . . . well, you know what happens!

Improper or negative socialization is even worse than no socialization at all. Any traumatic experience or physical punishment that occurs between 3 and 12 weeks of age could permanently scar a cat's personality towards a specific group or species for life. This is one reason why all physical punishment should be avoided during this time in your kitten's life. Such activity could damage the kitten's relationship with the punisher for life!

SOLVING PROBLEM BEHAVIORS IN CATS

When searching for the leading cause of dissatisfaction among cat owners, problem behaviors top the list. Each year, a multitude of cats are abandoned, evicted from their homes, or even put to sleep because of annoying behavioral activity. However, by understanding why these behaviors happen and by employing special training techniques or therapy to correct such vices, cat owners can often avert such drastic actions as those mentioned above.

House soiling

Cats exhibit two types of normal elimination behavior. The first involves urine spraying to delineate territories (the typical feline territory encompasses over one-tenth of a square mile) and to attract members of the opposite sex. The second type is called *covering behavior*, in which a cat digs a hole in the soil (or litter), eliminates in it, and then covers it to mask the scent. Most inappropriate house soilings that occur with cats involve indulgences or deviations in one or the other.

The most frequent cause of house soiling deals with the first type, territoriality and sexual instincts. Both male and female cats, neutered or not, can exhibit such urine spraying behavior (FIG. 20-3).

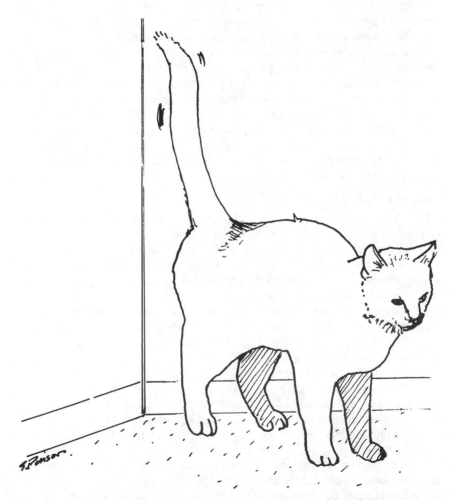

20-3 *Urine spraying is an annoying problem behavior.*

A new cat in the neighborhood or a female in heat can quickly set off instinctive behavior in a male cat kept indoors and lead to inappropriate markings. Even moving into a new house or apartment in which a cat previously lived might entice your cat to go around the house and mark those areas in which a scent from the previous inhabitant is picked up.

Neutering might help control urine spraying in the repeat offender, yet as mentioned before, it is not necessarily a cure-all. If there is a particular area in the house that your cat fancies the most for its spraying activities, prevent its access to that part of the house, or catch it in the act and punish it using a water sprayer or a blast of air from a compressed air canister. Then leave the sprayer or canister sitting beside the object or in the room in question for a few days. Chances are, your cat will get the drift and will abandon the desire to repeat the action.

Feline odor neutralizers used on carpets and furniture can help eliminate those lingering odors that might be originating the problem behavior. They should also be used anytime an elimination accident occurs outside of the litter box. These odor neutralizers are available from your veterinarian or your favorite pet supply. Household cleaners designed to simply mask odors or those containing ammonia are of no use; in fact, the latter might actually attract your cat back to the same spot.

For those tough cases of urine spraying in which nothing seems to work, special hormone therapy prescribed by your veterinarian might provide a satisfactory solution to the problem. Like any medications, these hormones are not sometimes without their side effects, and these should only be employed as a last resort.

Refusal to use the litter box

What about the cat that has stopped using the litter box? There could be a number of reasons for this unexpected refusal. Some of these cats don't like the type of litter that was put in the box. Have you changed brands lately? If so, switch back to the brand you were using before the house soiling started. Remember that litter filled with scents designed to mask cat-box odors might turn a cat off.

Some cats become upset if there is too much litter being placed in their box. Cats should be able to reach the bottom of their pan during their digging. If you have one of these fickle cats, restocking the box with a one-inch layer of litter might do the trick.

Still other cats will refuse to use a litter box that, in their minds, is dirty. Check your frequency of litter changes; if the litter is not being replaced every day or two, this could be the problem. Be careful not to use strong cleansers when doing your weekly litter box cleaning, as these too might be just enough to send your cat off searching for another place to do its business.

Another reason your cat might stop using the litter box might be traced to some traumatic incident, emotionally or physically, that occurred while it was using the box on a previous occasion. Because of this, it now associates the box or, more commonly, its location with the unpleasant incident. Obviously, the best way to find out if this is indeed the cause is to move the litter box to a different location, one that is quiet and away from disturbances. For those cats who are especially emotional, changing litter boxes might be required as well.

Not all causes of house soiling are psychological. The presence of feline urologic syndrome or other types of urinary tract diseases can be the underlying cause of abnormal elimination behavior in felines. Since some of these health disorders, especially feline urologic syndrome, can be life-threatening, always let your veterinarian rule out any medical causes for the house soiling before concentrating on the mental solutions to the problem (see chapter 30).

Destructive scratching

Scratching comes naturally to cats, who use this behavior to keep their retractable claws manicured (since a dog's claws are not retractable, they are manicured by everyday contact with floors or other hard surfaces) and to mark territories. As a result, scratching, though it might become destructive and annoying, should be viewed as a perfectly natural behavior.

If your cat is engaged in destructive scratching, you haven't satisfied one of its needs. A scratching post is a required tool for anyone who owns a cat. In fact, it is preferable to train a cat on a scratching post right from the start instead of bringing one in to offset problem scratching activity. See chapter 19 for more information on choosing and employing a scratching post for your cat.

If your cat seems to fancy one or more particular pieces of furniture in your house, see if you can catch it in the act (FIG. 20-4). If you do, use a blast of water or compressed air from a sprayer or canister to reprimand it, then leave the sprayer or canister sitting beside or on top of the piece of furniture in question for a few days. Most cats will avoid that piece of furniture like the plague from that point on. Some folks recommend commercial cat repellents or vinegar be used on furniture to discourage scratching, but these can be messy and could stain the pieces.

For that feline who seems refractory to punishment, try placing the scratching post near its favorite piece of furniture and patiently attempt to accustom it to this desired alternative, using food rewards and praises. Adorning the post or its base with food, toys, or catnip can also be effective weapons at luring the reluctant cat to its new scratching post.

Regardless of where you put the post, reward your cat with treats or with compliments whenever and wherever you observe it using the post. Remember to reserve these rewards for afterwards. Do not disturb your cat while it is scratching and kneading at the post.

As a last resort for the refractory scratcher, surgical removal of its claws can be performed to spare your house from total destruction (see chapter 23).

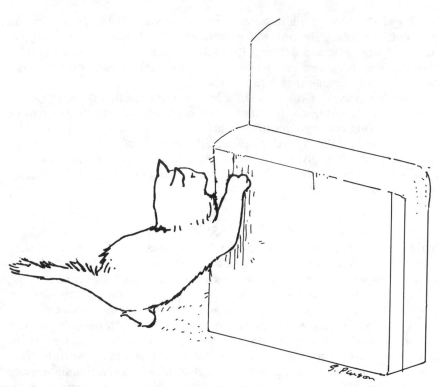

20-4 *Scratching anything other than a designated scratching post can prove to be quite destructive.*

Aggressiveness

Because of the fairly independent nature of the cat, a display of aggression towards another of its own species, especially if its territory is impinged upon, is not at all uncommon. Aggressiveness towards humans, on the other hand, can be influenced by a number of factors, including personality defects, fear, play activity, and medical disorders. Cats who have not been properly socialized to people can be expected to show some degree of aggressiveness when cornered; it is also a well-known fact that some of the more socialized cats just want to be left alone.

Personality defects

Personality defects can lead to true aggressive tendencies in cats. These are cats that have been properly socialized to humans, yet still exhibit aggressiveness towards them. An over domineering feline who might bite when petted near the base of the tail is such an example. Cats exhibiting this type of aggressiveness will flag their tail and twitch their ears against their head when approached or touched. A low-pitched growl or hiss is usually heard as well.

Fear-induced aggression

Aggressive felines such as these rarely respond to training or reprimand efforts; in fact, such attempts could lead to serious owner injury. Treatment should be aimed at neutering if this has not previously been done. In those cats that have been neutered and are still aggressive, special medical therapy prescribed by your veterinarian might help eliminate some of these aggressive tendencies.

The self-defense posture caused by fear-induced aggressive behavior is characterized by *piloerection* (hair standing on end), arched back, flattened ears, and hissing or spitting. Cats who feel threatened will lash out with their claws, and make short, sharp lunges at their adversary. If they really sense danger, they often roll over on their back, and assume a defense posture which will allow them to utilize the claws on all four feet.

People might be injured accidentally if they attempt to handle a fearful cat. Obviously the best way to treat this type of aggression is to eliminate the source of the fear if possible. This might be difficult if that source is a person or another pet within your household. In these instances, neutering with or without medical therapy might be required to take the edge off of these fearful cats.

Playful aggression

Playful aggression must be differentiated from the other two, since it is by far the easiest to treat. This type of aggression is seen especially in younger cats filled with the energy of youth (FIG. 20-5). You might have heard

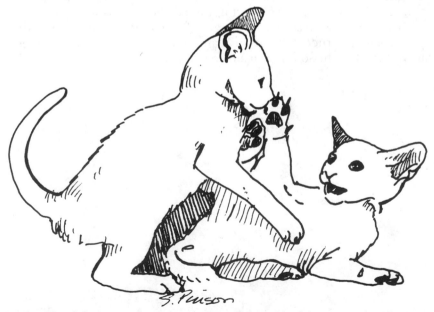

20-5   *Playful aggression is usually exhibited by kittens and is the easiest form of aggression to amend.*

of cats stalking house guests or ambushing unexpected owners when they arrive home. Most of these cases involve playful aggression on the cat's part. It provides them a way to release excess energy in an instinctive manner. Most bites inflicted during this play aren't meant to purposely break the skin; however, this is certainly a function of the game's intensity. One physical characteristic of a mischievous cat or kitten is that they often carry their tail arched up over their back or in an inverted U position during these "playful" times.

Playful aggression can be managed by allowing your cat more access to active toys, such as paper bags, ping pong balls, or wind-up, moving figures. If you play action games with your cat using string attached to toys, be sure to remove the string after the play session. Finally, taking your cat out for more walks during the day can help release some of its pent-up energy.

Negative reinforcement utilizing water sprayers or compressed air canisters can also be a helpful tool if your house guest has just become prey for your cat. In these situations, however, simply isolating your rambunctious feline in another room during your guest's stay is probably the simplest solution.

Medical causes

Let us not forget about medical causes for increased aggressiveness. Cats that don't feel good often just want to be left alone; if they are disturbed, an aggressive reaction could result. Diseases that affect the nervous system (including rabies), metabolic disorders, and, of course, any type of pain, can all have a negative effect upon a cat's personality.

If your cat has experienced a gradual or sudden change in personality, it would be prudent to have it examined by a veterinarian in order to rule out medical reasons for an adverse temperament.

21

Preventative Health Care

ENSURING THAT YOUR CAT remains healthy and happy should be your foremost goal as an owner. To accomplish this, you must implement a well-defined preventative health care program. Both you and your veterinarian will play vital roles in its success. Immunizations, parasite control, grooming, exercise, and proper nutrition are all preventative health care measures that are important to your pet's health (FIG. 21-1).

AT-HOME PHYSICAL EXAM

An important diagnostic tool used by veterinarians to evaluate the health status of their patients is the physical exam. With a consistent and systematic approach, he/she can detect signs of disease and anatomical abnormalities early, greatly increasing the chances of successful treatment.

You can learn how to give your cat a physical exam very similar to the one performed by your veterinarian. Though not as thorough as the one done by your vet, this physical exam is easy to administer and does not require any elaborate training, diagnostic tools, tests or instruments.

When and how often should you perform the exam? For starters, you should always examine your pet during or immediately after its annual veterinary checkup. Watch how your veterinarian performs the exam, and ask to actively participate in the process (FIG. 21-2). Don't be afraid to ask questions concerning the actual procedure or about any health problems that it may uncover in your pet. After all, what better way to learn how to distinguish normal from abnormal than by actual hands-on experience with a trained professional?

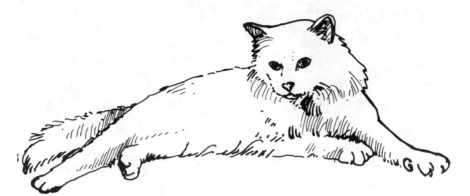

21-1 *Preventative health care is vital if your cat is to remain healthy and happy.*

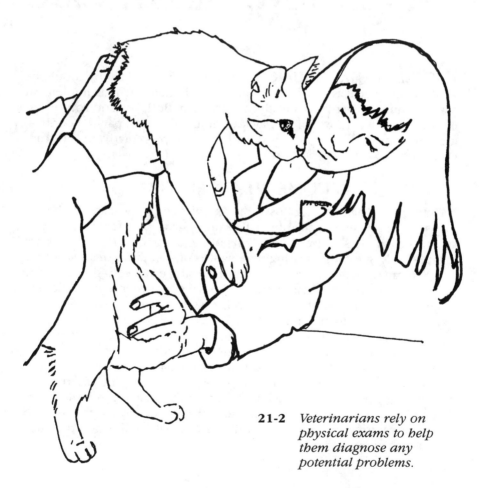

21-2 *Veterinarians rely on physical exams to help them diagnose any potential problems.*

Between these annual checkups, an at-home exam should be performed every three months for animals less than 8 years of age. Because geriatric cats are more prone to disease, particularly cancer, cats over 8 should be examined on a monthly basis. In addition, a physical exam should be performed whenever an injury or illness occurs.

You will find that the exam, in most instances, will help you determine if your cat needs first aid, immediate veterinary care or both. Always remember that the exam itself might not be a top priority in certain situations. For instance, if your cat is bleeding from a wound, your first priority is to attempt to stop the bleeding (using direct pressure), not to perform the physical exam.

1. Observe your cat

Begin the exam by taking a few steps back and getting a feel for your cat's overall appearance and attitude. Does it seem alert, active, and friendly, or do you note lethargy, depression, irritation, or aggressiveness? (Remember that animals that are ill or in pain might show aggressive behavior; therefore, handle them with caution.) Try to judge your own cat's attitude, keeping in mind that normal behavior will vary among individual animals and in different situations.

Next, does your cat's fur appear healthy and well-groomed, or does it appear greasy, matted, and unkempt? The latter will often occur in cats suffering from some underlying illness.

Finally, observe the cat's gait and posture. An abnormal gait without obvious limping or lameness could indicate cardiovascular, neurological or musculoskeletal problems. If a limp is involved, the source could be a sprain, a fracture, arthritis, or a localized infection. An abnormal posture, such as a wide stance with the neck extended or an arching of the back could signify a breathing difficulty or abdominal pain, respectively.

Certainly any suspicions that arise out of this initial overall assessment should be brought to the attention of your veterinarian as soon as possible.

2. Take your cat's temperature

To continue with the physical exam, carefully obtain a temperature using a nonbreakable rectal thermometer. First, lubricate the tip with petroleum jelly. Leave only the tip of the thermometer (no more than an inch) within the rectum for at least two minutes before taking a reading. (If your pet becomes unruly or upset, abort your attempt to get a temperature in order to avoid serious injury to your cat, as well at to yourself!).

While you're waiting for a reading, observe the external genitalia for any sores or discharges. This is also a good time to look for tapeworm segments around the rear end and tail. The segments often look like small white or brown grains of rice that might be moving. Cats most commonly acquire these worms during grooming activities, when they ingest fleas infected with tapeworm larvae.

When two minutes are finally up, remove the thermometer. Normal temperature for a cat should range anywhere from 100 to 102.2 degrees Fahrenheit. Remember, though, that an excited or nervous animal might have an elevated temperature, but this should rarely exceed 103.5 degrees (TABLE 21-1).

Table 21-1 Causes of Elevated Body Temperature in Cats

Fear/excitement
High environmental temperature
Exercise
Infection
Tissue inflammation/trauma
Autoimmune disease
Cancer
Drug reactions (e.g., tetracycline antibiotics)
Endocrine disorders (e.g., hyperthyroidism)

3. Weigh your cat

You can use your bathroom scale to obtain your pet's weight. If your cat will not stay on the scale long enough for you to determine its weight, try this technique. Hold the cat while you step on the scale, and determine what the two of you together weigh. Then put the cat down and step on the scale again. Subtract your weight from the combined weight of you and your cat. The difference is your cat's weight.

Be sure to use the same scale every time you weigh your cat. Compare your cat's present weight to a previous measurement taken three months before (or one month before in the case of a geriatric cat). Any loss or gain greater than 1 1/2 pounds, or any pattern of continual weight gain or weight loss, should prompt you to contact your veterinarian. Emaciation and weight loss are common signs in seriously ill cats. In contrast, obesity poses the same health hazards in animals that it does in humans. As a result, an obese cat should be put on a diet program formulated or prescribed by your veterinarian.

4. Observe the head region

Once you have obtained a weight and temperature, as well as an overall assessment of your cat's physical condition, focus your attention on its head region.

Eyes Abnormalities to look for include redness, cloudiness, discharge or drainage, squinting, and unequal pupil sizes. If one or both of the third eyelids are protruding, the cat could have a localized eye irritation, or more seriously, a generalized illness.

The whites of the eyes (called the *sclera*) should be just that—white. If inflammation is present, the sclera of the eye is usually reddened. Furthermore, a yellow-tinged sclera could mean that your cat is jaundiced. Regardless of apparent severity, any abnormalities you detect in the eyes should be brought to the immediate attention of your veterinarian. Your pet's sight and health could depend on it!

Ears   Inspect the ears for any foul smell or discharge. A black to brown discharge could mean ear mites. Conversely, a yellowish, creamy discharge indicates the presence of a bacterial infection. Other signs of ear disease include constant scratching at the ears, head shaking, and head tilting. Though ear problems are less common in cats than in dogs, they can still occur and actually become severe if not detected early. Be on the lookout for them!

Nose   Once the eyes and ears have been checked, observe your cat's nose. First, look for tumors and ulcerations affecting the mucous membranes of the nose.

Any discharge coming from the nostrils should alert you to a potential disease condition. Clear discharges usually indicate either allergies or viral infections. In these instances, the eyes tend to be runny, also. If the discharge is green and mucoid, a bacterial infection or foreign body could be involved.

Finally, actual bleeding from the nose could be the result of trauma, tumors, foreign bodies, or a blood-clotting disorder. It is important to realize that a nasal discharge in cats is often accompanied by a loss of appetite, because cats will not eat what they cannot smell. This might seem harmless enough; however, serious malnutrition can occur in certain cases unless the underlying disease condition is diagnosed and treated.

Mouth   Next, gently open your cat's mouth by grasping the head and upper jaw with one hand, tilting the head back and using your other hand to separate the lower jaw from the upper jaw. The gums and mucous membranes should be pink and moist. Pale, dry mucous membranes might indicate anemia, dehydration or shock, especially if the animal has been injured or is showing signs of illness.

If you suspect a problem, try to obtain what is called a *capillary refill time* (CRT). A CRT is done by pressing on a portion of the upper gum with your index finger. The gum region under your finger should turn white. Now release the pressure applied by your finger. The gum's color should return to pink within one to two seconds. If it takes longer, your suspicion that a health problem exists could be verified.

To continue your inspection of the mouth, look for swollen gums, foreign objects, tumors and sores. Using the blunt end of a pencil or similar object, lift up the tongue to get a good look underneath. This is a common lodging site for needles, strings and other items that cats might put in their mouths.

If you notice a bad mouth odor, it could be resulting from excessive dental tartar and gingivitis, as well as from tumors or infections involving the membranes lining the mouth. Dental tartar and gingivitis warrant a thorough teeth cleaning performed by your veterinarian. Loose teeth and any broken teeth should be professionally evaluated and possibly extracted.

5. Inspect the body

The next step in the physical exam is to run your hands over your cat's entire body to feel for any lumps or bumps. If you think you feel an abnormal bump or mass, compare the location of the bump to the comparable location on the other side of the cat's body. Is the bump present there, too? If it is, it might be a normal anatomical structure. If you have any doubt as to whether or not it is normal, let your veterinarian examine it.

An abnormal bump or mass might be an indication of cancer (only a veterinarian can determine this for sure), and the earlier the cancer is detected and treated, the better the chances for recovery. Other conditions to think about when you palpate a lump or bump include enlarged lymph nodes, cysts, foreign bodies and soft tissue swellings, such as hernias, bruises and abscesses.

6. Evaluate the skin and coat

Evaluate your cat's skin and coat carefully. Signs of skin problems can include constant licking or scratching, hair loss, redness, oiliness, scaliness, crustiness, or infection. Look closely for skin parasites, such as fleas and ticks. Is the coat dull and unkempt? This could be caused by poor nutrition or by, as mentioned previously, some underlying illness.

Remember that allergies and parasites aren't the only things that cause skin problems in cats. In fact, the potential causes of skin and coat disorders are so numerous that, to be safe, all such disorders should be properly diagnosed by your veterinarian.

7. Other observations

Direct evaluation of the heart and lungs is difficult to do at home unless you are trained in the use of a stethoscope. All cat owners, however, should be aware of certain clinical signs that could signify a heart or lung problem. The clinical signs can include weakness, shortness of breath, coughing, a wide-based stance, or labored breathing. Pale blue or purple tongue color or gum color means poor tissue oxygenation, which is often the result of heart failure.

Obtain a pulse by gently pressing your fingers against the upper, inner portion of the cat's rear leg. Normal resting pulse for a cat should be anywhere from 100 to 140 beats per minute. In the case of an abnormal pulse or any of the above clinical signs, your veterinarian should be notified. Radiographs and laboratory tests might be needed to accurately make a diagnosis of heart or lung disease.

Lastly, to complete the exam, gently press in on both sides of the cat's abdomen just behind the cat's rib cage. Slowly work your way back to the hip region, gently pressing as you go. Don't expect to know exactly what you are feeling. The purpose of doing this in the first place is to detect any swelling, tenderness, or pain involving the abdomen of your pet. If you do have any questions about what you are feeling, ask your veterinarian.

Congratulations! You have just performed a physical exam on your cat. Now that you have seen the wealth of information that can be obtained concerning a pet's health status, it is clear why every cat owner should perform these periodic physical exams on his or her cat. You will also find that with experience, you will be able to do the entire exam within a matter of minutes. Start practicing today!

THE ABCs OF IMMUNIZATION

The theory behind vaccinating any pet is to artificially provide that initial exposure to certain disease-causing agents, thereby priming the body's immune system before natural exposure occurs. Doing so will allow for a rapid, effective immune response if this exposure does happen, without the lag time associated with a first exposure.

If the queen has been properly vaccinated prior to pregnancy, most kittens receive protective antibodies from her through nursing, primarily during the first 24 hours of life. These passive antibodies are important, since the immune system of a neonate under 6 weeks of age is incapable of mounting an effective response to any *antigen* (foreign invader). Around 8 weeks of age, levels of these antibodies begin to taper off, leaving the kitten to fend for itself.

If a kitten that still has adequate levels of passive antibodies present in its system gets immunized, the vaccination will be rendered ineffective. For this reason, initial vaccinations for kittens are usually given around 8 weeks of age, when levels of passive antibodies are low. Vaccination as early as 6 weeks of age is warranted in those instances where the mother was not current on vaccinations, or if lack of passive antibody absorption is a possibility (such as in cases of inadequate nursing during the first hours of life).

Those feline diseases which are commonly vaccinated against include:

- Panleukopenia (parvovirus)
- Rhinotracheitis
- Calicivirus
- Feline leukemia
- Rabies
- Feline infectious peritonitis (FIP)

The first, second, and third vaccines are normally given as one injection, with the feline leukemia and the rabies vaccines administered as separate injections (FIG. 21-3). The FIP vaccine is administered intranasally. In addition to the above-mentioned vaccines, a vaccine is available against the *Chlamydia* organism, which can cause upper respiratory disease. Depending upon the prevalence of this organism in your area, your cat might or might not have received this immunization.

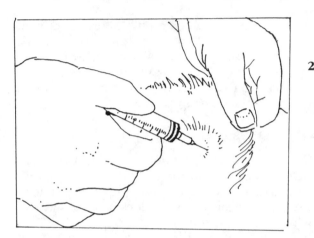

21-3 *Immunizations are an important line of defense against disease.*

Depending upon the type of vaccination that is being given, booster immunizations are normally given every three weeks until the kitten reaches 16 weeks of age. One exception to this is the FIP vaccine, which is first given at 16 weeks of age and then boostered again in three weeks. The purpose of these schedules is to successively prime the immune response to a higher level with each booster given to ensure that, if the kitten ever meets up with one of these diseases, a maximum immune response will be achieved.

The rabies vaccine does not require these three-week boosters to be given, since the immune response it stimulates after one injection is deemed adequate. However, a booster is certainly a good idea if contact with this deadly disease is suspected or confirmed.

Cats should receive boosters on all vaccines (even rabies) on a yearly basis to ensure that the immune system stays alert and ready at all times. Timely booster vaccinations are exceptionally important as cats get older, since an aging immune system needs constant priming for maximum effectiveness. Don't be lulled into a false sense of security simply because your pet is "never around other cats" or "never goes outside." If its immune system is caught loafing by one of these diseases you could easily track in on your shoe, the results could be disastrous.

STAYING ONE STEP
AHEAD OF INTERNAL PARASITES

Left undetected, intestinal parasites can rob your cat of much-needed nutrients, can cause severe gastrointestinal upset, and can predispose to secondary disease, such as panleukopenia. To make matters worse, many internal parasites of cats are also classified as *zoonotic* diseases; that is, they can be directly communicable to humans, especially children. As a result, controlling feline intestinal parasites is a vital part of any preventative health care program.

Management of feline internal parasites should begin in kittens as early as 3 weeks of age. At this age, kittens might harbor immature hookworms, roundworms, or coccidia without any evidence of eggs shed in the stool. Dewormings should be given again at 6 and 9 weeks of age. More treatments might be necessary if parasite eggs are found on stool exams during later visits. Stool examinations on these kittens should be performed by a veterinarian at 6, 9, and 12 weeks of age to ensure that they are indeed free of these parasites and are not shedding eggs into the environment.

Although cats over 1 year do not necessarily need routine dewormings, their stools should be examined for parasite eggs on a semi-annual or annual basis. Stool exams should also be conducted on any ill animal, regardless of clinical signs. Even when the illness is not directly caused by the worms, their mere presence and effect on the host's immune system can exacerbate any disease, regardless of cause.

Aside from routine stool checks, good environmental sanitation is another way to lessen the impact of feline intestinal parasites. Many parasite eggs that are shed into the environment via feces take days of sitting in the sun or in the right environmental conditions before becoming infective to other cats or to people. As a result, keeping that litter box cleaned on a daily basis is a very effective way of protecting your pet (and yourself) from these worms.

STAYING ONE STEP
AHEAD OF EXTERNAL PARASITES

Much confusion exists in the proper approaches to external parasite control and/or prevention in cats. Many different approved product types are available for external parasite control. The key to successful control is choosing and properly utilizing the safest products that provide the best possible results for the specific external parasite and environment involved.

External parasites such as fleas and ticks require both environmental and pet treatment. Since cats can be quite sensitive to insecticides, consultation with your veterinarian and exterminator is advised in choosing insecticidal products safe and effective for your specific needs (FIG. 21-4). Control measures for the individual parasites are listed below.

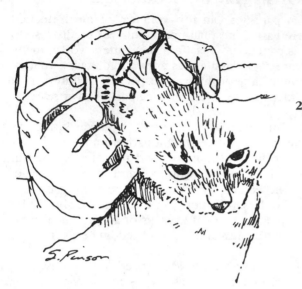

21-4   *Medicating for ear mites.*

PRECAUTION: Young kittens are ultra-sensitive to insecticides. Use only products recommended by your veterinarian on any pet under four months of age.

Insecticidal sprays

Flea and tick sprays are available in both liquid and aerosol forms. Sprays containing natural chemicals called *pyrethrins,* derived from chrysanthemums, are the preferred products over others for flea control due to their safety and efficacy if utilized properly. The big advantage of natural pyrethrins is that they are relatively safe for use on cats of all ages; the disadvantage is that they have poor residual flea-fighting activity, lasting only a day or so. Newer, synthetic pyrethrin products available on the market today have improved this residual activity while still maintaining a good safety margin. However, be sure to check the label for safety precautions when used on cats.

If you use pyrethrin products, frequent spray application is imperative for effective flea control. In some instances, this means on a daily basis. Just be sure before doing so to check the label on the particular product you are using to confirm the safety of this practice. If in doubt, follow label directions! Remember to always wear hand protection anytime you are using any type of insecticidal product.

You should begin application of the spray at the head region and progress toward the rear and tail of the cat. Pull the hair forward to ensure good penetration down to the skin, and try to achieve a light yet thorough application. You might notice some salivation after application.

Insecticidal powders

As with the sprays, pyrethrin-containing powders are preferred over others due to their low toxicity potentials. Powders do not evaporate like liquid products; therefore, under dry conditions, these stay active on the hair and skin somewhat longer than sprays. Again, frequent application is required for best results. Three to seven weekly applications are advised. Exposure to water inactivates most insecticidal powders.

As with sprays, application should begin at the head with progression toward the rear and tail of the pet and should provide good penetration down to the skin. The amount of powder applied to one specific area should be similar to that applied when salting a steak.

Powders should always be applied to a dry pet. Pyrethrin powders, like sprays, might also be applied to your cat's sleeping quarters to aid in essential environmental control.

Some pyrethrin powders contain another chemical called *carbaryl*, which belongs to the class of insecticides known as carbamates. Carbaryl is much stronger than pyrethrins and affords a better residual activity. It is also relatively safe when used according to label directions. It tends to have better activity against ticks than just pyrethrins alone.

Insecticidal shampoos

Insecticidal shampoos are common items in both retail stores as well as in most veterinary clinics. Many different insecticides in many different formulations can be found in the various shampoos. Flea shampoos, like flea dips, are best utilized as quick-kill measures for pet flea infestation episodes. Shampoos with relatively safe insecticides, such as pyrethrins and/or carbaryl, offer flea and tick-killing activity with low pet toxicity potential.

Shampooing too frequently can lead to excessively dry skin, so alternate application of flea sprays or powders are advised over shampooing for routine flea control on your pet.

Insecticidal dips

Dips are nothing more than highly concentrated preparations of insecticides. Chemicals such as pyrethrins, carbaryl, dl-limonene, and rotenone are all generally available in a dip formulation for use against external parasites. However, for severe flea and tick infestations, or for mange infestations, a more potent dip formulation might be required. Dips containing *organophosphate* compounds should NOT be used on cats due to their high toxicity. As alternatives, pyrethrin or rotenone dips are sometimes used. In any event, ask you veterinarian for his/her recommendations as to a dip safe for felines.

As a flea control technique, dipping is generally advised only as a quick-kill measure in cases of severe infestation. For routine control and/or prevention, milder products (sprays or powders) are safer and allow for

for more frequent usage. Always confer with your veterinarian in choosing a dip that suits your pet's particular problem. And always check on the label of the dip you are using for precautions concerning safe ages for use, frequency of application, and other pertinent facts.

You should always wear rubber gloves when applying the dip. After shampooing or wetting the cat thoroughly with water, dips are best applied by sponging the properly mixed product into the animal's hair coat, making sure that it penetrates down to the skin.

Insecticidal collars

Insecticidal collars act via time release of insecticide vapors or powders. In general, the effectiveness of such collars is inversely proportional to pet size, environmental area involved, and amount of flea exposure. Quality insecticidal collars can help reduce the overall flea and tick load on the pet but seldom produce adequate control of these pests if employed as the sole control measure. The best results with flea and tick collars have been seen in those cats that experience relatively low environmental exposure to external parasites. Water reduces collar efficiency on powder type collars.

The chemicals contained within the collar belong to any number of the classes of insecticides we have discussed so far. As a result, consult with your veterinarian before putting such a collar on your cat to be sure that it is safely compatible with the other products you are using for parasite control. In addition, flea collars used on cats should be the "breakaway" variety, designed to snap apart in case it gets caught on something.

Internal insecticides

Because of the toxicity, insecticidal tablets and liquids designed to be taken internally should **not** be used on cats owing to their toxicity.

Natural remedies

Throughout the years, countless natural remedies for parasite control have been touted as effective alternatives to insecticides. Some of these substances or devices are worn or applied externally; some designed to be taken internally.

Products such as brewer's yeast, garlic, and B-vitamins have all been implicated at one time or another as flea control remedies. Unfortunately, no proven efficacy exists for such products. Controlled scientific studies indicate little to no benefit in flea control with these products.

Certain products containing abrasive ingredients (i.e., silica gel, diatomaceous earth) are available for external flea control. These noninsecticidal products act by damaging the chitin exoskeleton of the flea. Desiccation and death of the flea might result. Moderate success has been reported with abrasive-type products. Drying and/or mild irritation of the pet's skin might occur with these products. Frequent application (four to seven times weekly) is required if these are to be used.

Electronic flea collars

Electronic flea collars have become quite popular in recent years as well. Although many manufacturers and pet owners will stand by their efficacy, scientific studies have shown that their worth in controlling external parasites is minimal. The idea behind them is that the device emits a high-pitched sound that can't be heard by humans or cats, yet it drives fleas away.

Unfortunately, aside from their relative ineffectiveness, some models might indeed deliver an audible pitch that can be heard and be quite discomforting to the cat wearing the collar.

Summary of flea and tick control

It is important to understand that fleas spend the vast majority of their time off of the cat, reproducing and maturing in the surrounding environment. As a result, effective environmental control measures are essential for successful flea control.

A complete approach to flea control should always involve three steps: Treating the home, then treating the yard, and finally, treating your cat. Because fleas, on the average, will only spend about 10% of their time on your pet, treating the surrounding environment is probably more important than treating the actual pet. Remember: For every one flea you see on your cat, there's nine more in the house or yard.

Start by fogging the house or having it professionally exterminated to kill the existing flea population. Thoroughly vacuum the carpet, draperies, furniture, and your pet's bedding to help remove any adult and immature fleas from these areas. After treating the house, spray or dust the yard with an appropriate insecticide to kill the fleas there. Then, in two to three weeks, repeat both the house and yard treatment to eliminate any newly hatched fleas.

As far as your cat is concerned, there are a number of flea shampoos, dips, and sprays available that are effective at fighting fleas. Because felines can be very sensitive to insecticides, *be sure* that the product you are using is safe for cats. Flea baths and/or dips should be given at least every two weeks during flea season. Between baths, pyrethrin sprays or powders can and should be used daily if needed. Again, before using any flea control product on your pet, be sure to always read and follow the label directions closely, and, to be on the safe side, consult your veterinarian before using any flea-control product combinations.

Note: Ticks tend to be more resistant to the milder type insecticides than fleas, and might remain temporarily attached to the skin after dying. Dipping or spraying with appropriate products is advised as the best measure in killing ticks on your cat. Veterinary advice is imperative in choosing both a safe and effective product for tick infestations. The ticks should be allowed to fall off the pet without manipulation since pulling might result in abscess formation at the attachment site.

Environmental measures are essential if your cat's tick infestation occurred in the home environment. Professional exterminators are recommended for dealing with such problems.

KEEPING YOUR CAT'S
TEETH AND GUMS HEALTHY

Periodontal disease, or tooth and gum disease, is one of the most common diseases affecting cats today. Signs can include tender, swollen gums, excessive drooling, loss of appetite, and, most commonly, bad breath. More importantly though, plaque and calculus build-up on the teeth can lead to heart and kidney disease if left untreated.

A complete dental exam should be performed on all cats at least once a year. If dental calculus is present at the gum line, the teeth should be professionally cleaned by your veterinarian. Because this cleaning can be a painful procedure, especially if periodontal disease already exists, a short-acting sedative or anesthetic is essential for your cat's comfort and safety. An ultrasonic dental scaler, combined with manual scaling instruments, is used to break apart and remove the hard calculus and deposits from the tooth surfaces. Afterwards, the teeth are polished with a special paste to restore their natural smooth surfaces.

Your pet's dental care doesn't stop there, though! At-home after care is a vital part of your cat's dental health. Toothpastes formulated for use in felines are readily available from pet stores or from veterinary offices. Human toothpastes should not be used, as these can cause stomach upset if swallowed by your cat. A soft-bristled pediatric toothbrush can be used to apply the dental paste to the teeth of a cat. Brush as you would your own teeth, concentrating on outsides of the large premolars and canine teeth. No rinsing is necessary.

As an alternative or supplement to pastes, specially formulated mouth rinses are also available which can help slow the buildup of dental plaque and calculus. Choose one that contains *chlorhexidine;* this antibacterial compound can remain effective for hours after application.

Remember: Good dental hygiene is important to the health of your cat. In fact, it can help it live a longer, happier life. If you have any questions concerning your cat's dental health, don't hesitate to confer with your veterinarian.

FEEDING YOUR CAT

There can be little doubt that proper nutrition is the cornerstone of a long, healthy life for all pets. As our understanding of the link between diet and health increases each day, so does the quality of foods that are available to feed your pet. Not long ago, the diet of most cats consisted primarily of table scraps, supplemented by whatever other foods they could find while roaming freely on ranches, farms and the like. Today, our pets more often live indoors with us, and it is much more practical to feed commercially prepared food that is complete and balanced for the particular stage of life of each pet.

While the quality of nutrition for cats has improved considerably with the increasing use of prepared pet foods, there remains a great deal you should know about choosing the proper diet for your pet from among the many thousands of brands available in this country alone. Because cats, like dogs, move through several "life stages" as they age, it is easiest to discuss the nutritional needs of these different life stages separately and in the order in which the cat experiences them.

Nutrition for kittens

For most cats, kittenhood lasts for about the first year of life. During this time, the kitten requires higher levels of minerals like calcium and phosphorus, protein, vitamins, and energy (calories) than it will as an adult. Therefore, foods fed to young, growing kittens should contain these higher levels in balance with each other and with all other dietary nutrients. Such a pet food will carry a designation such as "feline growth," "kitten food," etc. to distinguish it from diets that contain levels of nutrients that are right for some other life stage, like adult maintenance.

The commonly held belief that if "a little is good, more must be better" is not true when it comes to feeding pets. Diets that contain very high levels of minerals, protein, and some vitamins are not superior to those that contain the amounts required for growth, but not large excesses beyond the pet's requirement. Such excesses might actually be harmful to the growing kitten, as can the practice of supplementing a good growth diet with various human foods or vitamin/mineral preparations. To be sure your kitten gets all the good nutrition it needs for good growth and development, but never too much, follow these simple guidelines:

1. Feed a high-quality, balanced commercial cat food that specifically states on the label that it is intended for growth in cats. Your veterinarian—who should examine, vaccinate and deworm your kitten—can recommend a brand that is appropriate. Remember that your kitten's start in life will influence its lifelong health and happiness. It is very important that you invest in good nutrition at this crucial life stage.

2. Do not supplement a quality, balanced food; since you will almost certainly unbalance your pet's diet if you do. Avoid giving table food, table scraps, or treats and snacks to your kitten for the same reason.

3. Do not leave unlimited amounts of food out at all times unless your kitten is very small or a very finicky eater. Many kittens can be very eager eaters and will tend to overeat a high quality, highly *palatable* (good tasting) diet. It is much better to put down a large amount of food for a limited time, usually 15-20 minutes, allow

your pet to eat all it wishes to eat in that time, and then remove the food entirely until the next meal. Most kittens should be offered 2-4 of these meal feedings per day. If your pet starts to become overweight, reduce the number of these feedings or the time the food is available per feeding. Remember, overweight kittens tend to become permanently overweight adult cats, with all the serious health risks that come with excessive body fat.

4. Keep fresh, clean water available at all times.

Nutrition for adult cats

Once your kitten is grown (after 12 months of age), its needs for nutrition are considerably reduced from those of which supported the rapid development of that first year. Continuing to feed levels of minerals, particularly calcium and phosphorus, protein, and energy (calories) that are optimum for the kitten but are much higher than the adult needs might lead to problems later in life.

Just as we are finding that excess intake of certain dietary nutrients (like phosphorus, sodium, and fat) are harmful for humans over long periods, certain excesses might also contribute to diseases like kidney failure, heart failure, obesity, and diabetes in adult and older cats. Also, we know that reducing the level of key nutrients in the adult's diet to meet but not greatly exceed its needs is never harmful. Good-quality, scientifically designed adult maintenance diets always contain these reduced and balanced nutrient levels.

Guidelines for feeding adult cats include:

1. Feed a high-quality, complete, and balanced diet that is specifically designed for adult cat maintenance. Be aware that foods that are labeled "complete and balanced for all life stages" are actually kitten foods since they have been formulated to meet the needs of the most demanding life stage, growth. They contain excesses of most nutrients for the adult or older cat.

2. It is best not to give supplements or treats to your adult cat. If you must give an occasional food snack, either use a small amount of the regular food, or fresh unsalted vegetables cut up in bite-size pieces.

3. Do not feed bones of any kind to your cat. They can shatter, splinter, or become lodged in the mouth, throat, stomach, or intestines. They might also add unwanted amount of minerals to the diet.

4. Most cats should be fed their food in two or more equal meals per day, although many cat owners prefer to leave portions out all day long. Use the manufacturer's recommended feeding amounts as a starting point only. If your pet gains weight, reduce the portion per meal. If your pet starts to lose weight, increase the amount you feed. Your veterinarian can help you decide what your pet's

optimum weight is. Once you decide this, weigh your pet every week or so to prevent weight loss or gain from becoming a problem.

5. Some cats show a pronounced tendency to gain weight, especially around their midsection, as they grow older despite eating only moderate amounts of an adult-maintenance diet. Further reducing the portion size for these pets usually results in an unhappy, hungry cat that cries, rubs, raids garbage, and otherwise protests the unpleasant side effects of a diet. Once your cat is overweight, it should be placed on a medically supervised weight-loss program under your veterinarian's care using a specially prescribed diet developed for this purpose. If your pet is only beginning to show signs of becoming overweight, consider using a reduced-calorie, high-fiber, maintenance diet to help your cat keep trim and active throughout adulthood.

6. The pregnant queen will need extra nutrition in the last few weeks of her pregnancy and throughout the time she nurses her kittens. Actually, she requires a good growth diet again, the same one she needed when she was young. Feed such a food starting in the last 1/3 of pregnancy and continue until all kittens are weaned. Feed her free-choice, as much as she will eat, and do not add vitamin/mineral supplements unless your veterinarian recommends it. As the kittens grow and begin to investigate their surroundings they can be offered some of the mother's food which they will gradually start to eat. This makes the transition to a kitten-food-only diet much easier at weaning.

7. Keep fresh, clean water available at all times.

Nutrition for the older cat

Once your pet is about 7 years old, another dietary change might become necessary. As people and animals age, many organ systems begin to show the effects of wear and tear. The kidneys especially begin to lose the ability to handle waste material that must be removed from the bloodstream and excreted in the urine. Even older cats that appear to be in perfect health might have kidneys that are much less effective than they used to be.

Your veterinarian can advise you of any special health problems that your cat might already have and any other dietary adjustments that might be necessary. In many cases of "old age" diseases, special foods might be prescribed along with medication to help manage these conditions.

Dietary management of disease

For years, medical research has been telling us about the benefits of eating a well-balanced diet for good health. In addition, we also know that special modification of the dietary intake in the presence of a disease state can be helpful in the treatment and/or long-term management of the condition.

This same nutritional health concept can be applied to cats as well. Many disease conditions in cats, such as obesity (yes, obesity is a disease!), feline urologic syndrome, and gastrointestinal disease can be effectively controlled, and sometimes even cured, just through diet modulation alone. For example, obesity, constipation (such as seen with feline megacolon), certain types of colitis, and diabetes mellitus all warrant an increase in the amount of fiber present in the ration.

Cats suffering from feline urologic syndrome benefit from diets that acidify the urine and contain low levels of magnesium and other trace minerals. Finally, recommended management of cats suffering from heart and/or kidney disease includes diets low in sodium and containing restricted amounts of high quality protein.

These special diets or rations aimed at fighting or counteracting feline diseases can be purchased through your veterinarian, or can be prepared at home using special recipes. In general, the commercially available products are preferred over the homemade rations. The cost of these diets is negligible when compared to continuing veterinary bills and the poor quality of life that would result by not feeding them. Just remember to follow your veterinarian's directions closely as to amounts and frequency of feeding of these diets if they are indeed used.

BATTLING OBESITY IN CATS

Obesity is certainly one of the most prevalent diseases affecting the cat population today. For years, the frequency of this health disorder was skyrocketing at an alarming pace, owing primarily to improper feeding practices. Unfortunately, owners might not realize that by encouraging their cat to get fat, they are at the same time endangering its health and unfairly reducing its quality of life.

The health-related ramifications in cats are the same as they are in people. Although cats don't suffer from atherosclerosis and heart attacks like we do, obesity does place a great strain on their cardiovascular systems. Other internal organs suffer the consequences as well. Obese cats seem to suffer from more skin ailments and coat disorders than do their slim and trim counterparts. In addition, musculoskeletal disorders, including joint injuries sustained when jumping, occur with greater frequency in cats carrying around excessive baggage.

In summary, it is safe to say that the overall quality of and length of life for these cats is reduced, owing to these side effects of obesity.

Causes of obesity

The potential causes of obesity in cats are numerous, yet the most common of all of them is overfeeding. Because it can be difficult to force a cat to exercise regularly, many owners miscalculate their cat's caloric needs and feed too much. Also, feeding a higher calorie food to a less active or older cat that requires less energy can promote obesity as well (see the feeding instructions in this chapter). Furthermore, keep in mind that cats spending much of their time outdoors might have access to food elsewhere in the neighborhood.

Proper diet

If your cat is overweight, simply cutting back on the amount you feed will not do the trick. In fact, doing so could conceivably lead to a mild state of malnutrition and will cause your cat to be constantly hungry and hunting for food. Instead of cutting back the ration, switch to a diet that is specially formulated for weight loss. These diets are readily available from your veterinarian. They might cost a bit more than what you are accustomed to paying for cat food, but the switch is only temporary and the benefits to your pet immense.

These special foods have a high fiber content, which allows for calorie reduction while giving your cat that feeling of fullness after eating. Your veterinarian can assist you as far as how much to feed and how often to feed. Keeping a daily portion of food available in a bowl throughout the day might help satisfy your pet even more. Be patient with the results. You might not realize it but even one pound of weight loss is significant in a cat. It is vital that during the weight-reduction period that you remain consistent with the feedings and avoid giving any snacks (a few kibbles of the special diet now and then can make for an excellent snack substitute).

Exercise

As with people, lack of exercise does its part to promote obesity. Cats kept indoors rarely get enough exercise, unless, of course, they are leash-trained and can be taken for daily walks (see chapter 20). Simply playing with your cat more when you get home from work can do its part at combating obesity.

MAINTAINING A HEALTHY SKIN AND COAT

Routine skin care for cats with normal, healthy hair coats and skin should include brushing and bathing.

Brushing

Whether your cat has short hair or long hair, brushing the coat thoroughly on a regular basis will aid in its appearance as well as promote healthy skin. It does this by:

○ Removing *telogen* (dead) hairs from the coat, making way for new ones to grow in.

○ Preventing tangles and mats.

○ Stimulating sebaceous gland activity, which keeps the skin moisturized and the hair coat shiny. Brushing also helps to spread these oils across the entire skin and coat.

○ Removing scale (excess keratin), which could lead to itching.

○ Increasing owner awareness of the presence of external parasites or other skin-related problems.

In addition, frequent brushing will help prevent gastrointestinal problems related to the ingestion of hairballs by removing the source of the problem.

Long- or thick-coated breeds require more diligent brushing than shorter-coated cats due to high shedding and matting tendencies. Minor shedding is normal year round in all breeds. However, because the shedding cycle in cats is stimulated by changes in day length, most will occur during the spring and fall months, when the days are getting longer and shorter respectively.

During maximum shedding times, long-coated cats should be brushed four to seven (4-7) times weekly using a wire-pin brush or bristle brush. For short-haired cats, one to four weekly brushings with a bristle-type brush or rubber curry comb might be adequate during maximum shedding periods.

Always use firm, short strokes when brushing, never forcing the brush through the coat. If you encounter a mat, don't try to forcefully remove it with the brush. Instead, try to work it free with your fingers, using one hand to free the tangle and the other to stabilize the tuft of hair to keep it from pulling the skin.

If the mat or tangle still can't be freed, insert a comb between the mat and the skin surface, then take a pair of blunt-nosed scissors and snip as much of the mat off as you can between the comb and the free end of the hair. Don't worry about cosmetic appearances. It will grow back! Mats that are left in place can promote infection involving the skin beneath. And always remember: If you brush your cat as often as you should, you won't have a problem with matting!

Be aware that excessive matting could indicate that your cat has a problem with external parasites or with some type of skin disorder.

Bathing

Cats with normal, healthy skin and hair coats really do not require routine bathing. It's a good thing, too, since most cats abhor bathing! Actually, indiscriminate bathing can dry out the skin and predispose an otherwise healthy integument to disease. So when is bathing necessary? Our feline friends do need it when the following circumstances develop:

○ Accumulation of excessive dirt, grease, or other foreign substances on the skin and coat.

○ Build-up of waxy *sebum* (seborrhea), which often leads to body odor.

○ Accumulation of skin scale (dandruff).

○ Infestation with external parasites, such as fleas and ticks.

○ Skin infection.

Hypoallergenic or other mild shampoos are ideal for bathing cats with otherwise healthy skin and coats. Shampoos containing insecticides are necessary if external parasites are a problem. For medical conditions involving skin infections and seborrhea, only use those shampoos prescribed by your veterinarian. Using the wrong type of shampoo on such skin disorders will yield poor results and might exacerbate the disorder in some instances.

Even if your cat appears to have perfectly healthy skin, it is still prudent to consult your veterinarian in choosing a specific shampoo for your feline friend. He or she will be able to recommend products and give you valuable tips on how to keep your cat's integument in the top shape that it's already in.

Prior to putting your cat into the tub or laundry sink, brush the coat thoroughly and remove any mats and tangles. In addition, always apply some type of protection to both eyes to prevent accidental soap burns. Mineral oil has been used for this purpose; however, a sterile ophthalmic ointment is preferred. Such ointment is readily available from your veterinarian or favorite pet store, and it provides greater eye protection than does plain mineral oil.

Once these preparatory measures have been taken, you can proceed with the shampoo and rinse. If a medicated shampoo is to be used, plan on allowing it to lather and remain in contact with the skin for a good 10 minutes before rinsing. After rinsing, a towel or chamois cloth can be used for drying. Blow dryers are not recommended for cats.

Finally, if you have not had your cat declawed, its nails might need to be trimmed occasionally. Refer to chapter 23 for information on this procedure (FIG. 21-5).

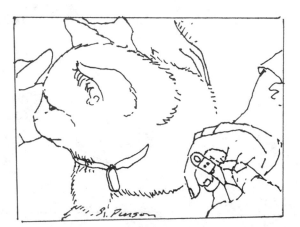

21-5 *Trimming the nails before a bath.*

GERIATRICS: CARING FOR YOUR OLDER CAT

It is estimated that in the United States alone, over 30% of all pets owned can be considered "geriatric status." Cats, like dogs, are considered geriatric when they reach 7 years of age. However, factors such as breed, genetics, nutrition, and environmental influences will all ultimately affect the aging process in a particular cat.

The overall care that a cat receives throughout its life will also have a great impact on the rate of aging. Cats that are well cared for throughout kittenhood and adult life tend to suffer fewer infirmities as they grow old. Furthermore, through diligent preventative health-care measures, age-related health problems can be detected early, thus greatly diminishing their impact. In contrast, neglecting a pet in husbandry or in preventative health care will greatly accelerate the aging process.

Cats tend to age most rapidly in their first years, which allows for early maturity and ability to breed. This might be a holdover from primitive times when their wild ancestors were subject to early death from fights, disease, and the harshness of pack life. An early puberty allowed young cats to raise litters and thus ensure speedy propagation of the species.

Not a great deal is known about the comparative aging of cats to man. However, since the life spans of both cats and dogs seem to run in similar patterns, it is safe to assume that the aging process of both species can be compared as well (TABLE 21- 2).

Table 21-2
Chronological vs Biological
Age of Cats as Compared to Man

Age of Cat (years)	Age of Man (years)
1	12
2	22
3	30
4	35
5	40
6	45
7	50
8	55
9	60
10	65
11	70
12	75
13	80
14	85
15	90

Physical problems in older cats

Physical changes noted as cats age are related to wear and tear on all body systems. Again, these are variable between individuals and breeds, and can be greatly influenced by an owner who provides good environment, proper nutrition, and routine veterinary care throughout the cat's life.

As with people, the overall metabolism of a pet has a tendency to slow as the years advance. This, combined with a decrease in the amount of exercise, can easily predispose a geriatric pet to obesity and all of its dangerous ramifications.

As dogs age, they don't suffer from many of the cardiovascular problems that humans do, such as hardening of the arteries and atherosclerosis. Yet as your cat matures, its heart does become less efficient at pumping blood during exercise or stressful situations that can arise. In addition, cardiomyopathies can increase in frequency in older cats (see chapter 27).

Bone and joint problems　Arthritis of the joints due to wear and tear can occur in cats as they mature. However, because most cats are light-weight compared to most dogs, arthritis does not seem to be as great a problem in cats as in their canine counterparts.

Muscular problems　The muscles of older cats tend to atrophy due to a decrease in muscle activity and due to age-related protein loss from the body. A loss in flexibility can also occur, causing cats that normally like to jump up and down off of high places to think twice about such maneuvers.

Disorders of the skin and hair　Disorders of the skin and hair can increase in prevalence in the geriatric cat due to aging effects upon the hair cycle and due to metabolic and endocrine upsets.

Aging kidneys　It is a well-known fact that as a cat matures, its kidneys become less and less efficient at filtering the blood and ridding the body of waste products. Incredibly enough, however, it would take a loss of over 75% of the functioning capacity of both kidneys to lead to signs of kidney failure in cats. As a result, care taken early to help ease the burden placed on the aging kidneys and keep them out of this percentage range will greatly enhance the longevity of a cat.

Reproductive problems　Also as one might expect, fertility and reproductive performance tend to decrease with advancing age. Female cats that were not spayed at an early age are also more prone to uterine infections and other disorders of the reproductive tract.

Intestinal problems　The aging digestive tract might begin to show signs of reduced efficiency and intolerance to excesses. For this reason, flare-ups of gastritis, colitis, and constipation can become more prevalent as a pet enters into the geriatric years. At the same time, liver function can decrease, making it more difficult to metabolize nutrients and detoxify wastes than it was during the younger years.

Weakened immune systems　It is well documented that the efficiency and activity of the immune system is compromised with age. As a result, geriatric pets are more susceptible to disease, especially viruses and cancer. For this reason, preventative health care takes on even more importance in these pets.

Endocrine problems　As cats mature, the activity of the glands within the body start to wear out, leaving the pet with hormone-related problems. For example, diabetes mellitus can occur secondarily to aging of the insulin-producing cells within the pancreas. In contrast, age-related tumors affecting glands within the body can lead to over-secretion of hormones, resulting in illness. Hyperthyroidism is a prime example of this (see chapter 36).

Sensory impairment　Older dogs can suffer from decreased vision, hearing, and/or smell. Fortunately, the incidence of such age-related sensory impairment is much less in geriatric cats.

The changes that occur with aging warrant special consideration when it comes to husbandry practices and preventative health care for geriatric pets. The following are five steps you can take to be sure your pet's geriatric years are filled with health and happiness:

1. Adjust your cat's diet to match its health needs. Your veterinarian can assist you with this switch. If your pet suffers from a specific ailment, such as heart disease, special diets can be prescribed to reduce the wear and tear on the affected organ systems. For the otherwise healthy cat, feed a diet that is higher in fiber and reduced in calories. Don't forget to weigh your cat on a monthly basis. Obesity is an enemy, and can significantly shorten your cat's life.

2. Be sure to groom and brush your pet daily. Skin and coat changes secondary to metabolic slow-down or adjustments within the body can often be managed with a stepped-up home-grooming program.

3. Along with grooming and brushing, be sure to give your geriatric pet plenty of attention each day. As the senses start to fail, pets can become frightened by the gradual loss of sensory contact with their owners. As a result, you need to reinforce the care and companionship you are offering.

4. Semiannual veterinary check-ups and periodic at-home physical examinations for aging pets are a must. Remember: Early detection of a disease condition is the key to curing or managing the disorder. Also, because of the effects aging has on the immune system, be sure to keep your pet current on its vaccinations.

22

Breeding Your Cat

A SOUND KNOWLEDGE of feline reproductive principles constitutes the livelihood of the professional cat breeder. But professional breeders are not the only ones that need to know about these matters; all cat owners desiring to breed their pet should do their homework first prior to proceeding with such plans. And because of the importance of preventative health care for kittens, be sure your female cat is up to date with all immunizations and stool exams prior to breeding (FIG. 22-1).

For an overview of the anatomical and functional features of the reproductive system, both male and female, see chapter 31.

PUBERTY AND THE REPRODUCTIVE CYCLE

Puberty is defined as the age in which the queen first comes into heat, or when the male testicle first begins to produce spermatozoa. It varies with each breed, but generally occurs anywhere between 6 to 12 months.

As a general rule, owners should wait until a male cat (*tomcat*) reaches at least 12 to 14 months of age before using it for breeding purposes; for females (*queens*), breeding attempts should not be made until the second or third heat cycle. Even these guidelines can vary some, depending on the cat's level of maturity, both mentally and physically.

The optimum breeding age for female cats is between 3 to 6 years. Kittens born to females in these age groups tend to be healthier at birth, faster growers, and wean much easier when compared to others. After six years, reproductive performance in the queen begins a steady decline.

Tomcats, on the other hand, have greater sexual longevity than do females, yet this too begins to decline over the years.

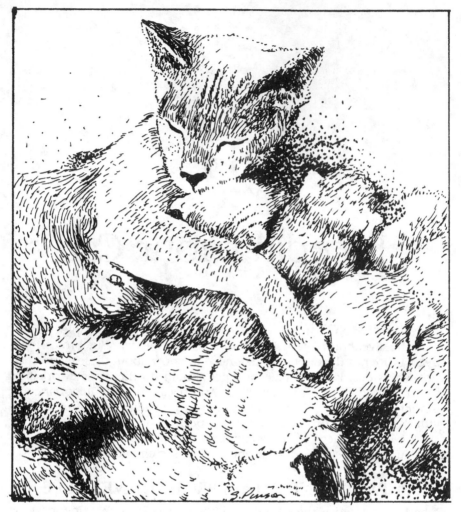

22-1   *A queen and her litter.*

The female estrous cycle

Estrous cycle is the term used to describe a series of events that occurs within the female reproductive tract between actual heat periods. Cats are considered seasonal breeders; that is, sexual activity becomes more active in the early spring and early fall. There are four phases to the feline estrous cycle:

1. Anestrus
2. Proestrus
3. Estrus
4. Metestrus-Diestrus

Anestrus　　This is the period of time in which there is no reproductive activity going on in the ovaries at all. The duration of anestrus is typically two to three months in the average cat.

Proestrus　　From anestrus, the reproductive cycle enters the period of proestrus. Signs seen during proestrus are minimal, although an increased frequency in urinary activity might be seen.

Estrus　　From proestrus, the queen enters into estrus, or true heat. This is the time receptivity to the male tom occurs. Marked behavioral changes also occur, such as increased vocalizations, loss of appetite, and elevation of the hindquarters into the air when the cat is petted (FIG. 22-2).

22-2　*A queen in heat will often elevate her hindquarters when touched.*

　　　Queens in heat often roll around the floor and rub up to anything they can find. The duration of estrus is 10 days to two weeks if mating does not occur. However, since queens are *induced ovulators*— that is, mating stimulates the egg to be ovulated from the ovary—estrus and its associated signs end within 48 hours after a mating occurs.

Metestrus-Diestrus　　Following estrus, the metestrus-diestrus period marks the end of sexual receptivity by the queen if nonmated, or the beginning of pregnancy if a successful mating takes place. False pregnancies can occur during this period in cats, just as they do in dogs. These are influenced by the progesterone secreted from the ovary where the ovulation occurred. False pregnancies can sometimes mimic the real thing, yet as the progesterone levels taper off due to the unsuccessful fertilization, the signs associated with false pregnancies will slowly abate. This can take anywhere from 30 to 40 days to happen.

　　　Tomcats sensing a queen in heat will start vocalizing to attract the female to its "territory." When the female approaches, the tom will grip the skin of the queen's neck in his mouth, a move properly termed the *neck grip*. After this, mounting and copulation will usually take place.

GESTATION

The gestation period for cats ranges from 58 to 70 days, with the average being 63 days. Unfortunately, there are no simple blood tests that can confirm whether or not a cat is pregnant. As a result, alternate means of pregnancy diagnosis must be utilized.

Ultrasonography provides a reliable way to confirm pregnancy status as early as 28 days. If an ultrasound is not available, abdominal palpation by trained hands can often achieve similar results. Abdominal enlargement and mammary development usually becomes noticeable after the first month of pregnancy. If an uncertainty still exists, radiographic X-rays can be used to confirm pregnancies as early as 45 days.

Care of the pregnant cat

Care of the pregnant cat consists of maintaining a good plane of nutrition and reducing stress as much as possible. Expectant queens should be put on a growth-type ration, similar to those used for kittens throughout the gestation and lactation periods. Because *eclampsia,* or milk fever, is rare in cats, mineral supplements are usually not required.

During your cat's pregnancy, administer all medications only upon your veterinarian's direct consent or under his/her direct supervision. Many drugs can harm both mother and unborn kittens if given during pregnancy. Always check the labels on insecticidal products used for flea and tick control before applying to pregnant pets. The label should state whether or not that product is safe to use on pregnant pets. If it doesn't say anything about it at all, play it safe: Don't use it.

THE BIRTHING PROCESS

One of the most fascinating and rewarding experiences associated with cat ownership occurs when a queen undergoes *parturition* (the birthing process). In most instances, you need only to sit back and let nature take its course.

While *dystocia* (difficult parturition) is not especially common in cats, it is important to be able to recognize problem situations that may arise in order to protect the health of both mother and offspring. Dystocia can occur in any type of cat, yet the more exotic breeds might be at higher risk than others. Those cats that have suffered a prior traumatic injury to their pelvis are at higher risk as well.

As you've learned, the average length of pregnancy in the cat is 63 days. If the cat is not already acquainted with the surroundings, be sure to allow it up to three weeks prior to the delivery date to become familiar and comfortable with its new environment. You may choose to provide it with bedding or a delivery box, yet chances are, it will seek out a birthing area of its own. Popular spots include bed (on or beneath), drawers, and closets.

Enlargements of the queen's mammary glands are often noted 48 to

72 hours prior to delivery. A mucoid discharge coming from the vulva might also be seen at that time. Although in the majority of instances, your assistance in the parturition process is not needed, some cats will seek out their owners as the time approaches. If this is the case, plan on staying with your cat until parturition is complete. However, it is important to let nature take its course and avoid interruptions during labor. Some queens have been known to delay labor for days if they feel uncomfortable with outside interference!

As the queen enters true labor and contractions become more frequent, the first placental sac will soon come into view. Following a normal birth, a greenish discharge is often seen. After delivery, the queen will clean the membranes off the kittens and sever the umbilical cord. Do not be alarmed if the queen eats the afterbirth. This is normal behavior. The expected interval between deliveries is five to 40 minutes. There have been some incidents in which the entire delivery process took one to two days to complete, with no ill effects to either mother or offspring!

Guidelines for parturition in cats

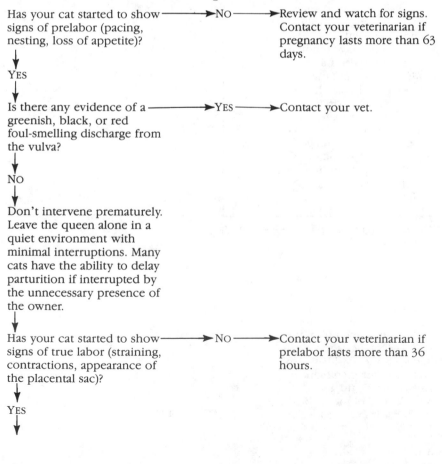

Has your cat started to show signs of prelabor (pacing, nesting, loss of appetite)? ———►NO———►Review and watch for signs. Contact your veterinarian if pregnancy lasts more than 63 days.

↓

YES

↓

Is there any evidence of a greenish, black, or red foul-smelling discharge from the vulva? ———►YES———►Contact your vet.

↓

NO

↓

Don't intervene prematurely. Leave the queen alone in a quiet environment with minimal interruptions. Many cats have the ability to delay parturition if interrupted by the unnecessary presence of the owner.

↓

Has your cat started to show signs of true labor (straining, contractions, appearance of the placental sac)? ———►NO———►Contact your veterinarian if prelabor lasts more than 36 hours.

↓

YES

↓

Has a kitten been born
within 2 hours after the onset ──────────►No──────►Contact your veterinarian
of true 2 labor?

│
▼
YES
│
▼

Immediately after giving─────►No──────►Remove the membranes.
birth, has the queen removed
the placental membranes
surrounding the newborn?

│
▼
YES
│
▼

Has the kitten started──────────►YES
breathing within one minute
after birth?

│
▼
NO
│
▼

Hold the kitten upside-down
to allow the fluid to drain
from its lungs, and
vigorously massage the skin.
A bulb syringe can be used to
suction excess fluid out of
the mouth and nose. If this
approach is not working
within two to three minutes,
institute artificial respiration
(see CPR pg. 646), and gently
expand the lungs, taking care
not to blow too hard into the
nostril. Avoid over-inflating
the lungs.

│
▼ ◄──────

Has the queen severed the─────►YES
umbilical cord?

│
▼
NO
│
▼

Tie off the cord with thin
gauze or thread by making a
knot about 1/2 inch from the
body wall of the newborn,
then sever the cord between
the tie and the membranes.
Discard the membranes.
Treat the end of the umbilical
stump with tamed iodine.

│
▼

Has greater than three hours ——————▶YES——————▶Contact your veterinarian
elapsed between births?

↓

Do you suspect a rejection of ——————▶NO
a newborn?

↓

YES

↓

Try warming the kitten with
a blanket or covered heating
pad (use the low setting!),
then place it back with
mother and the rest of the
litter. If this does not work,
you might need to hand-feed
the kitten yourself.

It is wise to have your cat examined by your veterinarian as soon as you think that all kittens have been delivered.

CARE OF NEONATAL KITTENS

This section is included to alert you to potential health problems that might arise in neonatal kittens. If you suspect something is wrong, consult your veterinarian immediately. Normally, healthy kittens should be doing one of three things: eating, playing, or sleeping. Crying usually indicates hunger, and should cease when the kitten is allowed to nurse. If it doesn't, something might be wrong (FIG. 22-3).

Hypoglycemia

Hypoglycemia (low blood sugar) can result from lack of adequate intake of the mother's milk. It is often seen in orphaned kittens too weak to nurse. This condition requires immediate attention, for it can lead to profound weakness, convulsions, and death. Commercial formulas available at your veterinarian or pet store are ideal milk substitutes. The amounts needed by the kitten are printed on the label.

In emergency situations, you can prepare and use a homemade formula that consists of one large egg yolk and enough homogenized milk to make 4 to 6 ounces of formula. The mixture might be sweetened by adding 1 teaspoon of honey to 8 ounces of formula.

This homemade formula can be fed according to the willingness of the kitten to accept the formula. A general rule of thumb is 1 tablespoon of formula for each 2 ounces of the animal's body weight per 24 hours. For example, a 6-ounce kitten would get 3 tablespoons of formula in 24 hours. Feedings should be performed every two hours.

You can obtain a feeding syringe or pet nurser from your veterinarian or local pet store. If the neonate simply refuses to eat, tube feeding might

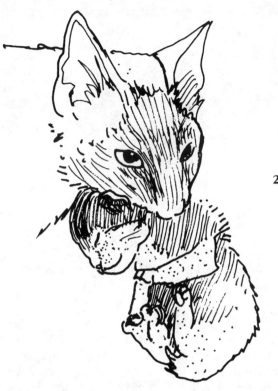

22-3 *Mother cats are very protective of their kittens.*

be required. Ask your veterinarian for details. It should be emphasized this formula is only for emergencies, and the commercial formula should be started as soon as possible.

Diarrhea

Diarrhea is another dangerous condition in newborn kittens. Sometimes, the only sign of diarrhea you'll notice is an inflamed anal opening, since mothers are so good at cleaning up after their young. *Toxic-milk syndrome* is one of the diseases that can cause diarrhea in neonates. ''Bad'' milk might result if *mastitis* (mammary gland infection) or uterine infection exists in the queen.

Affected neonates often bloat suddenly, cry frequently, run a fever, and are restless. When toxic-milk syndrome is suspected, kittens must be prevented from nursing the mother, and your veterinarian should be contacted. Oxygen, special fluids, and antibiotic injections might be necessary for treatment.

A newborn's hydration status might be easily evaluated by testing the elasticity of the skin over its back. If the skin fails to fall back to its natural position after being pulled up with your fingers, the kitten is most likely dehydrated. Since kittens can dehydrate seven times faster than adults, this condition can prove to be rapidly fatal if not managed immediately.

Hypothermia

Another major cause of death in neonates is *hypothermia* (loss of body temperature). This condition is often seen in kittens rejected by their mothers. To help prevent hypothermia, the air temperature in the kittens' environment should be maintained at or around 80 at all times, and care should be taken to prevent the young from being exposed to drafts and to cold floors.

Retained urine and feces

Orphaned or neglected kittens less than 3 to 4 weeks of age can suffer from retained urine and feces, since they normally need to be stimulated by their mother to eliminate. Kittens should be gently massaged in the genital area with a cotton ball soaked with warm water in order to stimulate these necessary functions. This should be done after each feeding and at least once between feedings.

Kitten Mortality Complex (KMC)

This condition is not uncommon in certain breeds of cats, especially the Himalayan. Queens predisposed to KMC often exhibit apparent infertility even after repeated attempts at breeding, abortions, and stillbirths. For those kittens that survive parturition, most are extremely weak and poor "doers," with the end results being death within hours to days after delivery.

The precise cause of KMC is not known; however, certain disease conditions—including feline leukemia, upper respiratory viruses, and feline infectious peritonitis—are all suspect of being able to initiate KMC in a newborn litter.

Unfortunately, because the cause remains unknown, there is no way to specifically treat KMC. Supportive care is certainly warranted for those individuals affected. As far as prevention is concerned, it is recommended that all queens that are prone to kitten mortality complex not be used for breeding purposes.

23

Elective Surgeries in Cats

TWO OF THE MORE common *elective* surgeries (surgeries not resulting from disease or illness) performed in cats include neutering (ovariohysterectomy, castration) and declawing. The latter procedure has come under much public scrutiny as to its necessity and humaneness. Whether or not you decide to have such a procedure performed on your cat is entirely up to you (and current laws governing such practices), but you are encouraged to communicate with your veterinarian before making a final decision. He/she will be able to answer your questions regarding benefits, risks, and controversy surrounding any particular elective surgery.

THE FACTS CONCERNING ANESTHESIA

Anesthesia is a word that tends to inspire uneasiness and fear in many people. In actuality, though, anesthesia is an indispensable tool in veterinary medicine (and human medicine, as well!) It is required for the painless performance of many important procedures, including surgery, dentistry, diagnostics, and restraint.

There are two types of anesthetics that are used alone or in combination in elective and nonelective surgeries. *Injectable anesthetics* are used quite often for procedures lasting for only a short period of time. For longer procedures, *inhalation* (gas) *anesthesia* is used for maintenance.

Isoflurane is the name of the newest, safest anesthetic gas available for use in pets. Because of its safety, most veterinary hospitals now employ this agent in their anesthetic routines. Regardless of the type of anesthetic agent used, it is important to remember that none, even isoflurane, are risk-free. It is difficult to predict how each pet will react while under anesthesia, yet with strict monitoring and adherence to basic anesthetic principles, many problems can be avoided.

Ideally, animals should be as healthy as possible prior to undergoing anesthesia. For this reason, laboratory work is often required to confirm the health status of your pet. Of course, certain situations will require the use of anesthesia in sick animals. It is easy to see how the risks of anesthesia tend to be greater in these patients. Older animals also tend to be at greater risk. Yet, again, with the proper laboratory work-up and a good physical exam performed by your veterinarian prior to anesthesia, the risks associated with the anesthesia can be greatly minimized.

Owners, too, have a responsibility to help ensure the safety of a pet undergoing anesthesia. Be sure to inform your veterinarian of any medications your pet is currently taking, as well as any changes you have noted regarding your pet's behavior (such as more frequent urinations, exercise intolerance, etc.). Don't hesitate to review your pet's past medical history with your veterinarian and to ask questions concerning the anesthesia to be used.

If the pet is to stay at home the night before the surgery, it is imperative that all food be taken away at least 12-18 hours prior to the scheduled procedure. Water, on the other hand, may usually be offered up to 4 hours before the scheduled anesthesia. Be sure to check with your veterinarian regarding this subject. If for some reason your pet does eat food or drink water when it's not supposed to, it is important that you relate this information to your veterinarian.

OVARIOHYSTERECTOMY

Ovariohysterectomy (OHE) involves the surgical removal of the ovaries and uterus from an intact female cat. The common term assigned to this procedure is *spaying*. OHE is a preferred method of birth control in cats, since it is easy to do and ensures 100% sterility. Most veterinarians require a cat to be at least 6 months of age before undergoing such an operation.

Aside from birth control, there are many other reasons for performing an OHE on your female cat. For instance, it can be lifesaving as treatment for or prevention of *pyometra* (accumulation of pus within the uterus) as an animal matures. In addition, it has been used as a behavioral modification tool to calm excited or overly aggressive cats.

Finally, and very importantly, spaying a cat at an early age might reduce the risks of that individual developing mammary cancer in the future.

The operation

The operation involves making a small incision just under the navel. The abdomen is entered, and the uterus is retrieved with the help of a special spay hook. The veterinary surgeon must then manually break down a strong, fibrous ligament that attaches each ovary to the inner abdominal wall. Once this ligament is broken, the ovaries can be easily exteriorized. The blood vessels leading to the ovaries are then tied off (ligated) using suture material, and the ovaries are detached from their blood supply.

Next, suture material is again used to ligate the blood vessels supplying the uterus and the actual body of the uterus itself. Once accomplished, the uterus is excised just above the ligatures, and uterus, along with the ovaries, are removed. The abdomen and skin are then sutured closed.

The entire process takes anywhere from 10 to 20 minutes, depending upon the skill of the surgeon and upon certain patient factors. For instance, the procedure normally takes longer if the cat is in heat at the time of surgery, owing to an increased blood supply to the reproductive tract, requiring additional care and ligatures. The same holds true for pregnant cats. Cats that are excessively overweight are more difficult to spay because increased fatty tissue within the abdomen obstructing the surgeon's view. Finally, in the case of an OHE because of pyometra, the operation can take two to three times as long as it normally would, as the surgeon must use delicate care not to rupture the pus-filled uterus.

For whatever reasons, veterinarians often get asked if they can just remove the ovaries and leave the uterus (or vice-versa). While the intentions of such a request might be good, the medical reasoning that condones such a move is not. Cats that have their ovaries removed without the uterus are still at risk of developing pyometra in the future. Similarly, cats that have had their ovaries left intact, but have had their uterus removed, can still develop a pyometra in the stump of the uterus left behind. In addition, such an operation does little to reduce the risk of mammary cancer in that particular individual.

Common misconceptions about OHEs

One common misconception about spaying a cat is the belief that a cat needs to go through at least one heat cycle or have at least one box of kittens before the deed is performed. Many incorrectly feel that this is necessary for the proper emotional development of their cat; it isn't.

Another false notion is that cats that are spayed will get fat. Research has basically disproved this theory; most conclude that the obesity is due to poor feeding practices, lack of exercise, or certain medical conditions. Since most kittens are spayed at an early age, there is no sure way to tell whether or not these kittens would have been obese as adults regardless of the surgery.

CASTRATION

The technical term for *neutering* a tomcat is *castration*, which involves the surgical removal of the testicles. This procedure is commonly employed for birth control, and for reducing territoriality and aggressiveness in male cats (FIG. 23-1). In general, castrations can be safely performed on a cat as early as 6 months of age.

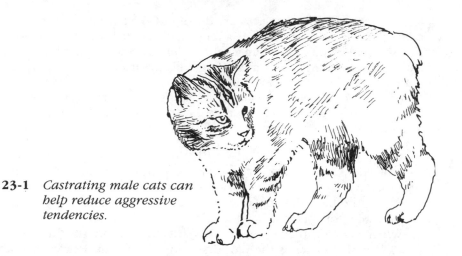

23-1 *Castrating male cats can help reduce aggressive tendencies.*

The operation

The surgeon makes a small incision on each side of the scrotum, and each testicle is pushed forward and out through the incision. Once exteriorized, the blood vessels and associated structures leading to the testicles are tied off and incised, allowing the testicle to be completely removed. After both testicles have been removed, the skin incision is usually left open to heal.

Currently, studies are being performed on a new, nonsurgical method of castration in dogs that might be seen applied to their feline counterparts. This method involves an injection of a sterilizing substance directly into the testicles, effectively rendering the cat sterile. If approved, it could make surgical castration obsolete.

Common misconceptions

The same misconceptions about ovariohysterectomies in female cats exist for castrations in male. Yet, as with the former, these claims are without foundation.

DECLAWING

The decision on whether or not to have a cat declawed is certainly a controversial one, yet it is one that needs to be made based on individual circumstances. For indoor cats that refuse to stick to their scratching post, declawing is certainly a better solution that drug therapy or—worse yet— eviction from the home. Also, for predominately outdoor cats who spend their time indoors destroying the furniture with their claws, declawing might be the answer. It is important to remember, however, that cats without their front claws cannot climb as well (although they can still climb!) as they could with them, and they might have trouble avoiding hostile dogs or fellow cats that they might encounter.

Contrary to popular myth, cats devoid of their front claws can still defend themselves. What renders a feline truly defenseless is the removal of those hind claws, which are vital for defense and for climbing. As a result, removal of the back claws along with the front ones is highly discouraged!

Before the decision is made to declaw your cat, try to train it to a scratching post first. If done correctly, you might find that it just may solve the problem (see chapter 20).

Nail clipping

Also, consider keeping your cat's nails clipped short to minimize the damage caused by its scratching activity. Since the nails of cats are somewhat fragile, be sure the nail clippers you use are sharp. Guillotine-type clippers available from pet stores work best.

When clipping the nail back, be sure to stop short of the pink "quick," which contains the blood supply to the nail. However, if an accident does happen, the bleeding can be controlled with direct pressure to the site through the use of clotting powder, again available at your favorite pet store.

If these options don't work, however, then removal of the front claws might be the only option left to secure that happy owner-pet relationship.

The operation

Declawing can be performed as early as 12 weeks of age. In fact, younger cats seem to recover much faster from the surgery than do older cats, primarily due to the immature development of the blood supply and other supporting structures to the nails at those young ages.

The procedure involves nothing more than the surgical removal of the third phalanx or bone containing the nail itself from each digit. This is accomplished with the cat under anesthesia using a surgical scalpel blade or a sharp pair of sterilized guillotine-type nail trimmers (FIG. 23-2). After the removal of the nails, the skin of each digit is closed using a special tissue glue instead of sutures, as were used in the past. The advantage of using the adhesive over sutures is that it is associated with a lower risk of secondary infections.

Following the procedure, your cat's paws usually remain wrapped in bandages for 12 to 24 hours to discourage use and to control any bleeding. After the operation, it is imperative that you replace normal box material with shredded newspaper for a week or so to prevent contamination of the surgical sites. The wounds usually heal within 7 to 10 days, with normal function returning soon afterwards.

POST-SURGICAL CARE FOR CATS

For cats undergoing surgery, there are a few guidelines you should always follow once your furry friend comes home from the hospital.

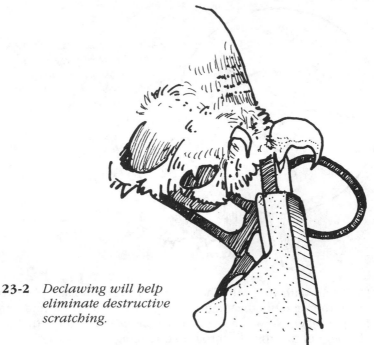

23-2 *Declawing will help eliminate destructive scratching.*

○ Do not give your cat food or water for 30 minutes after arriving at home. To do so can cause nausea and subsequent vomiting.

○ Restrict your pet's activity for 8 to 10 days, or until the sutures, if present, are removed. Protect your pet from stressors, such as extreme exertion, excitement, temperature fluctuations, and drafts (FIG. 23-3). Traveling should be kept to a minimum.

○ Check the incision site twice daily for any swelling and/or discharge. Keep the incision site clean and dry at all times. Avoid bathing your pet until all sutures have been removed. Replace the litter in the litter box with shredded newspaper to prevent inadvertent contamination of the incision site.

○ Unless otherwise instructed, return to your veterinarian in 8 to 10 days for suture removal.

○ If medications are dispensed, follow all label directions closely. (See also instructions regarding oral medications, below.)

○ Don't hesitate to call your veterinarian if any problems arise or if you have any questions regarding your pet's recovery.

If you are required to give your pet oral medications, here's how:

Oral tablets Open your pet's mouth by placing your hand over the muzzle and your thumb and fingers behind the canine teeth. Now tilt the head back, and press inward and upwards with your thumb and fin-

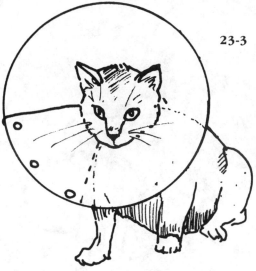

23-3 *Special Elizabethan collars may be needed post-surgically to prevent self-trauma to the suture line.*

gers (FIG. 23-4). With your other hand, separate the jaws and place the pill far back on the center of the tongue, using your fingers or a commercially available pet-piller. Now close your pet's mouth and lower the head. It might be helpful to stroke its throat to encourage swallowing.

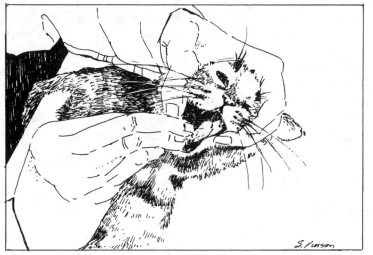

23-4 *To give your cat oral medication, tilt the head back and press inward and upward with your thumb and fingers.*

Oral liquids Simply "tent" the skin of the cheek out away from the gum line, and insert the syringe or spoon in the pocket formed. Now point your pet's muzzle upwards and deliver the medication. Keep the head pointed up until the medication has been swallowed. Do not deliver liquid medications directly onto the tongue or into the back of the throat. To do so could cause choking.

24

Infectious Diseases

INFECTIOUS DISEASES are among the most common feline illnesses seen by veterinarians. Organisms responsible for diseases in cats include a multitude of viruses, bacteria and bacteria-like organisms, and fungi, and they can affect any number of different areas of the body (FIG. 24-1).

VIRAL DISEASES

Viruses account for a high number of infectious illnesses seen in cats. Because of the lack of specific treatment measures for most viruses, prevention of these diseases through vaccinations is essential. The following are the most prevalent viral diseases seen in cats.

Parvovirus (panleukopenia; feline distemper)

The feline parvovirus is found worldwide, affecting cats in much the same way as parvovirus affects their canine counterparts. The feline parvovirus causes severe gastroenteritis in affected cats, and can be fatal unless treated with haste. This highly contagious disease primarily affects unvaccinated cats less than a year old.

Symptoms

Spread by oral contact with infective feces, urine, or saliva, the feline parvovirus strikes the intestines with a fury, causing fever, depression, vomiting, diarrhea, abdominal pain, and dehydration. The disease can be complicated even further as bacteria within the gut proliferate as a result of the virus and release toxins into the bloodstream. The virus itself can

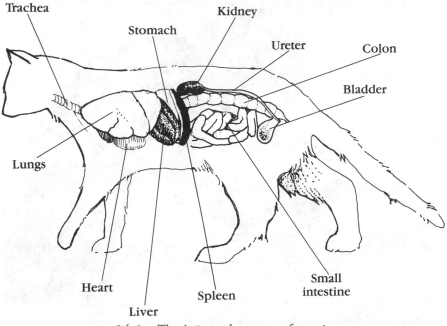

Trachea
Kidney
Stomach
Ureter
Colon
Bladder
Lungs
Heart
Spleen
Small intestine
Liver

24-1 *The internal organs of a cat.*

even spread to the bone marrow and interfere with the body's ability to mount an effective immune response to the disease. If a queen becomes infected with the parvovirus while pregnant, abortions or weak kittens could result. In many instances, these newborn kittens suffer from under-developed brains, causing permanent incoordination.

Diagnosis & treatment

Diagnosis of a parvovirus infection in cats is based upon history, clinical signs, and a marked reduction in the circulating number of white blood cells (FIG. 24-2).

Treatment is supportive, involving antivomiting drugs and intrave-nous fluids to correct and prevent further dehydration, and antibiotics to keep the secondary bacterial infections at bay. Recovery will depend upon how rapidly this supportive treatment is instituted.

Prevention

Feline parvovirus can be prevented through vaccination. The vaccines available are very effective, and they should be given to kittens every three weeks starting at 6 to 8 weeks of age up to 16 weeks of age, then once annually. Queens should be current on vaccinations prior to becom-ing pregnant to protect unborn offspring from the virus.

Finally, this virus is relatively stable in the environment, so it is a good idea to wait three to four weeks before introducing any new kittens or cats into a house where the parvovirus has been.

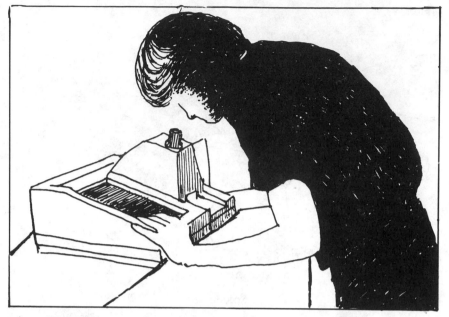

24-2   *The hallmark of parvovirus infection (panleukopenia) in cats is a low white blood cell count.*

Feline infectious peritonitis

Feline infectious peritonitis (FIP) is a unique viral disease of cats—unique in that the actual organ damage resulting from infection is not directly caused by the virus itself, but from the immune response to the invader.

The FIP organism is classified as a coronavirus, belonging to same group of viruses that cause gastrointestinal disease in dogs. Cats actually can be infected with two types of coronavirus—the *feline enteric coronavirus* and the *feline infectious peritonitis coronavirus.* Although the former can cause severe gastroenteritis in affected cats, most cases are subclinical; that is, there are no apparent clinical signs caused by the infection. The importance of these enteric coronaviruses is that their presence in a feline can interfere with some standard testing procedures designed to diagnose FIP.

Cats under 4 and over 12 seem to have a higher preponderance for this disease than other age groups. Inhalation or ingestion of infective secretions and excretions is the primary way in which this highly contagious disease is spread from cat to cat. The virus can even be passed via the uterus from an infected queen to her kittens.

Symptoms

Interestingly enough, most cats that contract this potentially deadly viral disease rarely show signs of infection, and may actually eliminate the infection soon after exposure occurs. If they are to appear, clinical signs usually show up two to three weeks after exposure, although this can vary by months to years. Upper respiratory signs can appear for a few days, then subside without any further problems until other clinical signs appear years later. Many researchers feel that although these cats might not be showing any clinical signs, they are active carriers of the disease and, in this capacity, pose a threat to other cats.

Another interesting fact about cats infected with FIP is that many are also concurrently infected with the feline leukemia virus. Since the leukemia virus suppresses the immune system, this paves the way for clinical FIP if exposure occurs.

FIP infections are unique in that the actual virus itself does not cause specific damage to the body's organs or tissues. It is the cat's exaggerated immune response to the virus that damages the organs, tissues, and blood vessels within the body. Clinical signs seen depend upon where this damage is done. Almost all affected cats run persistent, low-grade fevers. Insidious weight loss and appetite loss are not uncommon as well.

Clinical FIP presents itself in three forms:

1. Wet or Effusive FIP
2. Dry or Non-effusive FIP
3. A combination of 1 and 2

Wet FIP   When the immune system attacks the blood vessels in response to FIP, wet FIP results. Fluid that leaks out of the damaged vessels accumulates within the chest and/or abdomen, causing nonpainful abdominal distension and/or breathing difficulties.

Dry FIP   With dry FIP, many small nodules and regions of inflammation appear in various areas of the body, including the gastrointestinal tract, the lungs and heart, the brain and spinal cord, kidneys, and/or the eyes. Obviously, with so many organ systems potentially affected, a wide variety of clinical signs, including coughing, vomiting, diarrhea, seizures, and blindness, can result.

Diagnosis and treatment

In an effort to diagnose a suspected case of FIP, a veterinarian will rely initially on clinical signs seen, physical exam, blood samples, and perhaps microscopic examination of any abnormal fluids within the chest or abdomen. A persistent nonresponsive fever in a cat may point to FIP infection.

As mentioned, diagnosis of the FIP coronavirus using certain tests designed to detect antibodies to FIP can be obscured by the presence or absence of the enteric coronavirus. However, newer, more specific tests that will be able to overcome this dilemma have recently been developed and will soon be on the market.

Unfortunately, to date, there are no effective treatments aimed at eliminating the FIP virus from the body. Modulating the immune response with steroids and certain chemotherapy drugs can help temporarily provide relief from clinical signs, but will do nothing to afford a cure.

Survival time for cats exhibiting clinical signs can vary from days to weeks, depending on the degree of organ involvement.

Prevention

Because of the lack of an effective treatment, prevention is the key with this disease. A vaccine is now available against FIP, and it should certainly be incorporated into a cat's preventative health-care program. Given intranasally, it affords protection along mucous membranes and airways, preventing the FIP virus from gaining entrance into the body should exposure occur (FIG. 24-3).

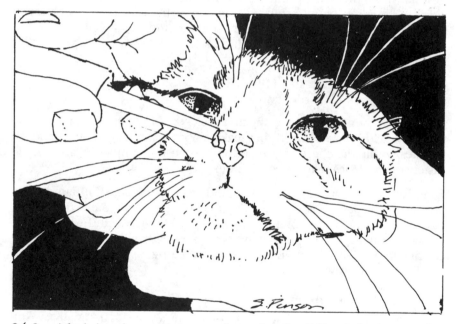

24-3   *Administering an intranasal vaccine for feline infectious peritonitis.*

Apart from vaccination, there are measures owners can take to protect their cats from the deleterious effects of FIP. Because FIP can gain a foothold in cats with unhealthy immune systems, it is important to keep the immune system in top-notch shape. It is imperative that cats be kept on a good plane of nutrition and current on all other vaccinations, especially the one for feline leukemia. Restricting the contact your cat has with strays or free-roaming felines in the neighborhood by confining it indoors is also an excellent way to afford protection against this disease.

Enteric coronavirus (EC)

As a disease entity itself, EC can cause fever, vomiting, and diarrhea in kittens; however, if supportive care is provided, the gastrointestinal tract of these kittens usually recovers in a few days. Yet, the primary importance of this virus, which is almost identical to virus that causes feline infectious peritonitis, is not in the disease it causes, but in the confusion it often generates when trying to diagnose a case of feline infectious peritonitis. (See the section in this chapter about feline infectious peritonitis for more information.)

Feline upper respiratory disease (URD)

There are at least six infectious agents that are responsible for upper respiratory disease in cats. The primary agents in the majority of cases include the *feline herpes virus* (rhinotracheitis) and the *feline calicivirus*. Vaccinations against these two organisms are routinely administered to cats at the time of their yearly checkup. In many parts of the country, veterinarians also routinely vaccinate for *Chlamydia psittaci*, a bacterial agent that causes a condition known as *feline pneumonitis*. However, because there are other less common organisms which can cause feline respiratory problems besides these three, vaccination is not a guarantee against a cat coming down with respiratory disease (FIG. 24-4).

24-4 *Conjunctivitis caused by an upper respiratory virus.*

Feline rhinotracheitis

Feline rhinotracheitis is caused by a herpes virus that infects the nasal passages and upper airways of the affected individual. The virus itself is very contagious, with the *incubation period* (the period from exposure to the appearance of clinical signs) ranging from 2 to 20 days. Kittens are usually more severely affected by acute disease than are adults. The presence of the feline leukemia or AIDS viruses can also significantly increase the susceptibility to rhinotracheitis.

Clinical signs associated with rhinotracheitis include sneezing, loss of appetite, conjunctivitis, oral ulcers, and nasal discharge. The discharges might start out as clear, but then they turn thick and mucous-like as secondary bacterial infection sets in. Severe infections can result in corneal ulcers of the eye, and pregnant queens might even abort their fetuses. Rhinotracheitis in newborn kittens can be deadly, with infected kittens dying within hours to days after birth. This syndrome is better known as *fading kitten syndrome.*

Many cats, especially those infected when young, will suffer continued recurrences of this disease as they mature if the virus decides to set up housekeeping within the bones of the nasal passages. Purebreds such as Siamese and Himalayan are especially predisposed to these chronic, recurring infections and become effective carriers of the virus. Recurring episodes are brought on by stress due to shipping or boarding, pregnancy, or other illnesses.

Feline calicivirus

As with rhinotracheitis, the feline calicivirus is a very contagious organism that can create both acute upper respiratory disease and chronic carriers in all ages. The incubation period of the calicivirus is anywhere from 2 to 10 days. Sneezing, fever, nasal discharge, oral ulcers, and conjunctivitis are all characteristic signs of the acute disease; the chronic disease can be responsible for recurring gingivitis and oral infections in infected individuals.

The feline calicivirus has also been implicated in the disease syndrome of kittens known as *limping kitten syndrome* (LKS). LKS is seen in kittens less than 14 weeks of age and appears as a generalized arthritis (hence the name), especially affecting the back legs. This presentation of the disease will usually run its course without causing any permanent joint damage.

Chlamydia psittaci

Chlamydia psittaci does not limit itself to the airways of cats; humans and birds are also susceptible to infection by this organism as well. Although this organism is not a virus, Chlamydia behaves very similar to the herpes virus and the calcivirus in causing disease and clinical signs. The incubation period for this organism is approximately the same as that for the calcivirus.

Chlamydia psittaci is susceptible to antibiotic therapy and can be brought under control with rapid treatment. Unfortunately, as with the viruses, carrier states can occur, and recurrence of clinical signs might result secondary to stress.

Diagnosis and treatment of upper respiratory disease

Because viruses cannot be readily identified microscopically or cultured, diagnosis of URD in cats is reliant upon history of occurrence and clinical signs seen. Laboratory findings from blood samples are usually nonspecific as well. If Chlamydia is suspected, microscopic examination of some of the cells lining the conjunctiva and/or nasal passages might reveal characteristic inclusions created by this organism. And because of its effect upon the immune system, all cats suffering from URD should be concurrently tested for feline leukemia.

Any sign suggestive of upper respiratory disease in cats warrants prompt veterinary examination and treatment to prevent serious sequela from forming. In the case of rhinotracheitis and calicivirus, there are no specific drugs to combat these agents; however, with good supportive care, life-threatening situations can be avoided. Antibiotic therapy is usually implemented to prevent any secondary infections from setting up; antibiotics are also indicated for combating chlamydia infections. If eye manifestations are present, antibiotic-containing eye drops or ointment will help protect the eyes and speed healing.

In addition to oral and, if needed, ophthalmic antibiotics, it is vital that the nose and airways be cleared of discharge and fluid as soon as possible. Because a feline's appetite is dependent upon its ability to smell its food, cats with URD will show a marked reduction in appetite, which could conceivably lead to secondary complications from malnutrition and dehydration.

Nasal discharges should be manually removed as often as possible. Human nasal decongestant sprays might be used to help break up any mucus buildup that might be present (contact a veterinarian as to types and frequencies).

Humidifying the cat's room air using a vaporizer or by placing it in a misty bathroom made that way by running hot water in the shower will also assist in the break-up of mucus within the airways. If dehydration is a factor, intravenous fluid replacement performed by a veterinarian might be necessary.

Finally, good nursing care can do wonders to assure a positive outcome. Keep the ill cat warm and dry and free from stress. If required, force feeding or tube feeding can help boost the effectiveness of the cat's own immune system and shorten the convalescent period.

Prevention of URD

Owners can help prevent URD in their cats by making sure they remain current on vaccinations. Both intranasal and injectable vaccines are available to combat respiratory viruses; the latter seems to be the method of choice with most veterinarians. Vaccination affords good immunity against the respiratory viruses and, if a combination vaccine is employed, only fair immunity against Chlamydia. In multi-cat households, prompt isolation of sick and sneezing cats might help prevent its rapid spread to other cats in the household.

Feline leukemia virus (FeLV)

Certainly one of the most devastating diseases affecting cat populations around the world is feline leukemia. The feline leukemia virus belongs to a group of infectious agents known as *retroviruses,* and it shares some characteristics with the human AIDS virus. It can occur by itself, or in combination with the Feline Immunodeficiency Virus, a new, deadly AIDS virus which in itself has been spreading at an alarming rate in cats in recent years.

Like the human AIDS virus, both of these feline diseases wreak havoc upon the cat's immune system, predisposing it to a wide variety of infectious diseases and to cancer.

The feline leukemia virus can be transmitted via all bodily excretions from an infected cat. Infected queens can transmit the disease to their offspring through the placenta prior to birth or through the milk during lactation. As a result, even newborn kittens can test positive for this disease.

For other cats, close contact is required for effective transmission (FIG. 24-5). As a result, feline leukemia is most prevalent in multiple-cat households and catteries.

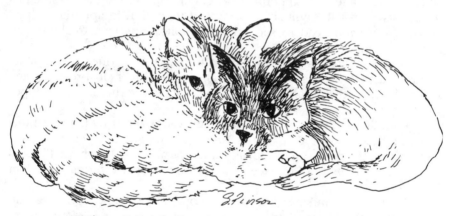

24-5 *Feline leukemia is spread by close contact.*

Symptoms

Because of the ability of the feline leukemia virus to suppress the cat's immune system, infected felines are prone to cancer (especially lymphosarcoma and leukemia), anemia, kidney disease, and a wide variety of secondary infections such as feline infectious peritonitis, hemobartonellosis, cryptococcosis, and upper respiratory viruses. Pregnant queens might abort their kittens, or give birth to weak, unthrifty offspring that die soon after.

Even cats suffering from seemingly innocent lesions on their skin and mucous membranes could actually be suffering from an underlying infection with feline leukemia. Finally, in some affected individuals, the only apparent signs might be lethargy, weight loss, and/or chronic gingivitis.

Diagnosis and treatment

Diagnosis of feline leukemia is accomplished by a simple test that can be performed right in a veterinarian's office. Tears and saliva can be used for initial screening purposes, but for definitive answers, a blood test should be performed.

The most common blood test used in-house is the *ELISA (enzyme-linked immunosorbent assay)*, which will detect the presence of virus particles in the serum. If a cat is found to be positive using ELISA, an *indirect fluorescent antibody (IFA)* test is also performed. The IFA assists in determining how long the infection has been present and whether or not it has reached the bone marrow.

As a rule, cats showing signs of illness that test positive for FeLV on ELISA, or seemingly healthy cats that test positive on both ELISA and the IFA test, are permanently infected with the virus. However, if a seemingly healthy cat tests positive for the leukemia virus on ELISA and negative on the IFA test, it might not be permanently FeLV-infected. In fact, many of these felines can successfully fight off and eliminate early infections by FeLV if their immune systems are functioning up to par.

Because of this, such cats should have the ELISA repeated at one month, and, if still positive at this time, again at three months. If still positive after three months, the virus has undoubtedly outsmarted the cat's immune system and has set up housekeeping within the bone marrow. An IFA test at this time will usually confirm this.

When bone marrow penetration like this has occurred, permanent infection is likely, and the majority of these individuals will become active carriers and shedders of the disease. FeLV has the ability to incorporate itself into the genetic material within host cells and remain dormant (not causing disease) for long periods of time. As a result, an infected cat might not show any adverse signs for years. However, if the immune system becomes stressed in any way, the FeLV will become active, and clinical signs appear. In general, cats with permanent FeLV infections usually succumb to FeLV-related disease within three to five years after initial exposure.

Currently, there is no cure for the FeLV virus. Treatment is directed at relieving any clinical signs seen and eliminating secondary infections or managing cancerous conditions present. Unfortunately, however, recurrence of such diseases are common after treatment. Many experimental agents, such as interferon, antiviral drugs, and medications designed to modulate the immune system, have been employed in an attempt to eliminate the feline leukemia virus itself. Unfortunately, to date, these have met with poor results. Bone marrow transplant, though helpful in some experimental instances, are not as yet a proven or practical means of treatment. The bottom line: The best treatment for feline leukemia is prevention!

Prevention

Vaccines that can help protect a pet against this deadly disease are available from veterinarians. In recent years, there has been much controversy as to the effectiveness of such vaccines at protecting cats from infection. While it is true that the FeLV vaccine (as with other vaccines) cannot be deemed 100% effective in all cases, it is also true that a cat has zero chance of protection if it is not vaccinated at all. As a result, it makes sense to have all cats immunized. Kittens can be vaccinated as early as 8 weeks of age. All kittens and those adult cats who have yet to be immunized should receive two initial boosters three weeks apart, followed by a booster vaccination annually.

Prior to receiving the vaccine, all cats should be tested for the leukemia virus. While such testing is not mandatory before the vaccine is given, it is always a good idea to prevent a false sense of security in an owner's mind. Remember: Because they can be born with this disease, even kittens that have no other history of exposure should be tested.

There are other control measures that you can implement to protect cats from FeLV. Testing all new cats before introducing them into a household is one. In addition, when boarding a feline or taking one to cat shows, be certain that the facility or event requires that all cats be tested free of leukemia and vaccinated prior to admission. Finally, keeping a cat indoors at night and, if it is a male, having it neutered, will help reduce potential interactions with neighborhood carriers of the disease.

A question frequently asked by an owner whose cat has tested positive for FeLV is, "Is feline leukemia transmissible to humans?" To date, no antibodies to FeLV have ever been found in human individuals in high-exposure-risk groups such as veterinarians, cat breeders, and laboratory handlers. In addition, the incidence of cancer in humans seems to show no correlation with exposure or nonexposure to FeLV-positive cats.

However, the ultimate decision governing whether or not a FeLV-positive cat is to be kept in a household rests upon the cat owner. Many veterinarians and researchers do recommend segregating children, pregnant women, the elderly, and other persons, who might for one reason or another have a immune system that is not functioning up to par from cats that are actively shedding the feline leukemia virus. Certainly other cats within the household, even if fully vaccinated, are at risk of contracting the disease from an infected cat. However, in those situations in which none of the above apply, the difficult decision on whether or not to keep a FeLV positive feline is a personal one, and should be influenced by an owner's individual feelings on the matter and upon the cat's overall health status.

Feline immunodeficiency virus (feline AIDS)

Until the late 1980s, the feline leukemia virus was the only agent linked to acquired immunodeficiency syndrome in cats—that is, it was until the feline immunodeficiency virus (FIV) was identified. This organism is unlike the feline leukemia virus in that it belongs to the same subfamily of retroviruses as the human AIDS virus (HIV). It has actually been around since the 1960s, yet it had never been identified. Today, through advanced laboratory testing procedures, FIV is now known to be widespread among the cat population across the United States and around the world.

FIV behaves the same way in cats that HIV does in humans; that is, it attacks the host's immune system and debilitates it, leaving the body wide open to secondary invaders and disease. The disease does not appear to be readily sexually transmitted between cats, and rarely is it passed on through casual contact with saliva, urine, or other bodily fluids, as the feline leukemia virus can be.

Instead, the main mode of transmission of FIV between cats is through penetrating bite wounds which introduce infected saliva deep into the tissues. This method of transmission is said to be analogous to the use of a dirty hypodermic needle in humans as a means of spreading HIV between people. Needless to say, unneutered male cats between the ages of 3 and 10 years who are allowed to roam about the neighborhood and fight with other cats are at greatest risk of contracting this deadly disease.

Symptoms

Clinical signs associated with FIV in cats can be quite variable due to the immunosuppressive nature of the diseases. Some cats might be carriers of the disease, not showing any clinical signs of illness whatsoever. In others, the only subtle signs noticed might be recurring infections (abscesses and skin infections, respiratory infections, bladder infections, etc.), weight loss, or chronic gingivitis and bad breath. Chronic, unresponsive diarrhea is another sign commonly seen in cats harboring FIV. Lymph node enlargement, loss of appetite, cancerous growths, and/or bizarre behavioral changes might also be present in an active infection.

Finally, FIV makes the affected cat more susceptible to parasitic infections, such as toxoplasmosis, hemobartonellosis, and demodecosis, and their associated disease syndromes.

Diagnosis and treatment

Diagnosis of FIV can be made by a veterinarian right in his/her own office using a quick, easy test similar to the one used to test for feline leukemia. In fact, it is common to test for both diseases at the same time, since they can occur concurrently.

All cats presented with acute illnesses or those with chronic, recurring disorders, are prime candidates for testing. In addition, all new cats should be tested for both feline leukemia and FIV prior to their introduction into the household.

As with feline leukemia, there is no known cure for FIV in cats. In the early stages of the disease, many infected individuals will respond well to treatments geared specifically towards any secondary problems of infections, yet as the disease progresses, even these treatments become less and less effective.

Felines exhibiting pronounced clinical signs are usually in the terminal stages of the illness, yet even then they might live months to years in slow deterioration. Euthanasia should be a consideration in these instances.

Prevention

There is no vaccine currently available for FIV, yet veterinary researchers are working diligently to find one. The best ways to protect a cat from the ravages of FIV are to have it neutered and to keep the cat indoors during the evening hours (the time when it is most likely to get into a fight with another cat). Cat owners should report all stray cats in the neighborhood to animal control because such animals are the most likely carriers. Finally, as mentioned above, have all new cats tested for the disease prior to their induction into a household.

As with feline leukemia, the question arises, "Is FIV transmissible to humans?" The general consensus of veterinary and medical researchers is that it is not; however, most agree that more research needs to be done to come to a definitive conclusion. Studies analyzing individuals at high risk of exposure to FIV (veterinarians, lab technicians, multi-cat owners) have failed to show any link between FIV and human illness. Furthermore, viruses belonging to the same subfamily as HIV and FIV are quite species-specific, rarely crossing species lines.

The decision governing whether or not a FIV-positive cat is to be kept in a household rests upon the cat owner. Many veterinarians and researchers agree that owners should consider segregating children, pregnant women, the elderly, and other people who might for one reason or another have an imperfect immune system from cats that are carriers of FIV. Whether or not such action is justified is still debatable, but until more research data is in, owners should not hesitate to consult with a veterinarian if ever faced with such a decision. The insight gained should make the process easier.

Rabies

If there was ever a disease to strike fear into the hearts and minds of pet owners everywhere, this is it. Rabies is a deadly viral disease that can infect any warm-blooded mammal, including the cat. As a disease to be avoided, rabies is one of the earliest ever to be recorded, dating back to almost 2000 B.C. It is found worldwide, except in a few countries, such as Great Britain and Japan, who have strict laws designed to keep the countries rabies-free.

The incidence of rabies within the United States varies with each state, depending upon the normal fauna found in that state, and on existing vaccination laws. On the average, the United States experiences over 300 cases of rabies each just in dogs and cats alone. These account for over fifty percent of all persons receiving prophylactic rabies treatment each year.

It is estimated that 86% of all rabies cases occur in wildlife species of animals, with about 14% spilling over into the domestic pet and livestock population. It is certainly these latter groups that pose the greatest threat to public health.

Species that are commonly culprits of spreading wildlife rabies include skunks, raccoons, foxes, and bats. Opossums are noted for their resistance to this virus, and rarely become infected. Rodents, such as rats and mice, are not significant carriers of the disease either, since most don't survive encounters with rabid animals in the first place.

Skunk rabies is most prevalent in the Midwest, Southwest, and California; raccoon rabies in the Mid-Atlantic and Southeastern US, fox rabies in the Eastern states; and bat rabies—well, it's found in all states. Most cases seem to occur during the spring and fall months of the year.

The rabies virus is transmitted via the infected saliva of affected animals, usually through a bite wound or contamination therewith of an open wound or mucous membranes. Contrary to popular belief, however, this isn't the only way. Aerosol transmission has been known to occur as well, though certainly the incidence of this is very low. In addition, in skunks, oral ingestion of the virus leading to an active infection has been demonstrated. Regardless of route of transmission, the disease is almost uniformly fatal once contracted.

The incidence of rabies in cats has increased in recent years, actually surpassing that in dogs in 1988 (FIG. 24-6). In fact, the majority of prophylactic rabies treatments in humans result from exposure to rabid cats. Reasons for this include poor vaccination compliance on the part of cat owners, increases in the number of stray or roaming cats, and the propensity of cats afflicted with rabies to exhibit the "furious," biting form of the disease.

Symptoms

Traditionally, when rabies is spoken of, most people visualize a snarling, frothing cat snapping at anything in sight. While this is true in some instances, pet owners should understand that this represents only one of three stages that are part of the overall disease process. Depending upon each individual case, viciousness might take on a prominent role, or might not occur at all. These three stages of rabies include the *prodromal* stage, the *furious* stage, and the *dumb* or *paralytic* stage.

The first stage, which might last from one to three days, is characterized by a change in the overall behavior of the animal. Normally friendly cats might suddenly exhibit aggressive tendencies towards their owners or towards other pets in the household. Affected individuals might also hide a lot, preferring to be left alone, and becoming upset when disturbed. Loss of appetite might become apparent, and owners might notice an increased sexual arousal and/or frequency of urinations.

Once the prodromal stage is complete, the victim then enters into the furious stage. This is the stage most persons equate with a traditional rabies presentation. Cats in this stage often become quite restless, excitatory, and aggressive, losing fear of natural enemies. They might wander about aimlessly, snapping and biting at anything that moves. The charac-

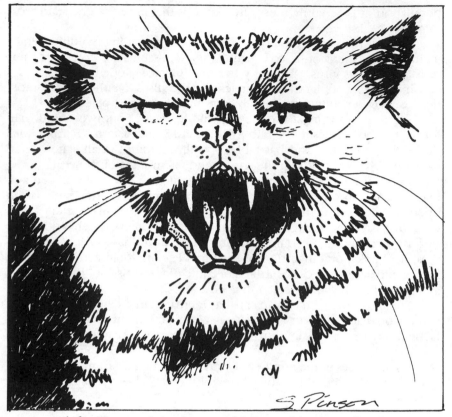

24-6 *The number of cases of feline rabies is on the rise.*

ter of the animal's vocalizations might noticeably change. *Pica,* or an abnormal desire to eat anything within reach (i.e. rocks, wire, dirt, feces, etc.), might become apparent as well.

As the disease enters the third stage, the swallowing reflex becomes paralyzed, making it impossible to eat, drink, or swallow saliva. This is what accounts for the excessive drooling seen in rabid animals.

The furious stage might last for up to a week before progressing into stage 3, the paralytic stage. Pet owners should be aware of the fact that some cats might skip the furious stage entirely, going directly from the prodromal stage into the paralytic stage. When this happens, the disease can be easily mistaken for other nervous system disorders if the diagnostician is not careful. Because this quick transition can occur, the risk of human exposure is greatly increased. The paralytic stage presents itself as a general loss of coordination and paralysis. A droopy lower jaw with the mouth just hanging open is often characteristic. A general paralysis and death usually overtakes the unfortunate animal in a matter of hours.

Diagnosis

Rabies should be suspected anytime a cat exhibits behavioral changes with unexplained, abnormal nervous system signs. Unfortunately, the only way to definitively diagnose a case of rabies is to have a laboratory analysis performed on the animal's brain tissue, which means of course, euthanasia of the animal in question.

Treatment

There is no known treatment for this fatal disease; as a result, stringent control and vaccination measures are a must.

All kittens should receive a rabies immunization between 3 and 4 months of age. In most states, this vaccine must be administered by a licensed veterinarian. Depending on the vaccine used and on the state in which you live, a booster immunization is required every one to three years. Owing to the public health implications of this disease, cat owners who fail to keep their pets current on this immunization are putting their own health at risk!

Other preventative control measures that can be taken include discouraging night roaming and keeping all pets restrained on a leash when walking outside. Repairing or constructing fences and enclosures to help keep wild animals out of a pet's play area will also help reduce chances of exposure.

If a cat is bitten by a stray or wild animal, the wound needs to be seen immediately by a veterinarian, and, depending on when the last one was given, a booster rabies immunization should be administered. The animal should also be placed in quarantine for a minimum of 90 days, unless the particular animal that did the biting can be found and its rabies status confirmed as negative.

If the cat that was bitten by a known carrier of rabies has never been vaccinated before, immediate euthanasia is warranted. If an owner of such a pet refuses to do so, then, for safety sake, the pet should be quarantined for at least six months before it is declared uninfected.

Laws in most states spell out regulations concerning vaccinations, bites involving humans, and the ownership of wildlife in order to curb the impact of this disease. Any vaccinated cat that bites a human being needs to be placed in quarantine for a minimum of ten days to observe for signs of rabies. If suspicious signs appear, the animal is then euthanized, and samples are sent to the laboratory. If there is no history of the cat ever having a rabies vaccine in the past, or if a wild animal is involved, euthanasia and prompt laboratory examination of the brain tissue is warranted to expedite the diagnostic process.

Euthanasia should be carried out only by veterinarians or other public health and/or wildlife officials to ensure that the sample that reaches the lab has been properly handled and stored. Certainly any person bitten by an animal should contact his/her physician immediately. If the situation warrants it, prophylactic rabies treatment will be started on the bitten

individual until the quarantine period is over or until the specific laboratory tests are in.

It is interesting to note that because the concentration of the rabies
virus in the infected cat might be low or even absent in some cases, less
than 50% of all bites from rabies-positive animals will result in the transmission of the disease. Yet because there is no way of knowing which fall
into this category, prophylactic treatment is a must, just to be on the safe
side!

Finally, ownership of wild animals, especially skunks (de-scented or
not) and raccoons, should be avoided for a number of reasons. First, there
are no licensed vaccines available for these wild pets. Secondly, because
the incubation period of rabies can last for months, owners might be
exposing themselves to rabies right from the start without knowing it.
Finally, in many states, it is outright against the law to own such pets without a permit.

Parents should always discourage children from interacting with stray
animals or wildlife. Their natural curiosity could lead to a serious bite
wound and much anxiety, especially if the offender is not found.

BACTERIAL DISEASES

Infections in cats caused by bacterial organisms often occur secondarily
to other disease conditions or trauma, such as bite wounds, stress, viral
infections and/or parasites. For this reason, whenever a bacterial disease
is present, treatments should be directed also against any existing underlying problems.

Bacterial infections of the skin and underlying tissues comprise the
majority of cases seen by veterinarians. For more information on such
infections and their treatment, see chapter 32.

FUNGI AND YEAST

Along with viruses and bacteria, fungal organisms can produce infectious
disease (*mycoses*) in cats. Probably the most common one pet owners are
familiar with and have heard about is *dermatophytosis*, or *ringworm*. In
addition, yeast infections can be a common problem in the ears of cats.
These types of yeast and fungi that affect mainly the outer skin surfaces
are termed *superficial mycoses.*

Ringworm

The most prevalent fungal organism that afflicts felines is ringworm. Ringworm can actually be caused by three different organisms, *Microsporum
canis*, *Trichophyton mentagrophytes*, or *Microsporum gypseum*. The first
two are contracted from infected animals, the third from contaminated
soil.

Microsporum canis is the most common variety affecting cats. In
fact, ringworm-infected cats might not show any external signs whatso-

ever, making them ideal transmitters of the disease to other pets in the household and to people! In some cats, the ringworm causes a circular patch of hair loss with or without an accompanying lesion on the skin beneath (FIG. 24-7).

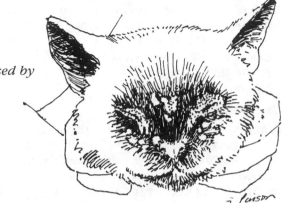

24-7 *Facial lesions caused by ringworm.*

Diagnosis of ringworm is confirmed by a fungal culture performed by a veterinarian. In many cats, ringworm infections are self-limiting and will go away on their own. However, because of the potential threat to humans, all cats found to be positive for ringworm should be treated. This treatment consists of chlorhexidine shampoos, topical antifungal medications (such as miconazole), and oral antifungal medications, such as griseofulvin. It should be strongly emphasized that griseofulvin can cause birth defects and should not be given to pregnant cats.

Subcutaneous or deep mycoses

In contrast to ringworm, fungal and yeast infections involving the deeper tissues of the body are termed subcutaneous or deep mycoses, depending upon the level of tissue involvement. These organisms, including sporotrichosis, aspergillosis, blastomycosis, histoplasmosis, cryptococcosis, and coccidioidomycosis, can be quite severe, and even life-threatening at times. Others exist as well, yet their importance is minor.

Inhalation of fungal spores from infected soil through the respiratory tract is the primary mode of transmission for the majority of these deeper fungi and yeast (with the exception of sporotrichosis). As a result, often the first clinical signs seen relate to some type of respiratory problem. Many of these cats just seem to do poorly and often suffer from chronic weight loss. Others are presented to the veterinarian for a skin disorder or abscess, when in fact the skin problem is being caused by underlying drainage from the deeper fungal involvement.

Sporotrichosis

The fungus that causes sporotrichosis in cats, *Sporothrix schenckii*, can gain entrance into the body via a direct injury to the skin or by inhalation. It then spreads throughout the body by way of the lymphatic system. Cats afflicted with this soil-borne organism can exhibit numerous, tender lumps, nodules, and/or ulcerations anywhere on the body surface, but particularly on the extremities. Some of these lumps might actually resemble warts. In severe instances, liver, lungs, and other body organs can become involved as well. Rhinitis, or inflammation of the nasal passages, is also known to occur in cats suffering from sporotrichosis. Sneezing, nasal discharge, and facial swellings can result from such involvement.

Blastomycosis

Blastomyces dermatitidis is the organism responsible for this disease in cats. Eighty percent of cats affected will show some type of respiratory signs, such as a nonproductive cough. Skin involvement can occur with numerous draining lesions and abscesses, along with lymph node enlargement. Other organ systems can be affected as well. Blindness can result if the organisms spread to the eyes, and lameness, especially in the hind legs, occurs secondary to bony involvement.

Histoplasmosis

Histoplasmosis is caused by the organism *Histoplasma capsulatum*. Soil contaminated with the droppings of starlings and other birds appear to be an important source of this disease in cats. Like blastomycosis, histoplasmosis can strike the respiratory systems of affected cats, leading to coughing and breathing difficulties. The gastrointestinal tract is often involved as well, resulting in chronic diarrhea. Bone, eye, and skin lesions can also result from a histoplasmosis infection.

Coccidioidomycosis

Infections with the fungus *Coccidioides immitis* are associated more with the soil from the dry, desert regions of North America. As with other deep fungi, these spores are inhaled into the lungs, where the organisms set up housekeeping. If the disease remains localized in the lungs, the clinical signs usually reflect this respiratory involvement. Coughing and breathing difficulties result from invasion of the lung tissue and from enlargement of lymph nodes within the chest cavity. If the coccidioidomycosis disseminates throughout the body via the blood and lymphatics, bone infection is common. Lameness, pain, and joint swelling usually occur as a result. Oftentimes, one or more draining tracts originating from the bone infection break through the skin and create unsightly lesions.

Cryptococcosis

Unlike the three conditions mentioned above, this disease is caused by a yeast organism, *Cryptococcus neoformans*, rather than a fungus. Soil contaminated with pigeon and bat feces is a main source of these yeast organisms. Cryptococcosis in cats is mainly an upper respiratory and nasal problem. A thick, copious, continuous nasal discharge usually results, and sneezing can be a clinical sign. From the nasal passages, cryptococcosis can spread throughout the body and cause lameness, enlarged lymph nodes, nervous system impairment (seizures, coma), blindness, and skin infections.

History, physical exam findings, and laboratory tests, including radiographic X-rays and biopsies of affected regions can lead the veterinary practitioner to a tentative diagnosis of a fungal infection within the body. Microscopic examination of body fluids or drainages for fungal spores or yeast can also be helpful. In most cases, a definitive diagnosis is made by testing a blood serum sample for antibodies against the fungal organisms in question, or, less commonly, by culturing for growth.

Medications commonly used to treat fungal infections in cats include amphotericin B, ketoconazole, and 5-flucytosine. Depending upon which agents are used (many are used in combination with one another), duration of treatment required is often one to three months to afford a complete cure for these infections. Radiographs and special immunologic tests can be used to monitor the response to treatment. In many cases, surgical excision of those regions infected with the fungus can afford faster recovery. The prognosis for cats is good when fungal infections are detected and treated in their early stages; guarded to poor if dissemination throughout the body has occurred.

25

Parasitic Diseases

ALONG WITH INFECTIOUS diseases, internal and external parasites are responsible for the vast majority of illnesses and disorders seen in cats. As a result, timely diagnosis and treatment for these pests is vital to the health of the cat.

FLEAS

Fleas are by far the most common external parasite that afflict cats. Aside from the relentless chewing and scratching they cause, fleas are also carriers of such diseases as bubonic plaque and tapeworms. As a result, the development of a good control program to combat these irritating pests is a must.

The flea life cycle includes four major stages: egg, larva; pupa, and adult stages. Both the egg and pupa stages are very resistant to insecticides, which can make complete flea control difficult. During summer months, the entire flea cycle (egg to adult) can be completed in 16−21 days. Heat and humidity tend to shorten this cycle period. In addition, fleas are most prolific during hot humid weather.

TICKS

Ticks, unlike fleas, attach themselves to the pet's skin via their mouth parts. Ticks generally remain attached in one spot for long periods. The head, neck, and interdigital (between toes) areas of the pet are the most common sites of severe infestation (FIG. 25-1). Ticks produce local irritation and even anemia in heavy infestations. They can also serve as inter-

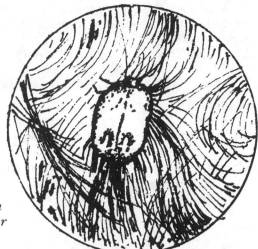

25-1   *Ticks generally remain attached to one spot for long periods of time.*

mediate hosts for disease producing microorganisms and may transmit such illnesses to the infested pet.

For more information on flea and tick control, see chapter 20.

MITES

Mite infestation is commonly known as *mange* and requires the expertise of a veterinarian for diagnosis and treatment.

Notoedres mange

The most common mange mite infecting cats, *Notoedres cati*, is microscopic, and it requires special skin scrapes for its detection. Direct exposure to an infected animal is required for its transmission.

The major symptom of notoedres mange is a sudden onset of severe itching. As the mite burrows into the host's epidermis, itching, hair loss, and scaly skin result, initially on the face, neck, and ears, and then to other areas on the body. The hair coat on these cats often takes on a "mousy" odor as well.

Treatment for notoedres mange consists of special miticidal dipping. These dips should only be performed by a veterinarian, since toxicity can be a problem if they are not used correctly. Total cure can generally be achieved with one to three dippings. All other cats in the household should also be treated due to the highly contagious nature of this mite.

Demodex mange

The *Demodex* mange mite can also affect cats as it does dogs, yet its occurrence rate in the former is quite low. If present, it causes scaly, bald regions on the skin of the head, legs, and feet.

As in dogs, this type of mange infestation is thought to be caused by a poorly functioning immune system. This, combined with the fact that there are no safe, effective medications or dips available to treat this disease in cats, makes a complete cure unlikely.

Cheyletiella mange (walking dandruff)

The third type of mange that can be seen in cats is *Cheyletiella*, or "walking dandruff." This type of mange presents itself as dry, flaky skin with variable amounts of itching. Upon close inspection of the skin flakes, they will appear to be actually moving, hence the name. Microscopic examination of the flakes or of a skin scraping will afford a diagnosis (FIG. 25-2). Once diagnosed, treatment with any one of the common topical insecticidal sprays or powders will usually take care of an infestation.

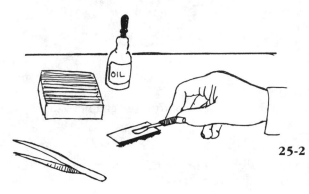

25-2 *Skin scrapings can be used to detect mite infestations in cats.*

WARBLES

Warbles (*Cutrebra*) are an unusual type of parasite that can be found on, or rather in, the skin of cats. They usually appear as nodules or lumps around the head or neck region of affected cats. Oftentimes, these nodules are mistaken for plain abscesses, yet upon close inspection inside, an actual worm, sometimes the size of a grape, will be visible (FIG. 25-3).

Needless to say, such unwelcome guests need to be manually extracted by a veterinarian. In addition, the open cavity left over in the skin after extraction will usually require antibiotics in order for fast healing to take place.

TAPEWORMS

By far, the most prevalent species of tapeworm seen in cats is called *Dipylidium caninum*; the double-pored tapeworm. The reasons it is so common are:

○ It uses the flea as an intermediate host.

○ Because cats are so efficient at grooming themselves, they are likely to accidentally ingest fleas if they are present on the coat.

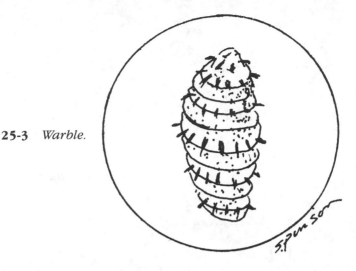

25-3   *Warble.*

Segments from the tapeworm are passed in the feces, or actually "crawl" out onto the hair coat of the infested animal. Once outside, the segments dry out and release egg baskets into the environment. These eggs are then ingested by flea larvae looking for food, and a new tapeworm begins its development inside of the flea. If the flea happens to be ingested by the cat during chewing or self-grooming episodes, the tapeworm larvae will continue its development into an adult worm within the pet's small intestine (FIG. 25-4).

Though less frequent, cats can become infected with other types of tapeworms besides *Dipylidium*. For instance, the hunting habits of some felines put them at high risk of exposure to *Echinococcus granulosus*, the tapeworm responsible for hydatid cyst disease in humans (see chapter 53).

Symptoms

Cats infested with adult tapeworms may or may not exhibit the typical signs associated with gastroenteritis, such as vomiting and diarrhea. Weight loss certainly can occur as the worms absorb nutrients from within the gut.

Diagnosis of a tapeworm infestation can be confirmed by actually seeing the white, moving, worm-like segments in fresh fecal material or on the hair coat around the hind region. Segments might also be seen upon anal sac expression. If dried, the segments will take on a brownish, "rice-like" appearance. Microscopic examination of the stool may be helpful as well; however, because the shedding of the segments is sporadic, a negative finding cannot totally rule out an infestation.

Treatment

Tapeworms can be difficult pests to treat and totally eliminate. Praziquantel and epsiprantel are two effective medications used by veterinarians to

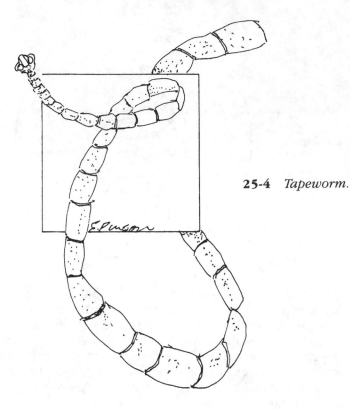

25-4   *Tapeworm.*

eliminate tapeworms from the intestines. Other drugs, such as niclo-samide and bunamidine, have also been used as well. Repeating the treatment in two to three weeks helps ensure thorough elimination.

Flea control is the best way to prevent *Dipyldium caninum*. Daily brushing is an additional means of preventing repeat infestations from occurring. Other tapeworms, including *Echinococcus*, can be prevented by curbing a feline hunting habits via confinement indoors.

ROUNDWORMS

Roundworms, known as ascarids or spool worms, are thick-bodied, whitish- to cream-colored worms that can inhabit the small intestine of cats. Adult worms exist unattached within the intestinal lumen, and can grow up to 8 inches in length.

Symptoms

If present in large enough numbers, roundworms can cause prominent malnutrition and gastroenteritis, with associated vomiting and diarrhea. In addition, larval forms of the worms have the ability to migrate through the tissues when ingested and, in rare instances, cause neurological disease (FIG. 25-5).

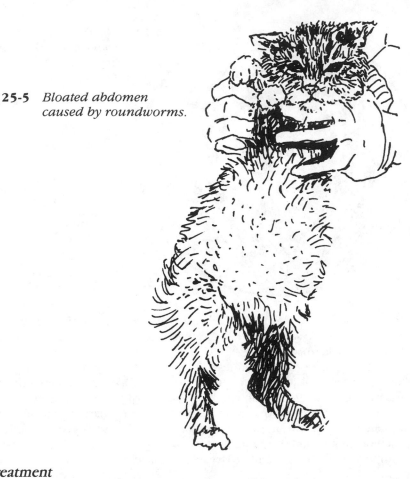

25-5 *Bloated abdomen caused by roundworms.*

Treatment

Veterinarians can diagnose roundworms by using a microscope to look for eggs in a sample of stool from a cat. If diagnosed, there are a wide variety of deworming drugs effective at removing roundworms from the intestines. Relatively inexpensive dewormers can be obtained at grocery stores and pet supplies. Owners should be sure, however, to consult a veterinarian before using one of these to be certain that it contains the correct ingredients for the pet's particular problem. Repeat dewormings should be performed three weeks later to ensure a complete kill has been achieved.

HOOKWORMS

The hookworm is another type of parasite that can inhabit the small intestine of cats. Unlike the roundworm, which floats unattached within the intestinal lumen, absorbing nutrients through its skin, the hookworm actually uses teeth to attach itself to the wall of the intestine (FIG. 25-6).

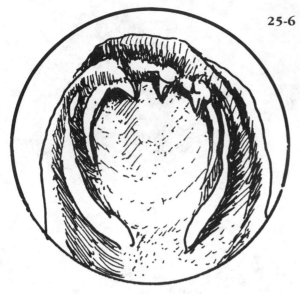

25-6 *The mouth of a hookworm is designed for grasping and sucking.*

Once attached, it begins to suck blood from vessels within the wall. In fact, it can become so severe that the resulting anemia and gastroenteritis could lead to death!

Fortunately, hookworm infestations are not very common in cats. Diagnosis of a hookworm infestation is based upon an examination of a stool sample by a veterinarian for the presence of hookworm eggs. There are a number of safe dewormers available from veterinarians that can help eliminate a hookworm infection. After the initial dose is given, a follow-up deworming should be administered two to three weeks later to ensure a complete kill. Any migrating larvae that have since reached the intestines.

LUNGWORMS

Lungworm infections in cats are uncommon, yet worth mentioning. *Aleurostrongylus abstrusus* and *Capillaria aerophila* are two parasites that can live within the respiratory tract of affected felines, causing weight loss, chronic coughing, and difficulty breathing (FIG. 25-7).

Because eggs or larvae from these lung parasites are passed in the stool, fecal examinations can be used by veterinarians to diagnose an infection. Radiographic X-rays, microscopic examination of respiratory fluids, and direct examination of the airways using an endoscope can also lead to a diagnosis. Once this is confirmed, dewormers such as levamisole or fenbendazole can be used to tackle lungworm infestations in cats.

Paragonimus kellicotti, the lung fluke, can also infest the airways of cats, causing disease very similar to lungworms. Diagnosis and treatment are the same as for lungworms. Fortunately, this parasite is quite rare in cats.

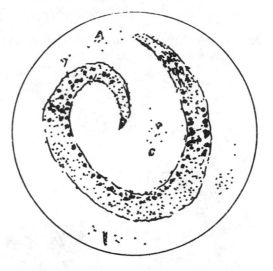

25-7 *Cat lungworm.*

HEARTWORMS

As frightening as it might seem, the incidence of this disease, once thought limited to canines, is on the rise in cats as well.

Symptoms

Dirofilaria immitis, the same mosquito-borne organism that causes canine heartworm disease also causes the feline disease. Most cats that become infested with heartworms develop less than ten worms within the heart, yet even this low number can damage the heart and lead to lung and kidney disease as they do in the dog.

Male cats allowed to roam outdoors are at greatest risk of contracting this disease. Many cats infested with heartworms will show no clinical signs whatsoever, with the disease being identified incidentally when these cats are brought to the veterinarian for other reasons. In more advanced cases, lethargy, breathing difficulties, coughing, vomiting, and sometimes even blindness can occur.

Treatment

Similar testing procedures used to diagnose canine heartworm disease can be used in an attempt to diagnose the condition in cats, yet because the worm burden in these felines is often very low, some cases may not be picked up by such tests. As a result, many veterinarians base their diagnosis on clinical signs and chest radiographs (X-rays), which usually reveal changes in the heart and lungs characteristic of heartworms. Treatment is basically the same as that used for dogs, with thiacetarsamide sodium given intravenously in a hospital setting for several days.

Although it might be on the horizon, administering preventative heartworm medication to cats as it is done so in dogs is not common practice at this time.

COCCIDIA

Coccidia are microscopic protozoan parasites that inhabit the small intestine of affected cats (FIG. 25-8).

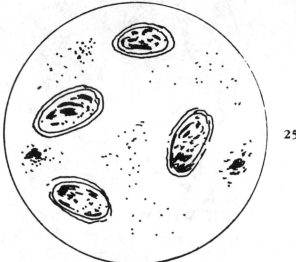

25-8   *Coccidia.*

Symptoms

The disease caused by coccidia (coccidiosis) is characterized by diarrhea, which can rapidly dehydrate a young kitten if not brought under control.

Overcrowding and poor sanitation greatly contribute to the spread of these organisms with a group of cats or kittens. Eggs passed in fecal material can be directly ingested by another feline, leading to the development and maturation of the organisms within the gut of the new host.

Occasionally, tissue migration can occur, especially with the coccidian parasite, *Toxoplasma*, leading to fever, muscle pain, and/or convulsions. Fortunately, this presentation is quite uncommon in cats.

Treatment

Blood tests might be necessary for a diagnosis of toxoplasmosis; however, for most coccidian parasites, a microscopic examination of a stool specimen for eggs is all that it takes. If coccidia are present, treatment then consists of administering an anticoccidia drug in proper dosages. Sulfa drugs and nitrofurazone have been used by veterinarians to eliminate active coccidia infections in cats.

If *Toxoplasma* is involved, more extensive treatment utilizing different types of medications might be required. Certainly if dehydration or other signs are noticed, supportive hospital treatment will be needed

Good sanitation practices are the best ways to prevent exposure to coccidiosis. Routine stool checks performed by a veterinarian should also be utilized to ensure cats remains parasite-free.

As a zoonotic disease, toxoplasmosis is of quite significance, especially in pregnant women. For more information, see chapter 53.

CYTAUXZOONOSIS

Cytauxzoonosis is found mainly across the southeastern portion of the United States in cats allowed to roam in heavily wooded areas.

Symptoms

Ticks are thought to transmit this protozoal organism, which attacks the host's red blood cells and causes anemia. As a result, clinical signs associated with cytauxzoonosis include those related to anemia, such as loss of appetite, lethargy, breathing difficulties, and pale mucous membranes.

Treatment

Veterinarians can diagnose this disorder by observing specially stained blood smears under the microscope. Unfortunately, once a diagnosis is made, there is no known effective treatment and infected cats invariably die from the disease. Good tick control and limiting access to high risk environmental areas are the two best ways to protect a cat from this fatal disease.

HAEMOBARTONELLOSIS

Haemobartonellosis in cats is caused by the bacterial organism *Haemobartonella felis*. This disease, which causes a profound anemia, occurs most often in young, male cats around 4 to 6 years old. Insects are thought to be the mode of transmission between these organisms and cats.

Symptoms

Clinical signs of haemobartonellosis include a sudden onset of depression, loss of appetite, and fever. Because of the anemia the disease causes, the gums and mucous membranes of these cats are often quite pale. In addition, the skin and whites of the eyes may appear jaundiced as well.

Treatment

Diagnosis of this disease in cats can be made in a veterinary setting from the microscopic examination of fresh blood from suspected cats. Many felines suffering from haemobartonellosis also concurrently have feline leukemia. As a result, a feline leukemia test should be preformed on all cats with haemobartonellosis. Haemobartonellosis is treated with blood transfusions if the anemia caused by it is severe, and with special antibiotics, including tetracycline. Thiacetarasamide sodium, the antiheartworm drug, has also been used with some effectiveness in tough cases.

The prognosis for recovery from the anemia and associated symptoms is good if treatment is instituted quickly. Unfortunately, a total cure is rarely possible with this disease, and owners should be on the lookout for stress-induced relapses, and seek prompt treatment for their felines if such should happen.

26

The Immune System

WITHOUT A FUNCTIONING immune system, our pets (and ourselves) would fall easy prey to every hostile organism that came around. Immunity is designed to protect against such infectious invaders and eliminate any foreign matter or cells that somehow gain entrance into the body. Preventing the growth of cancer cells and tumors is also in its job description.

The immune system itself is a complex network of cells, organs, and special chemicals. No one division overshadows another; each team member relies on the others for support. In this way, they all work in unison towards a common goal. Since the immune system of the cat is essentially identical to that of dogs, see chapter 8 for more details as to the cells, organs and functions of the immune system.

IMMUNOSUPPRESSION

Although the immune system serves a rough and rugged function, a delicate balance does exist as far as its activity is concerned. Stress, poor nutrition, and hormone fluctuations are but some of the many factors which can deleteriously alter this activity, leading to a weakened defense system. As if this weren't enough, certain viruses, such as the feline leukemia and feline AIDS viruses, also have the ability to suppress the very system designed to defend against them. Overcoming the body's natural defense mechanisms can only lead to one outcome, and it isn't good.

AUTOIMMUNE DISEASE

In contrast to immunosuppression, an overactive immune system can actually harm its hosts by damaging its internal organs. *Lupus erythematosus* and *pemphigus* are two autoimmune disorders that result from an overactive immune system. These two diseases often cause notable skin lesions, aside from affecting other organs of the body. *Autoimmune hemolytic anemia* is another disease caused by an overactive immune system. In this instance, the immune system actually destroys the body's own red blood cells, leading to anemia.

Finally, the classic example in cats of an immune system gone awry is *feline infectious peritonitis.* In this disease, it is not the virus itself but rather the exaggerated immune response to it that actually proves fatal to the cat.

Autoimmune reactions are controlled with high doses of corticosteroid medication, which has a suppressive effect on the immune system. However, because these steroids can have significant side effects at these high doses, such treatments should only be performed under the close, continual supervision of a veterinarian.

27

The Cardiovascular & Hemolymphatic Systems

THE SYSTEMS RESPONSIBLE for the effective transmission of oxygen and nutrition to all organs and tissues of the body. This system is comprised of the heart, the vessels which carry blood to and from the heart, the blood itself, and the lymphatic channels, which transport lymph within the body (FIG. 27-1).

For a more in-depth discussion regarding the anatomy and function of cardiovascular/hemolymphatic systems, see chapter 9 in the *Dogs* section.

FELINE CARDIOMYOPATHY

Changes in the thickness and/or contractility of the muscles making up the heart are termed *cardiomyopathies*. Cardiomyopathies are known to occur in the feline species. The two main types of cardiomyopathies that cats can suffer from are *hypertrophic cardiomyopathy* and *dilated cardiomyopathy*.

In hypertrophic cardiomyopathy, the muscular heart walls become excessively thickened, shrinking the chambers of the heart and disrupting normal filling of the heart with blood. With dilated cardiomyopathy, the opposite occurs: The heart walls become thinned and weak, making normal contractions difficult. Regardless of the type, a cardiomyopathy can lead to overt heart failure if progression occurs.

Cardiomyopathies seem to be more prevalent in middle-aged cats; males seem to have a greater preponderance than do females. In addition, Siamese, Burmese, and Abyssinian cats appear to have a higher incidence of this disorder than do other breeds. The causes of hypertrophic cardiomyopathy in cats remain unknown; however, researchers have found a

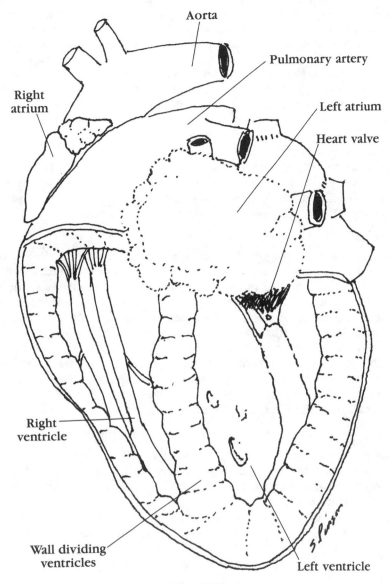

Aorta

Pulmonary artery

Right atrium

Left atrium

Heart valve

Right ventricle

Wall dividing ventricles

Left ventricle

27-1 *The feline heart.*

link between dilated cardiomyopathy and dietary deficiencies in the amino acid taurine.

Symptoms

An increased lethargy and loss of appetite might be the initial signs seen in cats with cardiomyopathies. Other more advanced clinical signs can include coughing, difficulty in breathing, and overt "collapsing." Vomiting can also become a factor, especially if there is secondary kidney damage caused by poor blood circulation. In addition, hind-end weakness and muscular pain due to aortic thromboembolism can be seen in these affected individuals.

Such clinical signs can help lead a veterinarian to a diagnosis of cardiomyopathy in a cat. Using a stethoscope, the veterinarian can often detect rapid heart rates, abnormal rhythms, and heart murmurs as well. Radiographic X-rays and ultrasound often show abnormal heart shapes, abnormal heart wall thickness, and, if heart failure is present, fluid buildup within the thorax in these cats.

Electrocardiograms are useful to determine the extent of any heart enlargement and to assess the electrical conduction occurring within the heart walls. If a taurine deficiency is suspected, measuring blood levels of this amino acid can prove or disprove such suspicions.

Treatment

Treatment of cardiomyopathies consists of medications designed to reduce blood pressure and to increase the efficiency of heart contractions. Drugs designed to move fluids out of the lungs may also be prescribed if such a condition exists. In those cats with advanced heart failure, oxygen therapy might be necessary. Obviously, for those cats with taurine-deficiency cardiomyopathy, taurine supplementation should also be used to normalize cardiac function.

Unfortunately, there is little that can be done to reverse the anatomic changes to the heart afforded by most cardiomyopathies. With supportive treatment, however, the quality of life for affected felines can be maintained at a good level for months, even years.

Taurine and feline cardiomyopathy

Taurine is an amino acid that plays several important roles within the body. It is used to help inactivate toxins within the liver and—more importantly in terms of cardiomyopathy—assists in the normal contraction of heart muscle cells.

Taurine is normally synthesized within the bodies of most mammals—most, that is, except the cat. As a result, felines need to obtain their taurine through dietary means. If a diet contains subnormal levels of the amino acid, then a taurine deficiency and dilated cardiomyopathy can result.

Heart disease is not the only syndrome that can result from deficient levels of taurine. Another, called *feline central retinal degeneration,* involves the retina of the eye and can eventually lead to blindness.

Less commonly, taurine deficiencies can produce other neurologic problems, abortions in pregnant queens and neuromuscular disease in kittens, and immunosuppression.

To ward off deficiencies in this vital amino acid, cat foods should contain over 1000 ppm taurine in dry varieties, and greater than 2000 ppm taurine in the moist types. Until just recently, many commercial diets designed for feline consumption were deficient in taurine levels. However, since the link between taurine and cardiomyopathy in cats has been discovered, most pet food companies have reformulated their products to include adequate amounts of taurine. As a result, taurine-deficiency-induced cardiomyopathy is not seen as often as it once was.

Taurine deficiencies can also be caused by gastrointestinal disturbances impeding the proper absorption of taurine from the intestines. This can become significant in those cats suffering from chronic inflammatory bowel disease. It is vital that these cats be fed a taurine-rich diet, and that they have heart function monitored periodically by a veterinarian. Needless to say, any cat that is suspected of having a cardiomyopathy should have blood taurine levels checked, even if the diet it is on is adequate in the amino acid.

For those instances in which taurine supplementation is warranted, taurine supplementation can be accomplished through taurine capsules prescribed by veterinarians. As far as natural food substances go, minced clams and tuna are both good sources of taurine and can be used as substitutes for the capsules if desired. Owners should ask a veterinarian for feeding amounts.

ARTERIAL THROMBOEMBOLISM

Cats afflicted with cardiomyopathy suffer from impaired circulation, which in turn can lead to a condition known as *arterial thromboembolism*. This disorder is characterized by large blood clots that form within the left side of the heart and pass into circulation, only to lodge within one or more blood vessels within the body. The most common region for this lodging to occur is where the large aorta divides into two smaller arteries that supply the hind end.

Symptoms

When such a clot restricts blood flow to the back legs, pronounced end limb weakness results. The hind paws might feel cold to the touch, and the clear nails might take on a bluish tinge. As the muscles of the hind end are deprived of blood and oxygen, they become firm and painful to the touch.

Diagnosis of arterial thromboembolism is based upon clinical signs seen and a physical exam. A total absence or partial reduction in hind-limb pulse is diagnostic as well (FIG. 27-2).

Treatment

Treatment for arterial thromboembolism is difficult at best. Surgery is usually unrewarding, and the existing heart disease in these cats makes them high anesthetic risks. Medical therapy can be somewhat effective if instituted within a few hours of onset. This involves administering drugs designed to dissolve the blood clot and restore normal blood flow.

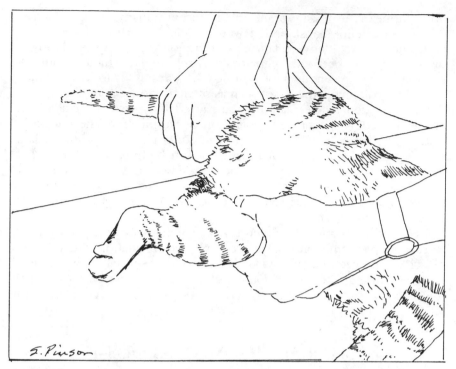

27-2   *Cats with thromboembolism often lack a pulse in the hind limbs.*

Prognosis for a full recovery is guarded, simply because of the pre-existing heart disease and because of chronic pain and tissue damage caused by the temporary loss of oxygen. However, with physical therapy and attentive nursing care, many cats can obtain at least partial functional restoration in one to two months.

ANEMIA

Anemia is defined as an overall reduction in the number of red blood cells within the bloodstream relative to normal levels. This reduction can occur from a number of processes, including an increased destruction or decreased production of red blood cells within the body. TABLE 27-1 lists some of the major causes of anemia in cats. The overall consequence of anemia is the inability of the blood to supply desired levels of oxygen to the tissues.

Symptoms

Signs seen in an anemic cat include intense lethargy, weakness, increased respiratory and heart rates, and a pallor of the mucous membranes. Depending upon the cause of the anemia, signs related to a blood clotting disorder might be seen as well. Finally, if red blood cells are being

Table 27-1   Potential Causes of Anemia in Cats

Iron/B_{12} deficiency
Kidney disease
Addison's disease
Liver disease
Toxins (e.g., lead poisoning)
Cancer
Feline leukemia
Haemobartonella
Trauma—blood loss
Hookworms
External parasites (fleas, ticks)
Blood clotting disorders
Gastric ulcers
Drug reactions (e.g., aspirin)
Autoimmune hemolytic anemia

destroyed within the body, the skin and mucous membranes might become jaundiced.

Treatment

Treatment of anemia depends upon the underlying cause. In severe cases, blood transfusions and oxygen therapy might be required to save the pet's life until the cause can be identified and treated.

BLEEDING DISORDERS

Whenever an injury or illness compromises a blood vessel and leads to bleeding out of that vessel, a remarkable mechanism or chain reaction begins within the body in an effort to stop the leakage of blood from the damaged vessel and prevent the individual from bleeding to death. This mechanism is known as *hemostasis*.

When a blood vessel is compromised, the first reaction that occurs is constriction of the vessel to help slow blood loss. Following this, special blood cells called *platelets* begin to adhere to the injured vessel wall, forming a temporary plug. At the same time, a *coagulation* (clotting) pathway is activated within the body, involving a complex interaction of blood and tissue components, as well as calcium and vitamin K. The end result of this pathway is the formation of a more permanent clot at the site of injury.

Bleeding disorders can occur whenever any part of the clotting mechanism is interfered with. Platelet numbers or function can be interfered with by diseases or substances such as toxins, drugs, cancers, autoimmune hemolytic anemia, and infectious agents such as feline infectious peritonitis. In addition, kidney disease and certain congenital defects can also lead to poor platelet function and secondary bleeding.

Any disruptions of the coagulation pathway also spell trouble for hemostasis. For instance, most mouse and rat poisons contain substances that interfere with the vitamin K component of the coagulation pathway. If these are accidentally ingested by a cat, the cat's coagulation pathway will be effectively disrupted. Liver disease can lead to bleeding disorders because many of the components used in blood clotting are manufactured in that organ. Inherited defects in the coagulation pathway, such as hemophilia, are rare in cats.

Serious diseases or injuries such as feline infectious peritonitis, heat stroke, or massive trauma (such as that caused by a car) can lead to a secondary condition known as *disseminated intravascular coagulation* (DIC). In DIC, tiny blood clots form all throughout the body. Not only are these clots detrimental to the health of the animal, but DIC also leads to a depletion of the body's clotting components. This, in turn, predisposes the cat to a bleeding disorder. DIC is invariably fatal to a pet unless rapid supportive treatment is instituted.

Symptoms

Clinical signs of a bleeding disorder usually include noticeable bruising of the skin and mucous membranes. Blood in the urine or feces, nosebleeds, joint pain, abdominal pain, and breathing difficulties might be seen as well. Because of the variety of potential causes, a veterinarian will need to run a series of tests to determine the exact cause and to formulate a proper treatment regimen.

Treatment

Initial treatment for any bleeding disorder entails blood transfusions until the exact cause is discerned. If rodenticide poisoning is suspected, vitamin K injections, followed by oral vitamin K tablets, will help reverse the effects of the poison. These tablets should be given daily for a minimum of four weeks, since the ingested poison could linger within the body and exert its effects for this length of time.

28

The Respiratory System

THE RESPIRATORY system works in conjunction with the circulatory system to provide oxygen to and remove carbon dioxide from the body tissues. Oxygen is the driving force behind all chemical reactions that occur internally; obviously, without it, life could not exist. As a result, the function of all body systems, including the respiratory system itself, depends first upon the ability of this system to deliver its product.

In addition to this vital function, the respiratory system also serves as a means of *thermoregulation*, or body heat exchange, in the cat. Since cats can't sweat in the conventional way, they rely upon heat transfer out of the body through exhaled air. That is why cats pant when they get hot.

For more information on the anatomy of the respiratory system, see chapter 10.

NASAL FOREIGN BODIES

Occasionally, foreign bodies can gain entrance into the nasal passageways of cats via the mouth, causing extreme irritation and rhinitis or sinusitis. The two biggest culprits in this category seem to be plant awns and blades of grass—not unusual since many cats love to chew on foliage.

Cats with nasal foreign bodies will exhibit sneezing and usually have a cloudy or bloody discharge coming from one or both nostrils. Veterinary inspection of the far reaches of the mouth and inner entrances into the nasal passages while the cat is sedated or anesthetized is often enough to identify and extract the culprit (FIG. 28-1). If not, surgery might be required for removal and to prevent secondary complications associated with bacterial infections.

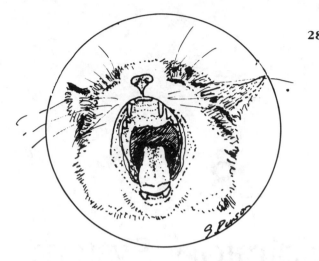

28-1 *A veterinarian's inspection of the far reaches of the mouth and inner entrances to the nasal passages are usually enough to determine whether or not the cat has a foreign body lodged in its nasal passages.*

FELINE ASTHMA

Felines can suffer from asthma attacks very similar to those seen in people. They are usually triggered by an allergic reaction to pollens and other allergens that are breathed into the lungs. The reaction caused by the immune system's response can be minor, or it can be quite severe, causing bronchitis and *pneumonitis* (inflammation of the lungs). This, in turn, can lead to severe breathing difficulties, coughing, and gagging in affected felines. Any cat can suffer from feline asthma, regardless of age.

Along with a good history of occurrence and clinical signs seen, diagnosis of feline asthma is aided by radiographic X-rays of the lungs. Long-standing, recurring cases can actually exhibit scarring or fibrosis of the lung tissue.

Treatment of feline asthma involves identifying, if possible, the source of the allergic reaction and the use of corticosteroids to reduce the allergic inflammation. When looking for the source, some experts recommend starting with and changing the cat litter, especially those that exude a dust when poured. Often, though, the source of the problem cannot be pinpointed, and symptomatic therapy will be needed each time a flare-up occurs.

PNEUMONIA AND PLEURAL EFFUSION

Any inflammation and/or infection involving the lungs is termed *pneumonia*. In cats, pneumonia can result from a variety of diseases and organisms.

Pleural effusion is not really a disease entity in itself; rather, it is a sign of disease in cats. The *pleural space* is an air-filled space located in the thoracic cavity between the inner thoracic wall and the thoracic organs themselves. Pleural effusion is a buildup of fluid—such as blood, pus, or serum—within this pleural space. This effectively interferes with the normal functioning of the heart and lungs.

Some of the potential causes of pleural effusions include infectious diseases (bacterial infections, FIP, feline leukemia), foreign bodies, rupture of lymphatic vessels, cardiomyopathy, or cancer.

Cats afflicted with pneumonia or a pleural effusion must fight for every breath, often exhibiting open-mouthed breathing with their necks extended forward. In severe instances, they can collapse from lack of oxygen. Emergency treatment is a must.

If pleural effusion is present, treatment will involve drainage of the fluid from the chest. This usually entails placement of a temporary drain tube within the chest to facilitate continued drainage as it is required until the exact cause of the problem can be discerned. The nature of the fluid removed from the pleural space will usually afford the veterinarian enough information as to pinpoint the exact cause of the effusion. Treatment is then directed accordingly.

The prognosis is poor for those cats exhibiting severe respiratory signs upon admission to the hospital, or for those suffering from FIP or feline leukemia.

29

The Digestive System

THE DIGESTIVE SYSTEM of the cat is made up of a collective network of organs designed to supply the body with the nutrition it needs for growth, maintenance, and repair. It also functions to rid the body of waste that it does not use. Because of this role in nutrition and waste management, diseases involving the digestive system can have a profound effect not just on the region so afflicted, but on the entire body as well.

For a more in-depth discussion regarding the anatomy and function of the digestive system, refer to chapter 11 in the *Dogs* section.

GASTROINTESTINAL RESPONSE TO DISEASE

Considering what they have to go through each day, the stomach and intestines (gastrointestinal tract) comprise a remarkable organ system. In the performance of their daily nutritional functions, they must be on constant guard to protect themselves from autodigestion by digestive acids and enzymes produced and must constantly battle foreign organisms and agents that are inadvertently taken in by mouth.

When the stomach and/or intestines become acutely diseased, three major factors come into play that can quickly turn a seemingly harmless situation into a life-threatening predicament. These are pain, secondary bacterial infection, and dehydration.

Pain

Any inflammation and/or excessive smooth muscle contractions occurring within the gastrointestinal system can be quite discomforting and painful. In fact, in severe cases of viral enteritis, intestinal obstructions, and intussusceptions, this pain can be so great that the patient goes into life-threatening shock. As a result, the sooner therapeutic measures are undertaken to correct the problem and stifle the pain associated with it, the less the chances are of complications from occurring.

Secondary bacterial invasion

The second factor to contend with is secondary bacterial invasion. Normally, the intestines are inhabited by billions of bacteria that peacefully reside within without causing any problems whatsoever. In fact, the very presence of these non-disease-causing bacteria actually helps to prevent the growth of *pathogenic,* or disease-causing, bacteria within the intestinal setting. However, if disease strikes the small or large intestines, these ''friendly'' bacteria can be wiped out, allowing pathogenic ones to proliferate and cause disease themselves. If the inflammation persists, or if an intestinal perforation occurs, these and any other bacteria within the intestines can leak out of the gut and even gain entrance into the bloodstream, causing a life-threatening systemic infection and shock.

For these reasons, it is obvious that antibiotics become very important in the treatment of moderate to severe cases of gastroenteritis, even if the original cause is nonbacterial in origin.

Dehydration

The final threatening factor that arises when acute gastroenteritis strikes a pet is dehydration. Pets suffering from vomiting and/or diarrhea can quickly become dehydrated due to water loss through the bowels. Since inflamed bowels cannot regulate water absorption as they do when they are healthy, any fluid intake that indeed occurs will usually pass right out of the body via vomiting and/or diarrhea without being absorbed.

In fact, the disruption of normal motility and distension occurring within the affected bowel can actually attract and draw water right out of the body and into the intestinal lumen. As a result, cats that have become dehydrated or are on the verge of dehydration due to gastroenteritis require intravenous fluids to correct the dehydration occurring within the body's cells, at least until the gut has healed sufficiently to resume these functions once again.

Treatment

Once the gastrointestinal system is on the mend, and all vomiting has been brought under control, a good plane of nutrition is required to counteract any malnutrition induced by the disease. Bland diets that are easily digested are prescribed until complete healing of the stomach and/or intestinal linings have taken place. Offering a convalescent cat some type of electrolyte replacement drinks during these first few days can also promote rapid recovery as well. Feeding plain yogurt is also helpful towards repopulating the gastrointestinal tract with nonpathogenic bacteria.

DISORDERS OF THE TEETH AND ORAL CAVITY

Diseases and disorders affecting the teeth and/or oral cavity interfere with a pet's ability to prehense and process food for digestion. In addition, other general signs associated with conditions involving these areas usually include increased salivation, swallowing difficulties, bad breath, gagging, and/or decreased appetite.

Periodontal disease

Periodontal disease, or tooth and gum disease, is one of the more prevalent health disorders in cats. Early signs of this disorder can include tender, swollen gums, and, most commonly, bad breath. More importantly though, left untreated, periodontal disease can lead to secondary disease conditions that can seriously threaten the health of affected cats.

Periodontal disease begins with the formation of plaque on tooth surfaces. This plaque is nothing more than a thin film of food particles and bacteria. Over time, however, plaque mineralizes and hardens to form calculus. Owners who lift up their cat's lip and glance at its teeth, especially near the gum line, might note a brownish to yellowish build-up of calculus on the inner and outer surface of the teeth.

Diet can play an important role in the development of periodontal disease in cats. For instance, moist cat foods tend to be high in sugar content, and they can promote plaque formation much more readily than do the dry varieties. In addition, diets containing too much phosphorus (such as all-meat rations) have been linked to periodontal disease.

Certain underlying disease conditions can also promote periodontal disease as a side effect. For example, both feline leukemia and feline AIDS are commonly manifested outwardly as swollen and infected gums. Periodontal disease can also occur incidentally to tumors involving the gum tissue and/or teeth.

Symptoms

Cats suffering from periodontal disease can exhibit a diverse selection of clinical signs. Early periodontal disease might be marked only by a decreased appetite due to swollen, painful gums. Cat owners often complain of bad breath in their pet, and they might notice signs of gagging or retching as secondary tonsillitis sets in. As the disease progresses, these signs might worsen, and other symptoms, such as gum recession, gum bleeding, and tooth loss, might arise. Infected teeth that do not fall out can form abscesses and can be marked by sinus infections, nasal discharges, or draining tracts appearing on the face.

But the damage caused by periodontal disease doesn't stop there. Bacteria can gain entrance into the bloodstream by way of the teeth and gums, seeding the body with infectious organisms. In advanced cases, these bacteria can overwhelm the host's immune system and set up housekeeping on the valves of the heart. The resulting *valvular endocarditis* in turn can lead to heart murmurs and eventual heart failure. The bacteria which gain access to the body because of periodontal disease can also lodge in the kidney, causing infection, inflammation, and acute damage. Over time, signs related to kidney failure might develop in affected cats.

Treatment

Early cases of periodontal disease can be treated by a thorough scaling and polishing of the teeth to remove the offending calculus. This scaling needs to be professionally performed under sedation or anesthesia to ensure complete removal of the calculus under the gum line. Using special instruments to hand scale a cat's teeth at home without anesthesia is not only dangerous, but highly ineffective at cleaning the teeth where it counts the most, up under the gum line. Furthermore, such scaling, if not followed by polishing, will leave etches in the enamel covering of the teeth, which serve as foci for future plaque and calculus buildup.

Antibiotics will also be prescribed for cats suffering from moderate to advanced periodontal disease to combat the associated bacterial infection. Teeth that are excessively loose within their sockets serve only to propagate infection and should be extracted. For infected teeth that are still deemed viable, root canals can be performed as salvage procedures.

See chapter 21 for prevention tips to help protect cats against the adverse effects of periodontal disease.

Cleft palate

The palate is a fleshy structure located at the roof of the mouth that separates the oral cavity from the nasal passages. The firm portion located forward-most in the mouth is termed the *hard palate*, whereas the softer, flexible portion towards the back of the mouth is called the *soft palate*. *Cleft palate* is a disease condition in which the palate fails to fully develop, leaving a communication gap between the mouth and the nasal passages.

This condition can be inherited, or it can be acquired secondary to foreign bodies puncturing the palate, or by burns caused by electrical cords.

Neonatal kittens born with cleft palates often die because they are unable to suckle properly. The ones that do survive initially can develop nasal infections and aspiration pneumonia if the problem is not surgically corrected in time. The recommended time of surgery for these kittens is around 6 weeks of age. Until then, daily feedings using a tube passed directly into the esophagus and bypassing the mouth altogether is indicated to prevent these secondary complications.

Plasma cell gingivitis

Plasma cell gingivitis is a condition of the oral cavity characterized by red, friable gums, which often grow over and cover the teeth.

Symptoms

Cats affected with this disorder often have difficulty chewing their food, have foul-smelling breath, and might even have cavities affecting the teeth. The inflammation associated with the disease can also spread to the back of the throat, making swallowing difficult.

The exact cause of this disorder in cats is unknown; however, conceivably any type of chronic inflammation that attracts special types of immune system cells, called *plasma cells*, could cause such a reaction.

Treatment

Diagnosis of plasma cell gingivitis is made by collecting a biopsy sample of the affected tissue. Treatment consists of surgically removing and/or cauterizing the excess gum tissue. If periodontal disease is present, it should be treated as well.

In especially severe cases, steroid anti-inflammatory medication might be indicated as well. Unfortunately, however, plasma cell gingivitis tends to reoccur frequently after treatment; a fact all cat owners should be aware of.

Oral ulcers

Although ulcerations affecting the feline mouth and tongue can be caused by chemical or electrical burns, many such ulcers occur secondary to some underlying health disorder (FIG. 29-1). For instance, infectious diseases such as feline calicivirus and feline leukemia might cause such ulcers and associated bad breath. Other serious internal disease conditions such

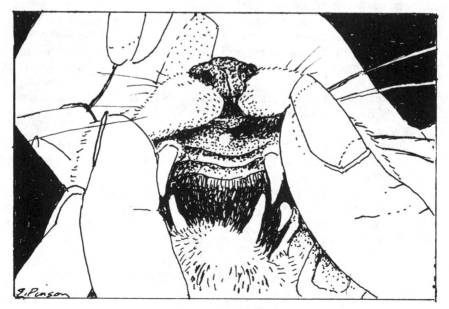

29-1 *Oral ulcer.*

as kidney failure, diabetes mellitus, or autoimmune disease can also be manifested in this fashion as well. In all of these instances, treatment is aimed at clearing up the underlying disease syndrome if possible.

Ulcerations affecting the lips of cats can be caused by a condition known as eosinophilic granuloma complex. These red, angry-looking lesions often lead to excessive salivation and a reluctance to eat. Treatment using anti-inflammatory or progestin medications can help clear up these types of ulcers; unfortunately, however, re-occurrence is common.

Oral foreign bodies

A cat's natural playful attraction to strings, threads, and ribbons could lead to health problems. As impossible as it might seem, such items can become wrapped around the base of the tongue and be partially swallowed, causing gagging, retching, salivation, and difficulty swallowing food and water. Other oral foreign bodies, such as fishhooks, needles, bones, and grass awns, can cause similar signs.

Symptoms
Many cats suffering from an oral foreign body will paw at their mouths or exhibit exaggerated licking motions in fruitless attempts to dislodge the unwelcome object. Depending on the length of time that the object has been there, *halitosis* (bad breath) might become an obvious sign as well.

Treatment
In most instances, a diagnosis of such a problem can be made upon an oral examination—assuming, of course, that the cat wants to cooperate. If it doesn't, sedation might be required first. Needles, fishhooks, and other metal objects will also show up on radiographic X-rays.

Removal of the offending foreign body will afford a cure. However, if a piece of string (for instance) is extending down into the esophagus, forceful removal should be avoided. In these instances, surgical removal might be required.

Finally, for those foreign bodies that penetrated any oral tissue, antibiotic therapy should be instituted following their removal to prevent secondary bacterial infections from setting up housekeeping within the mouth.

Oral tumors

Like other regions of the body, the oral cavity is not immune to its share of tumors and growths. A wide variety of tumors, including melanomas, sarcomas, and carcinomas, can arise within the oral cavity of cats. The most prevalent tumor occurring within the mouths of cats is the *squamous cell carcinoma*.

Signs associated with oral tumors in cats include halitosis (bad breath), oral bleeding, excessive salivation, and/or swallowing difficulties. In severe cases, actual facial deformities could occur secondary to the tumor growth.

Rapid recognition of the presence of an oral tumor and concurrent treatment are essential, since most oral tumors in cats, if malignant, will spread very rapidly to other areas of the body, including the lungs. For more information on oral tumors, see chapter 54.

ESOPHAGEAL DISORDERS

Disorders involving the esophagus will manifest themselves as difficulty in swallowing and regurgitation. Effortless regurgitation of solid food, which must be differentiated from vomiting and its associated abdominal spasms, often tips off the pet owner and veterinary practitioner to an existing problem with the esophagus. Due to the inability to properly swallow food, cats afflicted with esophageal disease are at high risk of accidentally aspirating food into their lungs, causing serious, life-threatening pneumonia.

Megaesophagus

Megaesophagus is the term given to the condition in which a generalized enlargement of the esophagus occurs, making it unable to push food into the stomach. This condition might be inherited, or seen secondary esophageal obstructions or to neuromuscular diseases.

Symptoms

Signs seen with megaesophagus include regurgitation minutes to hours after eating or drinking. Oftentimes, the undigested food will appear to be shaped like a tube or a sausage link. Certainly weight loss occurs as food is unable to enter the stomach, and, if the build-up of food and water within the esophagus is great enough, the pressure placed on the trachea can make breathing difficult as well.

Treatment

Diagnosis of megaesophagus is made by physical exam, analyzing clinical signs, and by taking radiographic X-rays of the esophagus or actually visualizing the enlargement with an endoscope inserted into the esophagus via the mouth.

Cats diagnosed with this disorder must be fed with their front end elevated on a chair or table to encourage gravity flow of food and water into the stomach. Feeding liquid or semisolid food will also help facilitate passage into the stomach.

Depending upon the cause, some individuals do improve with time. Yet for the most part, the condition is permanent, and cat owners must be on guard at all times for potential complications.

Esophagitis

Inflammation occurring anywhere along the esophagus is termed *esophagitis*. Esophagitis can be instituted by foreign bodies which injure the organ's lining, by ingestion of caustic substances, and by reflux of stomach contents and acids up into the esophagus. In keeping with the latter cause, chronic, long-term vomiting can also lead to esophagitis.

Symptoms

Regurgitation, inappetence, and weight loss are the most frequent signs seen. If left untreated, damage to the lining of the esophagus could occur, causing strictures and secondary megaesophagus.

Treatment

As with megaesophagus, diagnosis is made using clinical signs, physical exam findings, and endoscopic exam or radiographic X-rays of the esophagus using barium as a contrast media. Treatment of esophagitis consists of treating any primary problems that might be present, and, if stomach acid reflux is to blame, reducing the amount of stomach acid secretions and increasing the rate of gastric emptying.

Esophageal obstructions

Esophageal obstructions in the cat can occur secondary to tumors (squamous cell carcinoma), infections, strictures (as seen with chronic esophagitis), and to the ingestion of foreign objects, including bones, fishhooks, and strings (especially bones).

Symptoms

Again, regurgitation and weight loss are the two most common signs seen in cats afflicted with such a problem. However, if a foreign body has penetrated the esophageal wall, then more generalized signs, such as fever, loss of appetite, breathing difficulties, and vomiting might be seen due to secondary infection.

Treatment

Obstructions can be diagnosed using radiographs and/or endoscopy. Obviously, treatment is aimed at the surgical or endoscopic removal of the offending obstructor and at treating any secondary infection.

HAIRBALLS

The accumulation of hair within the stomach is the most common cause of vomiting in cats. Because of their self-grooming habits and the roughened nature of their tongues, cats in general—be they short-haired or long-haired—are prone to hairballs (FIG. 29-2). Incidence of this problem increases during the spring and fall months due to increased shedding.

Symptoms

When the hair is swallowed, it can coalesce into a ball within the stomach and act as a gastric foreign body, irritating the stomach lining. Vomiting, often right after eating, and gagging are usually the result when this happens; coughing might also be noticed.

Aside from these signs, those cats affected seem otherwise clinically normal.

29-2 *Self-grooming habits can lead to hairball formation in the stomach.*

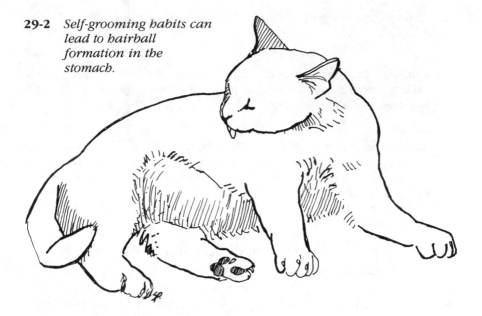

Treatment

Diagnosis of hairballs is based upon clinical signs (and the absence of other clinical signs) and physical examination. If the vomiting is continuous or severe, radiographs of the stomach or direct endoscopic examination might be required to rule out other gastric foreign bodies common to cats, such as cloth, strings, and plastic wrap.

Another way to make a diagnosis of hairballs is to monitor response to treatment. There are numerous "cat laxatives" on the market that can be given to a cat suspected of harboring hairballs. These agents, most of which are nothing more than flavored petroleum jelly, act to lubricate the hairball and facilitate its passage out of the stomach and into the stool. Once this occurs, the clinical signs seen should abate.

In severe instances, surgical removal of a prominent hairball might even be required to afford a cure.

Prevention

Pet owners can do their part to prevent hairballs in their cat. Giving laxative in a preventative manner once or twice weekly should help keep things moving smoothly through the gastrointestinal tract.

One word of caution: Mineral oil should never be used as a hairball laxative, primarily because this substance can be easily aspirated into the lungs. In addition to giving hairball laxative periodically, brushing a cat's hair coat on a daily basis will help reduce the amount of hair available for ingestion.

GASTROINTESTINAL ULCERS

An ulceration within the stomach or intestines occurs when the protective mucus barrier covering the inner surfaces of the gastrointestinal tract is lost or destroyed, allowing stomach acids and bile acids to erode the gastrointestinal lining.

Symptoms

The same type of heartburn humans can sometimes experience with this problem can affect cats as well, leading to inappetence, vomiting, and lethargy.

Gastrointestinal ulcers are actually a sign of disease rather than a distinct disease syndrome in themselves. Sharp foreign bodies or harsh chemicals that are swallowed can scrape, injure, and (in the case of the latter) burn the stomach or intestinal lining as to cause a primary ulceration. Ulcers occur secondary to stress, infectious diseases, intestinal parasites, and metabolic diseases such as kidney disease. Certain drugs, such as steroid anti-inflammatories, can also have a deleterious effect upon the stomach and intestinal lining.

Treatment

Diagnosis of an ulcer relies heavily upon clinical signs seen and the history or evidence of an underlying disorder.

Radiographs taken after the oral administration of barium can be used to pinpoint the exact location of an ulcer. In addition, direct visualization of the actual stomach and upper intestinal lining using an endoscope is another means of diagnosing ulcers in a cat.

Obviously, when formulating any treatment regimen for ulcers, any underlying source for the ulcerations must be identified and treated. Specific ulcer treatment is aimed at reducing the amount of stomach acid secretion, and providing a protective coating over the existing ulcer until it has time to heal. As with humans, cimetidine and ranitidine are both very effective medications for reducing the amount of stomach acid secretion in cats.

FOOD ALLERGIES

Allergies to foods can be a cause vomiting and diarrhea in cats. In many instances, it is not the natural food ingredients themselves that cause the problems, but the additives and fillers that are present in a ration.

Symptoms

In addition to vomiting and diarrhea, weight loss, abdominal pain, excess gas formation, and dermatitis might be seen as well. Allergies to food have also been implicated as a primary cause of lymphocytic-plasmacytic enteritis.

Treatment

Food allergies are often diagnosed after the fact—that is, after other common causes of the same signs have been ruled out. Food trials might also be conducted to determine if there is an abatement of signs either from withholding food altogether for a day or two, or by feeding a hypoallergenic diet. Cottage cheese and rice or certain types of baby food can be used in recipes for diets prepared at home. Better yet, special hypoallergenic prescription diets are available from veterinarians. If a cat does indeed have a food allergy, then it will need to remain on a hypoallergenic diet indefinitely.

EOSINOPHILIC GASTROENTERITIS

Eosinophilic gastoenteritis is characterized by a thickening and inflammation of the walls of the intestinal tract caused by an infiltration of special types of blood cells called *eosinophils*. These cells also infiltrate the liver, spleen, and lymph nodes around the gastrointestinal tract, causing marked enlargement of these organs. Cats so affected exhibit vomiting, diarrhea, and weight loss. The exact cause of this disorder remains unknown.

Diagnosis of eosinophilic gastroenteritis is made through examination of biopsy samples from affected organs. Treatment consists of corticosteroids to reduce the inflammatory response; however, because the nature of the disease, relapses are not uncommon and long-term medical and dietary management might be required.

LYMPHOCYTIC/PLASMACYTIC ENTERITIS (LPE)

Instead of an infiltration of the intestinal walls by eosinophils, LPE is characterized by intestinal infiltration by lymphocytes and plasma cells, similar to plasma cell gingivitis (see Plasma Cell Gingivitis in this chapter). This disease is seen in cats older than 1 year of age. Food allergies are thought to be the inciting cause of LPE.

Symptoms

The primary presenting sign in cats suffering from LPE is a chronic diarrhea that persists weeks to months and fails to respond to conventional treatments. This diarrhea is usually quite mucus-filled, with or without fresh blood.

Treatment

As with eosinophilic gastroenteritis, definitive diagnosis of LPE is reliant upon biopsy findings. If the disease is detected, those cats should be placed on special hypoallergenic diets until the symptoms subside. In many cases, these diets must be maintained indefinitely in order to prevent clinical signs from reoccurring.

LINEAR FOREIGN BODIES

Cats are notorious for playing with and swallowing linear items such as strings, threads, and ribbons. If, for instance, a string becomes wrapped around the tongue or remains trapped within the stomach while the remaining portion passes on into the intestine, normal intestinal peristalsis will cause the intestine to "bunch up" around the string, resulting in intestinal obstruction. Furthermore, as the intestine becomes more and more irritated, its motility will increase, creating a "sawing" action against the immobilized string. In this way, intestinal perforation and secondary peritonitis can result (FIG. 29-3).

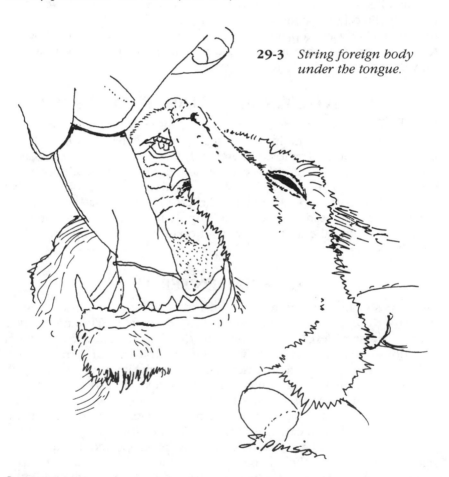

29-3 *String foreign body under the tongue.*

Symptoms

Cats suffering from a lodged linear foreign body have painful abdomens and exhibit persistent vomiting, with or without diarrhea. Fever and weight loss are also accompanying signs. If intestinal perforation occurs, septic shock could result.

Treatment

Diagnosis of a linear foreign body is made by physical examination and radiographic X-rays. Oftentimes, a diagnosis can be confirmed by finding a free end of the object wrapped around the base of the tongue. In these instances, however, manual extraction of the foreign body through the mouth should not be attempted. Instead, the string or foreign body should be freed from under the tongue and allowed to pass down into the stomach, and then into the stool.

Often, this provides enough relief from the tension placed on the intestines to allow intestinal function to return to normal. However, if radiographs show that the intestinal bunching has not been relieved, or if the cat's clinical signs continue, then surgical exploration with removal of the foreign body and repair of any intestinal perforations might be necessary. If perforations have indeed occurred, antibiotic therapy is indicated as well to combat infection.

INTESTINAL OBSTRUCTIONS

In addition to string foreign bodies, other items can obstruct normal flow through the gut and result in clinical signs, such as lethargy, vomiting, and black, tarry stools. Swallowed foreign bodies (such as bones, plastic wraps, cloth), tumors, fungal infections, and herniations are all capable of causing either partial or complete obstructions if large or extensive enough. Unless the obstruction is relieved in a timely fashion, usually through surgical means, loss of blood supply to the affected portion can occur, resulting in the death of that portion of bowel, systemic infection, and shock.

BACTERIAL ENTERITIS

Two types of bacteria are responsible for most cases of feline bacterial enteritis: *Campylobacter fetus jejuni* and *Salmonella*. Though rarely a primary cause of fever, depression, and diarrhea in cats, these bacterial infections often occur secondary to other gastrointestinal diseases (such as feline parvovirus) and to diseases that depress the immune system (such as feline leukemia). Severe salmonella infections can also spread to the liver and lungs, causing abscesses and associated clinical signs. On the other hand, a primary importance of Campylobacter lies in the fact that it is transmissible to and can cause diarrhea in humans.

Diagnosis of salmonella enteritis can be supported by finding a marked depression in the number of white blood cells in a blood sample. In most cases, however, a positive response to treatment with antibiotics provides the best method of diagnosis for most veterinary clinicians. Because bacterial enteritis can cause profound dehydration, intravenous fluids are a must during convalescence to protect against this deadly complication.

COLITIS

Problems involving the large intestine of cats are not uncommon in veterinary medicine. *Colitis* refers to the inflammation of the lining of the large intestine, resulting in diarrhea, with the feces often containing and abundance of blood and mucus. The blood seen with colitis is usually bright red, in contrast to small intestinal bleeding, which contributes a black tarry appearance to the feces. *Tenesmus*, or straining to defecate, is another prevalent sign with colitis that is often mistaken for constipation.

Symptoms

Acute colitis refers to a sudden onset of signs that usually lasts only a short period of time with proper treatment. Chronic colitis is a long-term, recurring condition that might last an entire lifetime of the cat. Parasites such as coccidia are common causes of colitis in cats; dietary indiscretions and stress factors are two other prevalent sources as well.

Feline leukemia and feline AIDS should be ruled out in any case of long-standing problems with the bowels. Less commonly, fungal infections, foreign bodies, intussusceptions, polyps, food allergies, immune system disorders, and tumors can all result in signs related to a chronic colitis.

In cats, a special type of colitis, called *idiopathic colitis,* has been known to occur. Although the exact cause of this is unknown, many researchers suspect food allergies. An unusual characteristic of idiopathic colitis is that diarrhea is rarely a clinical sign; instead, the stools appear relatively normal except for a small amount of blood and/or mucus coating the surface. Most of these cats show no other signs of apparent illness.

Treatment

Diagnosis of any type of colitis is made from a predisposing history (such as known dietary indiscretion), existing clinical signs, and physical examination. Stool examinations and other laboratory tests, especially feline leukemia and feline AIDS testing, should be performed in an attempt to identify the underlying cause of the colitis. Radiographs, including barium contrast studies are indicated in nonresponsive, recurring cases. Biopsies obtained using an endoscope or through exploratory surgery can also prove to be helpful for establishing a definitive diagnosis. In some cases, an exact cause of the inflammation can never be discerned, even with extensive laboratory testing.

Treatment of colitis is aimed at eliminating the inciting cause. Parasites should be treated using proper dewormers and antiparasitic medications. Antibiotics can be used to help remove any disease-causing bacteria within the colon, and steroid anti-inflammatories might prove to be helpful in abating clinical signs.

If polyps or tumors are presented, surgical removal might be necessary to afford a cure. However, understand that in many cases of chronic colitis, especially those caused by stress or by immune system disorders, a complete cure cannot be achieved. In these cats, treatment goals are aimed at managing flare-ups as they occur. Anti-inflammatories, antibiotics, and local protectants such as kaolin and pectin can help provide relief from these intermittent flare-ups.

Dietary management is an important component of colitis treatment. Acute cases of colitis caused by dietary indiscretion or some infectious process respond well to feeding an easily digestible diet.

Chronic, recurring bouts with colitis may be managed by increasing the fiber content in the diet to increase the bulk of the stool which helps normalize intestinal motility. Finally, for those cases caused by food allergies, a hypoallergenic diet composed of rice and mutton can help eliminate the effects of the allergy.

FELINE MEGACOLON

Feline megacolon is a disease condition marked by a large, distended colon that has lost its ability to contract and undergo peristalsis properly. When this occurs, feces build up within the affected segment and prevent normal flow of ingesta through the intestinal tract.

Megacolon is caused by a disruption of or lack of nerve innervation into the muscular walls of the colon. It might occur secondary to spinal cord trauma, other diseases affecting the nervous system, or, as in the case of some Manx cats, be an inheritable trait.

Symptoms

The clinical signs associated with feline megacolon can vary. Straining to defecate is certainly the most obvious sign; diarrhea can also be seen alongside of firm, hard stools. If the obstruction is severe, vomiting, dehydration, and loss of appetite can be seen as well.

Treatment

Diagnosis of feline megacolon can be made upon physical examination and, for confirmation, from radiographs. Treatment involves removing the fecal impaction using warm water enemas and by infusing the colon with mineral oil.

Enemas designed for use in humans should not be used in cats, as the components making these up can cause severe dehydration in cats. Severe cases might require surgical relief of the impaction.

There is no effective cure for this condition; as a result, preventative maintenance therapy should be used to prevent recurrences. Giving an oral hairball laxative on a daily basis will help keep fecal matter moving along nicely. Increasing the amount of fiber in the diet has also been shown to be helpful in preventing relapses.

FELINE LIVER DISEASE

Because of the important role the liver plays in the metabolism of nutrients and in the detoxification of poisonous substances, any malfunction or interference with its function can place the life of the pet in serious jeopardy. In the cat, liver damage can occur secondarily to infections elsewhere in the body (including the gastrointestinal tract), to internal diseases such as diabetes mellitus, heart disease, and cancer, and to the ingestion of toxic substances.

This latter cause becomes especially important when it is realized that the feline liver, unlike that of most other species, is deficient in a certain enzyme called *glucuronyl transferase* that is normally responsible for metabolizing and detoxifying certain therapeutic drugs that reach the liver. This is the reason cats are so sensitive to drugs such as aspirin and acetaminophen; even small doses can be deadly.

Hepatic lipidosis is a common type of liver dysfunction in cats that has baffled researchers for years. It is characterized by an extensive infiltration of the liver by fatty tissue that, in essence, crowds out the normal liver cells and interferes with normal liver function.

Symptoms

Seen in all ages of cats, the exact cause of the condition is unknown, yet obesity and/or prolonged periods of food deprivation due to loss of appetite are thought to increase the body's utilization of fats for energy, the metabolism of which is carried out in the liver.

Like so many other diseases, liver disorders can cause loss of appetite (often profound), vomiting, diarrhea, and fever in affected cats.

One unique sign often seen with liver disease, including hepatic lipidosis, is jaundice, or icterus. Jaundice is caused by elevated levels of bile pigments in the bloodstream and is characterized by a yellow discoloration of the skin, mucous membranes, and the blood serum.

Other clinical signs that can result from chronic, long-term liver disease include a fluid buildup within the abdominal cavity (*ascites*), due to increased resistance to blood flow through the liver bleeding tendencies, and anemia. Seizures, comas, and other neurologic disorders can also appear with advanced cases as ammonia and other toxins are allowed to build up within the bloodstream.

Treatment

Diagnosis of feline liver diseases is based upon clinical signs, physical exam findings, and upon demonstrating elevated levels of liver enzymes in a blood sample. Radiographic X-rays can be used to judge the size of the liver, which gives the veterinary practitioner some idea as to the duration of the problem. In many instances, a biopsy is required to determine the actual cause of the liver malfunction.

Treatment objectives for feline liver disease are aimed at eliminating any injurious agents that might be present, and to promote healing of the affected tissue. The liver is one of the few organs within the body that can actually regenerate itself after injury provided of course that the source of the injury is dealt with properly. Intravenous fluids are a must to prevent dehydration and its unpleasant side-effects.

It is vital for recovery that these cats be force-fed, especially in cases of hepatic lipidosis. This might require actual feedings through a stomach tube. An easily digestible, low-protein diet with high biological value is ideal for patients suffering from a liver disorder.

Antibiotics can be used if bacterial infection is suspected; for those cases exhibiting neurological signs caused by too much ammonia in the bloodstream, they can also be helpful for eliminating ammonia-forming organisms in the gastrointestinal tract. Ascites can be treated with diuretic drugs such as furosemide and by reducing the amount of sodium in the cat's diet.

Finally, in select instances only, steroids might be used to increase appetite and to counteract the loss of protein which can occur with liver disease.

30

The Urinary System

IN THE NORMAL, day-to-day functioning of the body, lots of waste material is formed as a result of metabolic activity. It is the function of the urinary system to handle and to rid the body of these waste products. In addition, through its ability to dilute or concentrate the urine, it serves to regulate fluid levels within the body.

Because of its vital function, any interference or alteration of urinary system function can quickly have serious health consequences. For this reason, prompt and proper diagnosis of urinary tract disorders in cats is essential. Periodic checkups by a veterinarian can help detect potential problems before they reach such a magnitude as to threaten the health of a pet.

For more information regarding anatomy and function of the urinary system, see chapter 12 in the *Dogs* section.

FELINE UROLOGIC SYNDROME

Feline Urologic Syndrome, or FUS, is a disease syndrome of cats characterized by the formation of crystals (termed *struvite crystals*) within the urinary bladder. These crystals in turn cause inflammation, urinary bleeding and straining, and sometimes life-threatening obstruction to the normal flow of urine out of the bladder (FIG. 30-1).

No one knows for sure why some cats get FUS and others don't; many potential causes have been hypothesized, including viruses, abnormal urinary retention, obesity, bladder defects, and—the most popular theory to date—improper diet. In reality, one or all of these factors might play a role in the occurrence of FUS.

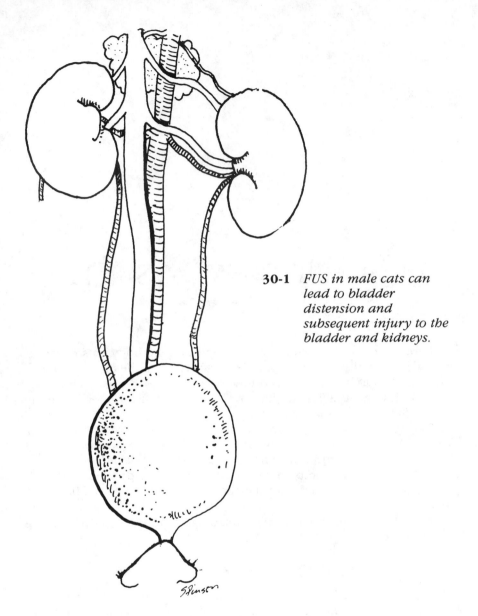

30-1 *FUS in male cats can lead to bladder distension and subsequent injury to the bladder and kidneys.*

   If a cat is prone to this disorder, it will usually show some signs of the disease by the time it is 3 years of age. Both male and female cats are at risk of developing FUS; however, males have a greater likelihood of developing a life-threatening obstruction simply because the male urethra is smaller in size than that of the female, and it can become plugged with crystals more easily. If such an obstruction occurs, urine can back flow back into the kidneys, causing damage to these organs and also causing toxins to begin building up in the bloodstream.

Symptoms

Early clinical signs of FUS result from the irritation that these crystals cause within the bladder itself. These can include inappropriate urinations in places other than the litter box or normal elimination areas, increased licking at the genital region, straining, and frequent attempts at urination with crying or vocalization, and blood in the urine (FIG. 30-2). Cats often lose their appetites and become more irritable as well. More seriously, male cats suffering from partial or complete obstruction of the urethra can exhibit vomiting, intense lethargy, and a distended, painful abdomen.

30-2 *Cats with FUS often lick excessively.*

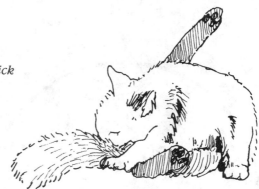

Diagnosis

Diagnosis of FUS is based upon clinical signs, physical examination, and a urinalysis. An enlarged, painful bladder can also be palpated in those cats suffering from some degree of obstruction. If a bladder infection is suspected, then urine cultures might also be performed.

The obstructed cat will usually have high levels of kidney enzymes (BUN, creatinine) present in its bloodstream, signifying the toxin buildup and kidney destruction that is occurring. Most veterinary hospitals are equipped to monitor these enzymes.

Treatment

If an actual obstruction is suspected, then rapid treatment is essential to save the life of the cat. Obstructed cats are immediately placed on intravenous fluids to help dilute the toxin levels within the bloodstream. A catheter is then inserted into the urethra to "unplug" it in order to re-establish urine flow (FIG. 30-3). Once this flow is re-established, the bladder is flushed repeatedly with sterile saline to remove any crystals that might be remaining within (FIG. 30-4).

It is up to the veterinarian's discretion as to whether or not to keep the urinary catheter in place for a few days. While catheterized, these cats are placed on antibiotics to prevent any secondary bladder infections

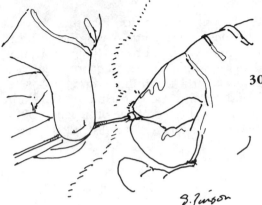

30-3 *Urinary catheterization is necessary to relieve FUS cats with obstructions.*

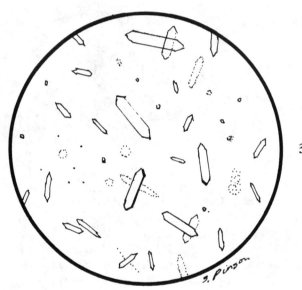

30-4 *Urinary crystals.*

from occurring as a result of the catheter. Intravenous fluids are continued in the hospital setting for two to three days after the obstruction is relieved.

For the cats that are not obstructed but still are showing signs of FUS, smooth muscle relaxants and anti-inflammatory medications can be used to help reduce the discomfort and urge associated with this disease. The use of antibiotics in such patients is still controversial; studies have shown that bacterial infections are present in less than 20 percent of the cases. However, if urine culture confirms the presence of such, of course antibiotics are indicated.

Acidifying the urine in order to dissolve any crystals present within the bladder is another important step in treating this disease in both obstructed and unobstructed felines. Crystal formation in cats with FUS is encouraged by an alkaline urine pH (pH > 7.5); on the contrary, making the urine more acidic will help dissolve existing crystals and help prevent the formation of new ones.

FUS and diet

In the past, special oral tablets designed to acidify the urine were pre-scribed, yet the preferred method of urinary acidification today is through diet, not through oral supplements. This is because the pH of the urine is less likely to fluctuate if it is maintained through dietary means. Veterinarians will prescribe a special diet not only designed to lower the pH of the cat's urine, but also one that is severely restricted in the miner-als that make up the crystals.

Following an acute attack of FUS, such diets are usually maintained from anywhere from one to three months. **Note:** Never feed such a diet to a cat for longer than three months without the prior consent of a veteri-narian.

Most veterinary researchers agree that diet plays the foremost role in the creation and in the treatment/prevention of this disease syndrome. Dry diets with high contents of magnesium and ash (mineral) levels are the biggest culprits in promoting FUS in cats. As a rule, those diets, either dry or moist, that have over .10% magnesium (dry matter) and/or over 5% ash content should be avoided.

Unfortunately, many of the commercial "grocery-store" brands of cat food exceed these limits. Most pet food manufacturers are now begin-ning to address the problem of too much magnesium and ash in their products, yet cat owners should still check all pet food labels to be sure of compliance.

Diets specially formulated for the prevention of feline urologic syn-drome can be obtained in both moist and dry forms from most veterinary offices. Because of its high calcium and mineral content, cow's milk should never be offered to those individuals prone to FUS.

Besides feeding a diet that acidifies the urine and is low in magne-sium and ash, providing cats free access to a fresh water supply is a must. Increased water consumption will help increase the number of urinations each day, effectively keeping the bladder flushed out. In fact, most com-mercial diets formulated for the prevention of FUS have an increased salt content to promote an increased water consumption. With these increased urinations comes the responsibility of keeping the litter box cleaned on a regular basis. Many cats refuse to urinate in a dirty litter box; a practice which encourages urine retention and FUS.

Although it might not seem important, regulating the frequency of meals fed can play a direct role in the prevention of FUS. After a cat con-sumes a meal, its urine undergoes a temporary rise in pH. For those cats allowed to eat and nibble all day long (such as those fed dry foods), this might promote a relatively constant alkaline urine, and thereby predispose to crystal formation. As a result, in terms of preventing FUS, offering one or two meals a day rather than free-choice meals is preferred.

Obese cats are more prone to FUS than their slimmer counterparts, so weight control is an important preventative measure to follow as well. Overweight felines, especially those who have exhibited signs of FUS in the past, should be placed on a reducing diet prescribed by their veterinarian and have their activity levels increased until the desired weight is reached. Once weight loss is accomplished, they can be switched back over to preventative-type rations.

Prognosis

Without proper dietary management, FUS can be expected to recur over 50% of the time. In some cats, however, FUS recurs over and over again, even with dietary management. In these instances, treating the symptoms when they first appear and continuing with prevention measures will usually keep such episodes from turning serious.

For those male cats that have had recurring obstruction, a special operation known as a perineal urethrostomy might be indicated to reduce the danger of death due to urinary blockage. This surgery involves the removal of the end of the penis and widening the urethral opening, effectively allowing for free passage out of any and all crystals. Keep in mind that such a procedure is not intended to cure the FUS; it merely lessens the risk of severe, life-threatening complications associated with it.

KIDNEY DISEASE

The kidneys are responsible for eliminating waste products produced by the body's normal metabolism. If they fail to perform this function adequately, the body will literally poison itself. For this reason, special attention must be directed at keeping the kidneys healthy, and—if a disease state already exists—at treating to prevent further functional deterioration.

Causes of kidney disease

In cats as in dogs, kidney disease is a common disorder associated with old age. In essence, through normal wear and tear, the kidneys become unable to perform their functions in the same way that they did when they were young. Worn-out kidney cells die and are replaced by scar tissue, which can't filter out toxins from the blood. When enough of these nephrons die and the buildup of toxins in the blood becomes great enough, then the pet begins to exhibit signs of kidney failure.

But don't get the idea that older cats are the only ones that can suffer from kidney impairment. Young cats might be born with inadequate kidney function. For instance, kittens can be born with inadequately developed kidneys, or with kidneys containing open cysts embedded within the normal tissue, a condition known as *polycystic kidneys*.

Cats of all ages might suffer from other diseases or toxic agent which kill nephrons and impair renal performance. For example, bacterial infections, feline leukemia, feline infectious peritonitis, heat stroke, heart disease, and cancer are but some of the acquired conditions that can lead to kidney disease and kidney failure.

Glomerulonephritis and renal amyloidosis are two types of kidney impairments caused by over-reactive immune systems in the affected cats, which actually destroy healthy kidney tissue in an attempt to eliminate infections or diseases elsewhere within the cat's body.

Next, many therapeutic drugs, such as aspirin and certain antibiotics, can be damaging to the kidneys if used indiscriminately. In addition, antifreeze, or ethylene glycol, is deadly to cats when ingested because of the profound damage to the kidneys it causes (FIG. 30-5). Finally, periodontal disease, with its associated complications, can predispose felines, both young and old, to kidney problems in the future.

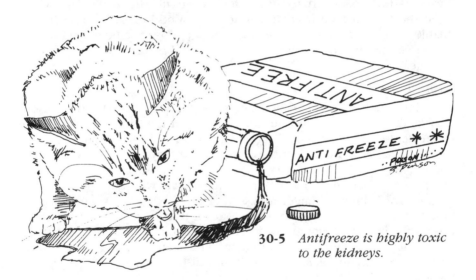

30-5 *Antifreeze is highly toxic to the kidneys.*

Symptoms

The clinical signs associated with kidney disease can be quite variable, depending on the extent of damage to the kidneys. Interestingly enough, cats rarely show outward signs of kidney disease until at least 75 percent of the function in both kidneys is lost! As a result, when signs do finally become apparent, it is vital that therapeutic measures be taken quickly to prevent the loss of the remaining 25 percent.

Sudden, acute kidney failure, the type that can result from the ingestion of a poison such as antifreeze, can lead directly into intense dehydration, shock, unconsciousness, and death without showing any other signs. Chronic, more long-term kidney disease and kidney failure rarely have such a dramatic presentation, yet such conditions can eventually turn into acute kidney failure if measures aren't instituted to prevent this progression.

Cats with chronic renal failure will exhibit an increased thirst and an increased desire to urinate. Depression and loss of appetite might also set in. In addition, since renal disease can cause stomach ulcers, vomiting might occur.

Diagnosis

Veterinarians can diagnose kidney disease through a series of laboratory tests performed on the blood and the urine. Two blood parameters or enzymes, blood urea nitrogen (BUN) and serum creatinine, will be elevated if the kidneys are failing.

The urine *specific gravity* is also an important parameter that helps the veterinary practitioner determine the extent of damage to the kidneys. Under normal circumstances, the specific gravity of the urine, which measures how concentrated the urine is, should fluctuate depending upon the body's own needs for water. Diseased kidneys, however, are unable to conserve water for the body, hence, this specific gravity of the urine in a cat with advanced kidney disease will be dilute, even if the pet is clinically dehydrated.

Treatment

Cats suffering from acute renal failure must be hospitalized and place on intravenous fluids to correct dehydration. Other medications designed to stimulate kidney function will be given as well. If the cat survives this acute attack, support measures for chronic kidney failure must then be implemented.

Stress reduction is of vital importance in cats with chronic renal disease and/or failure. Unlimited access to clean, fresh water should be provided at all times, since deprivation could lead to an acute kidney failure crisis. Special diets that are low in protein should be fed to help reduce toxin build-up within the bloodstream. These are available from veterinarians. Vitamin supplementation should also be considered to replace those lost in the increased urine flow.

Since renal disease can alter, among other things, the blood levels of calcium and phosphorus, medications designed to keep levels of these electrolytes constant are used as well. If a pet is having trouble with vomiting, human anti-ulcer medications such as cimetidine can be employed to help settle the stomach.

Finally, since kidney disease places an incredible burden on the affected pet's immune system, all underlying disease processes and disorders (such as periodontal disease) need to be addressed and treated.

31

The Reproductive System

PROPAGATION OF THE species is the purpose for the reproductive system (FIG. 31-1). Because the anatomy and physiology of this system is similar to that in dogs, this chapter will only involve select disorders of the reproductive system in cats. See chapter 13 for more information on anatomy and physiology, and chapter 22 for more information concerning breeding cats.

ACCIDENTAL MATINGS (MISMATINGS)

The question about what to do with the female cat who is accidentally bred is not an easy one to answer. In the old days, all that cat owners needed to do was to take their pet to the veterinarian for a "mismating shot or pill." Yet because of potential undesirable side effects from using such drugs for aborting pregnancies, their use is now discouraged. Instead, the queen should be allowed to have the litter of kittens if the mating was indeed a successful one, or an ovariohysterectomy should be performed.

REPRODUCTIVE TRACT INFECTIONS

Infections can occur within the female reproductive tract whether a cat becomes pregnant or not.

Vaginitis/Metritis

If the infection involves the uterus, it is called *metritis* or *pyometra*. If it involves the lower portions of the reproductive tract, it is properly

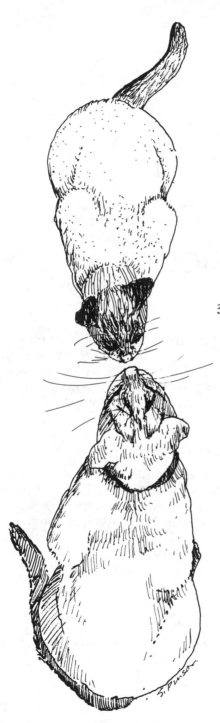

31-1 *Accidental matings are not uncommon in cats allowed to roam outdoors.*

termed *vaginitis*. Both vaginitis and metritis can occur independently of each other or together. Causes of vaginitis/metritis can include such things as venereally transmitted organisms, metabolic diseases like diabetes mellitus, and retained fetuses or placentas.

Symptoms

Classic signs of vaginitis/metritis include a thick, yellow-to-green discharge seen coming from the vagina. Owners might notice their pets licking excessively around this area. In especially dour metritis cases, loss of appetite with an increased water intake, fever, and abdominal pain can become apparent. The discharge might also become discernibly blood-tinged.

Because of the intimacy of the urinary tract with the reproductive tract in females, bladder infections that occur secondary to the vaginitis/metritis are also not uncommon.

Treatment

The type of treatment used for reproductive tract infections depends upon which portions are involved. For instance, in mild cases of vaginitis, direct infusion of the vagina with antibiotics or chlorhexidine douches provides effective results. If the vaginitis is severe or if the uterus is involved, high doses of antibiotics given orally or by injection are required. To determine which antibiotics will work the best, a bacterial culture is taken. Certainly if there are any kittens nursing on the affected queen, they should be removed and placed on formula.

In critical metritis cases, intravenous fluids might even be required for support. Unless the queen is a valuable breeding animal, an ovariohysterectomy should be performed on these cats to directly eliminate the source of the problem and to prevent metritis from reoccurring at a later date. For those cats considered too valuable to be spayed, special medications called prostaglandins can be utilized to help the uterus contract and empty. These, however, must be used with extreme care under the direct supervision of a veterinarian, and even then, only as a last resort.

Pyometra

Pyometra in cats is characterized by a grossly enlarged uterus filled with pus. Signs seen include depression, loss of appetite with a markedly increased thirst, and abdominal pain. Unless an ovariohysterectomy is performed immediately, uterine rupture is possible.

32

The Skin and Hair Coat

THE SKIN, OR *integument*, functions to protect the body from outside foreign invaders and from loss of water. It provides a focus for the sense of touch and assists in the regulation of the temperature within the body. In addition, special modifications of the skin, such as claws and pads, provide a means of defense as well as shock absorbency.

For more information on the anatomy and function of the skin and hair, see chapter 14 in the *Dogs* section.

THE ITCHY CAT

Many disease conditions can produce itching in the cat (TABLE 32-1). However, only a few disorders result in severe and/or prolonged itching. The primary symptoms of the itchy cat is scratching, biting, and/or licking at the involved skin (FIG. 32-1). Early signs often noticed include wet hairs, reddened skin, miliary dermatitis, and hair loss in the affected areas. Prolonged itching results in further hair loss, excessive scaling, thickening, and discoloration of the involved skin. Secondary skin infection is not uncommon in these situations.

Severe and/or prolonged itching is most always a symptom of an underlying skin disorder, such as fleas or allergies. As a result, correction of the underlying problem is imperative if the symptom of itching is to be successfully controlled. Topping the list as causes of itching in cats are the following:

Flea allergy

Aside from the discomfort caused by the actual bite of a flea, cats can develop an allergic response to the flea's saliva deposited in the skin dur-

Table 32-1   Causes of Itching or Hair Loss in Cats

Fleas
Neurodermatitis
Food allergy
Inhalant allergies
Anal sac impaction
Feline endocrine alopecia
Ringworm
Mange

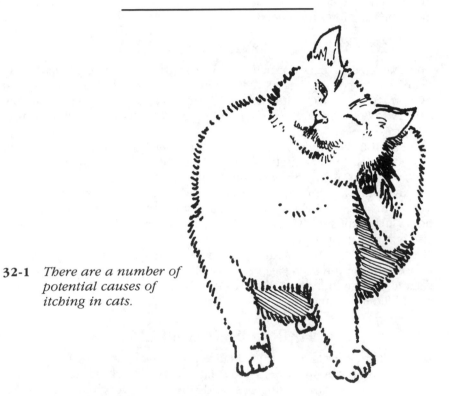

32-1 *There are a number of potential causes of itching in cats.*

ing feeding. *Miliary dermatitis* with moderate to severe itching and hair loss usually results, especially around the head and neck and along the back near the tail. As one might guess, successful treatment of a flea allergy is heavily dependent on the ability to control fleas on the pet and in the environment.

Food hypersensitivity (food allergies)

Food allergies are another potential cause of itching and miliary dermatitis in cats. Skin lesions related to such an allergy generally involve the head and neck, although other areas can also be affected. Food-related allergies have also been implicated in numerous gastrointestinal disorders as well. Fortunately, food allergies are relatively rare in occurrence.

Food allergies should be suspected any time a recent change in diet has led to the appearance of a skin condition, or if itching starts soon after eating. A definitive diagnosis of food hypersensitivity requires the exclusive feeding of a hypoallergenic diet for two to four weeks. A veterinarian can prescribe such a diet. If a positive diagnosis is made, the cat will need to remain on the hypoallergenic diet indefinitely. Simply changing food brands or types seldom benefit food allergy cases because most commercial foods contain similar ingredients. If you're feeding your cat a homemade blend, be sure it has the added taurine and vitamins necessary to meet the cat's long-term needs.

Contact allergies

The hair coat of cats normally offers an efficient protective barrier to many substances and agents that could produce an allergic reaction just by coming in contact with the skin. Unfortunately, when people step in and try to help, they can inadvertently cause problems related to contact allergies.

For instance, the most common contact allergy-producing agents are flea collars, shampoos, pet sprays, insecticides, etc., all which are generally applied or used with good intentions.

Symptoms of a contact allergy include redness and swelling of the skin, with intense itching. These signs will generally develop 24 to 72 hours after exposure. Hair loss, especially with allergies to flea collars, is also a common finding.

Many times, treatment of contact allergies simply requires the removal of the offending agent. In tougher cases, administration of topical and/or systemic corticosteroids may be needed as well to reduce the associated inflammation.

HAIR LOSS (ALOPECIA)

Loss of hair either locally or generalized over the coat of a cat is another type of skin problem owners could face. As with itching, the causes of hair loss can be quite numerous, and sometimes very complex (TABLE 32-2). A proper diagnosis is essential for restoring the full-bodied hair coat that once was. Here are some of the potential causes of alopecia in cats.

Shedding

The normal shedding cycles for cats tend to occur in the spring and fall, yet if the cat is kept indoors, shedding could occur year-round. If normal shedding is truly the cause of the hair loss, rarely do raw spots or patches of exposed skin appear. If they do, another cause of the hair loss should

Table 32-2   Diagnostic Aids for Dermatopathies in Cats

Test	Purpose
Skin scraping	Detects mange mites, one of the most common causes of itching and hair loss in cats.
DTM (Dermatophyte test medium)	Tests for the presence of the ringworm fungus, another common cause of hair loss and secondary skin infection.
Woods lamp (ultraviolet light)	A screening test for ringworm; may not detect up to 90% of actual cases; if negative, must be accompanied by a DTM
Thyroid testing and other hormonal assays	Detects hypothyroidism and hormonally-related dermatopathies
Blood and stool parasite checks	Detects internal parasitic organisms, some of which can cause itchy skin reactions
Cytology	This microscopic examination of fluid or cells from skin lesions is also used as a preliminary test for cancer
Biopsy	This microscopic examination of a tissue sample is the definitive test for cancer and autoimmune diseases
Bacterial culture/sensitivity	Used to identify which bacteria are causing the skin lesions and which antibiotics they are sensitive to
CBC/biochemical profile	Blood test used to identify internal diseases such as diabetes, which can outwardly manifest themselves as a skin and coat disorder
Allergy testing (skin test or blood test)	Helps identify which substances a pet is actually allergic to

be suspected. If a cat sheds excessively, brushing its coat daily will help remove the dead hairs and make way for the new ones. Failure to do this can predispose your feline to itchy skin and infections.

Any event that is associated with abnormally high amounts of stress can cause increases in shedding activity and in some cases, overt alopecia. A good example of this is the queen undergoing pregnancy or lactation. The physiologic and nutritional stress placed on the cat's body can lead to accelerated hair loss. Fortunately, in most instances, the hair will return once the stress abates.

Malnutrition

The hair cycle in cats is dynamic and active, with new hairs constantly growing in to replace old, dead hairs that are naturally shed. These new hairs require a bounty of protein and other nutrients for their proper formation and development. If these are not supplied, replacement hairs might not grow in at all, or they might be weak, brittle, and easily broken. As a result, cats suffering from poor nutrition often have scanty, lackluster hair coats, not to mention unhealthy skin. Since the source of the problem is internal in nature, the distribution of this hair loss tends to be symmetrical over the entire body.

The wrong type of diet is not the only cause of nutritionally related hair loss. Internal parasites can also lead to malnutrition because intestinal parasites can steal vital nutrients from the cat, causing the hair coat to bear the brunt of the consequences.

Obviously, providing a good plane of nutrition and correcting any internal parasite problems that might exist are the two key means of restoring normal hair growth in these cases.

Itching

As might be expected, incessant itching and scratching can cause loss of hair as well. This hair loss might be due to self trauma from licking, chewing, and/or scratching, or it could be secondary to inflammation affecting the hair follicles themselves. The distribution of the hair loss can be localized or diffuse, symmetrical or asymmetrical, depending on the extent of the causative disorder. For instance, if hormonal disorders are to blame, the resulting hair loss is often symmetrical, affecting both sides equally. On the other hand, hair loss caused by mange or ringworm usually appears localized to certain portions of the body at first, although this hair loss can spread to other parts if the disease is left unchecked.

Identifying and correcting the underlying problem is the most important step to take for restoring the scanty coat. Realize that in many conditions involving inflammation of the hair follicle, the coat might look worse with treatment before it gets better due to treatment-induced shedding of already dead or damaged hair. A good plane of nutrition, one that is adequate in protein and fatty acids, will also speed replacement of the lost hair in recovered pets.

Feline endocrine alopecia

Traditionally, otherwise unexplained hair loss affecting neutered male and female cats has been attributed to a hormonal disorder known as feline endocrine alopecia. This condition is characterized by a nonitchy, symmetrical hair loss affecting the abdomen, thighs, and posterior region; however, the underlying skin in these areas appears healthy and unaffected.

Diagnosis of this disorder is based on ruling out other potential causes of hair loss and upon experiencing a positive response to therapy. Treatment using progestin compounds is usually sufficient to stimulate hair regrowth in these cats.

Ringworm

Fungal infections involving the skin and hair can cause hair loss without associated itching. The most prevalent fungal infection affecting the integument of felines is ringworm.

For more information regarding ringworm in cats, see chapter 24.

FELINE MILIARY DERMATITIS

Miliary dermatitis is a term that refers to a specific way in which feline skin responds to inflammation and/or irritation. Such a skin reaction is characterized by the formation of tiny, seed-like crusts that frequent the head, neck, and tail regions of the body. In extensive cases, the entire body might be involved. Furthermore, the miliary reaction is quite itchy, and leads to scratching, rubbing, and licking of the affected skin. Hair loss often results due to these activities. Oftentimes the irritation miliary dermatitis causes is so great that the affected cat becomes easily agitated and twitches its skin when disturbed or touched.

The potential causes of miliary dermatitis are numerous. Irritation caused by external parasites is the most common cause of localized miliary reactions. Allergies—including food, inhalant, and contact allergies—are other potential causes. In addition, adverse reactions to medications and drugs, and fatty acid deficiencies in the diet have also been implicated as inciting feline miliary dermatitis.

Treatment for feline miliary dermatitis is aimed at correcting the underlying cause for the disorder, if this is known. For those cases in which an underlying cause cannot be identified, treatment with corticosteroids or progestin compounds can provide relief from the clinical signs. Antibiotics are rarely necessary, since bacterial infection is rarely a component of this disorder.

EOSINOPHILIC GRANULOMA COMPLEX

This dermatopathy of cats is characterized by the unexplained appearance of red to yellow-brown ulcerated lesions with associated hair loss occurring at various locations around the body. On the average, it tends to strike female cats that are under 6 years of age.

When the raised, well-demarcated reddish ulcers appear on the lips of affected felines, they are termed *eosinophilic ulcers* or *rodent ulcers* (FIG. 32-2). *Linear granulomas* are eosinophilic granulomas that can occur anywhere on the body, but especially frequent the back portion of the hind legs. These ulcerations are yellowish to pink in appearance, and, as the name implies, they tend to run in a straight line down the affected portion of skin.

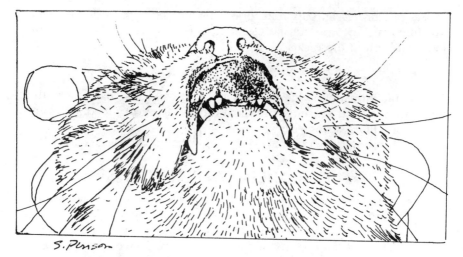

S. Penson

32-2   *Eosinophilic lip ulcer.*

With both eosinophilic ulcers and linear granulomas, pain and itching do not appear to be significant factors. However, prompt treatment is still important, since some of these lesions, especially eosinophilic ulcers, can evolve to skin cancer if left alone.

Eosinophilic plaques are types of eosinophilic granuloma that are associated with intense itching. These well demarcated, raised ulcers are often bright red in appearance and show up primarily on the abdomen and on the upper, inside portions of the back legs. Cats so affected will often lick constantly at the lesions due to the irritation and itching caused by them.

Diagnosis of eosinophilic granuloma complex in cats is routinely made upon physical exam and upon microscopic examination of cells or tissues from the lesions. Treatment employs corticosteroids given orally or by injection for three to four weeks. Progestin compounds can also be effective at resolving the ulcers within weeks after treatment is instituted. In cases that don't respond to either, radiation therapy might be necessary to bring the lesions under control. As with miliary dermatitis, antibiotics are rarely necessary to afford a cure.

STUD TAIL

This skin disease is seen in purebred, intact, male cats who are sexually active. It is caused by overactive sebaceous glands near the base of the tail which cause a greasy, waxy deposit to be laid down over the skin and coat in this region. Although unsightly, this condition usually causes no pain or itching in affected tomcats.

Treatment consists of periodic cleansing of the region with a mild, hypoallergenic shampoo or soap, being sure to dry the area well after doing so. More extensive treatment regimens are usually not necessary.

BACTERIAL INFECTIONS

Healthy skin has several mechanisms by which it resists infectious organisms. A dry, outer layer of *keratin*, combined with periodic shedding of dead skin cells, helps to discourage population of the skin surface with harmful bacteria. Even *sebum*, produced by the sebaceous glands of the skin, is antibacterial at normal concentrations. Finally, a normal population of bacteria that resides on the skin surface and in the hair follicles competitively inhibit the growth of disease-causing bacteria (FIG. 32-3).

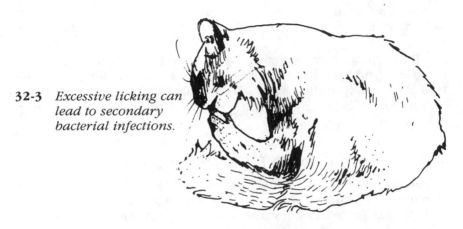

32-3 *Excessive licking can lead to secondary bacterial infections.*

Problems can start to occur when the integument becomes traumatized, or when underlying disease alters the normal integrity of the skin. If the skin's defenses are penetrated in such a way, disease-causing bacteria found naturally on the skin (or on the teeth of other felines) can set up housekeeping.

Superficial bacterial skin disease

Superficial bacterial skin disease in cats can take on a number of appearances. *Feline acne* is perhaps the most common type seen in veterinary circles. This disease is characterized by infection of the hair follicles and the appearance of blackheads and/or pustules on the chins of affected cats. Although the exact cause for this disorder remains unknown, many researchers feel that it is due to the cat's inability to adequately groom this area.

Treatment for feline acne consists of clipping the hair away from the chin and scrubbing the chin daily with a mild antibacterial solution containing benzoyl peroxide or chlorhexidine. Afterwards, a drying agent such as alcohol or ear-cleansing solution should be applied to the chin. In severe instances, systemic antibiotics might be required to completely clear up an infection.

As far as other superficial skin infections are concerned, any at-home treatment that uses topical antibacterial creams or ointments should be first approved by a veterinarian. Avoid those preparations containing hydrocortisone or other steroid compounds. In cases where the infection is spreading or is not responding to topical medications, then oral antibiotics will be required.

Cellulitis and abscessation

Cellulitis and abscessation are types of deep infections that occur secondary to tissue injury, usually from bite wounds. Cellulitis involves a poorly defined region of inflammation involving the deeper layers of the skin with no apparent rim or border, whereas abscesses do have a well-demarcated line of surrounding inflammatory cells that make them stand out.

Both can be characterized by a painful build-up of pus, and usually cause fever and depression. Both can also lead to blood poisoning if not treated in a timely manner with high doses of antibiotics. Because of their isolated nature, veterinarians often lance and flush out abscesses to help speed the healing process.

FELINE NEURODERMATITIS

Feline neurodermatitis results in hair loss and/or skin irritation due to nervous licking and chewing (FIG. 32-4). The highly emotional breeds of cats, such as Siamese and Himalayan, are more prone to this disease than others.

This nervous licking and chewing can be triggered by any disruption or stress in the cat's normal daily routine, such as moving into a new home or introducing a new addition to the family. The lesions caused by this abnormal grooming activity can resemble eosinophilic ulcers, or it might present itself as a "stripe" of hair loss on the back or sides of the body. Often the hair loss looks similar to that seen with ringworm.

A diagnosis of neurodermatitis is made after carefully examining the history of occurrence, plus ruling out other causes of similar dermatologic signs. If possible, eliminating or correcting the inciting cause is the best way to treat neurodermatitis. In difficult cases, therapy using progestins or tranquilizers might be necessary to calm the nervous feline and prevent the self trauma to the skin and coat.

FELINE SOLAR DERMATITIS

Initiated by the ultraviolet rays of the sun, *feline solar dermatitis* can occur in cats with insufficient skin pigmentation to block the harmful effects of the sunlight. Cats with white hair coats, especially in the ear or facial region, that live in hot, sunny climates are most prone to this dermatopathy.

Lesions usually begin at the tips and margins of the ears, yet they can also appear on the eyelids, nose, and/or lips. Hair loss, scabs, and ulcera-

32-4   *Neurodermatitis.*

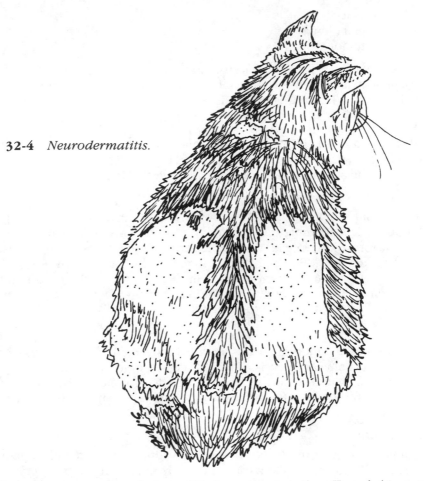

tions characterize these lesions. If left unattended, the affected skin can eventually become cancerous, and metastasize to other parts of the body.

Diagnosis of solar dermatitis is confirmed through surgically obtaining a biopsy sample of the affected areas. Treatment is geared towards reducing exposure to the sun's rays via indoor confinement and through the use of commercial sunscreen products. Corticosteroids applied topically can also help reduce any associated inflammation. For those lesions suspect of becoming cancerous, surgical removal (if possible) and/or radiation therapy is needed to prevent its spread.

SKIN LUMPS AND MASSES

Whenever a lump or mass appears on or beneath the skin of a cat, five possibilities exist as to its source:

1. An abscess
2. A hematoma/seroma

3. A cyst
4. A granuloma
5. A tumor

Obviously, because the cause can vary, a veterinary diagnosis is essential. A fine needle aspirate of the mass, or an actual biopsy sample will assist him/her in this diagnosis.

Abscesses

Abscesses are usually painful to the touch and are often associated with other signs, such as fever, depression, and loss of appetite. They also tend to be fluctuant when direct pressure is applied to them.

Hematomas and seromas

These result from leakage of blood or serum, respectively, from damaged blood vessels. Traumatic blows to the skin can result in hematoma or seroma formation beneath the affected area of skin. The swellings caused by these are also fluctuant; due to the traumatic nature of their occurrence, they can be painful as well. In most cases, the swellings caused by hematomas and seromas will resolve on their own with time, assuming infection does not set in in the meantime.

Cysts

A cyst is nothing more than a well defined pocket filled with fluid, secretion, or inflammatory debris. Unlike abscesses, cysts are usually not filled with pus or painful to the touch. Although they normally pose no specific danger to the health of a cat, especially large cysts should be surgically excised.

Granulomas

Granulomas are firm, raised masses consisting chiefly of inflammatory cells sent to the particular area by the body in response to skin penetration by a foreign substance or infectious agent. In essence, the body attempts to quickly surround and ward off the foreign invader before it can spread to other parts of the body. Thorns, insect stingers, vaccines, fungal organisms, and certain bacteria are but a few of the things that can incite granuloma formation. If a cat develops one of these growths, an attempt should be made to determine the cause of its appearance. If an infectious agent is suspected, appropriate antimicrobial therapy is indicated to prevent further development of the granuloma. Granulomas may or may not recede with time, depending upon the cause. In some cases, surgical removal of the mass gets rid of the unsightly lump and its inciting cause all at the same time.

Tumors

Skin tumors or cancers can appear in a variety of types, sizes, and shapes. Common tumors that appear as a lump or mass on or beneath the skin of a cat include *squamous cell carcinoma, basal cell tumors, fibrosarco-*

mas, and *mast cell tumors.* It is imperative that a biopsy is performed in all instances to determine whether the tumor is malignant or benign. For more information on skin tumors in cats, see chapter 54.

Mammary tumors

Mammary tumors in cats are serious, since the vast majority of these are malignant or cancerous. Most common in older, intact queens, these tumors can spread throughout the body quite rapidly unless diagnosed and treated early.

Treatment involves surgical removal of the affected gland(s). For extensive tumors, chemotherapy might also be employed (see chapter 54.)

33

The Eyes and Ears

THE EYES

The sense of vision is important to nocturnal hunters such as the cat, more so than in their canine counterparts. Unique adaptations of the feline eye allow for this greater visual acuity. For instance, the unique slit-shaped design of the feline pupil allows it to dilate exceptionally wide in dimly lit or dark surroundings. In addition, the ability to focus in on objects and to detect even the slightest of movements is highly refined (FIG. 33-1).

Certainly such visual characteristics account for the effectiveness of the feline as a hunter. As with dogs, cats, too, possess in their eyes those structures necessary to perceive their world in color. Whether they actually take advantage of their presence is doubtful.

Except for the shape of the iris and pupil, the anatomy of the feline eye is essentially the same as that of the dog. For more information concerning visual anatomy and function, see chapter 15.

The Siamese perception

As far as visual capabilities are concerned, one interesting breed to take note of is the Siamese cat. Although anatomically their eyes differ little if at all from their brethren, nevertheless research has revealed that they might perceive their world a little bit differently. While *binocular vision* (visualizing one scene with both eyes) is the standard for humans and most animals, Siamese cats might actually visualize two different presentations for the same scene—one for each eye.

Confusing? Imagine a set of keys sitting on a countertop. That is what a person would see, a set of keys. A Siamese cat, on the other hand, might

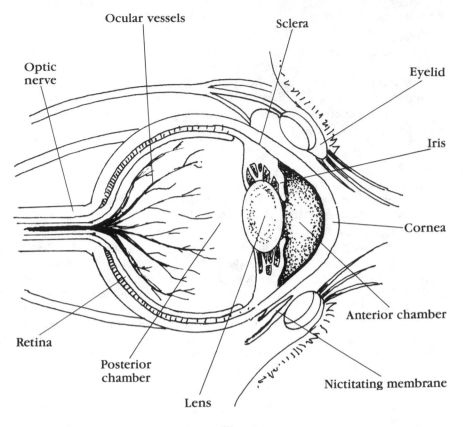

33-1 *The eye.*

visualize two sets of keys because each eye is focusing in on the set separately. Because of this apparent lack of binocular vision, depth perception is not as refined in this breed as with others. Could all this explain the unique behavior exhibited by this fanciful breed?

Corneal ulcers and scratches

The transparent cornea enclosing the front portion of the eye is a remarkable organ in itself. Responsible for gathering light and directing it into the eye, healthy corneas are essential for proper vision. It stands to reason, then, that ulcerations (loss of surface epithelium) or scratches involving one or more corneal surfaces can seriously threaten eyesight if not managed promptly.

Corneal scratches and ulcerations in cats can occur secondary to skirmishes with other cats, dust and foreign debris entering the eyes, and other types of direct trauma. Ulcerations can also occur through improper eye protection applied when bathing or dipping.

Symptoms

Clinical signs of a corneal ulcer include squinting and aversion to light, ocular discharge, and obvious discomfort, often signified by pawing at or rubbing the affected eye. A change in the normal color or transparency of the corneal surface is also an indicator that something is wrong. Definitive diagnosis of a corneal ulcer is made by a veterinarian using a special fluorescein dye to stain the corneal surfaces. Dead, diseased corneal tissue will readily take up such stain whereas healthy tissue will not.

Treatment

Luckily, the cornea is one organ that will heal quite rapidly if treatment is administered vigorously and in a timely fashion. For ulcers involving only the superficial layers of the cornea, topical antibiotic ointments or solutions designed for use in the eyes and applied three to six times daily will help speed healing. Special drops or solutions are sometimes used to reduce pain and discomfort associated with the ulceration by dilating the pupil. Doing so also prevents adhesions from forming between the iris and the lens or cornea should any inflammation spread into the interior of the eye itself.

Of course, if an underlying cause, such as a piece of nail, still exists in the eye, it must be removed before proper healing can take place. Superficial ulcers can heal within 36 to 48 hours with proper treatment applied.

Deep corneal ulcerations

Deep corneal ulcerations are treated the same way that superficial ulcerations are, yet deep ulcerations require close observation for progression or worsening of the ulcer. Bacterial cultures of such ulcers are necessary to be certain that the antibiotics being used are effective against the organisms involved, if any.

For deep ulcers that worsen, or even fail to respond to conventional treatment, additional procedures might be necessary to speed healing or to prevent the cornea from actually rupturing. A new procedure being used by many veterinarians consists of surgically freeing and extending a portion of the thin conjunctiva over the ulcer and actually tacking it down against the ulcer using suture material (*conjunctival flap*). The flap of conjunctiva provides nutrition and speeds healing to the ulcer, and also allows any medications applied directly to the eye(s) to reach the ulcer without hindrance. Once healing has been accomplished, the flap is released, and excess conjunctival tissue is trimmed away from the healed surface.

Conjunctivitis

Inflammation of the thin, transparent mucous membrane lining the inner portion of the eyelids and front part of the sclera is termed *conjunctivitis*.

Symptoms

Conjunctivitis is the most common cause of "red eyes" in cats. Other signs seen with conjunctivitis include discharge, swelling, and, if other eye structures are involved, pain. The type of discharge present can sometimes give a clue as to the underlying cause of the conjunctivitis. For instance, a watery discharge can indicate irritation from an allergy, virus (such as feline rhinotracheitis), or contact with dirt or dust. In contrast, a cloudy discharge often links the problem to a bacterial infection, either primary or secondary to any of the causes previously mentioned.

Treatment

Because conjunctivitis can be secondary to other problems, diagnostic tests performed by a veterinarian should be directed at identifying any underlying causes. Corneal staining using a fluorescent stain is usually performed to determine whether or not the cornea is concurrently affected.

Treatment of conjunctivitis is aimed at treating or eliminating any inciting causes, and at controlling the localized inflammation. If dust or pollens are the source of the conjunctivitis, daily flushing of the eyes with a sterile saline solution designed for use in the eyes or daily application of a sterile ophthalmic lubricant can help reduce the irritation caused by these offenders.

Ophthalmic drops or ointments containing antibiotics are warranted if a bacterial infection is present. In addition, ophthalmic preparations containing steroids can be used to reduce the inflammation present, provided that the surface of the cornea is intact. Preparations containing both antibiotics and steroid compounds for use in the eyes are readily available for pets through a prescription from a veterinarian.

In cases of conjunctivitis that don't respond to conventional therapy, a bacterial culture/sensitivity test and an eye-pressure test should be performed. The first can help determine if the type of antibiotic ointment or solution being used is indeed the right choice; the second will help identify any underlying problems with the eyes themselves (such as glaucoma) that might be contributing to the lingering conjunctivitis.

Cataracts

Fortunately, the incidence of cataract formation in cats is much less than that in dogs. When it does occur, the most common underlying cause is diabetes mellitus. As a result, any change in a cat's visual responsiveness or any obvious changes in the lens color warrants a complete veterinary medical work-up.

Glaucoma

Glaucoma is a condition characterized by an increase in fluid pressure from the aqueous humor within the eye(s). In the normal eye, pressure and aqueous levels are maintained at a constant level by the continual drainage of excess aqueous humor out of the eye through tiny ports (*drainage angles*) located where the edge of the iris meets the cornea. If for any reason this drainage is obstructed or altered in any way, a rise in pressure within the eye can result. Unfortunately, even short-term rises in this pressure can lead to irreversible damage if not detected and treated in a timely fashion.

Conditions such as a buildup of inflammatory material within the eye secondary to FIP or feline leukemia, luxation of the lens due to trauma or cataracts, and *synechia* (where the iris ''sticks'' to the lens or cornea), can all effectively prevent the normal drainage of the aqueous humor from the eye.

Symptoms

Clinical signs of a glaucomatous eye include a marked redness both affecting the conjunctival tissue and the sclera; a blue, hazy cornea; a dilated, unresponsive pupil; and apparent blindness due to the increased pressure the fluid is placing on the optic nerve. In instances where the glaucoma has been present for quite some time, enlargement of the affected eyeball might become noticeable, and actual rupture of the cornea could occur.

Treatment

Diagnosis of glaucoma can be easily confirmed by a veterinarian through the use of an instrument called a *tonometer*. This instrument, which is placed directly upon the surface of the cornea, measures the exact pressure occurring within that eye. If the pressure reading is indeed elevated, then treatment should be instituted immediately to prevent lasting damage to the eye.

Treatment for glaucoma is aimed at decreasing the pressure within the eye to an acceptable level as quickly as possible, and then stabilizing this pressure to prevent increases in the future. Drugs designed to quickly draw fluid out of the eye and into the bloodstream will initially be used by a veterinarian to reduce the pressure within the pet's eye(s); other drugs that act by decreasing the production of aqueous humor and by increasing the size of the drainage angles are then prescribed and given for the long-term management and prevention of recurrence. At the same time, anti-inflammatory medications can be used topically on the eye to clear up any primary or secondary inflammation that might be aggravating the glaucoma.

Entropion/Ectropion

Entropion is an ophthalmic condition in which the eyelids roll inward, allowing lashes and hair to irritate the surface of the eyes. *Ectropion* is the opposite: One or more lids roll outward, exposing conjunctival tissue and predisposing it to irritation. In both instances, the surface of the affected eye(s) become irritated and damaged, and inflammation results. Kittens can be born with either of these eyelid defects, or they can acquire them later in life, usually as a result of trauma to the lid(s). Fortunately, the incidence of both conditions is quite low in cats. When it occurs, surgical correction is required to prevent permanent damage to the eyes.

Masses involving the eyelids

The integrity of the eyelids is vital for the protection of the eyes from environmental hazards. Any disruption or alteration in the normal lid anatomy can place vision in jeopardy. And certain masses involving the lids can do just that if they become disruptive enough.

Tumors are the most common types of eyelid masses seen in cats. The presence of an eyelid tumor can be very serious because it is impossible to remove one surgically without disrupting the integrity of the lid. Squamous cell carcinomas are frequently involved in this location.

As alternatives to the potential complications afforded by eyelid surgery, radiation therapy, chemotherapy, and cryotherapy (freezing) might all be employed for treatment, depending upon the type of tumor is involved.

THE EARS

The sense of hearing in the cat is much more fine-tuned than that in a human, allowing the cat to detect much higher sound pitches that might be emitted by potential prey. Like the dog, its hearing apparatus can be divided into three portions: the inner ear, the middle ear, and the external ear canal and associated structures (FIG. 33-2). For more information on anatomy and function of the ear, see chapter 15.

Otitis Externa

Inflammation involving the external ear canal is called *otitis externa*. Although it occurs only infrequently in the cat, it can conceivably result from allergies, infections, foreign bodies, and ear mite infestations. Otitis externa can also lead to secondary infections within the ear canal if the inflammation persists for long enough.

Symptoms

Signs of otitis externa involving one or both ears include head shaking, itching, painful ears, personality changes, and/or odiferous discharges coming from the ear canal(s). Hair loss might be noticed around the pinnae due to scratching.

Treatment

Diagnosis of this condition is based on clinical signs and direct examination of the ear canals by a veterinarian. Once the exact nature of the problem is identified, then specific treatment can be instituted (FIG. 33-3).

Ear mites

Otodectes cynotis is the name of the ear mite commonly found in the feline ear canal. These tiny parasites, which are transmitted by close con-

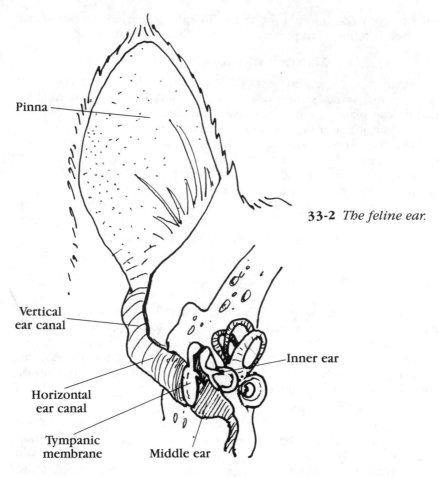

Pinna

Vertical
ear canal

Horizontal
ear canal

Tympanic
membrane

Middle ear

Inner ear

33-2 *The feline ear.*

tact with other infected animals, live on the skin surface within the ear canal and feed on body fluids. Their presence irritates the glands lining the ear canal, leading to an increased cerumen production.

Symptoms

Secondary yeast infections within the ear often occur because of them, leading to the brown, crusty discharge so often seen with ear mite infestations. In isolated cases, intense allergic reactions to ear mites can occur, causing severe inflammation and secondary bacterial infection.

Treatment

Diagnosis of an ear mite infestation is confirmed by identification of the mites directly on otoscopic exam or through a microscopic examination of an ear swab. Treatment involves the use of medications containing antiparasitic compounds, such as pyrethrins, rotenone, and/or thiabendazole. Mineral oil has also been employed as a home remedy for killing mites by suffocation. Since secondary yeast infections are commonly

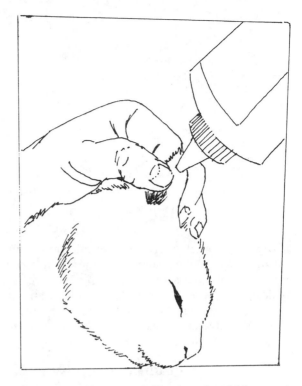

33-3 *Treating the ears.*

found with ear mite infestations, an anti-yeast medication should be used concurrently with anti-mite preparations.

Ear mites can be difficult pests to eliminate. Daily treatment for three to four weeks might be needed to ensure a complete kill. All pets in the household, regardless of whether or not they are exhibiting signs of infestation, should be treated at the same time. In addition, to prevent re-infestation from the hair coat, an insecticidal spray or shampoo should used on the coat at least twice during the treatment period.

Otitis media

Otitis media, infection involving the middle ear, usually results from a chronic, untreated or recurring otitis externa. In such cases, the ear drum might become so diseased that it tears or ruptures completely, allowing direct access of infectious organisms into the middle ear chamber.

The clinical signs of otitis media are essentially the same as those for otitis externa, with a few notable additions. Cats so afflicted will usually exhibit a head tilt towards the side of the affected ear (FIG. 33-4). In severe cases, paralysis of the facial muscles on the side of the lesion might be seen as the nerves passing through the middle ear become involved. This can result in a characteristic drooping of the eyelids, cheeks, and lips. In addition, a decreased tear production, pinpoint pupil, and protrusion of the third eyelid might be noted in the eye on the affected side.

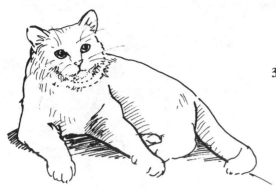

33-4 *Middle ear infections can cause a head tilt towards the affected side.*

Otitis interna

If the infection extends from the middle ear into the inner ear apparatus (*otitus interna*), the signs become even more pronounced. Since the inner ear functions in maintaining balance and equilibrium as well as hearing, cats suffering from otitis interna tend to become very uncoordinated and might fall down frequently or move in circles to the affected side. A characteristic twitching of the eyeball, called nystagmus, also becomes noticeable.

Treatment of otitis media/interna

Although the clinical signs seen are often diagnostic, radiographs of the skull are quite helpful in confirming a diagnosis of otitis media/interna and determining the extent of the disorder.

Therapy for otitis media/interna must be instituted promptly to prevent permanent damage to the hearing apparatus. Oral antibiotics should be started immediately. In cases of otitis interna, continued treatment with antibiotics might be required for up to thirty days to afford a complete cure. In select cases, anti-inflammatory medications have been used to reduce signs associated with inflammation.

If it is not already ruptured, the ear drum on the affected side will usually be punctured to allow for thorough drainage of the middle ear cavity and to allow for the direct infusion of medications. Of course, such treatment steps must be carried out in a veterinary hospital under heavy sedation or anesthesia.

In tough, refractory cases, surgical placement of a drain in the bony tympanic bulla affords excellent exposure to the middle and inner ear spaces.

Ruptured ear drums

Ear drums can tear or rupture as the result of direct trauma from a foreign body (such as a twig, cotton-tip applicator), sudden pressure changes, or most commonly, as a secondary complication due to otitis externa.

Though a serious and painful condition, a torn ear drum will heal quite quickly provided the underlying cause of the perforation is eliminated.

Medications designed for use in the ears must be used with caution if a cat suffers from a ruptured eardrum. Not only can their application be painful, but, as mentioned previously, certain antibiotics and solutions, if allowed direct access into the middle and inner ear chambers, can cause damage to the auditory nerve endings, resulting in deafness. As a result, owners must be certain to follow their veterinarian's recommendations closely.

Deafness

Veterinarians are often confronted by frustrated owners claiming that their cat is going deaf! A cat's apparent inability to perceive sounds can result from a number of reasons.

First, there might be impedance to the sound waves traveling through the ear. An external ear canal clogged with wax and debris secondary to ear mites can certainly be the culprit.

The effective transmission of sound waves to the middle and inner ears can also be diminished by torn or ruptured eardrums or by inflammation in these regions.

Besides interference with the transmission of sound waves, deafness in cats can also be caused by developmental defects of damage involving the actual nerve endings within the inner ear. For instance, congenital (inherited) nerve deafness is known to occur in white-haired, blued-eyed Angora cats. Certain drugs, such as the aminoglycoside antibiotics, are well-known for their adverse effects upon the hearing function in cats. Furthermore, chronic, untreated bacterial and fungal infections within the middle and inner ears can undoubtedly lead to nerve deafness as well.

Symptoms

One way you can test for hearing function in a cat is to stealthily approach it in a manner that it is not immediately aware of your presence. Then using a hand clap or a whistle, observe it for a response. It should either turn to face you, or you should notice a twitching of the ears as the sound is evoked. You should stand a good distance away from the cat when this is done to be sure that air currents created by your actions or your scent won't inadvertently alert the pet to your presence.

If you are still not sure as to the status of a pet's hearing, let a veterinarian take a look. As mentioned before, a simple otoscopic examination might reveal a simple solution to the hearing problem. Special instruments are even available at universities and teaching hospitals across the country that can measure the amount of nerve activity taking place within the inner ear.

Treatment

Treatment for deafness obviously depends upon the inciting cause. Hearing loss caused by impedance of sound waves through the ear is usually reversible once the underlying condition is addressed. Unfortunately, this optimism is lost when it comes to actual nerve deafness. In most cases, the injury sustained by infections or toxic medications is irreversible.

There is no reason why cats that are deaf can't lead normal lives. However, owners of such pets must be aware of the limitations and dangers that this loss or absence of hearing can place on a pet that is allowed outdoors. As a result, these cats should be confined to the house to keep them out of harm's way.

34

The Musculoskeletal System

THE MUSCULOSKELETAL system in mammals is responsible for locomotion and support, not to mention protection of vital internal organs. The components of this system include muscles, bones, and a variety of supportive structures, including ligaments, tendons, and cartilage. Disorders of the musculoskeletal system can be quite debilitating to a cat and be accompanied by a lot of pain.

For more information on the anatomy and function of the musculoskeletal system, see chapter 16.

ARTHRITIS & DEGENERATIVE JOINT DISEASE

Arthritis is the term used in both human and veterinary medicine to describe any type of joint inflammation. *Polyarthritis* describes inflammation involving multiple joints throughout the body. This inflammation could be accompanied by loss of cartilage or bony changes within the joint(s) in question.

Causes of arthritis in cats include infections, autoimmune diseases, and trauma. Even certain drugs, such as sulfa antibiotics, can promote joint inflammation if used indiscriminately.

Osteoarthrosis, or degenerative joint disease, describes the condition in which a cartilage defect or cartilage erosion occurs within a given joint. Though not considered a true inflammatory condition, many people use the term interchangeably with arthritis. Osteoarthrosis usually strikes older cats as a result of normal wear-and-tear associated with aging.

Stiffness or lameness involving one or more limbs is often the most obvious sign of a joint problem. In many instances, this lameness is aggravated by colder weather and prolonged periods of rest or overexertion. Affected cats might be reluctant to play or jump, and they could become more irritable when touched due to pain. Joints might also be noticeably swollen and painful to the touch.

Diagnosis of a joint disorder is based upon physical palpation of the joint(s) in question, observing the abnormal gait or movement associated with the disorder, and by obtaining radiographic X-rays of the joints.

Treatment approaches for osteoarthrosis include forced rest, weight loss, and anti-inflammatory medication if needed for pain. Since aspirin and acetaminophen can be highly toxic to cats, corticosteroids such as prednisone are prescribed instead for their anti-inflammatory activity.

Infectious arthritis

Apart from the normal wear-and-tear due to aging, joint inflammation can be secondary to an infectious process. Bacteria that gain entrance into the body's blood stream can circulate to one or more joints of the body, setting up housekeeping within the joint fluid. Bite wounds resulting from fights with other cats is an important cause of infectious arthritis in felines.

Symptoms

Fever, depression, and painful, swollen joints, with accompanying lameness, are prominent clinical signs seen in most cases of infectious arthritis. If allowed to fulminate untreated, actual degeneration of the bones making up the joint can occur, causing actual joint collapse.

Treatment

Laboratory testing, including cultures of the fluid within the joint, might be needed to positively identify the offender. Once this is accomplished, specific treatment, usually involving high doses of antibiotics for four to six weeks, can then be instituted. Hot packs applied to the affected joints can also be used to help relieve some of the swelling and pain associated with the arthritis.

Limping kitten syndrome

Young kittens under 14 weeks of age can be afflicted with a form of infectious arthritis called *Limping Kitten Syndrome*. Caused by the calicivirus, this syndrome presents as fever, generalized lameness and pain, and hot, swollen joints.

With the severity of signs being as they are, one would expect these kittens to suffer long-term ill effects from such a disease. Interestingly enough, however, prognosis for a complete recovery is excellent, since the disease is self-limiting and will go away with time even without treatment.

Immune-mediated polyarthritis

Sometimes, an overactive immune system can lead to an arthritic condition. In these instances immune complexes consisting of antibodies coalesce within the joints of the body, causing inflammation. The resultant *polyarthritis* (arthritis affecting more than one joint) can be very painful and debilitating.

Symptoms

Many cats that suffer from immune-related polyarthritis are also infected with the feline leukemia virus. As a result, other symptoms not related to the arthritis might be seen. Fever and a generalized depression are two of these that are seen quite consistently.

Treatment

Special blood tests and/or tests on joint fluid are used to diagnose autoimmune disorders in cats. Treatment usually consists of high dosages of steroid anti-inflammatory medications designed to curb the body's overactive immune response. Life-long therapy might be required.

Hip dysplasia

Hip dysplasia refers to a hereditary arthritic condition involving one or both hip joints of affected cats. It presents itself as a partial dislocation, or in severe cases, a complete dislocation of the hip joints. With time, the cartilages lining the joint surfaces wear down due to the abnormal stress and strain placed on the joint, and arthritis results.

Symptoms

Because of its inherited nature, signs associated with hip dysplasia can appear at any age. These clinical signs consist of posterior pain, unsteadiness on the hind limbs, difficulty in rising from a prone position, and a reluctance to move or exercise. Manipulation of the hip joints will reveal obvious pain. In less severe cases, signs might only appear after intense activity and exercise.

Treatment

Diagnosis of hip dysplasia in a cat is based upon the history, clinical signs, and physical exam findings. A definitive diagnosis can only be made by having radiographic X-rays taken of the hip joints to confirm their involvement.

For those cats suffering from a mild case of hip dysplasia, anti-inflammatory medications such as prednisone can be used to temporarily decrease pain and discomfort associated with the disease. A program of regular exercise and weight loss can also benefit these patients.

In severe cases, a surgical procedure called *femoral head and neck ostectomy* can be performed. This involves the surgical removal of the ends of the femur bones which normally fit into the pelvic sockets, making up the hip joints. Surprisingly enough, these cats do quite well after surgery, and often show no signs of lameness or locomotion deficits within weeks after the procedure is performed!

HIP LUXATION

One common sequela to car accidents involving cats is dislocation, or *luxation*, of one or both hip joints. These cats are rarely able to move and experience pain in the affected regions.

Diagnosis can be made with a physical examination and radiographic X-rays of the hips and pelvis. Treatment involves realigning the hip joints under sedation, and strict cage confinement for a period of three to four weeks as healing takes place. In severe cases, a femoral head and neck ostectomy might be required.

FRACTURES

Most bone fractures in cats are trauma-related. In isolated instances, metabolic diseases such as nutritional osteodystrophy and bone cancers can also be underlying causes as well.

Symptoms

A fracture will present itself as a non-weight-bearing lameness, with noticeable swelling and pain in the region of the affected bone. *Crepitus* (the grinding feel made by broken ends of bone rubbing together) and an anatomical distortion of the site, such as a shortening of an affected limb, might also be seen.

Treatment

Diagnosis of a fracture is based upon physical exam findings and radiographic X-rays. Treatment depends upon the type of fracture and region involved, and consists of any combination of cage rest, bandaging/splinting, and surgery to reduce and stabilize the fracture. For instance, fractures involving the pelvis will often heal up nicely with cage rest alone; whereas malaligned fractures of one or more limbs might require surgical fixation using orthopedic pins, screws, or plates. In general, properly managed fractures usually heal quite fast in cats with minimal complications.

TORN KNEE LIGAMENTS (CRUCIATE INJURIES)

The knee joints of cats are held together by a fibrous joint capsule and number of ligaments, the most prominent of these being the *cruciate ligaments*. Because of their configuration, the range of motion allowed the knee joint is limited to simple flexion and extension. If an abnormal force is placed upon the joint, usually from a traumatic incident, these ligaments could tear or rupture, leading to instability and pain within the affected knee joint. This instability, if not corrected in a timely fashion, will lead to arthritic changes and permanent pain within the joint.

Symptoms

Acute ruptures or tears involving the cruciate ligaments usually result in a sudden, non-weight-bearing lameness in cats. Over time, a gradual return to function might occur even if not treated, yet the lameness will undoubtedly return as the activity level of the cat increases or as arthritis strikes the joint.

Treatment

A diagnosis of torn knee ligaments is made if a veterinarian can demonstrate an obvious laxity within the affected knee joint. Due to the pain involved with such a diagnostic procedure, sedation might be necessary in order to obtain an accurate assessment. Radiographs might be helpful, depending upon the duration of the problem.

Treatment of this condition involves surgical repair and reconstruction of the torn ligaments in an effort to restore normal knee joint stability. Many techniques for such repair are available for use, depending upon the extent of the injury and other circumstances involved. In general, cats are excellent candidates for surgery, due to their light body weight not placing extraordinary stress on the repaired knee(s).

OSTEOMYELITIS

Infections involving bony tissue within the body are termed *osteomyelitis*. Bacterial osteomyelitis in cats usually occurs secondary to a deep bite wound or some other type of penetrating trauma. Open fractures can also predispose a cat to bone infections. Furthermore, fungal organisms such as histoplasmosis and blastomycosis can also spread from other areas of the body via the blood and infect bony tissue in cats.

Symptoms

Cats with osteomyelitis are lame and feverish. The affected site is usually quite painful. These signs, combined with the localized swelling that often occurs, might be mistaken for a fracture, and indeed, must be differentiated from one. To do this, radiographic X-rays should be taken of the suspected skeletal region. In addition, bone biopsies might even be necessary to differentiate some cases of osteomyelitis from bone tumors, and to collect samples for bacterial or fungal cultures.

Treatment

Because infections that become embedded in bone can be difficult to clear up with antibiotics alone, surgery is usually needed to actually remove those portions of bone severely affected. Drain tubes are placed as well to allow for post-surgical drainage and flushing of the site with medicated solutions.

Following surgery, antibiotic therapy might be required for one to two months; if a fungal organism is involved, medications might need to be given for four to six months.

MUCOPOLYSACCHARIDOSIS

Mucopolysaccharidosis is an inherited disorder that has been documented in Siamese cats. It results from an enzyme deficiency that allows polysaccharide carbohydrates to accumulate within the cells of the body.

Symptoms

The skeletal system is particularly affected, with stricken cats suffering from bony spurs on the vertebrae, arthritis and abnormal formation of the joints, and a generalized osteoporosis, or thinning of the bones themselves. These cats also have a characteristic "flattening" of the face, resulting from a widening of the facial structure, and, at an early age, can suffer from opacities or cloudiness involving the corneas of both eyes.

Treatment

Diagnosis of mucopolysaccharidosis is made by physical examination, blood tests, and radiographic X-rays of the skeletal system. A special test that detects mucopolysaccharides in the urine can also be employed in the diagnosis of this disorder.

Unfortunately, because of the congenital nature of this disease, there is no known treatment. Future generations should be protected by neutering those pets affected to prevent passage of the trait.

MYOSITIS

Myositis is inflammation of muscle tissue which results in pain, weakness, and muscle *atrophy* (shrinking).

Symptoms

Cats suffering from severe bouts of myositis are reluctant to move and can actually appear as if they are paralyzed due to the inflammatory effects on the muscles. Myositis in felines can be caused by a number of different disease entities, including toxoplasmosis, bacterial infections (abscesses), hypokalemia (low blood potassium) and, rarely, autoimmune disease.

Treatment

Myositis is diagnosed using clinical signs and blood tests designed to detect increased levels in muscle enzymes within the blood. In especially elusive cases, biopsy samples taken from suspected muscle tissue can help a veterinarian obtain a definitive diagnosis.

Treatment for myositis is aimed at the underlying cause. For instance, if infections are to blame, appropriate antimicrobial or antiparasitic therapy will help relieve the myositis. Anti-inflammatory medications can also be used to relieve the pain and discomfort associated with the inflammation until the underlying cause is treated.

HERNIAS

A *hernia* results from a tear or defect in a muscular wall, allowing the contents contained behind the wall to protrude through the opening in the muscle. In cats, two common types of hernias include *inguinal hernias* and *diaphragmatic hernias*.

Inguinal hernias

Inguinal hernias occur in the inguinal region of the abdomen, or that region where the abdominal musculature meets that of the hind legs. They are seen as birth defects, or, more commonly, secondary to trauma.

These hernias can be serious, since the herniated material often includes intestines. As a result, normal digestive processes can be disrupted. Treatment involves surgical replacement of the herniated material back inside the abdomen and suturing the defective muscle.

Diaphragmatic hernias

By far the most serious type of hernia is the diaphragmatic hernia. The *diaphragm* is the thick wall of muscle which separates the thorax or chest cavity from the abdominal contents. Tears or ruptures occurring in this band of muscle, resulting either from congenital defects or from traumatic incidents, can allow liver, intestines, and other abdominal contents to herniate through into the chest cavity. When this happens, the pressure applied to the crowded lungs and heart results in, among other things, breathing difficulties, weakness, and gastrointestinal disturbances.

Definitive diagnosis of a diaphragmatic hernia can be made by coupling history, clinical signs, and a physical examination with radiographic X-ray findings. Surgical repair of the torn diaphragm will alleviate the signs and usually result in a complete recovery.

POTASSIUM DEPLETION

As an electrolyte within the body, potassium serves a variety of functions, including maintaining proper fluid volume and pH within the body. Potassium is also necessary for normal muscle contraction. Just recently, veterinarians have discovered that many illnesses in cats can also produce a state of *hypokalemia*, or low blood potassium, within their bodies (FIG. 34-1). This is especially true for those cats suffering from kidney disease, liver disease, or diabetes mellitus.

Still under investigation is a possible link between hypokalemia and low taurine levels seen in cardiomyopathies, and low potassium levels associated with long-term use of urinary acidifiers, such as those used to treat FUS in cats.

Symptoms

Actual signs of hypokalemia can include weight loss, loss of appetite, constipation (due to poor motility of the muscles lining the gastrointestinal tract), muscle weakness, muscle pain, and incoordination.

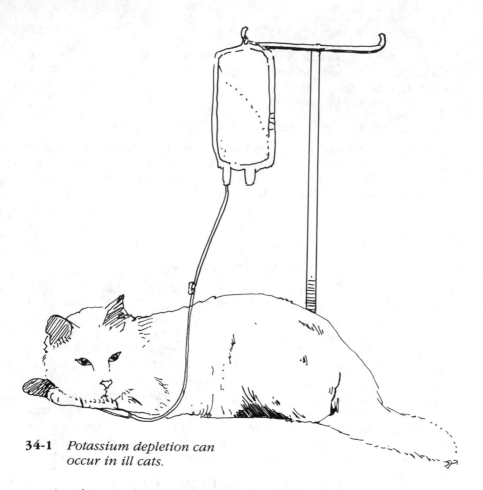

34-1 *Potassium depletion can
occur in ill cats.*

   As the condition progresses and respiratory muscles become
affected, breathing difficulties might be noted. In severe cases, death from
respiratory paralysis could result.

Treatment

Diagnosis of hypokalemia in a sick cat is based upon a history, clinical
signs, and measurements of blood potassium levels. If hypokalemia is
diagnosed, treatment consists of intravenous injections of a potassium
supplement to correct the immediate deficit, followed by oral supplementation with potassium gluconate as long as deemed necessary. Prognosis
for recovery is good if treated early.

35

The Nervous System

THE NERVOUS SYSTEM involves a complex interaction between special elements designed to originate or to carry unique electrochemical charges to and from the various organs within the body. Like its endocrine counterpart, the nervous system initiates and regulates bodily functions and ensures its owner of an awareness to its surrounding environment. For more information regarding the anatomy and function of the nervous system, see chapter 16.

PARALYSIS

Paralysis can be defined as a disruption of the nervous system leading to an impairment of motor function and/or feeling to a particular region or regions of the body. This impairment can be in the form of a spasticity of the muscles in the involved region, or these muscles might become completely limp. In either case, the muscles involved are unable to function in the manner they were intended.

Paralysis involving the sensory portion of the nervous system can result in an increased sensitivity to pain, or in a complete absence of it. Finally, paralysis resulting in the inefficient function of certain internal organs can occur as well if the nerves supplying these structures are disrupted in any way. If the bladder or colon are involved, this can lead to either urine and fecal retention or incontinence.

Any disease or disorder that traumatizes the brain, spinal cord, and nerves, or disrupts circulation to these regions, has the potential to cause paralysis. In cats, some of the more common causes seen by veterinarians include infectious diseases and parasites (such as feline leukemia), trauma (such as being hit by a car), and circulatory disturbances.

Treatment of paralysis is geared towards identifying and treating the underlying cause. If it is caused by trauma, anti-inflammatory agents combined with drugs designed to draw fluid out of the central nervous system can help reverse signs of paralysis, yet their usefulness is dependent upon the extent of the nervous injury and how quickly therapy is instituted.

Cats that have sensory paralysis in a limb might require limb amputation to prevent self-mutilation to the leg. In instances where an irreversible paralysis involves more than one limb, or involves the malfunction of internal organs, pet owners must seriously consider not only their cat's quality of life as a paralytic, but their own as well, before prolonged therapeutic or rehabilitative measures are undertaken.

SEIZURES

Owners who have a cat that suffers from seizures know first-hand how frightening these episodes can be. A *seizure* is defined as uncontrollable behavior or muscle activity caused by an abnormal increase in the brain's nervous activities. *Epilepsy* is the term used to describe recurring seizures.

What causes seizures? The following are some potential sources:

○ Viral infections (i.e., FeLV, FIP)
○ Toxoplasmosis
○ Trauma
○ Fungal infections
○ Cancer
○ Intestinal parasites
○ Low blood sugar
○ Insecticidal poisoning
○ Heat stroke

Because the causes are so numerous, a thorough examination and blood workup by a veterinarian is warranted anytime a cat exhibits seizures. In some cases, managing or eliminating an underlying cause will eliminate the seizures. In others, such as with *idiopathic epilepsy*, there is no known cause, yet by ruling out the other potential causes and establishing a pattern of occurrence, most cases can be effectively managed with anticonvulsant medications.

With idiopathic epilepsy, seizures can begin at any stage in life, yet, for the most part, begin around one to three years of age. As mentioned before, the cause of idiopathic epilepsy is unknown; however, if it occurs in young animals, it was probably inherited. In contrast, if it occurs in older cats, some traumatic cause, such as a stroke, should be considered.

Characteristics of seizures

Most seizures themselves are rarely life threatening, unless some physical harm comes to the cat as a result of the fit. However, there is one seizural presentation called *status epilepticus* which can prove fatal to a cat unfortunate enough to be afflicted with such. This condition is characterized by continual seizures occurring one right after the other. Unless appropriate emergency medication is administered intravenously to stop the seizures, these cats can lapse into a coma and die. As a result, prompt recognition and action on the part of the pet owner is essential.

The typical seizure or epileptic fit has three stages, or phases. The first of these, the *preictal phase*, is marked by anxiety and restlessness on the part of the pet. The actual period of the seizure activity, *ictus*, follows next. Its duration might be for only a few seconds or it might be minutes. Certainly the longer the seizure lasts, the more dangerous it is to the health of the pet.

The *postictal phase* following the seizure is characterized by an overall depression or confusion. Postictal cats can appear to be blind, running into walls and objects, or they might just sleep a lot. This phase can last for a few hours or for days, with the cat returning to its normal state after its conclusion.

Treatment

For cases other than idiopathic epilepsy, treatment is geared toward correcting or managing the underlying problem, be it kidney failure, poisoning, low blood sugar, etc. In instances in which idiopathic epilepsy is suspect, anticonvulsant medications can be used to control or even eliminate the seizural activity.

Cats suffering from idiopathic epilepsy do not necessarily need to be on any medication unless the seizures last for more than two minutes at a time or occur more often than every two months. For those cats that require medication, oral *phenobarbital* is the drug of choice (FIG. 35-1).

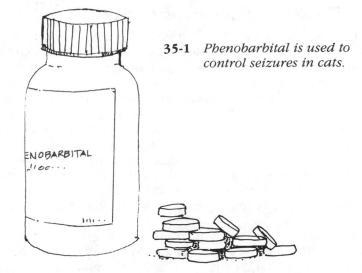

35-1   *Phenobarbital is used to control seizures in cats.*

Determining the exact dosages of any of these medications for a pet might require frequent adjustments at the start in order to accommodate its individual needs. Pets taking anticonvulsant medication should have liver-function tests performed at least annually, since some anticonvulsant medications can deteriously affect the liver over the long-term.

VESTIBULAR DISEASE

The vestibular portion of the nervous system is responsible for maintaining balance and coordinated muscle activity. Cats can suffer from a number of disorders affecting this vital area, resulting in clinical signs that include head tilting, rolling, falling, disorientation, vomiting, and/or nystagmus.

Potential causes include infectious diseases, trauma, and ear infections.

Vestibular ataxia syndrome is seen in kittens born of queens stricken with feline parvovirus during pregnancy. Owners often are alerted to a problem when these kittens seem to have trouble in attempting to walk. The condition will not improve as these kittens mature, nor will it usually worsen.

Congenital vestibular syndrome is seen in Siamese and Burmese cats, with signs appearing anywhere from 2 to 4 weeks of age. Many of the Siamese cats affected are deaf as well.

The prognosis for Siamese cats with congenital vestibular syndrome is good, with clinical signs usually abating by the time the cat is 6 months of age. In Burmese cats, however, the prognosis is not as good, and the poor quality of life for most of these individuals will usually warrant euthanasia.

FELINE HYPERESTHESIA SYNDROME

Feline Hyperesthesia Syndrome (Twitchy Skin Syndrome) is a condition characterized by some unique clinical signs. Cats so affected exhibit rippling of the skin on their back, especially when petted in the lower back region (FIG. 35-2). They might chew or lick at their tail incessantly, and appear to be "spaced out," spontaneously darting throughout a room or house and attacking objects and owners without provocation.

The exact cause of this condition remains unknown. Some researchers feel that it is a form of epilepsy. Because "emotional" breeds such as Siamese, Persians, and Himilayans seem most often affected, other researchers believe that it is actually a behavioral disorder brought about by an upsetting experience or circumstance. Even food preservatives used in cat foods have been accused of causing feline hyperesthesia syndrome.

Medical therapy for this disorder consists of the use of progestin compounds and/or sedatives in an attempt to modify the cat's behavior. Attempting to identify and correct any environmental upsets, including changing the food, that might have a possible link to the problem is also advocated.

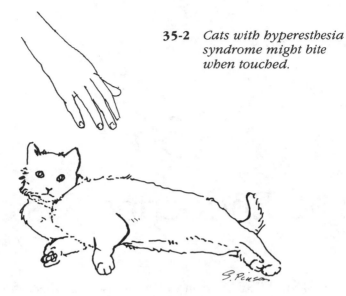

35-2 *Cats with hyperesthesia syndrome might bite when touched.*

FELINE ISCHEMIC ENCEPHALOPATHY (FIE)

Feline Ischemic Encephalopathy, or stroke, occurs when a blood clot prevents the normal supply of blood reaching a portion or portions of the brain, resulting in tissue death in that area. Cats that have suffered a stroke might exhibit incoordination, seizures, marked or subtle behavioral changes, depression, and/or blindness.

Treatment involves using high doses of anti-inflammatory steroids to help reduce the swelling caused by the infarction. Many cats will recover completely with time; others retain postural or behavioral deficits for the rest of their lives.

36

The Endocrine System

ENDOCRINE DISEASES in cats are those that affect hormones or hormone-producing glands within the body. Because of the importance of hormones in metabolic regulation and function within the body, diseases affecting endocrine glands within the body can lead to a wide variety of clinical signs. In addition, proper diagnosis and treatment is essential to prevent permanent damage to the body.

Those endocrine diseases that have the greatest prevalence in cats will be discussed subsequently. Keep in mind that other less-common ones do exist, which reinforces the importance of a proper diagnosis.

For more information on the anatony and function of the endocrine system see chapter 18 in the *Dogs* section.

HYPERTHYROIDISM

The thyroid gland, through production of thyroid hormones, functions to influence nutrient and oxygen utilization within the body, hence affecting overall metabolism. As a result, deficiencies in thyroid hormone or interference with its function can have profound effects on the body. For instance, in dogs, a state of hypothyroidism can lead to a multitude of health problems. Hypothyroidism itself is rare in cats; however, the same can't be said for *hyperthyroidism*, a condition characterized by an increase in circulating levels of thyroid hormone.

Symptoms

Hyperthyroidism in cats is usually caused by a tumor of the thyroid gland. It is more commonly seen in felines over 8 years of age. Clinical signs of an overactive thyroid include an increase in appetite with accompanying

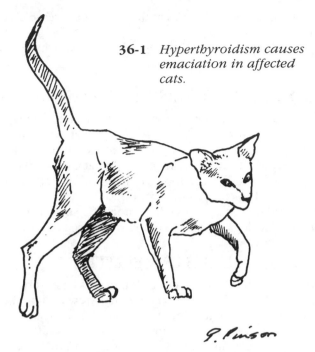

36-1 *Hyperthyroidism causes emaciation in affected cats.*

9. Pinson

weight loss (due to a rapid metabolic rate), nervousness, a rapid heart rate, soft stools, and a scruffy, ungroomed hair coat (FIG. 36-1). If the thyroid enlargement is great enough, difficulty in breathing might be noticed as well.

Treatment

Besides clinical signs and physical exam findings, diagnosis of hyperthyroidism can also be made by a simple blood test performed right in a veterinarian's office.

Treatment for hyperthyroidism is geared towards treating the tumor causing the over secretion of hormone. Surgical removal of the thyroid gland, with post-operative supplementation of thyroid hormone, is often used to treat this disorder.

As an alternative, cancer therapy utilizing radioactive iodine, which targets the thyroid gland and kills off malignant cells, is a newer approach to treatment. Other chemotherapy drugs have been employed, yet most give only temporary results, and can be associated with many unpleasant side-effects.

HYPERADRENOCORTICISM (CUSHING'S DISEASE)

Cushing's Disease is characterized by an overabundance of glucocorticosteroids circulating within the body. It is extremely rare in felines. When it does occur, increases in appetite, water consumption, and urinations usually result. In addition, the typical thinning of the skin, hair loss, and pot-bellied appearance seen in dogs with Cushing's disease can be seen in cats as well.

For more information on Cushing's Disease and its treatment, see chapter 18.

HYPOADRENOCORTICISM (ADDISON'S DISEASE)

Like Cushing's Disease, hypoadrenocorticism is rare in cats. Instead of being caused by too many corticosteroids circulating within the body, this disease is caused by the exact opposite: inadequate amounts of circulating corticosteroids. If this disease occurs in cats, it is usually the result of administration of drugs that suppress the immune system, such as synthetic corticosteroids or progestin compounds.

Diagnosis and treatment of hypoadrenocorticism in cats is essentially the same as that for dogs. For more information, see chapter 18.

DIABETES MELLITUS

Diabetes mellitus is an endocrine condition in cats caused by a deficiency in the hormone called *insulin*, which is normally created by the pancreas. Insulin is responsible for regulating the uptake of blood sugar, or glucose, into cells and tissues of the body for use as energy. Deficiencies in this hormone in cats are usually caused by a condition known as *pancreatic amyloidosis*, which destroys the tissue responsible for insulin production. Prolonged drug therapy with corticosteroids and progestins has also been implicated in causing feline diabetes. Finally, obesity is known to decrease the body's responsiveness to insulin and can promote high blood glucose levels.

When a deficiency in insulin does occur, this transfer of glucose from the bloodstream to the tissues does not occur; hence, blood glucose levels become elevated. At the same time, the cells, tissues, and organs of the body don't receive the proper nutrition needed to maintain their function, and start to look for other sources of energy in the body, namely proteins and fats. And this is where the problems start.

Symptoms

Cats with this disease will exhibit an increase in water consumption and, consequently, urinations. As the body calls on these alternate sources of energy, pronounced weight loss results as well. In addition, as bodily fat stores are called upon and metabolized for energy, an excess of ketone bodies, by-products of fatty breakdown, accumulate within the body. In large amounts, these ketone bodies have the ability to damage the liver and to depress the nervous system, leading to unusual stances and postures, depression, and coma.

Diabetic cats have a decreased resistance to infection; as a result, they often suffer from chronic skin and bladder infections. Damage to small capillaries within the body caused by diabetes mellitus can lead to secondary kidney disease, blindness, and gangrene of the skin and extremities.

The clinical signs associated with diabetes mellitus are similar to diseases such as Cushing's disease and kidney disease; therefore, a thorough laboratory workup is needed to ensure a correct diagnosis. Blood tests on cats with diabetes mellitus will consistently reveal elevated glucose levels, and evaluation of urine samples will reveal the same. Such findings, along with the ruling-out of other potential causes of the clinical signs, can lead to a definitive diagnosis of diabetes mellitus.

Diabetes mellitus can be classified as uncomplicated or complicated. Uncomplicated cases exhibit mild to moderate signs of the disease, yet none are truly life-threatening. In contrast, cats diagnosed with the disease and exhibiting marked depression, vomiting, diarrhea, heavy breathing, and/or severe weight loss should all be considered complicated cases. These cases should always be considered medical emergencies. In most of these cases, the high levels of ketone acids produced as a result of increased fat metabolism lower the pH of the blood significantly enough to cause the harmful effects represented by the clinical signs. These cats usually become severely dehydrated at the same time.

Treatment

Treatment consists of immediate hospitalization with intravenous infusion of replacement fluids, medications designed to increase the pH of the blood (if the pH is too low), and insulin. The insulin is either given as a large bolus or as a continuous drip in the replacement fluids. Regardless of how it is administered, the levels of insulin given and corresponding blood glucose must be monitored closely, since too much insulin is even worse than not enough. If excess insulin is given, the pet could quickly become hypoglycemic and go into convulsions. Good monitoring and careful planning on the part of the veterinarian will help prevent this.

Often cats are presented with complicated cases of diabetes mellitus because of some underlying disorder adding to the problem. For instance, many of these cats suffer from coexisting disorders such as obesity, kidney disease, and cardiomyopathy. In order to increase the chances of recovery from a complicated case of diabetes mellitus, these disorders must be addressed and treated at the same time.

For those cases of uncomplicated diabetes mellitus exhibiting no immediate life-threatening clinical signs, treatment is aimed at keeping blood glucose levels between 200 mg/dl just prior to insulin administration and 60 mg/dl at the peak of the insulin activity. Because of the danger of insulin shock (*hypoglycemia*) if too much insulin is given, the first few injections should be performed by a veterinarian in a hospital to help establish a proper starting dosage.

Pet owners should realize that there are different types of insulin. The type that should be used for maintaining blood glucose levels in cats is called *PZI insulin*, and it, along with insulin syringes for administration, are available at pharmacies with a prescription. This type of insulin reaches its peak action after administration in 14 to 20 hours and can last up to 36 hours total.

At-home care for diabetic cats

When a pet finally comes home, it will be the owner's job to ensure that a proper dose is given each day and that adjustments are made in the dosage if necessary. This is done by monitoring urine glucose levels using special test strips available from pharmacies.

Obviously, this requires the collection of urine each morning, which can get tricky with cats. Special, nonabsorptive litters are available which will allow capture of such a sample. Alternatively, styrofoam packing noodles can be used in the litter box to achieve the same objective.

The test strips used will represent urine glucose levels as either a percentage or as a number followed by a +. For example, each morning, a urine sample should be obtained and a urine glucose strip be run. Ideally, the strip should read 1 + ($^1/4$ %)to trace ($^1/10$%) just prior to the administration of the day's insulin. If it indeed does read this, then the same dose of insulin that was given the day before should be administered again. If the urine glucose strip reads **negative**, then the dosage of insulin used must be cut back. Along the same lines, if the reading is greater than 1 + ($^1/4$%) then the insulin dosage must be increased accordingly. The following is an insulin dosing schedule that should be used to help establish and maintain a proper insulin dose for a diabetic pet. All injections should be given under the skin in the neck or shoulder regions.

If the morning urine glucose levels are at **3 + − 4 +** (1-2%) *increase* the previous day's insulin dosage by *1 unit* and administer.

If the morning urine glucose levels are at **2 +** ($^1/2$%), then *increase* the previous day's insulin dosage by $^1/2$ unit and administer.

If the morning urine glucose levels are at 1 + ($^1/4$%) or trace ($^1/10$%), then give the *same* dose of insulin as was given the previous day.

If the morning urine glucose level is **negative**, then *decrease* the previous day's insulin dosage by *2 units* and administer.

Keep in mind that it is better to give too little insulin than to give too much. Adjustments to insulin dosages need to be made slowly and carefully in these uncomplicated cases. Giving too much insulin can cause insulin shock (hypoglycemia), which can be fatal. Signs of this can include trembling, weakness, incoordination, and, if it is not rapidly corrected, seizures. Owners of diabetic pets should always keep a bottle of corn syrup or honey around in case of insulin shock. Two tablespoons or more given orally should be used if such a reaction is suspected. If relief is not obtained within 10 minutes, contact the veterinarian.

Owners must keep accurate records each day as to their pet's morning urine glucose levels, insulin dosage, overall attitude and/or clinical signs that day, and appetite. These will not only come in useful in regulating insulin levels, but such records can provide a veterinarian with valuable information should a question or problem ever arise.

Strict feeding schedules for cats with diabetes mellitus must be followed. Rations high in fiber and protein with restricted fat and carbohydrates are ideal for maintaining the diabetic cat because they can help lower blood glucose levels and insulin requirements. They are also useful in preventing obesity, which can perpetuate the diabetes.

A veterinarian can assist in the calculation of a total daily ration to feed a diabetic pet. One-fourth of this calculated ration should be fed at the time the insulin injection is given; the rest of the ration should be offered 12 hours later. Owners must remain consistent in feeding practices and avoid between-meal snacks.

If you have any questions regarding dosage regulations, clinical signs seen, or any abnormalities you note in your records, don't hesitate to contact your veterinarian at once.

BIRDS

JUST A FEW SHORT YEARS ago, when one thought of a house pet, a dog or cat came to mind. Not so anymore. As a substitute for these furry companion animals, birds are ever increasing in popularity. In fact, the pet bird population in the United States now exceeds 12 million and is growing every year.

Birds certainly have their place in history, where they undoubtedly served as an important food source for early man. As man's appreciation for their beauty and unique personalities grew, birds were eventually tamed as pets and, in the case of raptors, as hunters in the households of Egyptian, Grecian, and Roman elite. Ever since Christopher Columbus introduced the first parrot into European community from one of his many voyages to the New World, their popularity as companions has been on the increase.

What accounts for this new-found popularity of birds as pets in our day and age? For starters, they are fascinating creatures to be around. Most people fail to realize how much personality and affection a pet bird is capable of exhibiting toward its owner. Any bird fancier will be able to verify this fact. And when was the last time you've carried on a conversation with your dog, and it has talked back to you!

A second reason sparking the popularity of birds as pets is the increase in the number of people who live in apartments and condominiums. Space and lease restrictions against dogs and cats in many of these locations have left potential pet owners seeking options, with a pet bird being one of them.

Many books and articles promote the virtue of birds as being fairly maintenance-free pets. Granted, maintaining a pair of finches might not require much expenditure of energy on your part, but keep in mind that husbandry for the average pet bird requires just as much—if not more—effort as for cats and dogs. For instance, cleanliness is a key word in bird husbandry, and daily attention to it must be given. Also, many birds, such as cockatoos and hand-raised birds, require a definite daily time commitment to satisfy their need for interaction with their owners. Failure to do so can lead to great emotional stress, upsetting behavioral problems, and even disease.

The bottom line is this: Don't purchase a bird with the idea of low maintenance in mind. Like a dog or a cat, it will require both time and effort on your part to ensure that your relationship with your bird is a happy and healthy one.

37

Choosing the Right Bird for You

WHEN PURCHASING or selecting a bird, there are a number of factors to consider. The first obviously is what variety of bird you want. You have many to choose from. Be sure to visit the library or your local bookstore to thoroughly research the variety of bird you are most drawn to prior to becoming an actual owner (FIGS. 37-1 and 37-2).

FACTORS TO CONSIDER

Popular pet birds come from two categories, or families of avians; Psittaciformes (*Psittacines*) and Passeriformes (*Passerines*). One way to differentiate members of the two groups is to observe their feet when at perch. Psittacines—which include budgerigars, cockatiels, cockatoos, parrots, conures, and macaws—will perch on a limb with two toes pointing forward and two pointing backwards. Passerines, on the other hand, perch with three toes pointing forward and one pointing back. Members of the passerine group include finches, canaries, and the soft-billed mynahs.

Budgerigars

Budgerigars, or budgies, are by far the most fancied bird in America, accounting for almost 45% of all pet birds purchased. They are referred to by most people as *parakeets*, yet in reality, the word parakeet pertains to any long-tailed parrot, including budgies, lorikeets, rosellas, and those birds belonging to the genus *Brotogeris*.

Budgerigars are hardy birds that, for the most part, have a gentle disposition. Their popularity also rests on the fact that they are inexpensive to purchase, require little space, and maintain a relatively low noise level.

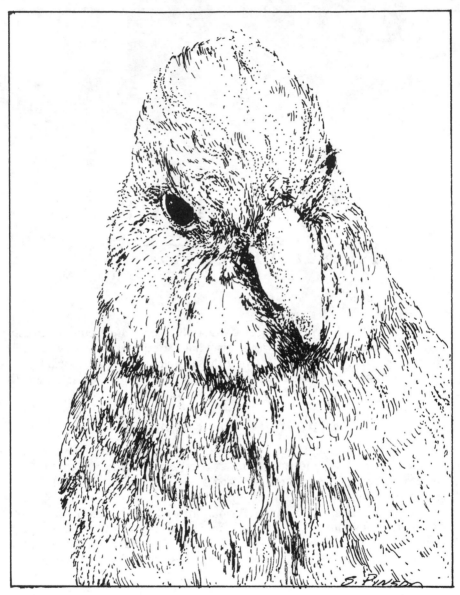

37-1   *Budgerigar.*

Budgerigars have the capability to live 15 to 20 years; unfortunately, because of poor husbandry practices on the part of many budgie owners, many of these birds fail to live past 6 years of age. As far as talking is concerned, budgerigars, especially males, have the ability to learn a broad vocabulary, and can actually vocalize entire phrases and sentences at a time.

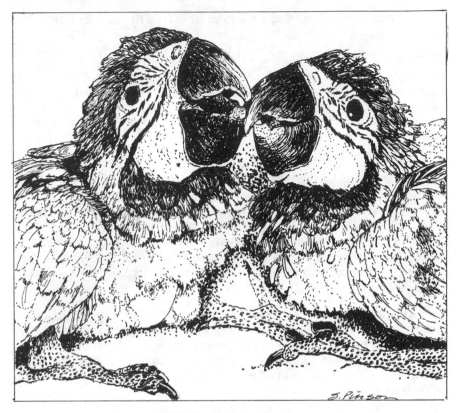

37-2   *Baby macaws.*

Cockatiels

The second most popular companion bird is the cockatiel. In fact, many experts feel that as a first bird for beginners, cockatiels rank among the best. Known for their affection towards their owners and their insatiable curiosity, these birds are relatively easy to maintain and can live as long as 20 years. Compared to budgies, their vocabulary is somewhat limited, yet they, especially males can be taught to talk. In addition, female cockatiels tend to have a more laid back personality than do their male counterparts.

Finches and canaries

Finches are small, lively birds. They make excellent pets, and just watching their busy activity can provide hours of enjoyment. The two most popular finch varieties for beginners include Zebra finches and Society finches. Because of their gregarious nature, finches should be kept in pairs.

Canaries, on the other hand, may be kept as singles and are easier to tame than finches. Another desired feature of canaries is that males have the ability to produce beautiful music and song, much to the delight of their owners. Finches can live anywhere from 6 to 10 years; canaries even longer.

Lovebirds

Lovebirds comprise about 5% of the pet bird population. These dwarf parrots originate from Africa and are tough to tame, requiring regular interaction with people to maintain any established trust between bird and owner. Energetic and active, lovebirds have a life span of 10 to 14 years.

Conures

Conures are a smaller variety of parrot that can make excellent starter-pets for the novice. Most have outgoing pleasant personalities and can be quite affectionate. The Half Moon Conure from Mexico is among the most popular.

Be forewarned however, that these birds like to vocalize and can be quite loud at times, much to the dismay of the neighbors. The average lifespan of a conure is anywhere from 15 to 30 years.

Parrots

The **African Gray Parrot** is the most popular of the larger psittacines. Fancied in ancient Rome for their outgoing personalities and impressive talking abilities, African Grays have proven to be faithful companions of man throughout history. When raised domestically and hand-fed when young, these birds enjoy and actively seek out the attention and affection of their owners.

One unique feature of African Grays is the vocal growl they won't hesitate to exhibit when surprised or stressed. The average lifespan of the African Gray is similar to that of their South American counterparts, 50 to 90 years. Their cost is usually not quite as high as the Amazon parrot, yet many factors, including whether or not the bird was hand-fed and tamed when young can influence purchase prices.

Like their African cousins, **Amazon parrots** are also a popular choice among bird fanciers, primarily due to their ready availability and to their social attraction to humans. They tend to be more expensive than the smaller psittacines and even the African Gray, with hand-fed birds bringing the highest prices.

Because the average life span of African parrots is 50 to 90 years, purchasers of these birds are truly accepting a lifelong responsibility. However, most owners will agree that the companionship and joy that these entertaining talkers offer is well worth the commitment.

Because of the danger of the disease *psittacosis* (see chapter 42) in birds that are illegally smuggled into the United States, potential buyers of Amazon parrots should only buy their pets from reputable sources.

Among the Amazon Parrots family, there are a variety from which to choose. **Yellow-Headed Amazons** are popular talkers, yet are also known for their somewhat temperamental dispositions. The **Blue-**

Fronted Amazon Parrot exhibits talking abilities that rival that of their yellow-headed counterparts.

Lilac-Crowned Amazon Parrots are a common species smuggled into the United States from Mexico. Potential purchasers of Yellow-Headed Amazons, especially from a shady source, should be on the look-out, since the heads of the less expensive Lilac Crowned parrots are sometimes dyed yellow to fool a potential buyer into thinking he is buying a more expensive bird.

Three other parrots from Mexico include the **Red-Headed Amazon**, the **Yellow-Cheeked Amazon**, and the smaller **White-Fronted Amazon**.

Cockatoos are magnificent birds and among the most intelligent and emotional of all the parrot family. Consequently, they tend to demand more social attention from their owners than do other psittacines.

Those who wish to obtain a cockatoo must be ready to devote lots of time to their pet in order to keep it satisfied. Cockatoos that feel neglected can become quite destructive and noisy, and can actually begin feather-picking as a result of emotional stress. However, as current cockatoo owners would agree, the high intelligence level and outgoing personalities of cockatoos rank them among the most entertaining and devoted of all psittacine pets. The average life span of these beautiful birds is 30 to 90 years.

Macaws

Macaws are the largest of the psittacines and among the most beautiful. Highly intelligent birds, they too enjoy interaction with people. Types include Blue and Gold Macaws, Scarlet Macaws, Green Wing Macaws, and Military Macaws. A fifth type, the Hyacinth Macaw, is the largest of all parrots.

Because of their size, macaws do have high space requirements; this factor, along with their high cost and high maintenance requirements, make macaws inappropriate choices for first-time bird owners. The incredible power of this bird's beak can quickly wreak havoc to household furnishings if allowed free access to them. Inexperienced handlers may also learn the hard way that macaws must be approached and handled with gentleness and care.

The loud shrill of these magnificent psittacines and its potential effects on the neighbors is another factor that must be taken into account by prospective buyers of these birds.

"Softbills"

Other types of birds that may be selected as pets include mynahs and toucans, both belonging to a special class of birds known as "softbills." **Mynahs** are probably the most prolific and expert of all talking birds; **toucans**, on the other hand, won't say a word. Both require fruit in their diets, which can make daily clean-up much more arduous than with parrots. **Thrushes** are also another popular type of softbill, especially due to the melodious song they produce.

Aside from cleanup, softbills require less social attention than most conventional psittacines, which can make them excellent choices for those owners who just enjoy having a bird in the house.

Purchase price

Cost of ownership undoubtedly comes into play when deciding which variety of bird to buy. Purchase prices can range from less than $20 for finches and budgies to over $10,000 for some hand-raised, domestic macaws. One can expect to pay more in food, housing, and veterinary care for the larger parrots and macaws, as well—and for a longer period of time.

Also, birds that are domestically hand-raised and hand-fed by breeders when young command higher prices than wilder imports, simply because they generally make tamer, more desirable pets. As a result, beginners especially should plan on paying a little extra for such a bird.

Beware of "special deals" and abnormally low prices advertised for some psittacines. These birds could have undesirable personalities or health problems, which accounts for their low price. In addition, psittacines that are smuggled into the United States can often be purchased at exceptional prices, yet these birds are often quite wild and can be carriers of psittacosis, a disease that can threaten human health as well as that of the bird. As a result, always be knowledgeable of the current price trends for the variety of bird in question, and always purchase your bird from a reputable breeder or pet store.

Time investment

Before you purchase a bird, you should consider how much time you are willing to invest in its care. Realize that acquiring a larger parrot or macaw generally constitutes a lifetime commitment on your part. If you have doubts about taking on such a responsibility, stick to the smaller varieties of birds with shorter life spans, such as budgerigars or cockatiels. Even with these birds, however, realize that you are still making a 10- to 15-year commitment!

The time you need to devote daily to a pet bird tends to increase with the size of the bird, with cockatoos generally leading the list of those requiring the most personal attention. Failure to devote daily attention and time to such birds can lead to many serious behavioral and health problems in the future (FIG. 37-3).

You must also consider if owning a pet bird will restrict or interfere with your ability to travel or go on vacation. This is an important factor that all potential buyers should consider.

Housing requirement

Housing and space requirements should also be figured into your purchase decision. Bird cages need to be roomy enough to provide for safe,

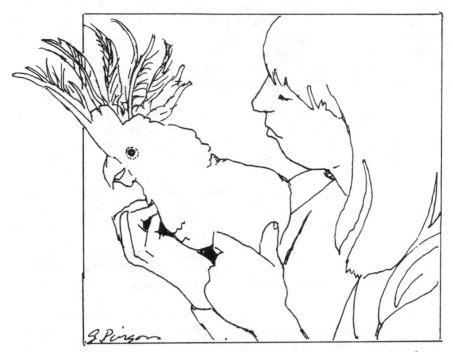

37-3 *Contrary to popular belief, many birds thrive on attention from their owners and could exhibit serious behavioral disorders if they don't receive it.*

adequate movement and exercise within. In addition, realize that most pet birds will require time outside of their cages, which can inevitably lead to abuses within your house or apartment. This is especially true with the larger parrots and macaws. Finally, conures, large parrots, and macaws can be quite noisy, which could pose a problem with your neighbors and your landlord.

Age of the bird

Consider the age of the bird you are going to buy. As a rule, younger birds are more desirable than older ones simply because they are more easily tamed and trained and are less likely to have difficult personality quirks. They are also more likely to develop into good talkers. If possible, purchase budgerigars and cockatiels before they are 3 months of age and larger psittacines before they are 1 year of age.

The eye color of African gray parrots, cockatoos, and macaws can be used as an age estimate. Younger birds tend to have darker eyes which turn grayish around 1 year, and then turn white to yellow around 3 to 4 years. The iris color of Amazon parrots turns from brown in young birds to a red-orange color as the bird matures.

Sex of the bird

The sex of a bird often determines its personality. For example, male psittacines tend to be better talkers than females of the same species, yet the latter are often less aggressive and more content.

Male budgies can be differentiated from females by the color of their ceres, or nostrils, and legs. The male budgie has a blue cere and a bluish hue to his legs; the female will have a tan cere and pinkish legs. Male cockatiels can be identified by yellow and orange markings on the head, in contrast to the grayish coloration of the female. Most cockatoos can be sexed based on the color of their eyes, with females having a red-brown tint to theirs. Male zebra finches can be identified apart from the female by red-orange patches on their cheeks and sides. On the contrary, male and female society finches and canaries are indistinguishable based on color. Male canaries, however, can be identified based on their ability to sing.

As far as conures, macaws, and the larger parrots, methods other than colorations and behavior must be used to determine sex. One of the most common methods used today is fiber-optic endoscopy to surgically sex these birds.

For those potential owners wishing to breed their bird at some point in the future, it is a good idea to have the bird sexed prior to purchase, as part of the pre-purchase screening, just so you can be sure of the sex and reproductive health status of your feathered friend.

TAMING AND TRAINING YOUR PET BIRD

Because of their highly intelligent nature, training a pet bird is not as difficult a task as it might seem. The first hurdle you must overcome, however, is the taming process. If you purchased a bird that was hand-reared, this taming no doubt has already been done for you. Your only job is to make friends with your new companion (FIG. 37-4).

When trying to win your way into your new friend's heart, you should go by way of the stomach! Use food, especially seed or pound cake, to entice your bird out of its cage and onto your hand or arm (FIG. 37-5). If you haven't already done so, get your bird's wings clipped to prevent it from flying away while you are trying to tame it.

Depending upon the previous socialization your bird has received, it might take some time for the bird to become comfortable with you, so be patient. Do this over and over each day. Keeping each session short and positive. Remember: This relationship is based on mutual trust.

Once tamed, birds can be taught to do a variety of tricks using food as reward. Be careful not to be overzealous when rewarding the food portions. You don't want your pet to get fat during the training process!

Talking

As far as talking is concerned, most psittacines have the uncanny ability to mimic what they hear, a skill that is natural and not learned. If you want to

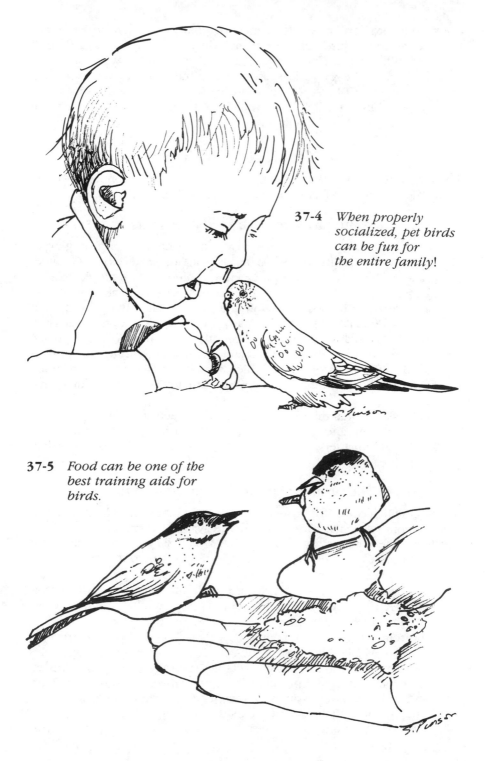

37-4 *When properly socialized, pet birds can be fun for the entire family!*

37-5 *Food can be one of the best training aids for birds.*

teach your bird certain words, names, or phrases, *repetition* is the key. Practice with your bird daily, even rewarding it with food for a desired response. When you are not there, a tape recording of the word or phrase repeated over and over again is an effective training tool you can leave with your bird. Just be sure you don't leave it on during the night, disturbing your bird's rest. With enough repetition and practice, you will soon find your bird talking like a pro!

PROPER NUTRITION

There is no doubt that, aside from good sanitation, nutrition leads the list as the most important factor in keeping pet birds healthy.

The problem with seed-only diets

The most common misconception held among novices regarding avian nutrition is that perching birds can be sustained on seeds alone. Granted, seeds add to the nutritional requirements of birds, yet an all-seed diet is inadequate for birds and will eventually lead to serious health problems.

Seeds are high in fat and carbohydrates, yet relatively low in protein and some essential amino acids. Many obese birds became that way because of too much seed, and consequently, too much fat, in their diets. Seeds alone are also deficient in certain vitamins, including vitamins A, D_3, and B_{12}. The hulls of seeds, which are rich in B vitamins, are often removed prior to consumption, thereby reducing the seed's nutritional value.

As far as essential minerals are concerned, seeds tend to be deficient in iodine, calcium, and other trace minerals, yet high in phosphorus. In birds fed seed-only diets, this high level of phosphorus can lead to musculoskeletal disease.

The proper diet mixture for your bird

Seeds should account for around 60% of your bird's diet. Mixtures suitable for your particular variety of bird are available commercially, or you can formulate your own mixture (TABLE 37-1). Ask your veterinarian for suggestions as to the best type of seeds to blend into your mixture, since this can vary between species of birds. Most bird seed mixtures often contain varying mixtures of canary seed, millet, and oats; sunflower seeds, pumpkin seeds, peanuts, and chili peppers can be added as well, especially for the larger psittacines.

The remaining 40% of your bird's diet should consist of protein sources, such as egg, high-protein dog food, or cheese; green vegetables such as bell peppers; green, leafy vegetables such as spinach, romaine lettuce, broccoli, and alfalfa sprouts; yellow vegetables like squash and carrots; and fruit, including apples, grapes, and bananas. This fruit should constitute no more than 25% of the psittacine diet.

If you don't want the hassle of preparing meals for your pet and wor-

Table 37-1   Seed Mixtures for Pet Birds

Canaries,	35%	Canary seed
Finches.	65%	Millet
Budgerigars.	35%	Canary seed
	60%	Millet
	5%	Hulled oats
Lovebirds,	25%	Canary seed
Cockatiels,	25%	Millet
Conures.	30%	Oats
	20%	Sunflower or safflower seeds
Large		
parrots,	25%	Canary seed
Cockatoos,	25%	Millet
Macaws.	30%	Oats
	20%	Sunflower or safflower seeds
	plus:	
	Peanuts	
	Pumpkin seeds	
	Chili peppers	

rying about seed to non-seed ratios, don't worry; you can substitute complete, nutritionally balanced foods in pellet form. These rations are readily available for most species of birds from your veterinarian or favorite pet store.

Supplements

All birds should also be fed a vitamin supplement containing vitamin D_3, and a mineral supplement that provides calcium to the diet. Cuttlebone, mineral blocks, or crushed oyster shells can be used as sources for calcium. As for vitamin supplements, these are readily available from pet stores and supplies and can be added to food or water.

The finicky eater

What happens if your bird appears to be hooked on seeds and refuses to eat its vegetables? The first thing to remember is that birds can become malnourished due to food refusal when abrupt changes in diet are made. For example, finches, who consume about one-third of their body weight per day, can die within 48 hours if they choose to go on a hunger strike! Since taste and smell are poorly developed in birds, sight recognition plays an important role in food desirability. Your bird might not like what it sees.

Any radical additions or deletions to your bird's diet should take place gradually over a seven to 10 day period.

If you are trying to get your bird to eat vegetables in addition to seeds, start by offering a vegetable mix with no seeds in the mornings, and then offering a small amount of seed in the evenings. Leave this seed in the cage for only a few hours; take it up after that. Keep repeating this exercise, gradually reducing the amount of seeds and increasing the vegetable portions that you are offering.

Another tool that can be used to entice a finicky bird into eating rations other than seeds is pound cake. Most birds will readily accept this tasty treat, which, when used to camouflage or cover up new types of foods, can be used to entice the bird into eating the varied rations. As the bird begins to accept the new rations, gradually reduce the amount of pound cake offered.

Pound cake is also useful as a vehicle for giving oral medications to birds.

Other nutritional requirements

For seed-eating birds, access to grit in another nutritional requirement. Grit does its work in the bird's gizzard, helping to crush and grind food, making it acceptable for digestion. Not much is needed for this purpose: only a few pieces over a week's time. Allowing access to too much grit at one time can actually cause serious health problems, especially in sick birds.

Twigs from apple, maple, oak, elm, or cherry trees should be offered to pet birds. Chewing on these will not only help keep their beaks in fine shape, but these also can add essential trace minerals to the diet.

Finally, fresh water should be offered at all times. Smaller birds consume anywhere from a teaspoon to tablespoon of water per day; larger birds up to 1 ounce (30 ml) per day. Filtered or purified water is ideal, and considering the small amount of water the average bird drinks in one day, it is relatively inexpensive.

HOUSING YOUR PET BIRD
Cages

The cage you select for your bird should be large enough that your bird will be able to fully extend its wings and will be able to perch without tail feathers touching the sides of the cage (FIG. 37-6). The larger the cage the better, for a large cage will allow your bird more opportunity for exercise (FIG. 37-7). In addition, many experts recommend bird cages with flat tops versus those with domed tops, since the latter has been implicated in toe and beak injuries from those regions on top where the metal bars converge.

If you plan to use an antique cage or a custom-made one, be certain there is no chance of exposure to lead-base paint and/or solder that might have been used in its construction.

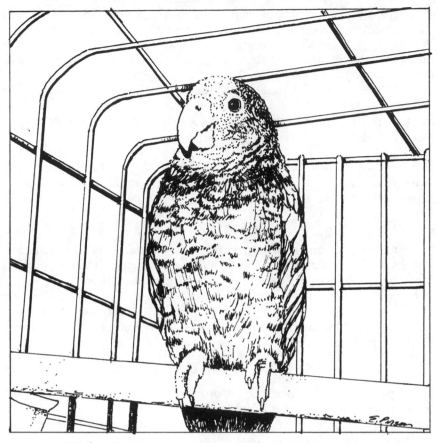

37-6   *The larger the cage, the better for your bird.*

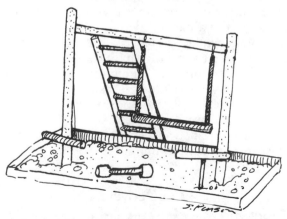

37-7   *When selecting toys for your pet, make sure they are suitable for the type of bird you own.*

Regardless of the type of cage you choose, be sure the metal bars of the cage are not spaced too wide that they predispose your pet to escape or—worse yet—to injury if it attempts to squeeze through. For smaller birds, this usually means a spacing no greater than 7/16 inch; for larger parrots, no greater than 1 inch.

For safety, the door leading into the cage should open out from the cage, not slide up and down. Also, if the door has a spring action, removing the spring and allowing the door to swing freely is another way to avoid accidents.

Finally, be sure that the cage you choose is constructed in such a way that it is easy to clean. Having to clean an entire cage through the small entry door can be difficult and tedious and is more likely to lead to neglect.

Cage lining

Paper towels or commercial cage pads can be used as covering for the bottom of the cage. Newspaper should not be used, since the news ink, if ingested, can be harmful to the bird. This lining should be cleaned daily to ensure good sanitation. However, always take note of the number and characteristics of the droppings on the liner before throwing it away. As will be pointed out later, these droppings can be useful indicators of subtle or unapparent disease (see chapter 41).

Perches

Every pet bird needs a perch to sit on, and choosing the right type will help prevent foot problems from developing later on. Ideally, more than one perch should be provided, each of a different diameter and hardness to provide variety for the bird's feet.

The best perches you can offer are simple tree branches. Be sure to wash, disinfect, and dry these before placing in the cage. Perches shaped like tree branches and made of nontoxic plastic are also available commercially. If you plan to use a painted perch, make certain that a lead-free paint was used. Avoid perches designed with a sandpaper covering (supposedly designed to keep the nails in shape) or those covered with ridges. These are hard on the feet, and can lead to foot problems, including bumblefoot (see chapter 42, Bacterial Infections).

For sanitary purposes, be sure to position the perches within the cage away from the food and water dishes. Like anything else, perches will need to be periodically cleaned and sanitized when they get dirty. Be sure to keep a few spares on hand to minimize the time you must spend on cage cleaning.

Cage covers

Pet birds need at least 12 hours of darkness per day in which to rest and sleep. As a result, a cage cover will be needed to help ensure that your bird gets the beauty sleep it needs. For greatest effectiveness, be sure the cover itself is made out of a dark fabric.

One word of caution: Be sure your bird is at perch before putting on the cage cover. If it is not, it could have difficulty finding the perch in the dark—many a bird has suffered injuries trying to do so.

Toys and accessories

When purchasing toys and accessories to place in the cage for your bird, select only those that are suitable for your variety of feathered pet (FIG. 37-10). Glass mirrors are not recommended for any bird, especially large ones. In addition, watch out for lead weights contained in some of these toys for birds. These can be an innocent source of lead poisoning. Finally, food and water dishes should be constructed durably and be easily accessible to the bird.

Sanitation

Apart from good nutrition, the cornerstone of bird husbandry is sanitation. Cages should be thoroughly cleaned from top to bottom and perches cleaned and rotated at least once a week. Food dishes and water dishes should be cleaned and disinfected on a daily basis. Toys should also be either cleaned or rotated on a daily basis.

Use nontoxic soap and water for cleaning, and apply a disinfectant. Quaternary ammonium disinfectants, available from most cleaning-supply stores, work well for this purpose. Mixing 2 teaspoons of the full-strength disinfectant into 1 gallon of water should give you the desired dilution to use when cleaning. You can use household bleach, diluted 1 tsp per gallon of water, as an alternative. Once you have applied the disinfectant, rinse well with tap water.

38

Basic Husbandry Techniques

BIRD FANCIERS SHOULD acquaint themselves with certain maintenance procedures that will help keep birds looking and feeling healthy. Four such procedures include nail trimming, wing clipping, beak care, and bathing. Before introducing these in more detail, the subject of restraint must be addressed.

RESTRAINT

When it comes to physical restraint of a bird, the ultimate goal is to cause the least amount of stress to your bird as possible. As a result, knowing how to properly—and gently—restrain your bird is a must!

There are three important principles with regards to bird restraint that owners must be aware of. First, birds have no muscular diaphragm to help them breathe, so they rely on active movements of the ribcage to draw and expel air to and from the lungs. Grasping a bird too tightly can severely restrict its breathing ability, and could lead to death through suffocation.

Secondly, birds, especially overweight budgerigars, can experience a phenomenon known as *cardiac racing* if they are extremely stressed or frightened. The heart rate in these birds increases to such a high rate that the heart itself can't pump blood properly, and death can result. As a result, certain measures should be taken to ease excitement as much as possible.

Finally, birds that are exhibiting signs of illness are not good candidates for any kind of restraint except for treatment by a veterinarian. These birds are already maximally stressed, and could succumb to even the slightest anxiety.

Proper procedure for restraint

Before reaching into a cage or carrier to capture a bird, be sure that all toys, perches, and bowls have been previously removed as to not impede your efforts. Also, make certain all doors and windows in the room are closed. For smaller birds, dimming the room lights can help immensely in their capture, since most are reluctant to fly in the dark.

Always camouflage your hand when capturing a bird to prevent it from becoming hand-shy in the future. A towel or a pair of gloves—the latter of which come in handy at protecting against the sharp beaks and nails of the larger psittacines—work just fine. Reach in slowly and intently, waiting until the bird grasps the cage bars with its beak as it tries to avoid your approach. Then grasp the bird's head between your thumb and forefinger. Let the bird chew on the towel if it chooses. Remember: The key to capturing and handling pet birds is to gain control of the head right from the start.

For smaller birds, gently cradle the body with your remaining fingers and the palm of your hand (FIG. 38-1). For larger birds, consider wrapping them up totally in a towel, leaving their head exposed, yet under the control of your hand (FIG. 38-2). Keeping the bird in an upright position will facilitate breathing.

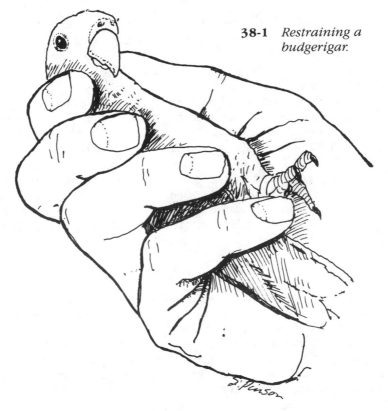

38-1 *Restraining a budgerigar.*

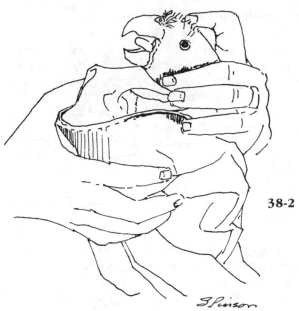

38-2 *A towel can be used to help restrain larger parrots.*

NAIL TRIMMING

The nails of birds should be kept at a proper length, since overgrowth can lead to broken tails, which can lead to significant bleeding. Worse yet, long toenails can get caught up in cages, and could lead to leg or foot injuries resulting from the bird's attempts to free itself.

You can trim the nails of a bird with a pair of dog or cat toenail clippers. For smaller birds, use a set of human nail trimmers. Before performing this procedure, always have clotting powder on hand in case you cut a nail too short. This is readily available from your veterinarian or favorite pet supply.

Simply capture and restrain the bird, then snip off the sharp ends to the nails (FIGS. 38-3 and 38-4). If one or more of the nails starts to bleed, apply clotting powder to the ends. Keep the bird restrained for a minute or two before putting it back in its cage to be certain the bleeding has stopped.

BEAK CARE

Birds usually keep their beaks in shape through normal eating habits and by chewing on soft woods and toys within their cages. The absence of such items within the cage, as well as injuries, various diseases, and poor nutrition, can all lead to uneven beak wear or overgrowth. Budgerigars seem to be the pet birds most in need of periodic beak trims (FIG. 38-5).

For minor overgrowths on smaller birds, use a pair of jeweler snips to trim off any excess portions, followed up with an emery board or finger-

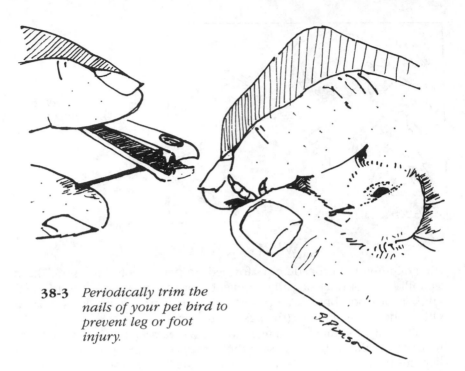

38-3 *Periodically trim the nails of your pet bird to prevent leg or foot injury.*

nail file to file down and shape the beak. Go slow and cautiously. Trim down only what is needed. If the beak starts bleeding, apply direct pressure to the end, followed by clotting powder. Apply the powder with a cotton swab, keeping it out of the mouth.

For severe overgrowth or if the bird is exhibiting signs of disease, don't attempt to trim the beak yourself. Enlist the help of your veterinarian.

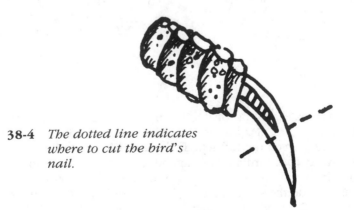

38-4 *The dotted line indicates where to cut the bird's nail.*

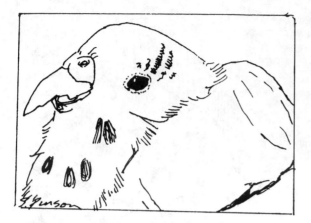

38-5 *Overgrown beak in a budgie.*

WING CLIPPING

Wing clipping is a procedure performed on pet birds to limit their flight capabilities. Not only does this prevent inadvertent escape out an open window or door, but it also protects the birds from hazards associated with flight within a house (such as ceiling fans).

The only instrument you need to clip wings is a pair of scissors. Starting from the tip of the wing, skip the first two or three primary feathers, then cut the remaining primaries down to the level of the covert feathers (FIG. 38-6). Secondary flight feathers may be left intact. Then, with your scissors, clip the very outer edges of the remaining flight feathers to prevent their adherence to one another.

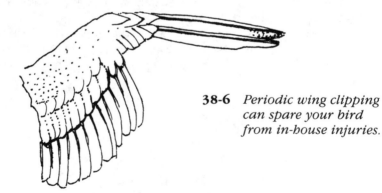

38-6 *Periodic wing clipping can spare your bird from in-house injuries.*

An alternate method of deflighting pet birds is to strip every other flight feather bare, leaving only a shaft. This will effectively eliminate adherence between the feathers, making it difficult to fly.

Evaluate your bird's flight capabilities after the clipping. If it is still able to fly well, consider clipping secondary feathers, too. You might even have to do the same to the opposite wing. In general, the smaller the bird, the harder it is to keep them from flying.

Wing clipping must usually be repeated every 6 to 8 months or so, after a new molt occurs. If clipping is to be performed soon after molting, use caution to avoid the new blood feathers that have come in. If you accidentally clip one of these and it begins to bleed, pluck the feather from its shaft and apply temporary pressure to the follicle to stop the blood flow. A new feather should replace it in 6 to 8 weeks.

BATHING

Most birds enjoy periodic water baths, so be sure to provide them with the opportunity. A shallow bowl filled with water can be placed in the cage for this purpose. Some birds would rather seek out the kitchen sink containing a small amount of water for their bath once allowed out of their cage. Other birds find toilet water attractive, which is fine as long as no detergents or automatic cleaners are present within the water (these can be highly toxic to the unsuspecting bird).

Many owners choose to use a spray bottle filled with water to give their bird a daily mist bath. If you use such a method, be sure the spray bottle you use did not previously contain any chemicals or residues that could harm your bird.

Finally, some birds enjoy showering with their owners. If this is the case, the water and surrounding temperature within the shower should not get too hot; to be safe, leave the bathroom door cracked to allow your bird to exit if the need arises.

39

Avian Anatomy and Physiology

IN ORDER TO BETTER understand the behavior that our pet birds exhibit, and the diseases and disorders that they may become afflicted with, we need to touch on a brief overview of avian anatomy and physiology.

Birds possess some unique features, both externally and internally, that set them apart from the rest of the animal kingdom. For the most part, these variations are geared towards making the bird's primary mode of transportation, flight, easier and more efficient (FIG. 39-1).

THE DIGESTIVE SYSTEM

Birds have a short, efficient digestive system. The beak is actually a lightweight substitute for the mammalian cheek, teeth, and lips. It can be used as an effective weapon; the strength contained in the jaws of the larger parrots and macaws is enormous and can lead to serious injuries if the inexperienced handler is not careful.

The tongue in birds, as in mammals, helps to manipulate food to the back of the throat, where it can enter the esophagus. As food passes down the esophagus, it enters the *crop*. The crop represents an out-pouching of esophagus at the point just before it enters the chest cavity. The crop serves as a temporary storage place for food. Canaries have no crop.

From the crop, food then passes into the *proventriculus,* or *glandular stomach*, and then into the *ventriculus*, or *gizzard*. Within the gizzard, strong muscular contractions, combined with ingested grit, serve to grind up food.

Digesta leaves the ventriculus and enters into the small intestine,

39-1   *Major organs of a bird.*

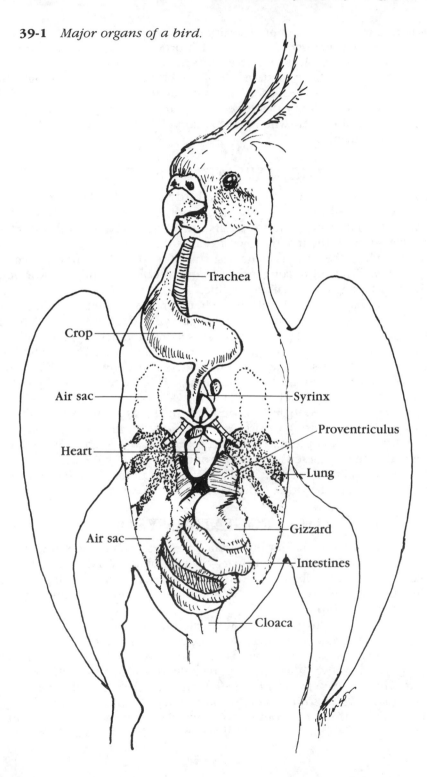

where most of the nutrient absorption takes place. Afterwards, it passes into the large intestine. The terminal portion of the large intestine is termed the *cloaca*. It is here that fecal matter is mixed with urates and urine from the urinary system, all of which then pass out through the external opening of the cloaca, called the *vent*.

As far as accessory digestive organs are concerned, the liver, pancreas, and gallbladder (when present) serve similar functions in birds as they do in mammals.

THE RESPIRATORY SYSTEM

The unique respiratory system of the bird begins with the *nares*, which are two small slits located in the upper portion of the beak. These mark the external entrances into the nasal cavity. The trachea extends from the back portion of the mouth down towards the chest cavity and splits off into two branches as it nears its destination. At this bifurcation is located the *syrinx*. This organ corresponds to our vocal cords and is responsible for a bird's singing and talking abilities.

From the syrinx, tube-like bronchi enter into the lungs. The lungs of birds are unique in that oxygen exchange within the lungs occurs during both inspiration and expiration (it occurs in inspiration only in mammals). Birds have no functional diaphragm that separates the chest and abdominal cavities; as a result, they rely on the active movement of the rib cage for expansion and contraction of the lungs. This is one reason why gentle restraint is a must when handling pet birds.

Finally, attached to and surrounding the lungs are unique structures called *air sacs*. Serving as large storage areas for air during respiratory activity, air sacs contribute to the aerodynamics of flight. Interestingly enough, some of these sacs actually communicate with the insides of certain bones, filling them with air. This is why a fractured bone can lead to inflammation of the air sacs, properly termed *airsacculitis*.

THE UROGENITAL SYSTEM

The kidneys and ureters of birds function in essentially the same way as do mammals. Birds have no urinary bladder, which would only serve to weigh them down in flight. Instead, the ureters empty their contents directly into the cloaca, which, as mentioned previously, communicates to the outside through the vent.

The reproductive system of the male bird, or cock, consists of testicles and associated structures, ductus deferens, and a copulatory apparatus. Female birds, or hens, have two ovaries, yet the left ovary is usually the only one active. When the egg, or *yolk*, is ovulated from the ovary, it enters the *oviduct*. In most birds, the left oviduct is the only one that is functional. Within the oviduct, the *albumin*, or "whites" of the final egg are added to the yolk. From the oviduct, the unfinished egg enters into the uterus. It is within the uterus that the hard shell is added. From here, the egg is transferred through the vagina to the cloaca, and from there is laid through the vent. Females lay eggs in groups known as *clutches*, the size of which depends upon the species involved.

ENDOCRINE, CIRCULATORY, & NERVOUS SYSTEMS

These three organ systems are very similar to those in dogs and cats (see parts I and II). Heart rates in birds can range anywhere from 175 beats per minute for large macaws to over 1,000 beats per minute for small finches and canaries. Birds do have lymphatic channels within their body which serve an immune capacity, yet they lack actual lymph nodes.

THE MUSCULOSKELETAL SYSTEM

As you might guess, the muscles and bones of birds are geared towards efficient flight. The skeleton of the typical bird is very light weight, making flying easier. In fact, some of the bones are actually air-filled, communicating directly with air sacs.

The muscles making up the breast of the bird, which are responsible for wing motion, are not surprisingly the largest and strongest in the body. Wasting of these muscles, which can occur secondary to disease, will cause the large *keel bone* or breast bone to protrude and become easily palpable.

THE INTEGUMENTARY SYSTEM

In contrast to most mammals, the skin of birds is very thin and has little blood supply or nerve innervation. In addition, this skin contains no glands per se, except for a special one located near the base of the tail called the *uropygial gland*. The oils produced by this gland are used by the bird during self-grooming, or *preening*, to lubricate and smooth the feathers (FIG. 39-2). Contrary to popular belief, these oils do not serve a water-proofing function.

The legs and feet of birds are covered in scales, a possible throwback, some feel, to a reptilian ancestry. The beak, which corresponds to teeth, cheeks, and lips seen in dogs and cats, is made up of a tough, horny material. The *cere* is a soft tissue structure located at the top portion of the beak. Often used to sex smaller psittacines, overgrowth of this structure could signify nutritional imbalances or parasitic infestations.

The feathers of birds are not only necessary for flight, but they play an important role in the regulation of body temperature and in courtship displays, as well. In addition, the overall structure and overlap of feathers helps waterproof the bird and protect it from the elements.

Two types of feathers

Contour feathers make up the majority of feathers seen on the head, wings, body, and tail of a bird. The flight feathers are contour feathers,

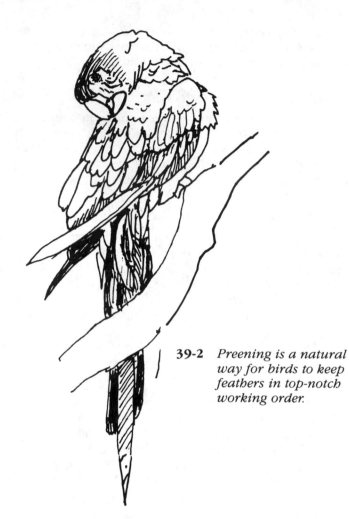

39-2 *Preening is a natural
way for birds to keep
feathers in top-notch
working order.*

and can be further broken down into the *remiges*, which include the primary and secondary flight feathers of the wings, and the *rectrices*, or those flight feathers making up the tail. *Semiplumes* are smaller contour feathers that blend in with the second main type of feathers, the down feathers.

Down feathers are the small, soft feathers found beneath the contour feathers. These serve as effective insulators against environmental temperature fluctuations. In addition, some species, such as cockatiels and cockatoos, have special down feathers called *powder down feathers*. These give off a fine powder that the bird uses when preening.

Molting

Birds go through molting periods in which feathers are lost and then replaced (similar to shedding in dogs and cats). Molting usually occurs seasonally, depending on species. Signs of an impending molt include an increase in preening activity, not to mention the increased number of feathers that will be noted at the bottom of the cage.

The new feathers that grow in after a molt are encased within feather sheaths, which are eventually shed once eruption is complete. These new feathers also have a rich blood supply, which will disappear when the feather reaches its mature length. If a growing feather is accidentally injured and begins to bleed, the entire feather should be plucked from its shaft. This will stop the bleeding, and allow for a new feather to replace the damaged one. On the other hand, mature feathers that are plucked will not be replaced until the next molt.

The molting period for birds is a very stressful one. Otherwise talkative birds might choose to remain silent during this time, and songbirds might stop singing. It is important that you take appropriate husbandry actions to ensure that other stressors are kept to an absolute minimum. Be sure to provide extra privacy and warmth during this time. Also, increasing the protein, fat and calcium in diets offered to birds in molt will help ensure that the molt is a successful one and that the new feathers are bright, shiny, and healthy.

Abnormal molting can result in new feathers that are ragged or incomplete, or that contain abnormal markings or streakings caused by improper feather development (*stress bars*). If you suspect that your bird has had an abnormal molt, contact your veterinarian right away.

VISION AND HEARING
Eyes

The bird's sense of vision is generally sharper and more acute than that of their furry household counterparts. This stands to reason, considering the maneuverability required for flight and the keen visual perception necessary for safe take-offs and landings. For example, the eyesight of birds of prey is so acute that they can pick up even the slightest movements on the ground from hundreds of feet up in the air! Researchers also believe that certain species of birds even have the ability to perceive and differentiate colors in their environment.

Anatomically, the eyes and ocular components of birds and those of cats and dogs are essentially the same (see chapters 15 and 33). There are, however, some unique features of the avian eye worth mentioning.

For starters, the muscles that control eye movement in birds are somewhat small and underdeveloped. As a result, birds must cock, tilt, and turn their heads when trying to focus in on a subject. Next, the iris of the bird eye is also unique in that its size can, at any time, be voluntarily controlled by the bird. This could account for the exceptional visual acuity displayed by birds, especially birds of prey while in flight. Finally, unlike the eyes of other companion animals, birds have small bones situated within the sclera of the eye, giving the bird's eye its characteristic shape.

Ears

The internal structure of the avian ear is also similar to that of dogs and cats, except for lack of ear pinnae and a much shorter ear canal (see chapters 15 and 33). Located just behind and below the eyes, the ears are rarely a source of health problems in birds. However, because of the ear's importance in maintaining balance and equilibrium, infections or injuries can seriously impair a bird's ability to fly and should be suspect in such cases.

40

Avian Reproduction and Breeding

FOR MANY, BREEDING PET birds represents the ultimate in fun and fulfillment when it comes to pet bird ownership. For others, it means a source of income, since offspring from a good breeding pair can demand attractive prices, depending on the species involved. Regardless of motives, breeding birds is not overly difficult if nutrition and husbandry practices are as they should be. Occasionally though, a bird may have trouble reproducing, and the potential causes for such are numerous. These and other breeding considerations are the focus of this chapter.

"SEXING" YOUR BIRD

Certainly the first item on a successful breeding agenda is to be sure you know the sex of your bird(s). This might sound funny, but for many birds, especially the larger psittacines, the sex can't be reliably determined by physical appearance.

Most smaller psittacines, finches, and canaries can be sexed using physical appearances and/or characteristic behavior. For instance, male **budgies** can be differentiated from females by the color of their ceres and their legs. The male budgie has a blue cere and a bluish hue to his legs; the female will have a tan cere and pinkish legs.

Similarly, male **cockatiels** can usually be identified by yellow and orange markings on the head, in contrast to the grayish coloration of the female. **Cockatoos** can often be sexed based on the color of their eyes, with females having a characteristic red-brown tint to theirs. Male **zebra finches** can be identified apart from the female of the species by characteristic red-orange patches on their cheeks and sides.

Not all finches can be differentiated sexually by their coloration. For instance, both male and female society finches look similar. However, behavior can be used to identify male society finches, who will often sing and dance in the presence of a female. The same holds true for male canaries, who can be distinguished by their unprecedented singing ability once spring is in the air.

For larger psittacines such as conures, macaws, African gray parrots, and Amazon parrots, special lab tests and/or surgical procedures are required to accurately determine the sex of these birds. One such test veterinarians can use is called a *fecal steroid analysis*, which tests for sex specific hormones within the bird's feces. This test is non-invasive, easy to perform, and fairly accurate.

Another sexing method that has become quite popular is the use of a fiber-optic endoscope to actually identify and view the reproductive organs within the bird's abdomen. With this method, a bird is placed under light anesthesia and a tiny incision is made in the bird's side into which the endoscope can be inserted. Once inside, the endoscope can reveal the ovaries or testes.

One main advantage endoscopy has over other methods of sexing psittacines is that while the endoscope is inside the abdomen, the veterinarian can also assess the overall health and breeding condition of the bird in question. Endoscopy can be used to detect excessive fat within the abdomen, abnormally developed reproductive organs, and infections— all of which can affect breeding performance. The disadvantage of this procedure, of course, is the risk associated with anesthetics used, although this is generally quite low in the hands of an experienced veterinarian. It is up to the bird owner to weigh the benefits and risks of having an endoscopy performed. It is a good idea for potential bird owners who are purchasing birds specifically for breeding purposes to arrange with the seller to have the procedure performed as part of the pre-purchase exam, if it has not been done so already.

PROPER BREEDING CONDITIONS

Because breeding can place much stress on pet birds, be sure to have your bird examined by a veterinarian before you begin breeding it. Breeding birds that are ill can endanger both their individual health and the collective health of their offspring. Also, because of the stress factors involved, birds should never be bred during a molting period.

The breeding cage and nesting box that you select should be spacious enough for two birds to move around in comfortably. The nesting box should be equipped with a perch or a ledge preceding the entryway into the box. Depending upon the species involved, you will also want to obtain appropriate material to place within the nest contained within the box to help keep the eggs from rolling around and to help absorb moisture and fecal matter. Food and water bowls should be kept spotless as usual, and a water bath should be provided, since many birds enjoy this activity during the incubation and pre-weaning periods.

BREEDING FINCHES AND CANARIES

The mating season for these passerines takes place in the spring. For purposes of introducing a new male to your existing female (or vice versa), a special breeding cage or nest box with a wire or wooden divider separating it into two compartments should be offered. Your local pet store should have such cages on hand. The male should be placed in one side of the cage; the female in the other. Keep the divider in place for seven to 10 days, allowing the two to get to know each other, then remove it to allow the two to interact.

A nest made of wicker or plastic needs to be provided as well (FIG. 40-1). Most pet stores will carry a suitable selection of these. In addition, dried grass, straw, cotton, or a thin blanket are all suitable nesting materials to place within the nest itself. String, thread, or hair should be avoided as nesting material, since these could wrap around a bird's toe, cutting off circulation and leading to toe loss.

40-1 *Breeding nest.*

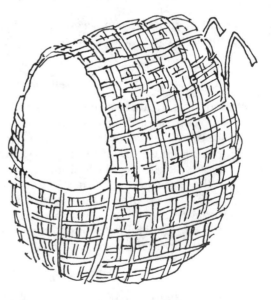

Incubation

Females will usually lay one egg per day over a period of two to seven days. Because it is less stressful and easier on the female to have the eggs in a clutch that all hatch at the same time, owners should carefully remove the first one or two eggs that are laid in the nest and replace them with fake or "dummy" eggs, available at most pet stores. The eggs that are removed should be kept in a cool environment and placed on soft cotton padding to prevent inadvertent damage. Once subsequent eggs are laid, the eggs that were originally removed can then be placed back into the nest to be incubated by the female and hatched. At the same time, you might want to again separate the male from the female to provide her with a more relaxed atmosphere.

The incubation period for the eggs after laying is approximately 14 days, give or take a few. During that time, the female will sit on them to provide the desired temperature for their development. To determine whether or not the eggs are fertile, you can hold them up to a bright light and observe their color. Fertile eggs will appear red within, which corresponds to developing blood vessels in the embryo. Non-fertile eggs will have no such appearance. If you know an egg is nonfertile, you can remove it from the nest and replace it with a dummy egg.

Hatching

Once the incubation period is completed, the eggs will begin to hatch. When this starts to occur, resist the temptation of assisting in the delivery. Mother Nature can do just fine on her own.

Baby finches and canaries are born featherless and unable to see. The eyes should open up after a week; feathering should be completed by week 2. By 4 weeks of age, they are ready to be weaned and leave the nest.

Nutrition

Throughout the incubation period and the pre-weaning period, the female should be kept on a high plane of nutrition in order to reduce stress. Egg biscuit or yolks from hard-boiled eggs provide an excellent source of nutrition for the mother with young, and should be fed twice daily in addition to her regular ration.

Once the eggs hatch, a soft nestling food should be added to the diet to provide the chicks with a source of nutrition. These nestling foods are available commercially, but if you can't find a commercial brand, use white bread dipped in boiled whole milk as a substitute. Keep your bird's food bowl filled with this food, and replace it daily with fresh supplies.

Foster parents

Sometimes, mother finches and canaries abandon their eggs or refuse to feed their young. In these cases, especially in canaries, remove the female from the nest and give the male a chance to rear and feed the young. If this doesn't seem to be working, a foster parent might be necessary. Finch lovers have discovered that society finches make ideal foster parents for such abandoned offspring, and can save you the time and effort associated with hand-raising the young.

BREEDING BUDGERIGARS

The mating season for budgerigars can occur year-round, with the spring being the most favorable time. Birds intended to be bred should be at least 1 year old, showing mature coloration. The female should be introduced into the breeding cage a few days prior to the male to allow her to become comfortable with the surroundings (FIG. 40-2). Males in courtship will try to impress the female by dancing around and bobbing their heads. As the couple becomes more and more comfortable with each other, they will start sharing food and feeding each other.

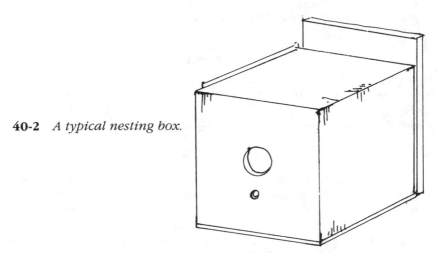

40-2   *A typical nesting box.*

After the two have had a week or two to become acquainted, a nesting box should be placed on the floor of the breeding cage. Within the nesting box, a wooden or plastic bowl or tray can be used as a nest, with a small amount of pine chips or straw used as nesting material.

Incubation

Female budgerigars will lay one egg every other day for a usual total of three to six. The incubation period for the eggs after laying is approximately 2^{1}/2 weeks, with the hen staying within the box the entire time. Once this period is completed, the eggs will begin to hatch.

Hatching

Baby budgerigars, like most birds, are born featherless and blind. The eyes of these chicks open up after a week; feathering should be completed by 4 weeks. By 6 weeks of age, they should be starting to fly and ready to leave the nest. Once they start to fly, young budgies should be separated from the parents and placed in separate cages.

Nutrition

Throughout the incubation period and the pre-weaning period, the female budgerigar should be kept on a high plane of nutrition in order to reduce stress. Egg biscuit or the yolks from hard-boiled eggs provide an excellent source of nutrition for the mother with young, and should be fed twice daily as a supplement to her regular ration.

Female budgies feed their young a special type of milk produced in the proventriculus of the digestive tract. This substance is rich in protein and other nutrients beneficial to the chicks. In addition, the male budgies will usually help in the feeding process as well, transferring partially digested food to the female, who in turn, feeds it to the hungry mouths of her offspring.

Foster parents

For especially large clutches, another budgie to serve as a foster parent can be used to ensure that the chicks are getting the proper attention and nutrition they need. Such foster parents can save you much time and effort, considering the hand-rearing alternative.

BREEDING COCKATIELS

Cockatiels are quite similar to budgerigars as far as reproductive management is concerned. Like budgies, the mating season for cockatiels is year-round, with springtime being optimal. Birds should be at least 2 years of age before attempting to breed. The female cockatiel should be introduced into a breeding cage a few days prior to the male to allow her to become comfortable with the surroundings. As the two become more acquainted with each other over a week's time, a nesting box can be introduced into the cage (FIG. 40-3). Within the nesting box, a wooden or plastic bowl or tray can be used as a nest, with a small amount of pine chips or straw provided as nesting material.

Incubation

Female cockatiels will lay one egg every other day for a total of four to ten eggs. The incubation period for the eggs after laying is approximately $2^{1}/_{2}$ weeks, with the male often taking turns with the female sitting on the eggs. For especially large clutches, eggs can be removed from the nest and placed with foster parents.

Hatching

Once the incubation period is completed, the eggs will begin to hatch. Baby cockatiels are born featherless and blind. The eyes of these chicks open up after a week; feathering should be completed by 4 to 5 weeks. At 6 weeks of age, they should be starting to fly and ready to leave the nest. Once they start to fly, young cockatiels should be separated from the parents and placed in separate cages.

40-3 *Breeding cockatiels.*

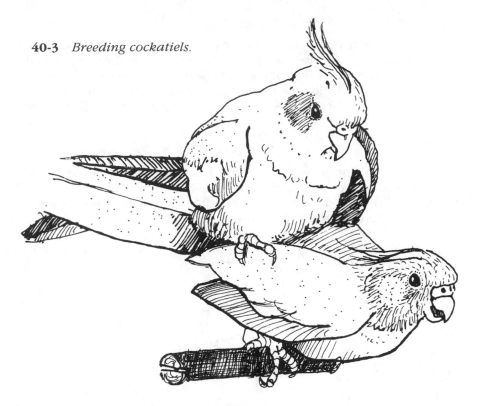

Nutrition

Throughout the incubation period and the preweaning period, the female cockatiels should be kept on a high plane of nutrition in order to reduce stress. Egg biscuit or the yolks from hard-boiled eggs provide an excellent source of nutrition for the mother with young, and should be fed twice daily along with her regular ration.

BREEDING PARROTS

The mating season for parrots such as Amazons and African grays is year-round, with springtime, as usual, being the most optimal time. Birds should be mature when bred, which means at least 2 years of age in smaller parrots and up to 6 years of age or more in larger varieties. The female parrot should be introduced into a breeding cage a few days prior to the male to allow her to become comfortable with her surroundings. The two should become acquainted with each other over a week's time; however, don't expect to see much courtship display by the male. A wooden nesting box with a portion of the floor concave can be introduced into the cage after the introductory period. Hard wood shavings can be offered as nesting material to absorb wastes and to keep eggs from rolling.

Incubation

Parrots will lay one egg every one to two days for a total of two to six eggs. The incubation period for the eggs after laying is on the average four weeks, with the male often taking turns with the female sitting on the eggs. For especially large clutches, eggs can be removed from the nest and placed with foster parents. Believe it or not, budgerigars can fill this role quite well!

Hatching

Once the incubation period is completed, the eggs will begin to hatch. Baby parrots are born featherless and blind. The eyes of these chicks open up in 10 to 14 days; feathering should be completed and weaning occurred by 12 to 14 weeks (FIG. 40-4).

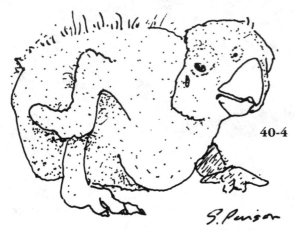

40-4 *Baby parrots receive their full compliment of feathers by 12 weeks of age.*

Nutrition

Throughout the incubation period and the preweaning period, the female parrot should be kept on a high plane of nutrition in order to reduce stress. Egg biscuit or the yolks from hard-boiled eggs provide an excellent source of nutrition for the mother with young, and should be fed twice daily along with her regular ration.

The male parrot will also sometimes assist in the feeding of the young, transferring softened food to the mouth of the female, who in turn, transfers it to the awaiting mouths of her hungry offspring.

REPRODUCTIVE PROBLEMS

As with other pets, birds can have their share of breeding problems. Infertile eggs, eggs with thin shells that crack easily, and fertile eggs that fail to hatch are often the product of poor nutrition and/or environmental conditions. *Egg binding* (see chapter 43) can occur secondary to obesity and other illnesses, or from sheer exhaustion from over-laying.

Improper or lack of mating between two birds can indicate that an overly stressful environment exists, perhaps due to lack of privacy. Occasionally, the personality of each mate might not be compatible with the other, causing them to ignore, or in especially tense cases, fight with each other. Also, in larger psittacines, be sure that each has been properly sexed, since this is not at all an uncommon cause of breeding failures.

41

Preventative Health Care

AS WITH DOGS AND CATS, the best treatment for any disease or injury when it comes to birds is prevention. With disease, this takes on a special importance when you consider that birds hide signs of disease quite effectively, and when evidence of illness does appear, subsequent treatment efforts are often futile. As a result, bird owners can and should play an active role in preventing disease in their pets. Listed below are 10 effective ways to do so:

1. Avoid overcrowding. Housing too many birds in a cage that is too small will not only lead to sanitation problems, but it will also increase the chances of physical trauma and injury.

2. Clean food and water bowls on a daily basis. Look at it this way: Would you like to eat and drink out of dirty dishes day after day?

3. Keep fresh food and water in the bowls at all times. This might mean replacing the food and water more than once a day. Use filtered or purified water if possible.

4. Provide adequate ventilation in and around your bird's living quarters. Environmental temperatures should be kept between 60 and 85 degrees Fahrenheit, and cages should be placed clear of any drafts in the room. If there are smokers in the household, be sure that such smoke is kept away from your bird.

5. Be sure your bird gets adequate amounts of sleep. Keep bedtimes constant and predictable.

6. Feed a well-balanced diet. What more can be said!

7. Prevent access of wild birds to your domesticated ones. It can happen, especially if a pet bird's wings aren't kept clipped. Wild birds can carry transmissible diseases such as avian pox and internal parasites.

8. Quarantine new birds brought into the household for six to eight weeks before introducing them to an existing bird in the house. A new-bird checkup by your veterinarian is also warranted to help detect any diseases or parasitism already present.

9. Minimize other sources of stress as much as possible. Avoid translocating your bird and its cage from place to place unless absolutely necessary. Keep the cage out of drafts, as these can quickly lead to stress and respiratory problems in exposed birds. Also, remember that dogs and cats in the household can place a great deal of stress on some birds; in these instances, it makes sense to bar access of the former to the latter. Also, other sources of stress such as loud noises and blaring music should be kept to a minimum.

10. Vaccines against some of the more common diseases seen in pet birds are being researched and developed, and could soon be in widespread use. For instance, vaccines against avian pox and Pacheco's disease have recently been introduced, and might be effective in preventing the spread of disease within aviaries, or in those instances in which access to wild birds cannot be controlled. Ask your veterinarian for details.

PREVENTING INJURY

Aside from preventing disease in pet birds, there are steps bird owners can take to minimize the chance of injury to their feathered pet within the home environment.

Flying hazards

To begin, to prevent your bird from embarking on an unexpected trip outdoors, get into the habit of keeping doors and windows closed. In addition, place stickers on clear glass doors and windows to help your bird avoid a mid-air collision with the glass.

Wing-clipping should also be performed periodically, including after each molting period, to help limit your bird's ability to fly, thereby reducing the chances of injury from flying about within the house (see chapter 38).

Other hazards that the average house can pose for pet birds include light bulbs, ceiling fans, and hot stove burners or ovens.

Other hazards

Toilet bowl cleaners that are hung within the tank can pose a special hazard to the innocent bird that sees the open toilet lid and decides it's bath time. Noxious fumes emitted from paint, cleaners, cigarettes, and even from the coating of certain cookware (such as Teflon) when heated can quickly overcome a bird if adequate ventilation is not provided. Jewelry and other small metal items may prompt a curious bird into a taste experiment, with unfortunate consequences.

Poisoning

Bird owners must also guard against and eliminate potential sources of lead poisoning in their pets, such as lead-based paint, caulking, ceramic glazing, linoleum, curtain weights, and even excess lead in the water supply caused by lead-lined water pipes.

The clinical signs of lead poisoning can vary, depending upon the amount consumed. General signs include lethargy, vomiting/diarrhea, and increased urinations. Neurologic signs, such as seizures, apparent blindness, tremors, excitability, and lack of coordination, are usually a tip-off to lead poisoning in birds.

Diagnosis can usually be made using radiographic X-rays, and actually seeing the lead particles within the gastrointestinal tract. Prompt therapy using the antidote EDTA can help relieve the clinical signs in these birds. Surgical removal of the remaining lead particles may also be necessary.

Finally, another source of poisoning that many bird owners may not realize exists is ornamental dough, such as that used to make Christmas tree decorations. This dough contains high levels of salt which, if consumed by an unsuspecting bird, can cause rapid dehydration, diarrhea, and neurologic signs in these individuals.

AT-HOME PHYSICAL EXAM

The physical exam is a useful tool that owners can use to assess the overall health of their bird. It can be performed prior to purchase and, thereafter, at periodic intervals, preferably at least four times per year. In addition, your bird should receive a professional check-up by a veterinarian at least twice a year (FIG. 41-1).

At-home or pre-purchase physical exams are easy to do and take little time. Owners should be cautioned, however, that if their pet is showing obvious signs of illness, veterinary attention is warranted at once. Here is the reason why.

In nature, birds have an incredible ability to mask signs of illness to protect them against predators looking for sick and wounded prey upon which to feast. However, such a tendency presents a problem in that birds kept as pets will also exhibit the same type of instinctive behavior, and illnesses might brew for months before a bird owner has any indication that something is wrong. Unfortunately, by the time the sickness overwhelms the bird's ability to mask its signs, subsequent treatment efforts often are unrewarding. Therefore, as an owner of one of these extremely

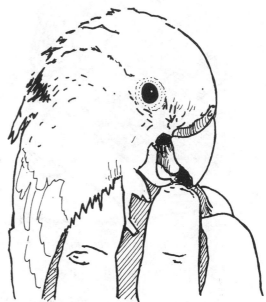

41-1 *Birds, like other pets, should have regular veterinary check-ups.*

stoic creatures, you must be constantly on the look-out for early, subtle clinical signs that can tip you off to an illness in your pet. Performing periodic at-home physical examinations on your bird will assist you in these efforts.

These exams can be and should be performed without physical restraint in the comfort of your bird's own surroundings. This same examination technique can also be used for your pre-purchase screening, and can alert you to any health problems before any cash exchanges hands.

If a particular problem or procedure warrants it, physical restraint might need to be employed on a pet bird (see chapter 38), yet try to avoid it if at all possible (FIG. 41-2). For a closer look, see if your bird won't stay perched on your hand or arm while you perform the exam, or, in the case of a pre-purchase exam, on the seller's arm.

Examine droppings

Every examination should start with a good look at your bird's droppings in the cage. Have they changed in color or consistency?

Normal bird droppings consist of three fractions:

1. A formed fecal fraction, which will appear green if the bird is eating seeds; brown if pellets are consumed
2. A white, creamy urate fraction
3. A liquid urine portion

Again, the consistency and color of the droppings can vary with the

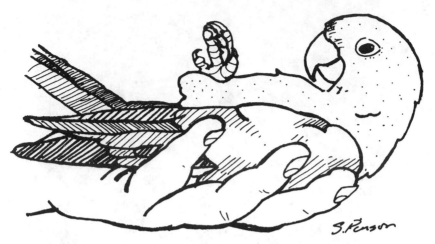

41-2 *Some birds need not be restrained for examinations.*

type of diet the bird is fed, so learn what is normal for your particular bird.

Abnormal droppings are characterized by changes in frequency, volume, color, and consistency. Birds can have anywhere from 20 to 40 droppings per day. A decrease in the frequency of elimination or in the volume of the fecal portion is a good indicator of a decrease in food consumption, which could be secondary to disease and stress. Keep in mind that birds can't go without food for more than two to three days without suffering serious health consequences.

Gastroenteritis usually causes the fecal portion to be liquid, whereas *pancreatic disease* can cause the feces to be bulky and gray in color due to inadequate digestion of food. On the other hand, undigested seed and/ or grit in the feces points to a potential problem in the gizzard region of the digestive tract. Pea-green stools are often seen with *psittacosis* or other serious infections. Finally, overt blood in the feces could signify a tumor or an ulcer.

Changes in the urate and urine fractions of the droppings can also result from underlying disease. Urates having a yellow-green tinge to them often reveal the presence of an underlying disorder of the liver. Also, increases in the amount of urate or urine produced can be caused by, among other things, kidney disease and diabetes mellitus. Finally, lead poisoning is one of the suspects if blood is ever noted in the urine.

Observe your bird

Observe the way your bird carries itself. Does it seem uncomfortable on the perch? Is it shifting its weight back and forth? If so, it could have sore feet or it could be acting restless because of an underlying illness. Are there any signs of lameness? Certainly musculoskeletal injuries and gout are two leading causes of lameness in birds. In addition, internal tumors can cause paralysis in one or both legs, resulting in apparent lameness.

How about your bird's posture—is it normal? Birds that are ill often appear sleepy and exhibit unsteadiness at perch. A decrease in singing or vocalization could also spell problems.

Weight   How is your bird's weight? For small birds, weight can be monitored using a small postal scale or food scale. Excessive weight gain is as undesirable and unhealthy in pet birds as it is in dogs and cats. Obesity tends to be a problem in budgerigars more than other species of birds. What is thought to be weight gain must be differentiated from internal masses or swellings that could cause a similar appearance. Have your veterinarian check it out. On the other hand, apparent weight loss could mean that your bird's appetite is off or it could mean dehydration, both signifying disease.

One key indicator of disease is the status of the large breast muscles. Disease often produces a wasting of these muscles, which results in a protruding keel (breast) bone that is easily palpable.

Eyes   The eyes should be bright and sharp. Look for signs of irritation and/or swelling. Greenish discharges coming from the eyes or crusty material surrounding the eye are good indicators of an eye infection. Clear discharges could indicate an allergy problem or a foreign body in the eye. Cataracts, which are not uncommon in older psittacines, will appear as a cloudy space within the pupil of one or both eyes. Are the eyelids droopy? This could be the result of a former eye infection, especially in cockatiels.

Facial area   The beak, nares, and cere should be smooth and free of growths and discharges. Discharges from the nares could indicate an active *airsacculitis*. Sneezing could be a sign of an early respiratory infection. Does the beak look like it is wearing evenly? How about its length? Overgrown beaks can be a sign of liver disease in birds. A scaly, flaky beak could be infected. The mite *Knemidokoptes* should also be suspected anytime the beak appears crusty and scaly.

Breathing   The breathing effort of a bird should be barely noticeable; also, healthy birds breathe with their mouths closed. Labored respirations with or without open-mouth breathing signify serious respiratory distress. A wheezing or clicking sound is also indicative of respiratory disease in birds, as is tail bobbing when at perch.

Wings and plumage   Observe the wings and plumage. Droopy wings might be injured or held that way due to sheer weakness. The feathers of a healthy bird should appear crisp and bright and should lie smoothly against the body. Ruffled feathers could indicate cool environmental temperatures or worse, illness. Are any feathers missing or broken? Broken tail feathers might mean that your bird's cage is too small. Missing or misshapen feathers can result from an abnormal molt or from feather picking.

Look at the feathers around the vent. Pasting of the feathers with fecal material should alert you to a potential gastrointestinal disorder. At the same time, observe the head feathers and those around the mouth for signs of matting and pasting, an indicator of previous regurgitation and/or vomiting.

Feet and legs   Check the feet and legs for signs of irritation, inflammation, or tissue proliferation. Keep in mind that poor perch selection and maintenance is one of the most common causes of foot problems in pet birds.

Overgrown nails can also adversely affect perching, and can pose a danger to the bird's health if they get caught in the cage. Overgrown nails could also signify underlying liver disease in these birds. Bands kept on the legs of pet birds can cause more harm than good and should be removed if not already done.

If your physical examination reveals any abnormalities, seek the advice of your veterinarian. Avoid further handling of your bird until you get it to your veterinarian, since unwarranted handling could have terminal consequences in the seriously ill bird.

Transport your bird to the veterinary hospital in its cage (very important!). Don't clean the cage before you go; your veterinarian will want to observe the character of your bird's droppings and all toys, food, and medicine that have been offered. However, you should empty water dishes and remove grit and perches from the cage prior to transport. Cover the cage for warmth and to minimize stress. If it's cold outside, warm your car up first before loading cage and bird.

42

Avian Diseases
and Disorders

THIS CHAPTER COVERS some of the more common afflictions seen in pet birds. When compared to dog and cat medicine, avian medicine is a relatively new endeavor for the veterinary profession. However, by using the new research data being generated on a continual basis, veterinary practitioners are learning and applying the knowledge to keep pet birds healthy.

Nonetheless, research still has much more to uncover about the prevention and treatment of disease in these fascinating creatures. For instance, diseases such as Macaw Wasting Disease continue to frustrate researchers and veterinarians searching for a cause at which a specific treatment can be directed. Hopefully, with continued research and persistence, this and other answers will be found to help treat or even eradicate such disease in birds.

Note: Most of the diseases discussed in this chapter will be grouped according to major organ systems affected. However, it is important to note that many of them, especially the infectious diseases, can affect multiple tissues and organs at a time, resulting in a potpourri of clinical signs. For this reason, the infectious diseases form their own section within this chapter and are not listed under the respective organ systems they affect.

RESPIRATORY TRACT DISEASES

Refer to chapter 39 for details regarding the anatomy and physiology of the avian respiratory system.

Respiratory tract disease is undoubtedly the number-one health disorder seen in birds. The causes are numerous, and can include viral, bacterial, and/or fungal etiologies (FIG. 42-1).

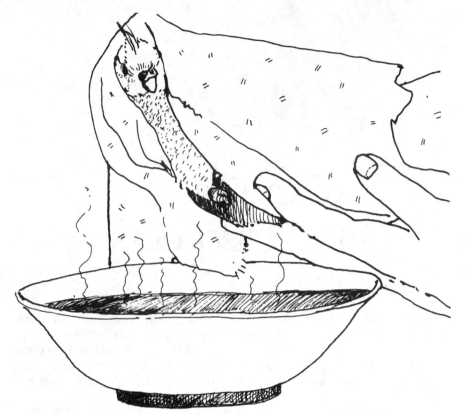

42-1   *One method of humidifying a bird with respiratory disease.*

Symptoms

Regardless of cause, clinical signs that indicate a respiratory problem in a bird include an increased breathing rate, tail-bobbing, labored breathing and abnormal respiratory sounds, nasal or eye discharge, and loss of voice. Other nonspecific signs—such as ruffled feathers, reluctance to fly, and a depressed, sleepy attitude—could also accompany these other signs.

Treatment

If respiratory disease is suspected, rapid diagnosis of the underlying cause and rapid treatment are imperative for a happy ending. Supportive care designed to reduce stress, combined with appropriate antibiotic therapy and, if needed, oxygen therapy are the hallmarks for treating respiratory disease in birds. Antibiotic therapy can be delivered through the process of nebulization to increase its effectiveness. (*Nebulizers* are devices that convert medications into a fine mist that can be inhaled directly into the respiratory tract.)

Aspergillosis

Aspergillosis is caused by a fungal organism that is normally found in the bird's environment. Because of this ubiquitous nature, disease caused by this organism is usually only seen in those birds that become highly stressed because of poor sanitation, nutrition, and overall husbandry.

Symptoms

The disease caused by aspergillosis is primarily respiratory in origin, with infected birds exhibiting clinical signs such as sneezing, nasal discharge, and breathing difficulties. Occasionally, the organism will spread to other organs within the body, leading to a wide variety of clinical signs seen.

Diagnosis of aspergillosis is based on history (i.e., poor husbandry), clinical signs seen, and physical examination. Radiographic X-rays can be used to confirm lung and/or air sac involvement, and cultures of respiratory secretions can help isolate and identify the causative organism.

Treatment

Treatment of aspergillosis is often successful if the disease is caught in its early stages. Antifungal medications can be employed solely or in combination with others to combat such an infection. Certainly a change in nutrition, sanitation, and other husbandry practices are warranted at the same time.

Airsacculitis

Airsacculitis is the term that refers to inflammation and functional impairment of the air sacs. The most frequent culprits causing airsacculitis include infectious diseases (bacteria, fungi, viruses), parasites such as air sac mites, and traumatic rupture of the sacs themselves. Diagnosis can be made using radiographic X-ray findings. Nebulization of antibiotics can be an effective mode of treatment for airsacculitis.

Gapeworms

The gapeworm, *Syngamus trachea* is a parasite that can inhabit the wall of the trachea in finches and canaries. Its nickname is derived from the clinical sign it causes in affected birds, namely an open-mouthed "gape" due to interference with normal air flow down the trachea.

The parasite gains entrance into the body through infected soil or, in some cases, via earthworms and insects harboring the worm larvae. From the gastrointestinal tract, the larvae migrate to the trachea. These migrating larvae can also lead to pneumonia.

A variety of medicines can be used to treat gapeworms. In fact, in larger birds, manual removal of the worms by a veterinarian can often be accomplished. Because of the damage and distress gapeworms cause in birds, early treatment is a must.

DIGESTIVE SYSTEM DISEASES

See chapter 39 for details on the anatomy and physiology of the digestive system in birds.

As far as accessory digestive organs are concerned, the liver, pancreas, and gall bladder (when present) serve similar functions in birds as they do in mammals.

Specific signs of gastrointestinal disease usually include regurgitation, vomiting, diarrhea, and/or weight loss. Some of the more prevalent diseases affecting this system in birds are as follows.

Candidiasis

Candidiasis is not a primary disease syndrome; rather, it is a disease seen secondarily to long-term antibiotic therapy, malnutrition, and overall poor husbandry. This yeast organism causes lesions and ulcers in the mouth, esophagus, crop, or even the proventriculus. A characteristic white film, or plaque, usually covers the ulcerated areas.

Symptoms

Birds afflicted with candidiasis often regurgitate food due to the irritation caused by the lesions. Others may exhibit only non-specific signs of illness, such as depression, ruffled feathers, and decreased appetite. Candidiasis is a serious disease in baby cockatiels, as it can quickly lead to death.

Treatment

Diagnosis of this disease can be made by your veterinarian by identifying the characteristic plaques within the mouth or throat, and by examining swabs taken from the mouth and other affected areas, and demonstrating the yeast organisms under the microscope. Once diagnosed, specific treatment using Nystatin can then be instituted. Correcting deficient husbandry practices is also a must to prevent recurrences.

Sour crop

Diseases affecting the crop invariably lead to one clinical sign common to all birds affected: Regurgitation. One of the more prevalent conditions affecting this region is known as *sour crop*.

Symptoms

Sour crop occurs when the crop becomes inflamed and ulcerated, usually secondary to bacterial or fungal overgrowth within. Spoiled or moldy feed is thought to play a role in the development of this condition. Continual tube feeding can also predispose the crop to infection.

Birds affected with sour crop will regurgitate foul-smelling food that has sat fermenting within the irritated crop.

Treatment

Treatment involves removing the crop contents using a feeding tube, and then repeatedly flushing out the crop using a special mixture:

> baking soda (1 tsp.)
> kaolin and pectin ($^1/_2$ tsp. mixed into 8 oz. of water)

Appropriate therapy for bacterial and/or fungal infection present is also necessary. Resuming feeding in small increments several times a day until the crop heals is also beneficial. Sour crop can be prevented by observing good hygiene when tube-feeding pet birds, by not overfeeding, and by feeding only fresh rations.

Crop and gizzard impaction

Impaction of the crop is another problem that can occur in pet birds. It can result when birds are allowed to gorge themselves on seed or grit, causing a grossly over-distended crop. Impaction can also occur secondary to infections, tumors, foreign bodies, and enlarged thyroid glands, all of which can affect the crop's contractility and ability to empty.

Palpation of the crop region will confirm a diagnosis of impaction. If diagnosed, treatment is aimed at emptying the crop of its contents, and treating any underlying disease condition present. In severe cases, surgical removal of the crop contents, and/or partial removal of the crop itself might become necessary.

Like crop impactions, impactions of the gizzard can be seen in birds that overfeed on grit or seeds. Sick birds have such a tendency to engorge themselves on grit that all grit should be removed from the cage of an ill bird.

Signs of a gizzard impaction include scant, bloody droppings that may have entire, undigested seeds in them. Radiographic X-rays can be used to reveal grit buildup within the gizzard. Surgery might be required to alleviate the impaction.

Macaw wasting disease

Probably the most infamous psittacine diseases affecting the gastrointestinal tract of birds is termed *Macaw Wasting Disease* (MWD). As the name implies, this condition, which is characterized by an abnormal distension of the proventriculus, is seen mostly in macaws, although other psittacines can be affected. The exact cause of this disease syndrome is still unknown, but researchers do know that it is a disorder characterized by poor nerve supply to the proventriculus and other organs, leading to muscular degeneration and weak contractions.

Once signs appear, the course of the disease is usually short. Sick birds will exhibit weight loss and muscle wasting, especially along the breast. Regurgitation can occur as the crop becomes affected, and as other normal digestive processes are disrupted, diarrhea containing undigested seed might be seen. Birds severely afflicted might exhibit incoordination and other nervous system signs. A radiographic X-ray that reveals a distended proventriculus is diagnostic for MWD.

Unfortunately, there is no treatment available. As a supportive measure, these birds should be put on a liquid-type diet to promote normal passage of nutrients through the gastrointestinal tract.

Gastrointestinal parasites

Ascarids

The most prevalent worm seen in the intestinal tract of psittacines is the *roundworm,* or *ascarid.* Affected birds often exhibit signs of unthriftiness, poor growth, weight loss, and sometimes diarrhea. Infestations are picked up in birds through contact with infected fecal material. In some cases, earthworms can act as an intermediate carrier of the parasite.

Diagnosis can be difficult, and repeated examinations of stool specimens under a microscope might be necessary to identify the characteristic eggs. Once diagnosed, treatment using a dewormer is usually effective. Thoroughly steam-cleaning the cage a few days after treatment will help prevent reinfestation originating from the bird's own droppings.

Threadworms

If ascarids are the most common internal parasite, the *Capillaria sp*, or threadworms, are the second most common. These hair-like worms live in the small intestines; in canaries and finches they can inhabit the esophagus and crop as well. Transmitted between birds through contact with infected soil or with earthworms, threadworms cause loss of appetite, weight loss, and profuse diarrhea, often bloody, in affected birds.

Microscopic examination of fluid from the crop or of a stool specimen can lead a veterinarian to a diagnosis of threadworms in a pet bird. Again, treatment for this parasite is similar to that of ascarids.

Other intestinal parasites

Other worms that can affect pet birds include *tapeworms* and *stomach worms*. Both have the ability to cause diarrhea and generalized unthriftiness in affected birds.

Tapeworms can be easily treated with special dewormers once identified in the stools. Stomach worms burrow into the lining of the proventriculus and gizzard, and can actually cause perforations if allowed to persist. As a result, expedient diagnosis and deworming can be lifesaving.

Other intestinal parasites that can adversely affect the health of a pet birds include *flagellates* (*Trichomonas*), *coccidia*, and *giardia*. The giardia organism can cause high mortality rates in baby budgerigars and cockatiels affected with the organism, and has been implicated as the cause of cockatiel feather syndrome.

All three of these parasites can cause pronounced unthriftiness, lethargy, and gastroenteritis. Trichomonas can also infect the throat, causing oral exudates and breathing difficulties (*frounce*). Microscopic examination of a fecal sample can help your veterinarian establish a definite diagnosis, and institute a proper treatment regimen.

Other intestinal diseases

While infectious and parasitic diseases can play a major role in gastrointestinal diseases, **poisonings**, such as lead poisoning or plant toxicity, can also cause their share of intestinal upset, and usually lead to profound diarrhea. A good history combined with microscopic examination of droppings can often reveal the cause of the problem, or at least rule some out. Once a diagnosis has been established, appropriate treatment measures can then be instituted.

Constipation can be a problem in dehydrated birds, overweight birds, or in those that eat too much grit. It can also affect females getting ready to lay eggs, due to pressure placed on the rectum from the maturing egg. Treatment consists of administering mineral oil or adding more fruit to the diet, and correcting any underlying problems.

Prolapse of the cloaca out of the vent can occur secondarily to egg laying and to straining, as seen with persistent diarrhea or constipation. Mild prolapses can often be replaced with minimal effort; more extensive ones might require surgery.

Liver disease

Liver impairment in birds can present itself in a variety of clinical signs, including weight loss, seizures, abdominal enlargement, diarrhea, regurgitation, and blindness. Various infectious diseases, such as psittacosis, Pacheco's Disease, and salmonellosis can all adversely affect the liver. In addition, ingestion of toxic substances can also impair liver function.

Diagnosis of a liver disorder can be made by demonstrating elevated levels of liver enzymes in a blood sample. Treatment is generally aimed at the underlying cause.

NEUROLOGIC DISORDERS

Disorders of the nervous system in birds can manifest themselves in the following clinical signs: Seizures, weakness, paralysis, incoordination and inability to perch, weight loss, vomiting, and abnormal posturing. Conditions that can induce such signs in pet birds include trauma, malnutrition, especially vitamin deficiencies, infectious diseases (such as Pacheco's Disease, psittacosis, Exotic Newcastle Disease), liver disease, proventricular wasting syndrome, parasites, and toxic substances such as lead or insecticides. Budgerigars suffering from tumors of the kidneys or pituitary gland can also exhibit neurological signs.

Seizures caused by epilepsy have been diagnosed in budgerigars and certain Amazon parrots. During an epileptic fit, these birds may fall off their perch, shiver, rock back and forth, and appear to be in a trance-like state. Some birds may even exhibit abnormal aggressive tendencies. Anticonvulsant medications, similar to those used in cats and dogs, can be administered to control such seizures.

Because of the wide possibilities that can be attributed to clinical signs related to the nervous system, proper diagnosis by a veterinarian is essential for establishing an exact cause. Once this has been done, an appropriate treatment, if available, can be formulated.

CARDIOVASCULAR DISEASES

Fortunately, noninfectious diseases affecting the heart are not seen much in pet birds. Certainly older birds can suffer from the wear-and-tear effects of aging, with chronic heart disease being one of them. The two clinical signs seen most in these birds include exercise intolerance and breathing difficulties.

Parasites

Interestingly enough, parasites that inhabit the bloodstream are not at all uncommon in birds. In fact, up to 50% of caged birds might be infested with some type of blood-borne organism! Types include microfilaria, trypanosomes, *Hemoproteus*, *Plasmodium*, and *Leukocytozoon*. Fortunately, most of the blood parasites seen in birds are harmless to their host, except when those birds are ill or highly stressed. In these, blood-borne parasites can cause clinical disease, usually due to anemia or due to impaired blood circulation, and will require specific treatment.

ENDOCRINE MALFUNCTIONS

Endocrine malfunctions resulting in diabetes mellitus, adrenal gland insufficiency, and hypothyroidism have been known to occur in pet birds. Because of the metabolic nature of these disorders, clinical signs associated with these disorders can be quite variable. Diagnosis can be achieved through the use of blood testing within the laboratory.

EYE DISORDERS

Eye disorders can afflict birds of all ages. Traumatic eye injuries resulting from flight injuries, fighting, foreign objects, and burns can disrupt the outer corneal surface of the eye, leading to corneal ulcerations and abrasions. Corneas so affected usually appear cloudy and opaque, with the bird reluctant to keep its eye open. Certainly such a condition can seriously threaten eyesight if not managed with ophthalmic antibiotics and other medications promptly. (See chapter 39 for details regarding the avian eye.)

Conjunctivitis is another source of eye problems in pet birds. Swelling and inflammation of one or both conjunctival membrane with or without discharge of one or both eyes is most often associated with respiratory infections in birds. In addition, cockatiels have been known to suffer from bacterial-induced conjunctivitis, which can cause ocular discharge and swollen, protruding conjunctival membranes. Such infections usually respond to antibiotic eye drops.

Inflammation of the internal structures of the eye, called **uveitis**, can be seen secondary to any generalized disease. If allowed to continue untreated, cataracts in the affected eye(s) could result. A **cataract** is an opacity of the lens within the eye that does not allow light to penetrate to the retina, which would ultimately result in vision loss. Not all cataracts are caused by inflammation or infections; they can be inherited as well, especially in canaries.

The **avian pox virus** has been known to cause serious eye disease in birds so affected. The eyelids of these birds often become scabbed shut, and corneal ulcers, conjunctivitis, and uveitis can result. Manual removal of these scabs can lead to intense scarring around the eyes and lids if the bird survives. Treatment is aimed at combating secondary infection with antibiotic ointments for the eyes, and at preventing the lids from becoming scabbed shut if at all possible using daily warm water washes. Vitamin A supplementation is thought to also be of some help in these birds.

Finally, parasites known as **conjunctival worms** have been known to set up housekeeping within the eyelids and conjunctival sacs of unfortunate cockatoos and macaws. Affected birds are seen constantly rubbing and scratching at the eye. The drug *ivermectin* can be used to get rid of these pesky parasites. However, if not treated promptly, these worms could actually penetrate into the eye itself, making removal all the more difficult and threatening vision in that eye.

EAR PROBLEMS

The ears are rarely a source of health problems in birds. However, because of the ear's importance in maintaining balance and equilibrium, infections or injuries can seriously impair a bird's ability to fly and should be suspect in such cases.

DISORDERS OF THE SKIN AND FEATHERS

Diseases of the skin and feathers are a major concern for most bird owners, not only for the health of their pet, but for cosmetic reasons as well. Disorders involving the integument and feathers are among the most frequent seen by veterinarians and can be among the most challenging to treat. Feather loss and skin involvement might signify a primary disorder, or they might occur incidentally to an unrelated disease process. The goal is to find out which it is!

External parasites

Dogs and cats are not the only ones that can suffer from external parasites; pet birds have their share as well.

Knemidokoptic mange is a skin and feather disease caused by a mite that burrows into the skin and feather follicles. In parrots and other psittacines, these parasites manifest themselves as deformities and overgrowth of the beak, and deformities of the legs, feet, and nails. In fact, severe infestations can actually lead to a sloughing of the toes and nails!

Canaries and finches can also be infested with this parasite, yet their legs and feet are affected more often than their beaks. Lesions caused by this mite have been known to take on a characteristic "honeycomb" appearance. Itching is not a symptom seen with this disease.

Your veterinarian can diagnose this condition by taking skin scrapings of affected skin and examining them under the microscope for the presence of the mange mite. Treatment using appropriate insecticides should be applied to the affected regions every three days for five treatments total, then repeated weekly until the lesions have cleared. The antiparasitic drug ivermectin, given orally or injected, has also been shown to be even more effective in eliminating these mites. During the treatment process, loosened scabs should be removed and the beak, if affected, should be kept trimmed.

Other mites that pester pet birds less frequently include red mites, feather mites, *Myialges*, and *Ornithonsyssus*, the northern mite. The tracheal mite, *Sternostoma tracheacolum*, can inhabit the upper airways of birds and can cause loss of voice and some breathing difficulties. Air sac mites can also cause breathing difficulties and coughing in affected birds; a characteristic "smacking" sound emitted from these birds should tip owners off to a potential problem involving these mites. Ivermectin administered by your veterinarian is the best treatment for these mites as well.

Feather-picking

Feather-picking is one of the most frustrating syndromes that can affect a pet bird. Characterized by a loss of or damage to the feathers from the neck down, the cosmetic effects this has on a prized pet can have devastating effect on the owner as well (FIGS. 42-2 and 42-3). It is important to realize that feather-picking is a sign of some other underlying problem, which must be addressed before the disfiguring habit can be stopped.

Possible causes

Medical illnesses can certainly play a role in the development of feather-picking. Diseases that need to be ruled out as a cause are numerous, and include the following:

○ Endocrine diseases (such as low thyroid levels)
○ Infectious diseases (pox virus, psittacosis)
○ Poor nutrition
○ Food allergies (especially to seeds)

Contrary to popular belief, external parasites such as feather mites are

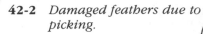

42-2   *Damaged feathers due to picking.*

42-3   *Feather-picking can have devastating effects.*

rarely a cause of feather-picking in pet birds. However, internal parasites such as roundworms and tapeworms can be, and must be ruled out as a cause. Giardia infections have been implicated as a cause of feather-picking in cockatiels and in budgerigars.

Another reason a bird might pick at its feathers is emotional upset and stress. Birds that have moved into a new home or those that are being handled excessively and unwillingly have been known to start feather-picking. Often, a new addition to the family will set off an emotional episode, resulting in feather loss. Finally, if not enough attention is being given to a bird on a daily basis, it might turn to feather-picking to relieve its frustration.

Treatment (underlying cause)

Treatment for feather-picking is directed at the underlying cause. If a medical reason exists, appropriate medications can be used to clear up both problems at the same time. Improved nutrition and husbandry are a must in all instances. In some birds, feather-picking might lead to secondary bacterial infections of the feather follicles; antibiotic therapy might be needed to treat this secondary problem.

Solutions for psychologically induced feather-picking

For those cases that are psychologically induced, there are a number of measures that an owner can take in an attempt to curb their bird's anxiety.

Sometimes moving the cage to a different location with more privacy is all that is necessary to calm an upset bird. Providing a larger cage with lots of safe toys and more room to move around also helps in some instances.

If lack of attention is the suspected cause, the obvious solution is to increase the amount of time you devote to your bird each day. Try leaving a radio or television on while you're not there; just hearing a familiar noise might be enough to emotionally satisfy your bird. If you haven't done so already, get your bird on a regular schedule of feeding, exercise, and sleep. This will help reduce its stress level.

Finally, if you are having difficulties fulfilling your time commitments to your bird, you might want to even go so far as to purchase your bird a feathered companion with which it can play and interact in your absence.

In especially tough feather-picking cases that are psychologically induced, your veterinarian might decide to prescribe tranquilizers for your bird to be given at regular intervals.

Special collars designed to prevent access of the bird to its feathers can also be used to temporarily spare remaining feathers from a similar fate while the underlying problem is being worked on. Please note that these collars should only be used for *temporary* relief and should not be relied upon long-term. Because birds wearing these collars cannot preen themselves, owners must be sure to remove the sheaths from the new feathers as they grow in. Feathers that have been previously traumatized and broken should be pulled to allow the new one to grow in.

Psittacine beak and feather disease

This disease, first seen in cockatoos years ago and then in other parrot species, is thought to be caused by a virus, but the exact agent remains a mystery.

Symptoms

Affected birds suffer from feather loss and concurrent deformities in new feathers attempting to replace those lost. The beaks and nails of these birds are also affected and often chip, split or slough as a result of the disease.

Diagnosis

Diagnosis of psittacine beak and feather disease is made by obtaining biopsy samples and performing microscopic examinations of deformed feathers and affected follicles. Unfortunately, an effective treatment for this disease is not available at this time. Affected birds eventually die as a result of complications associated with this disease.

French molt

Seen in budgerigars and other smaller psittacines, this condition is characterized by the abnormal development or overt absence of tail and flight feathers (FIG. 42-4). The exact cause is unknown, although a genetic viral etiology is suspected. Unfortunately, there is no effective treatment.

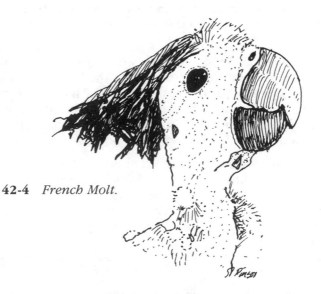

42-4 *French Molt.*

Feather cysts

Feather cysts are characterized by bulging nodules under the skin that contain abnormal feather shafts. Their exact cause is unknown, but they have been shown to be genetic in nature in canaries. Feather cysts must be differentiated from other lumps and bumps that can arise on the skin of a bird, such as abscesses, tumors, and cysts affecting the feather follicles themselves. Once a feather cyst is diagnosed, treatment consists of surgical lancing or removal of the cysts as they occur.

Hormone-induced feather loss

Feather loss can occur secondary to hormonal influences. In male canaries and budgies, a testosterone deficiency can cause such a loss. Accordingly, administration of testosterone hormone for four to six weeks will usually clear up these birds.

Deficiencies in thyroid hormone (*hypothyroidism*) due to iodine deficiencies or inflammation of the thyroid gland can, among other things, lead to feather loss. Treatment consisting of daily administration of a thyroid hormone supplement in the bird's water is usually quite rewarding.

Overgrown beak and cere changes

In a year's time, the beak of a healthy budgerigar should grow 2 to 3 inches; that of a larger psittacine should grow 1 to 1^{1}/2 inches. The normal length of the beak is usually well-maintained by the normal wear and tear placed on the beak from eating habits and from the manipulation of wood and other hard objects in the bird's cage. As a result, when a beak overgrowth occurs, it is usually a sign of an underlying disease problem. Genetic deformities can predispose a bird to beak overgrowth, as can other diseases such as malnutrition, bacterial and fungal infections, trauma, tumors, and liver disease.

Mites The *Knemidokoptes* mite is a common instigator of beak overgrowth in budgerigars. Characteristically, this mite causes proliferation and crusting not only of the beak, but also of the cere, face, neck, and legs (FIG. 42-5). Fortunately, these mites can be treated effectively, solving the overgrowth problem. The drug ivermectin is among the most efficacious at treating Knemidokoptes infestations.

Brown hypertrophy Unexpected changes in the color of the cere can be caused by a condition known as *brown hypertrophy* of the cere. This condition is seen primarily in budgerigars and is characterized by a brown, crusty thickening of the cere region, often becoming unicorn-like in appearance. The exact cause of brown hypertrophy is unknown. Removal of the crusts and application of a skin-softening cream to the region might help cosmetically, but you should count on the condition to reoccur.

Internal tumors Internal tumors can also cause a brownish discoloration of the cere in budgerigars. However, in most of these instances, other clinical signs, such as weight loss, neurological defects, and an apparent abdominal mass will be seen as well.

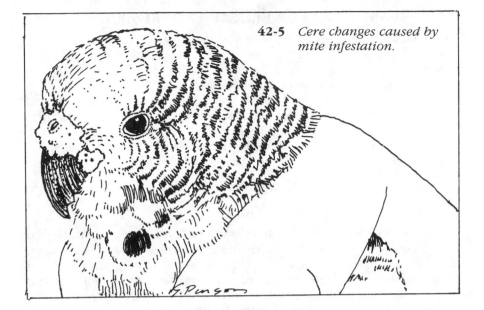

42-5   *Cere changes caused by mite infestation.*

Tumors of the integument

Lipomas and papillomas are the two most common types of tumors affecting the integument of pet birds.

Lipomas are fatty tumors that can appear on the breast, abdomen, wings, and neck of pet birds, especially budgerigars. These tumors can get so large that they interfere with flying, walking, and perching. Hypothyroidism is thought to be one of the predisposing causes of lipomas; diet might also play a role in their development. Feeding white millet on a regular basis has been shown to reduce the size of lipomas in a few select birds. Especially large and encumbering lipomas will need to be surgically removed.

Papillomas are warty-type proliferations that can affect many species of pet birds. The neck, toes, lower beak, and uropygial region are commonly affected. These pink to white growths are often covered with dry, brown crusts that themselves can be easily removed. As far as the papilloma is concerned, surgical removal will afford a cure.

Oiled feathers

We have all seen the devastating effects spilled oil can have on a bird. The harmful effects of such an oil coating are numerous. The bird's insulating mechanisms are lost, and the oral cavity and vent become clogged with oil, creating obvious problems. Oil is also toxic to birds and can quickly lead to organ failure, gout, and dehydration in birds so affected. Many of these birds also show signs of respiratory distress.

See chapter 43 for management of birds exposed to oil and other petroleum products.

MUSCULOSKELETAL DISORDERS

The hallmark of musculoskeletal disease, lameness, can result from a wide variety of illnesses and syndromes. Certainly one prevalent cause of lameness is sore feet due to poor perches. Perches that are too large or are covered with ridges or sandpaper are the biggest culprits.

Nutritional deficiencies, such as vitamin A deficiencies, can also lead to unhealthy skin on the bottom of the feet and, eventually, to lameness. Filthy living conditions and perches can lead to bacterial infections of the feet. Other causes of lameness can include arthritis, gout, Knemidokoptes, tight-fitting leg bands, abdominal and bone tumors, and bone fractures.

Gout

Gout is a condition leading to lameness in pet birds that is characterized by a deposition to uric acid in the tissues and joints. Diets high in protein, dehydration, kidney disease, and vitamin A deficiencies have all been implicated in causing gout. Besides obvious lameness, joint swellings, and flight difficulties, gout can also lead to weight loss, diarrhea, and breathing difficulties as other organs within the body are affected.

Diagnosis of gout is based on clinical signs seen and on laboratory detection of abnormal levels of uric acid within the tissues. Treatment consists of lowering protein levels and increasing vitamin A levels in the diet; providing low, soft perches; and adding allopurinol 10-15 mg/kg daily to the drinking water. Analgesics such as aspirin can be added to the drinking water, too, to reduce the discomfort. Unfortunately, not much can be done with the uric acid deposits that already exist within the tissues; therefore, the overall prognosis is poor.

Broken bones

Broken wings and legs are often the result of trauma from birds flying into sliding glass doors or windows that are not properly marked. Ceiling fans can also claim their share of broken bones in pet birds as well. Obviously, one of the best ways to protect your bird from such injuries is to keep its wings clipped to impair its flying abilities.

Poorly designed cages can also be implicated in many cases of broken bones. Cages that are too small for the bird or those that have narrowly spaced bars or convergences in which a nail or wing could get caught pose the biggest hazards.

Birds with broken wings will droop the affected wing or allow it to drag the ground when walking. If a break is suspected, immobilize the wing by pinning it against the bird's body using gauze wrap or a small towel. Be sure not to wrap it so tightly that you impair your bird's breathing. Transport the bird immediately to the veterinarian.

For leg fractures, a toothpick or pencil can be used as a temporary splint while you transport your bird to the veterinarian.

REPRODUCTIVE DISORDERS

Refer to chapter 39 for information about the workings of the reproductive system in pet birds.

Egg binding

Egg binding is the most prevalent problem seen involving the reproductive organ system. This condition is characterized by failure or inability of a maturing egg to be expelled from the reproductive tract. It occurs more frequently in smaller varieties of birds, such as budgerigars, canaries, and finches. Predisposing factors to egg binding include obesity (especially in budgerigars), exhaustion from repeat layings, and the presence of any underlying disease process. Also, calcium deficiency in the diet can lead to the formation of soft, thin-shelled eggs that can easily become bound.

Symptoms

Clinical signs of egg binding include tail wagging, swaying and unsteadiness while at perch, abdominal swelling, and a penguin-like stance, with the bird resting its weight on its tail with its legs spread apart. Some of these birds might show signs of leg paralysis due to the pressure the egg is placing on the nerve supply to one or both legs.

Diagnosis and treatment

Diagnosis of egg binding can be made using clinical signs, physical examination, and radiographic X-rays. Treatment involves removing the contents of the egg with needle and syringe prior to manual extraction. In some cases, actual surgical removal might be required.

New medical therapy can be instituted to help prevent future egg binding episodes in pet birds. Ask your veterinarian for details.

Tumors

Occasionally birds, especially budgerigars, can suffer from tumors affecting the structures of the reproductive tract. Signs associated with such growths include inability to fly, abdominal enlargement, breathing difficulties, and, characteristically, leg paralysis. Unfortunately, once clinical signs are manifested, surgical treatment is generally unrewarding.

INFECTIOUS DISEASES

Infectious agents account for many of the disease conditions seen in pet birds. These agents can occur as a primary disease entity (such as virus), or they can occur secondary to stress, poor nutrition, or poor sanitation (such as aspergillosis). Regardless of the organism involved, infectious diseases can be quite deadly to pet birds.

Psittacosis

Psittacosis, or *Chlamydiosis*, is a serious disease in birds that must be considered anytime a bird becomes ill. Not only can it become life-threatening if it is left undetected, but it also can pose a health threat to the owner. It is caused by the organism *Chlamydia psittaci*, which is transmitted from bird to bird (and from bird to man) via dried feces and nasal discharges. Birds become directly exposed by ingestion or inhalation of infected particles.

Many birds, especially cockatoos, can become carriers of the disease, not showing any outward signs until stress comes into the picture. Psittacines that are smuggled into the United States from Mexico and other countries without passing through a quarantine station are important sources of this zoonotic disease. Because of this, when purchasing a bird, always do so from a reputable source. If you do, the bird you choose will usually have already been tested for psittacosis, and should pose no health threat to your family.

Effect on humans

Psittacosis has been known to cause severe and sometimes fatal flu-like illness in people. The disease can be transmitted by both exotic birds and pigeons, and can be caught by humans breathing infective aerosols from dried bird droppings.

Symptoms in birds

The history of a bird affected with psittacosis usually involves recent exposure to other birds and to some stressful situation. Many will suffer from chronic, intermittent, low-grade illnesses and fail to fully regain their health.

The clinical signs of psittacosis include depression, muscle wasting, poor feathering, regurgitation, sneezing, nasal and eye discharges, and breathing difficulties. Psittacine birds will usually exhibit a classic sign in particular: Lime-green diarrhea. In addition, the urate portion of the dropping often takes on a yellow hue, signifying liver inflammation within. Heart disease can also occur secondarily to infection with the psittacosis organism.

Your veterinarian can diagnose psittacosis using laboratory tests. Increases in the number of white cells in the blood, evidence of anemia, and elevated liver enzymes in the blood can all point towards psittacosis. Specific diagnostic tests— including fecal cultures, selected antibody screens, and tissue stains—are also useful in pinpointing an exact diagnosis of psittacosis.

Treatment

Treatment of this disease involves the use of tetracycline antibiotics added to the bird's feed or water. Because some tetracyclines work better than others against psittacosis, antibiotics should be administered only under veterinary prescription. Treatment might be necessary for 30 to 45 days or, in some birds, for a lifetime.

During their convalescence, sick birds must be isolated from others to prevent inadvertent transmission of the disease and to reduce stress.

Because of its zoonotic potential, owners should always practice good hygiene when caring for a bird with psittacosis. Cages and utensils should be thoroughly disinfected on a daily basis, using a quaternary ammonium compound or a 1:10 dilution of bleach.

Prevention

Owners can prevent unwelcome surprises by having new birds examined and tested for psittacosis prior to bringing them into the household. This especially holds true for birds whose origins are uncertain. If you have other birds in your household, it is a good idea to keep any new birds away from these existing pets for two to three weeks before introducing it to the others. This will not only protect your existing birds from the threat of psittacosis, but from the threat of other diseases as well.

Exotic Newcastle's Disease (avian distemper)

Exotic Newcastle's Disease (END) has been effectively eradicated from the United States, but it bears mentioning, since not all new birds entering the country pass through quarantine stations like they should. This viral disease is spread by ingestion or inhalation of the infective virus in food, water, or on the hands of a handler. Among the psittacines, cockatoos and cockatiels are especially susceptible to END.

Symptoms

Clinical signs of the disease in affected birds include depression, loss of appetite and weight, breathing difficulties, nasal and eye discharge, diarrhea, and nervous system signs, such as incoordination, weakness, and paralysis.

If END is suspected in a pet bird from history and clinical signs, the United States Department of Agriculture is notified immediately, and the bird is placed in quarantine at a USDA facility. Unfortunately, there is no effective treatment for this disease.

Pox (avian diphtheria)

Avian Pox is a viral disease characterized by severe respiratory and skin disease. Almost all birds can be infected with a pox virus, the most likely candidates being canaries, finches, parrots, and pigeons. Cockatoos and cockatiels are relatively resistant to the disease. Exposure to the pox organism occurs via inhalation or by skin penetration, usually secondary to trauma. Insects, especially mosquitoes, can even spread the disease between susceptible birds. Pox seems to be an especially big problem in exotic bird quarantine stations.

Symptoms

The clinical signs associated with a pox infection include sneezing, breathing difficulties, discharges from the eyes and nose, ulcerated and/ or scabby lesions in the mouth, on the face, or on the extremities. The eyes of affected birds are often inflamed and painful. In severe involvement, death can ensue one to seven days after clinical signs appear.

Treatment

Diagnosis of a pox infection is based on clinical signs seen and microscopic examination of infected tissues and fluids. Unfortunately, not much can be done for treatment. Preventing secondary infections with antibiotics and treating any eye involvement is certainly warranted.

A vaccine that can be used to help protect canaries against the ravages of canary pox has recently been developed. In addition, owners can help reduce chances of transmission by preventing their pets' access to wild birds, by keeping mosquitoes under control, and by quarantining all new birds before introducing them into the household.

Papovavirus infection (budgie fledgling disease)

The *papovavirus* has been implicated as the cause of budgie fledgling disease, a highly fatal syndrome that affects young birds less than 4 weeks of age. The disease is transmitted through contact with infected droppings and other body fluids. Mother-to-egg transfer has also been documented. Fledglings stricken with this disease suffer from a severe gastroenteritis with accompanying diarrhea. Furthermore, the heart, liver, and kidney become additional targets for the virus as well.

Because of the disease's intensity and the lack of an effective treatment, these young birds usually die within one to two days after the onset of signs. Those rare birds that do survive often exhibit stunted growth and feather development.

Pacheco's Disease (inclusion body hepatitis)

Pacheco's Disease is caused by the psittacine herpes virus, which causes severe illness in affected birds. It is seen most often in newly imported and illegally smuggled birds. Transmission between birds occurs through contact with infected feces, usually from contaminated food and water bowls. Some birds can become carriers of this disease, with stress playing an important role in the appearance of clinical signs.

Symptoms

The clinical signs seen with Pacheco's Disease are a consequence of liver, spleen, gastrointestinal, and respiratory involvement. Bright yellow diarrhea, yellow-green urates, vomiting, breathing difficulties, nasal discharges, depression, and a generalized wasting are all signs that can be seen with this disease. Incoordination and head tilting can also occur if the nervous system becomes involved. In especially severe cases, sudden death might occur at any time.

Treatment

Diagnosis of Pacheco's Disease is based on history and clinical signs. Fecal cultures for the herpes virus can be performed as well. Unfortunately however, definitive diagnosis in most instances is made only after the bird has died.

There is currently no effective treatment for Pacheco's Disease, although the effectiveness of the new human antiviral drug *acyclovir* against this agent is being tested in the laboratory.

Prevention

A vaccine aimed at the prevention of Pacheco's disease does now exist and is available through your veterinarian. As with psittacosis, new birds should be quarantined and screened for Pacheco's before introduction into the household.

BACTERIAL INFECTIONS

The bacterial organism *Salmonella typhimurium* and others can cause significant disease in pet birds, particularly those stressed due to poor husbandry and nutrition. Pigeons are an effective carrier of Salmonellosis, yet rarely show any signs of infection. In contrast, pet birds other than pigeons that become infected can suffer from severe clinical signs and syndromes, some of which include depression, diarrhea, breathing difficulties, arthritis, and bone infections. Salmonellosis and other bacterial infections are spread from bird to bird via contact with infected fecal material. Rodents and certain insects such as cockroaches can also play a role in the active spread of some of these diseases.

43

General Treatment of Sick Birds

KEEP IN MIND THAT A SICK BIRD is fragile, and requires lots of attention and care to ensure that a proper recovery takes place. Because of the importance of minimizing stress, many veterinarians encourage convalescence at home in the environment that the bird is most comfortable with. As a result, owners should know how to best care for a sick or injured bird during that all-important recovery period.

CARE OF SICK BIRDS

The cornerstone of any treatment regimen for birds is to reduce stress as much as possible. For starters, this means that handling should be kept to a minimum at all times during the recovery period.

If applicable, remove other birds from the cage. Keeping the cage environment warm—between 80 degrees and 90 degrees Fahrenheit—is essential. A heating pad set on low may be placed beneath the cage (not in the cage!). Be sure a towel or blanket separates the pad from the metal of the cage.

An incandescent light bulb can also be installed to provide extra warmth. Avoid using white bulbs because the bright light they emit will interfere with sleep. Instead, use a 40- to 60-watt green bulb for this purpose. It can provide a source of heat, while at the same time, respect your bird's seclusion.

A cage cover should be used for the convalescing bird to help provide seclusion and warmth. The cover should encompass three-fourths of the cage during the day, and the entire cage at night. It is vital that convalescing birds receive at least 12 hours of undisturbed rest per day.

Since ill birds might overindulge in grit, remove all grit from the cage. Also, lower perches to ease access and to reduce the chances of injury from falling off. Place food and water within the bird's reach.

TUBE FEEDING

If a bird refuses to eat or drink on its own free will, then tube feeding might become necessary. Before doing this, however, try to hand-feed your bird.

Warmed baby food or oatmeal might prove be enticing enough to stimulate an appetite. To encourage drinking, add sugar or honey to the water, and offer it with a dropper or small syringe. This is especially helpful if medications are to be administered in the water. (If you decide to add sugar or honey to the water, be sure to change the water twice a day to prevent bacterial contamination.)

If tube feeding is the only solution, you will need some supplies.

A soft rubber feeding tube and plastic syringe are ideal for the job and can be obtained from your veterinarian. To allow for easier passage if only one pair of hands is available, keep the tube in the freezer between feedings. This will temporarily make the rubber tube more rigid, making it easier to pass down into the crop.

As an alternative, metal feeding tubes can be acquired and used for tube feeding purposes. The main advantage that the metal tube has over the rubber tube is its rigidity. However, a disadvantage is that too much pressure applied to a metal feeding tube during passage could actually damage or perforate the crop. They are also more expensive and not as readily available as rubber ones.

A speculum will be needed to keep the mouth open during the feeding and to prevent the bird from biting off the tubing. For small birds, a paper clip inserted into the mouth horizontally, and then turned vertically, works great. For larger birds, an empty syringe case with a hole big enough for tube passage made in the enclosed end functions as an effective mouth speculum. Again, your veterinarian can provide you with one of these.

Numerous **feeding formulas** are available for tube-feeding birds. A limited number of premixed commercial formulas are available on the market, yet they might be difficult to find. One home-made formula for tube feeding can be blended right at home includes the following:

Dog Food (Adult Formula)	1 Cup
High Protein Baby Cereal	1 Cup
Banana	1
Honey	1 tsp.
Vitamin-Mineral Supplement	1 tsp.

These ingredients should be blended with water to form a slurry that passes easily through the feeding tube. Feedings should be performed every six to eight hours. Consult your veterinarian as to amounts to feed your bird. As a general rule, canaries and budgies should receive $^1/_2$ to $^3/_4$ ml of the formula per feeding; cockatiels—3 ml of formula per feeding; small parrots—5 ml of formula per feeding; medium to large parrots—10 ml of formula per feeding; and macaws—15 ml of formula per feeding.

Refrigerate homemade formulas between feedings, and replace them every two days. Always warm the formula to room temperature and double-check the temperature before feeding; formula that is too hot could burn the esophagus and crop, whereas formula that is too cold could actually cause a detrimental drop in the bird's temperature.

Three steps to tube feeding

The steps involved in tube feeding are as follows:

1. Gently restrain the bird with one hand (see chapter 38); the other hand will control the speculum and the feeding tube. Measure the length of tubing it will take to pass from the bird's mouth to its crop (FIG. 43-1), and mark the stopping point directly on the tube using tape or a permanent ink marker.

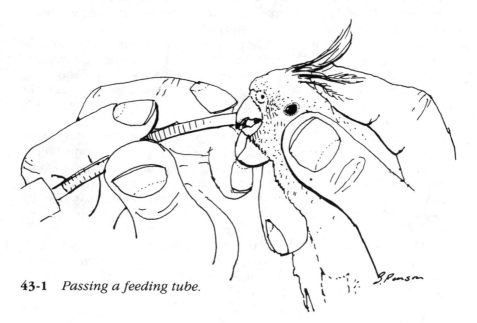

43-1   *Passing a feeding tube.*

2. Attach the feeding syringe filled with the desired amount of formula to the tube, and expel any air present within the tube. With the bird held upright, insert the speculum into its mouth. Pass the feeding tube through the speculum starting from the left side of the bird's mouth and progressing towards the right side of the throat. As you pass the tube, feel for the tube in the throat as it passes down. This will help ensure that the tube is in the correct

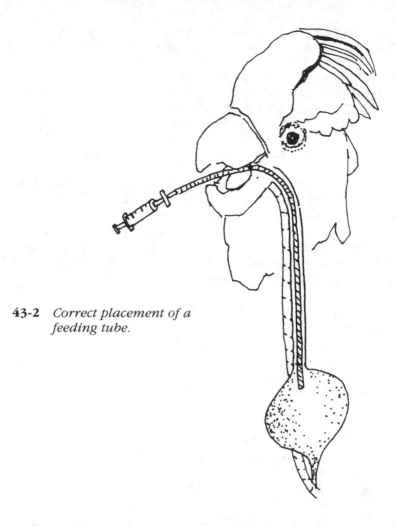

43-2   *Correct placement of a feeding tube.*

place and not in the airways. Insert the tube the premeasured distance (FIG. 43-2).

3. Slowly administer the desired amount of food. Palpate the crop for fullness. Do not overfill. Once finished, withdraw the tube. If the bird regurgitates food at any time during the feeding, withdraw the tube immediately. Be sure to clean and disinfect the equipment after each feeding, and put leftover formula back into the refrigerator.

HAND-RAISING BABY BIRDS

The time might come when you are faced with hand-raising a baby bird. It might be because the mother bird abandons the baby or is abusive towards it. Many bird breeders choose to hand-raise new offspring in order to stimulate the parents to produce more eggs. Finally, birds that are hand-raised as babies are tamer and generally make better pets.

Hand-reared baby birds must be kept warm, and a good way to do this is to either place a heating pad set on low under a portion of the box you are keeping the baby in, or by using a 75-watt light bulb hung overhead. For the first 10 days of the baby bird's life, the environmental temperature should be kept above 96 degrees; afterwards, it can be dropped to about 85 degrees for the next 30 days. Once the bird is feathered, maintaining an environmental temperature of around 75 degrees is ideal.

The floor of the box should be clean and spotless at all times. Paper towels or soft facial tissue can be used as floor covering. Wood shavings are not recommended, since birds might have a tendency to consume the shavings once they start eating on their own.

Feedings need to be performed at regular intervals, depending upon the age of the bird. An eyedropper or syringe, thoroughly cleaned and disinfected between feedings, can be used to deliver the food mixture. The following formula can be used:

Dog Food (High Protein)	1 Cup
Baby Food - including:	
High Protein Cereal	1 Cup
Vegetable (any type)	1 tsp.
Fruit (any type)	1 tsp.
Lowfat Milk (powder)	1/4 Cup

This formula should be blended and, at feeding time, mixed with warm water to form a mixture that can easily be fed using a syringe or dropper. The water used to prepare the feeding formula should not be soft water because high salt contents contained within can be harmful, especially to newborns. Purified or filtered water is the best. Additionally, a vitamin-mineral supplement can be added to the mixture, dosing according to the supplement's label instructions.

When feeding, give just enough to lightly distend the crop; don't overfill! The idea is to have the crop empty itself between feedings; if food sits too long in the crop, it can predispose to infections. If you are finding that the crop is not emptying between feedings, try cutting back on the amount you are feeding, or add more water to the formula. Also, recheck the temperature of the food you are feeding. If the formula is too cold, crop emptying might take longer.

Feed birds 1 to 7 days of age every two hours (feed only once or twice during the night so you do not disturb the bird's overnight rest). When the bird is 7 to 21 days old, feed it every four hours; at 3 to 6 weeks of age, feed three times daily. When the bird is 6 to 8 weeks of age, feed it twice daily. Birds over 8 weeks of age should not require more than one hand-fed meal, given at bedtime. At this age, they will usually start eating on their own without your assistance.

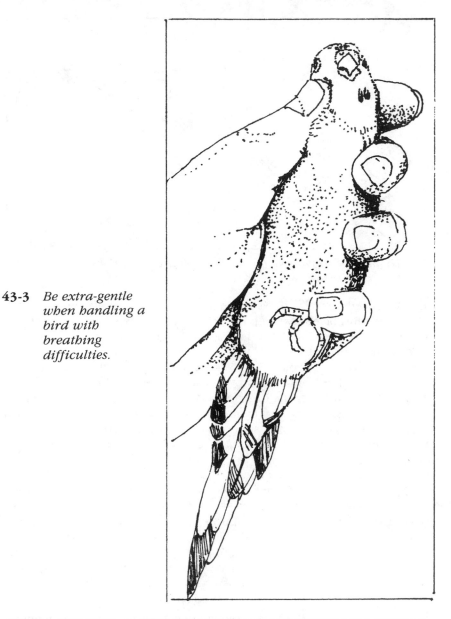

43-3 *Be extra-gentle when handling a bird with breathing difficulties.*

EMERGENCY & FIRST AID PROCEDURES IN BIRDS

Because any degree of injury or illness to a bird could lead to serious complications and even death, bird owners must be prepared in the event of an emergency. The more common situations that might arise include bleeding, broken bones, respiratory distress, and poisonings. As far as first aid is concerned, minor injuries such as bleeding toenails or minor lacerations can be effectively doctored at home. On the other hand, any

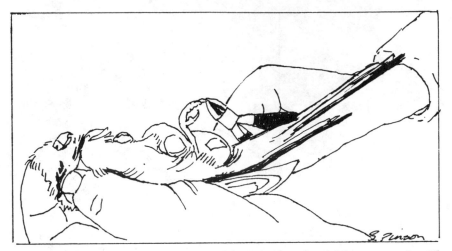

43-4   *Hemorrhage caused by nail trimming should be stopped with direct pressure.*

first aid procedures related to a more serious injury or illness are only palliative, and must be followed up immediately with a visit to a veterinarian. Remember: the life of an injured or ill bird is often fragile and could easily be lost unless prompt action is taken.

Ideally, transport your bird to the veterinary hospital in its original cage. Remove all perches and empty all water containers prior to moving. Also, place a cover over the cage for seclusion and warmth. If the bird is debilitated enough to where it cannot stand or balance, gently wrap it in a towel large enough to prevent spurious movement. Keep the environmental temperatures within the car warm enough to keep stress to a minimum.

Table 43-1   First Aid For Birds

Bleeding (hemorrhage)	Apply direct, firm pressure over the area for a minimum of five minutes using a cloth, towel, or even your hand. Be aware of how you are restraining your pet; don't grasp it so tightly that breathing is impaired (FIG. 43-3).
	After applying pressure for a few minutes, remove the covering and observe for further bleeding. Reapply pressure if necessary or apply a clotting cream or powder (toenails). Do not use clotting powders or creams on other open wounds (FIG. 43-4).

Table 43-1 Continued.

Bleeding (hemorrage) *continued*	Transport your bird to your veterinarian for an examination and additional medications if needed.
Cuts/wounds	Control bleeding.
	Wash the wound thoroughly with warm water only.
	Apply an antibiotic ointment to the wound. If large, cover the wound with a sterile dressing.
	Transport to your veterinarian.
Breathing difficulties/ *nasal discharge*	These two clinical symptoms signify respiratory disease, of which any type can be rapidly fatal if not treated promptly. Do not try to treat respiratory disease at home without first contacting your veterinarian.
Diarrhea/constipation	Bird owners should not attempt to treat diarrhea in pets at home, due to the high probability of infectious disease as being the cause.
	For the constipated bird, add mineral oil or fruit to the diet. If the problem persists for more than two days, veterinary attention is warranted.
Cloacal prolapse	Gently clean the prolapse with warm water and soap, rinsing well.
	Coat and lubricate the prolapsed region with petroleum jelly and attempt to gently push it back in. If it won't go back in easily, discontinue your attempts and let your veterinarian help you.
	Regardless of whether you reduce the prolapse or not, seek veterinary attention. These birds should be placed on antibiotics for a few days to prevent secondary problems.
Egg binding	There is no specific treatment that should be attempted at home. This condition requires immediate veterinary attention.

Table 43-1   Continued.

Oiled birds	Loosely tape the bird's mouth shut to prevent ingestion of the oil.
	Flush the bird's eyes, nose, and mouth to remove any oil present within.
	Using nontoxic mechanic's waterless hand cleanser or mild dishwashing liquid, wash the feathers thoroughly and rinse well. Repeat as necessary. Blot the feathers dry using a towel and take to your veterinarian.
	The environment these birds are placed in as they are recuperating should be warm and dark, minimizing stress as much as possible.
	Tube feed if deemed necessary by your veterinarian.
Poisonings	If the poison was ingested, rush both bird and poison container to your veterinarian as soon as possible.
	If the poison contacts the skin and feathers, rinse the bird well with copious amounts of warm water and blot dry with a towel. Transport to your veterinarian.
Seizures	Wrap the seizuring bird gently in a towel to prevent self-injury.
	Transport immediately to your veterinarian.
Eye injuries and disorders	Gently flush the eye liberally with an ophthalmic solution or tap water.
	Use a tissue or soft cloth to wipe away any discharge or foreign matter from around the eye.
	If available, apply a sterile petrolatum ophthalmic ointment to the affected eye.
	Transport to your veterinarian.
Heat stroke/smoke inhalation	Quickly remove the bird from the offending environment and provide free access to fresh air. Fan the bird to increase the surrounding air circulation.

Table 43-1   Continued.

Heat stroke/smoke *inhalation* *continued*	For heat stroke, wrap the bird in a cool (not cold) moistened towel and transport immediately to your veterinarian.
Fractures/broken bones	For broken wings, immobilize the wing by pinning it against the bird's body using gauze wrap or a small towel. Be sure not to wrap too tightly as to impair your bird's breathing. Transport immediately to your veterinarian. For leg fractures, a toothpick or pen can be used as a temporary splint while you transport your bird to the veterinarian.

EXOTIC PETS

DID YOU KNOW that improper handling of a rabbit can lead to spinal fractures? Or how about green iguanas—are you familiar with the special lighting requirements needed to keep these lizards healthy? Did you know that hamsters can go into hibernation and be easily mistaken for dead by their owners? Or that miniature pot-bellied pigs make great lap pets? If not, welcome to the world of exotic pets!

Any creature that doesn't bark, meow, or fly falls into the category of "exotic pet." In reality, most of these pets are not truly "exotic" or unconventional, owing to their ever-increasing popularity and numbers in households across the country. As American lifestyles change, so does it appear that pet preferences are changing as well.

Some of the more popular exotic pets being seen more and more by veterinarians include the small rodents (such as gerbils, hamsters, mice, and rats), guinea pigs, rabbits, ferrets, reptiles, fish, and the latest entry in this category—the miniature pot-bellied pig. Each of these pets has special husbandry, nutritional, and preventative health care requirements that are essential for health and happiness, and prospective owners must be sure to learn these before, NOT AFTER, obtaining such a pet. Veterinarians are becoming more specialized in exotic medicine, and can provide an excellent informational resource for first-time owners.

Maintaining an exotic pet is not difficult and can be loads of fun for owners. The following chapters are designed to touch on the main points concerning husbandry and care of the more popular exotic species seen today. If more in-depth information is needed, contact your veterinarian or pet health care professional.

44

Guinea Pigs

CAVIA PORCELLUS, THE guinea pig, has become quite popular as a pet in recent years. The guinea pig is a native of the South American continent, and there are a number of popular breeds from which to choose. Among them: the *English*, characterized by smooth, short hair; *Peruvians*, which have long, silky hair; *Abyssinians*, which sport short, coarse hair arranged in multiple whorls; *Crested*, which are similar to English guinea pigs but with a white crest on the head; and *Teddys*, characterized by coarse, kinky hair. Guinea pigs also come in a variety of colors, such as solids, agouti, Himalayan, and tortoise shell.

Like hamsters, guinea pigs have no tails. Good natured, they rarely bite, yet might emit a loud squeal when frightened or handled. Guinea pigs average about one to two pounds in weight when full-grown, and can live up to eight years when well-cared for (FIG. 44-1).

RESTRAINT

Restraint of the guinea pig is similar to that of rats. The chest region can be encircled with one hand and, if necessary, the head and neck can be controlled with the thumb and index finger of the same hand. At the same time, your free hand should control the guinea pig's hind feet and rump to prevent from being scratched.

HOUSING

Male guinea pigs can be housed with females, yet two males living together could turn to fighting. Housing for guinea pigs should consist of

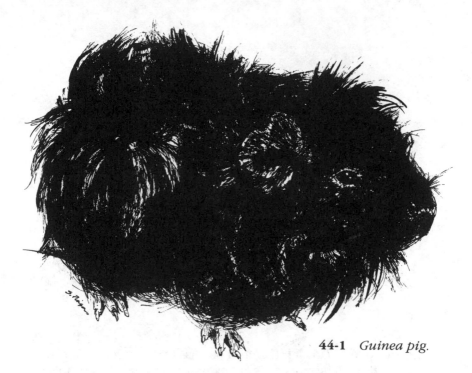

44-1 *Guinea pig.*

an open-top enclosure at least 12 inches high and providing at least 2 square feet of space for each pig. The smooth flooring of the cage can be lined with wood chips or shredded paper, and a small amount of hay can be used to provide material for burrowing. In addition, a ledge or ramp constructed of metal or plastic provides added enjoyment for most pigs to climb on or burrow beneath.

Both food and water delivery systems should be kept up off of the cage floor for sanitary purposes. Since some pigs might actually regurgitate food back up into the water sipper, be sure to check and maintain the patency of such devices on a daily basis. The cage itself should be thoroughly cleaned and sanitized at least twice weekly.

Guinea pigs cannot tolerate heat and humidity very well. Ideal environmental temperature for them is around 75 degrees. Temperatures exceeding 85 degrees can quickly lead to heat stroke if left unchecked.

NUTRITION

Guinea pigs must have adequate amounts of vitamin C in their diets, since their bodies are not capable of synthesizing the vitamin internally. Commercial guinea pig rations, in pellet form, can more than satisfy this requirement; just be certain that the pellets purchased are no more than six weeks old. After this amount of time, the vitamin C levels in such rations left sitting on the store or pantry shelf start to decrease, which could lead to dietary deficiencies.

Most guinea pigs enjoy fresh fruit and vegetables. You can offer fruits and vegetables along with the regular pelleted rations to ensure adequate amounts of vitamin C in the diet.

On an average, guinea pigs consume about 30 grams of feed per day. Be sure to provide plenty of clean, fresh water delivered through a bottle and sipper.

REPRODUCTION

Female guinea pigs cycle every 16 days and, if mated, will carry the developing offspring for an average of 68 days. Litter sizes usually range from one to eight pigs.

One unique feature of baby guinea pigs is that they, unlike other rodents, are born with hair and with eyes open. This enables them to be weaned almost immediately if the situation warrants it. However, allowing weaning to take place around 3 weeks of age affords better survival rates. Sexual maturity in these young pigs is reached at about 3 months of age.

Females that are not bred until after 6 months of age have a higher incidence of birthing complications than do those bred earlier in life. If a pig is not bred before this time, its pelvis might fuse together, making passage through the birth canal difficult. As a result, a Caesarean section operation might be necessary to deliver the litter. Also, pregnant guinea pigs are especially susceptible to heat stroke if environmental temperatures are not kept well-regulated.

DISEASES AND DISORDERS

TABLE 44-1 shows selected diseases and disorders seen in guinea pigs. Stress, overcrowding, improper nutrition, and poor sanitation all play important roles in the development of many diseases, especially the infectious ones. Remember that with the appearance of any clinical signs, a definitive diagnosis should only be made by a qualified veterinarian. Identifying and treating diseases in their early stages is the key to successful treatment and cure.

Table 44-1   Diseases & Disorders of Guinea Pigs

Disease	*Clinical Signs*	*Treatment/Comments*
	INFECTIOUS DISEASES	
Salmonellosis	Weight loss; conjunctivitis, diarrhea.	Often transmitted via contaminated food (greens). Treat with antibiotics; good sanitation: wash greens prior to feeding.
Streptococcosis	Enlarged lymph nodes ("lumps"). Variable signs and organ involvement; breathing difficulties.	Treat with antibiotics.
Bordatella bronchiseptica	Nasal discharge; breathing difficulties.	Same organism that causes canine cough. Treat with antibiotics.
Lymphocytic choriomeningitis virus	Poor growth; eye discharge; locomotion difficulties; seizures; breathing difficulties.	Transmitted by wild rodents. No treatment available. Zoonotic disease.

Table 44-1   Continued.

Disease	Clinical Signs	Treatment/Comments
Adenovirus	Breathing difficulties; nasal discharge; weight loss.	No treatment available.
Inclusion conjunctivitis	Eye crusting, discharge in young guinea pigs; swollen eyelids.	Treat with topical eye ointments. Will usually spontaneously clear up on its own.
DIGESTIVE SYSTEM DISEASES		
Malocclusion of teeth ("Slobbers")	Excessive salivation; inability to eat; weight loss.	Usually involves premolars and molars; causes include nutritional deficiencies, genetics. File down overgrown teeth—repeat every three weeks.
Hairballs	Loss of appetite; abdominal pain; palpable mass within abdomen.	Surgical removal necessary.
Coccidiosis	Abdominal pain and distension; loss of appetite; diarrhea; weight loss.	Associated with poor sanitary conditions. Treat with sulfa drugs.
Bacterial enteritis	Diarrhea; weight loss; abdominal pain.	Associated with poor sanitary conditions; also can be associated with improper antibiotic therapy. Treat using a select group of antimicrobial agents.
Hemorrhagic syndrome	Jaundice; diarrhea; blood clotting problems.	Seen in pregnant pigs; caused by uterus disrupting liver function. Treat by C-section; vitamin K therapy.
SKIN DISEASES		
Pododermatitis	Moist, ulcerated skin lesions on feet.	Caused by trauma from wire floors, environmental filth. Treat with antibiotics; change environmental conditions.
Hair loss	Can occur anywhere on the body.	Causes can include skin parasites, chewing ("barbering"), fighting, pregnancy, ringworm.
Ringworm	Hair loss; crusts on head, ears, back.	Treat with antifungal medications.
Mange (mites)	Intense itching; hair loss on face, ears; seizures.	Very contagious to other pigs. Treat with safe insecticidal shampoo or dip.
Fleas, ticks, lice	Itching; hair loss; anemia.	Treatment same as that for cats.
REPRODUCTIVE DISEASES		
Pregnancy toxemia	Loss of appetite; depression; seizures; breathing difficulties in pregnant or lactating pigs.	Obesity, genetics, stress, fasting can play a role. Treat with dextrose.
URINARY DISEASES		
Urethral obstruction	Inability to urinate; painful abdomen; irritable behavior; blood-tinged urine.	Seen in older males. Obstruction must be manually removed.
Kidney disease	Weight loss; loss of appetite; variable clinical signs.	Common in older pigs. Treatment generally unrewarding.
NERVOUS SYSTEM DISEASES		
Hind end paralysis	Inability to walk and support weight on hind legs.	Often due to spinal fracture or spinal cord damage secondary to pregnancy, vitamin C deficiency, arthritis. Treatment depends on severity.
MUSCULOSKELETAL DISEASES		
Hind leg fractures	Inability to bear weight on hind leg; dragging leg.	Caused by foot getting caught in flooring of wire cage, other trauma. Treatment depends on severity.
Myopathy	Reluctance to move; depression.	Due to vitamin E deficiency. Treat with vitamin E supplements.
"Stiff wrist syndrome"	Bone deformities; muscular stiffness; abnormal posture.	Due to magnesium deficiency. Treat by correcting ration.

45

Hamsters and Gerbils

THE MOST POPULAR species of pet hamster is by far the Golden (Syrian) hamster. Its smaller cousin, the Chinese (Striped-back) hamster is probably next in popularity. Hamsters are native to both the European and Asian continents. They are larger than gerbils, and unlike the latter, lack tails (FIG. 45-1).

As far as their status as pets is concerned, hamsters can be fun and loving pets, providing hours of enjoyment and fascination just watching their busy activity. Hamsters prefer to be most active at night (sometimes to the dismay of their owners!) and sleep during the day. During winter months, they might even go into hibernation if environmental conditions dictate it. These hamsters might even appear dead to an owner, but a little warmth and rousing will soon bring them back to life! The average life-span of a hamster is approximately two years.

Gerbils can be differentiated from hamsters by their smaller size and by the presence of a hairy tail (FIG. 45-2) The presence of hair on the tail can also be used to differentiate gerbils from mice, who have hairless tails.

The Mongolian gerbil, *Meriones unguiculatus*, is by far the most popular type. It is a native of the deserts of Mongolia and China. Because of their origin, gerbils possess many unique features, one being a very low daily water requirement. Like camels, gerbils can regulate their water reserves within their body quite efficiently, and can go days without water! Gerbils tend to be milder tempered than hamsters, rarely biting the hand that feeds them. They are curious creatures and rarely try to escape. Gerbils that are well cared for can have lifespans up to four years.

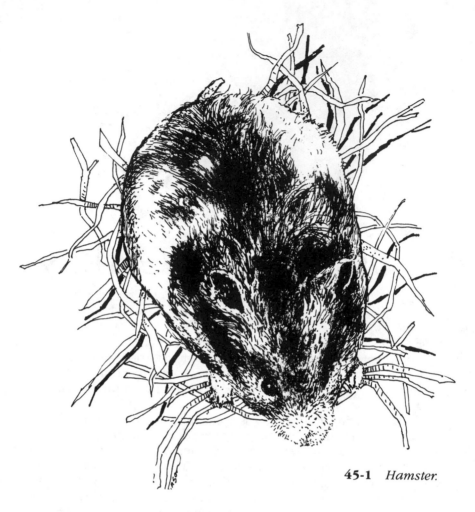

45-1   *Hamster.*

RESTRAINT

Hamsters

When handling or restraining hamsters, grasp the skin over the shoulder and neck region with the thumb and first two fingers of one hand and support the body with the other. For restraining hamsters that like to bite (this includes sick hamsters), be sure you grasp as much skin as you can. You can also use a paper towel or cloth to protect your hand as you grasp the neck region. In this way, if the hamster turns its head to bite, it won't be able to reach your fingers.

Gerbils

Gerbils are much easier to handle than hamsters, owing to their friendly and gentle dispositions. Most will climb right into an opened hand; others might need to be restrained similar to hamsters.

45-2 *Gerbil.*

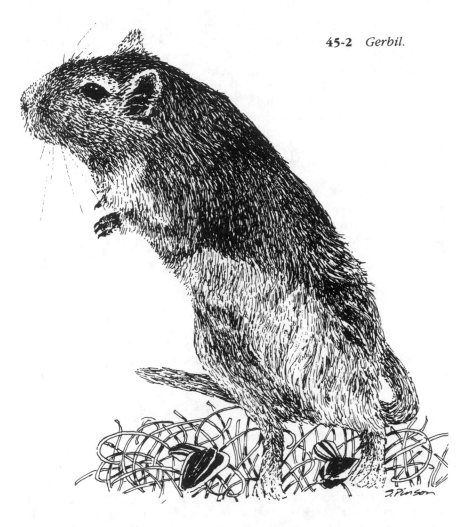

Never pick up a gerbil by its tail. By doing so, the skin covering the tail could come off in your hand, leaving your rodent friend in an unhealthy predicament! Also, frightened or stressed gerbils might undergo spontaneous epileptic seizures. This tendency to seizure is an inherited trait seen in some strains of gerbils—but don't be alarmed if this happens to your pet. The convulsions will subside on their own, and they require no specific management.

HOUSING

Hamsters, especially females, should be housed individually, owing to their preponderance for fighting. Gerbils, on the other hand, are happier when kept in pairs.

Housing accommodations for hamsters and gerbils can be readily purchased from your local pet store or pet supply. Cages with solid flooring and divided compartments connected with tunnels are preferred. This type of construction provides the pet(s) with a source of exercise, which helps curb boredom. Cages with wire mesh flooring should be avoided because they can be hard on the feet and, in the case of gerbils, be a source of tail injuries. Finally, hamsters are notorious escape artists, so be certain that cage outlets are secured at all times!

Commercial rodent flooring or litter can be used to line the bottom of the cage and help absorb waste material. It should be changed at least twice weekly. Be sure to provide bedding and nesting material (consisting of tissue or cotton).

Exercise wheels, toys, and makeshift huts or sleeping quarters should be installed for your pet's enjoyment. When choosing a wheel for gerbils, select one constructed of plastic. Avoid metal wheels with spaced slats or bars, since these can cause serious injuries to tails if they become intertwined in them.

NUTRITION

Rations for a hamster or gerbil should consist of commercial rodent pellets with a few vegetable or sunflower seed treats added. Don't overdo the latter; some pets will prefer to eat the seeds over their regular ration, leading to nutritional imbalances and obesity. At the same time, be careful not to overfeed regular rations as well. Obesity causes the same ill effects in these small animals as it does in larger ones. Hamsters are notorious for gathering food stores and even storing food in their immense cheek pouches for later use.

The average hamster or gerbil will consume about 5 grams of feed per day. Dispensers can be attached directly to the side of the cage and will dispense the allotted portion of food. This method of food delivery is much more sanitary than simply placing a food bowl on the floor of the cage. Water sippers can also be attached to the side of the cage. Just be sure that both the source of food and water are easily reachable and that the delivery end of the water sipper remains patent. Many hamsters and gerbils, especially, smaller, adolescent ones, die each year from water and food deprivation because these food and water sources are innocently placed out of reach or are inefficient at delivering their product!

REPRODUCTION

Hamsters

Male hamsters can be differentiated from females by the presence of two dark, pigmented spots on the hip regions of the male. These mark the location of hip glands used for marking territory and attracting females.

Female hamsters experience a heat cycle every four days. Towards the end of her heat period, a white discharge might be seen coming from the vagina. This is normal and should not be mistaken for an infection. Male hamsters should be introduced into the cage at this time.

Because it could take a few days for the female to become adjusted to the male, watch for aggressiveness on her part, and remove the male immediately if it occurs. Reintroduce him the next day, following the same precautions.

Once they are bred, the gestation period for the hamster is approximately 18 days. Litter size normally ranges from six to ten pups. They are born hairless and blind. Although not common, cannibalism of offspring by young females has been known to occur if the new mother becomes disturbed during the first week after giving birth. This can be aggravated by owners handling the young during the first week of life, improper nesting material, cage cleanings, and difficult access to food and water. As a result, be sure to leave the mother alone and undisturbed with her pups the first week, except of course to provide feed and water.

Hamster pups reach weaning age at 3 to 4 weeks and should be removed to their own housing at that time. Puberty is achieved around 8 weeks of age.

Gerbils

The breeding habits of gerbils are similar to those of hamsters. Interestingly, male and female breeding pairs form strong bonds that last a lifetime. Male gerbils can be differentiated from females by the distance between the anal opening and the genital opening—the distance for the male being much longer.

Females undergo a heat period every four to five days, and once bred, they experience a gestation period of approximately 24 days. Litter sizes usually range from four to five pups, which, like hamsters, are born hairless, blind, and helpless.

Cannibalism is not a problem in gerbils as it is in hamsters. Pups are weaned at 21 to 24 days, and will reach sexual maturity themselves at about 12 weeks of age.

DISEASES AND DISORDERS OF HAMSTERS

The following are some selected diseases and disorders seen in hamsters. Sick hamsters are generally very irritable and can bite! Stress, overcrowding, improper nutrition, and poor sanitation play important roles in the development of many diseases, especially infectious diseases. Remember that with the appearance of any clinical signs, a definitive diagnosis should only be made by a qualified veterinarian. Identifying and treating diseases in their early stages is the key to successful treatment and cure.

NOTE: Remember that hamsters undergoing hibernation might undergo behavioral changes and might appear lethargic or lifeless. Increasing the environmental temperature will restore such hamsters to normal behavior and activity.

Table 45-1   Diseases & Disorders of Hamsters

Disease	Clinical Signs	Treatment/Comments
	DIGESTIVE SYSTEM DISEASES	
Malocclusion of incisor teeth	Excessive salivation; inability to eat; weight loss; nasal discharge.	Trim incisors every 8-12 weeks as needed.
Salmonellosis	Weight loss; diarrhea; variable signs and organ involvement.	Often transmitted via contaminated food (greens). Treatment rarely helpful.
"Wet Tail"	Weight loss; diarrhea; ruffled fur; dehydration; rectal prolapse.	Can be rapidly fatal. Treat with antibiotics and fluids to correct dehydration.
Antibiotic-induced colitis	Severe diarrhea, dehydration, death.	Bacterial overgrowth in intestines caused by improper selection of antibiotic.
Tapeworms	Weight loss; poor appetite; diarrhea.	Rarely causes severe disease. Treat with anti-tapeworm medication.
	SKIN DISEASES	
Streptococcosis, staphylococcosis	Enlarged lymph nodes, abscesses.	Often secondary to fight wounds. Treat with antibiotics; lance.
Mange (Mites)	Hair loss, scaling, especially along back and face.	Often appears secondary to other diseases. Treat with insecticidal products as in cats.
	MUSCULOSKELETAL DISEASES	
Cage paralysis	Weakness; inability to move or lift head.	Caused by nutritional deficiency. Treat with vitamin supplementation.
	OTHER DISEASES	
Neoplasia	Variable signs, depending on organ systems involved; weight loss; loss of appetite.	Tumors are not uncommon in hamsters; often affect glands within the body. Treatment depends on organ system involved.
Amyloidosis	Weight loss, dehydration, loss of appetite.	Causes kidney failure in affected hamsters. Common disease.

DISEASES AND DISORDERS OF GERBILS

The following are some selected diseases and disorders seen in gerbils. Stress, overcrowding, improper nutrition, and poor sanitation play important roles in the development of many diseases, especially infectious diseases. Remember that with the appearance of any clinical signs, a definitive diagnosis should only be made by a qualified veterinarian. Identifying and treating diseases in their early stages is the key to successful treatment and cure.

Table 45-2 Diseases & Disorders of Gerbils

Disease	Clinical Signs	Treatment/Comments
DIGESTIVE SYSTEM DISEASES		
Malocclusion of incisor teeth	Depression; inability to eat; weight loss.	Trim incisors every 8-12 weeks as needed.
Tyzzer's disease ("Wet Tail")	Weight loss; diarrhea; ruffled fur; dehydration.	Can be rapidly fatal. Treatment generally unrewarding once signs appear.
Salmonellosis	Weight loss; diarrhea; ruffled fur; dehydration.	Treatment is generally unrewarding.
SKIN DISEASES		
Mange (Demodex)	Hair loss, scaling, especially at base of tail and rear legs.	Often appears secondary to other diseases. Treat with amitraz dip as in dogs.
Dermatitis	Moist skin lesions, abscesses; hair loss, abrasions on nose.	Usually secondary to poor husbandry and sanitation; self-induced trauma; parasites. Antibiotics might be needed for secondary bacterial infections.
RESPIRATORY SYSTEM DISEASES		
Upper respiratory infection/pneumonia	Sneezing; breathing difficulties; chattering; conjunctivitis.	Often caused by stress and poor husbandry. Treat with appropriate antibiotics.
URINARY SYSTEM DISEASES		
Kidney disease	Weight loss; increased water consumption; increased urination.	Common in older gerbils. No effective treatment.
NERVOUS SYSTEM DISEASES		
Epilepsy	Spontaneous seizures.	Certain strains of gerbils highly susceptible. No treatment necessary.
OTHER DISEASES		
Neoplasia	Variable signs, depending on organ systems involved; weight loss; loss of appetite.	Tumors are not uncommon in older gerbils. Treatment depends on organ system involved.

46

Mice and Rats

ALTHOUGH MORE POPULAR as laboratory research animals, mice and rats are occasionally kept as pets. They are relatively easy to care for, and most have gentle dispositions, making them easy to handle. The mouse, *Mus musculus*, and the rat, *Rattus norvegicus*, originated from the Asian continent, but soon spread with man throughout the world. They are both nocturnal creatures, becoming most active during the twilight hours. Both have hairless tails, a fact that helps differentiate the mouse from its rodent cousin, the gerbil. The average lifespan for mice and rats is around 2 to 5 years of age (FIG. 46-1).

RESTRAINT

Mice and rats are usually quite gentle and can be handled without much trouble. More feistier pets can be picked up and restrained by grasping the base of the tail with one hand and, as you lift, encircling the chest with the other hand. If necessary, use your thumb and index finger to control the head and neck. Be ready: Most will urinate and defecate when handled.

For mice and rats that like to bite, use of a paper towel or cloth to protect your hand as you grasp the skin over the neck and shoulder region. This cover will help prevent the rodent from turning its head and biting.

HOUSING

Mice and rats can be housed in any type of cage or container, provided there is enough room to maintain good sanitary conditions and to allow

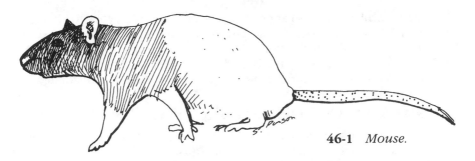

46-1   *Mouse.*

for free movement. Males and females can be housed together, but males should not be put together because of their tendency to fight.

You can buy cages for your pet mouse or rat at your favorite pet store; you could also use an aquarium for this purpose. Smooth floors are preferred over wire mesh; the latter can pose hazards to both feet and tails. The floor of the cage should be lined with wood shavings or commercially available bedding. This bedding should be changed at least twice weekly to maintain good sanitation.

Exercise wheels, toys, and makeshift huts or sleeping quarters can be installed for your pet's enjoyment. When choosing a wheel for mice and rats, select one constructed of plastic. Avoid metal wheels with spaced slats or bars, since they can cause serious injuries to tails that might become intertwined.

NUTRITION

Rations for mice and rats should consist of commercial rodent pellets with a few vegetables or fruit pieces added. Don't overdo these supplements. Some mice and rats will prefer to eat these treats instead of their regular ration, leading to nutritional imbalances. At the same time, be careful not to overfeed regular rations, since obesity causes the same ill effects in these small animals as it does in larger ones.

The average mouse will consume about 3 to 4 grams of food per day; rats will consume 10 to 20 grams. Dispensers that hang suspended from the side of the cage can be used to deliver water and the allotted portion of food. This method of delivery is much more sanitary than simply placing a food or water bowl on the floor of the cage.

Be sure the sources of food and water are easily reachable and that the delivery end of the water sipper remains patent. Failure to heed this advice could lead to death from starvation or dehydration, especially in small or weak animals.

REPRODUCTION

Male mice and rats can be differentiated from females on the basis of their external genitalia and by the longer distance between the anal and genital opening.

Female mice and rats experience a heat cycle every four to six days. Once they have been bred, the gestation period is approximately 21 days. Litter size normally ranges from six to twelve. Baby mice and rats, like other rodents, are born hairless and blind. Weaning occurs at 3 to 4 weeks, with sexual maturity being reached at 1 1/2 to 2 months of age.

DISEASES AND DISORDERS OF MICE AND RATS

The following are some selected diseases and disorders seen in mice and rats. Stress, overcrowding, improper nutrition, and poor sanitation play important roles in the development of many diseases, especially infectious diseases. Remember that with the appearance of any clinical signs, a definitive diagnosis should only be made by a qualified veterinarian. Identifying and treating diseases in their early stages is the key to successful treatment and cure.

Table 46-1   Diseases & Disorders of Mice & Rats

Disease	Clinical Signs	Treatment/Comments
INFECTIOUS DISEASES		
Bacterial infections	Enlarged lymph nodes; abscesses; breathing difficulties; conjunctivitis; weight loss; loss of appetite.	Treat with antibiotics. Lance abscesses.
Sialodacryoadenitis	Swelling in neck region due to inflamed salivary glands.	Seen in rats; caused by virus. Antibiotics for secondary infections.
Pox virus	Sloughing of tail and/or digits of feet.	No treatment available.
SKIN DISEASES		
Ringtail syndrome	Ulcerated lesion at base of tail.	Seen in mice; caused by low humidity. Treat by maintaining humidity at 50%.
Traumatic wounds	Sores and wounds on ear pinnae and tail.	Usually caused by fighting between males. Treat by separating males.
Mange	Hair loss, scratching especially around head and ears.	Seen primarily in mice. Treat with pyrethrin insecticide.
Ringworm	Hair loss; scaliness.	Treat with antifungal medications.
Mammary tumor	Lumps; ulcerated tissue in mammary region of females.	Must be surgically removed.
RESPIRATORY DISEASES		
Upper respiratory disease/pneumonia	Sneezing; chattering; nasal discharge; breathing difficulty; depression; eye discharge.	Can be viral or bacterial in origin. Treat with antibiotics.
GASTROINTESTINAL DISEASES		
Enteritis	Diarrhea; rectal prolapse.	Pinworms, protozoal organisms, bacteria can all cause. Treat according to source.
NERVOUS SYSTEM DISEASES		
Vestibular syndrome	Head tilt; circling.	Often seen secondary to respiratory infections. Treat with antibiotics.

47

Rabbits

THE DOMESTIC RABBIT we are all familiar with, *Oryctolagus cuniculus*, is actually a descendent of the European wild rabbit. Rabbits have been used for centuries for food and pelts, yet their importance and popularity as delightful house pets is rapidly increasing. Well over 50 breeds exist from which to choose, depending upon aesthetical preference. All rabbits come in three basic sizes: large, medium, and small, with body weights reaching as high as 15 pounds! As with other pets, the key to disease prevention and control in these creatures is good husbandry practices. Well maintained, the average rabbit can live to be 10 to 15 years old (FIG. 47-1).

RESTRAINT

When handling a rabbit, grasp the loose skin over the shoulder and neck region with one hand, and support the hind legs with the other. Not only will this help prevent you from being bitten or scratched, but it is also necessary to prevent inadvertent injury to the back and spine of the rabbit (FIG. 47-2). Rabbits that are restrained with their hind limbs unsupported might kick and struggle using their powerful hind legs, and have been known to actually break their back in their attempts!

HOUSING

Rabbits can be allowed free access to the house and can be readily litter-trained. One word of caution: Rabbits can be quite destructive with their teeth and nails unless closely supervised.

47-1 *Domestic rabbit.*

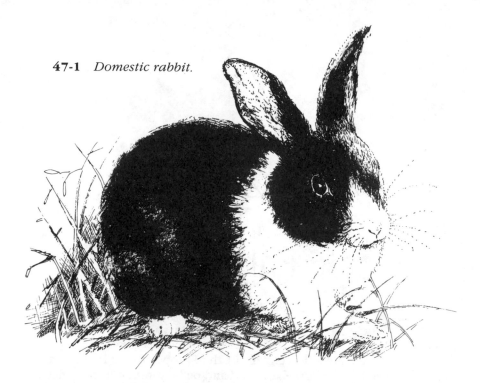

If your rabbit is to be kept in a cage, it should be housed individually in a suspended enclosure no smaller than 5 square feet and no less than 16 inches high. Cages can be purchased commercially or can be constructed out of wire mesh. This wire mesh should be 1 inch by 2 inches on the sides and no more than 1/2 inch by 1 inch for the floor.

Because wire mesh is hard on the rabbit's feet, many owners choose to place wooden or plastic resting boards on the cage floor. These are fine as long as feces and urine are not allowed to build up and the rabbit doesn't chew on the board. To ensure utmost sanitation, a tray filled with cat litter or gravel should be placed beneath the cage to capture urine and fecal material that passes through the wire mesh.

Cages should be placed in well ventilated areas to prevent buildups of ammonia fumes emitted from urine. In addition, rabbits enjoy environmental temperature that range between 65 and 80 degrees Fahrenheit. Temperatures exceeding 85 degrees are not tolerated well by rabbits.

Sipper bottles suspended from the cage side should be used in place of water bowls, since sippers prevent fecal contamination of the water supply and also reduce the chances of sore hock and other moisture-related diseases.

Cages, food bowls, and water suppliers should be cleaned and disinfected at least twice weekly. Household bleach or a quaternary ammonium compound diluted one (1) part to ten (10) parts water can be used as the disinfectant. Be sure to rinse well after application.

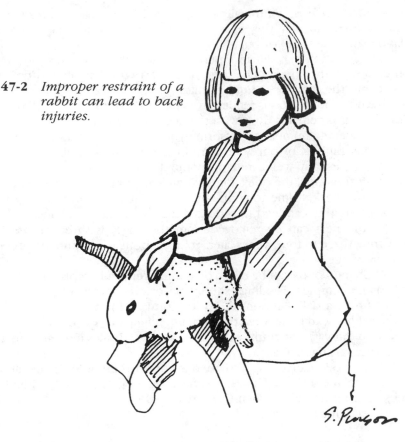

47-2 *Improper restraint of a rabbit can lead to back injuries.*

NUTRITION

Commercial rabbit pellets are available to use as a food source for your rabbit. For rabbits that appear overweight, look for a ration containing 25% or more of dietary fiber to help encourage weight loss.

The average rabbit consumes about 130 grams of food per day. Contrary to popular belief, rabbits do not need lettuce or carrots in order to sustain life. However, these do provide palatable treats for your bunny if you so desire.

One behavior of rabbits that might surprise new owners is *coprophagy*; that is, they might eat their own feces. This usually occurs during the morning hours. This practice shouldn't be frowned upon; it actually increases nutrient utilization and absorption within the rabbit's body.

REPRODUCTION

Justifiably, rabbits have been accused of being one of the most prolific breeders of all time. One reason for this is the female rabbit, or the doe, is *polyestrous*—that is, continually in heat. Rabbits are also *induced ovulators*, which means that the egg is released from the ovary only upon copulation with the male, or buck.

The gestation or pregnancy period for does is 28 to 34 days in length. Three weeks after breeding, a nest box filled with hay should be introduced into the cage for the doe to make final preparations for birth. Ideally, the box should be suspended from the floor of the cage such that the rim of the box remains flush with the floor of the cage.

The average number of offspring you can expect is around three to nine. Baby rabbits, or pups, are born in the nest naked, blind, and helpless, yet are usually well cared for by the doe.

After the birth, the doe's food allowance should be increased gradually over a week's time to compensate for lactation. Do not increase it suddenly, as this can lead to serious gastrointestinal problems. In three weeks, the nest can be removed from the cage, with actual weaning occurring three to four weeks later. Young rabbits reach puberty at 3 to 6 months of age.

Orphaned pups can be raised on commercial milk replacers intended for canine puppies. Feedings should be offered every eight to twelve hours, up to a daily amount of 10 to 20 ml of formula. Some of these young rabbits can be weaned onto commercial pellets as early as 3 weeks of age. As always, warmth, sanitation, and tender-loving care are vital whenever raising orphans.

Adult does can be spayed to prevent further pregnancies and to reduce the incidence of uterine cancer as they grow older. Similarly, bucks can be neutered when they are 8 to 12 months of age. Ask your veterinarian for more details.

DISEASES AND DISORDERS OF RABBITS

The following are some selected diseases and disorders seen in rabbits. Remember that others do exist, which is why a definitive diagnosis should only be made by a qualified veterinarian. Identifying and treating diseases in their early stages is the key to successful treatment and cure.

Table 47-1   Diseases & Disorders of Rabbits

Disease	Clinical Signs	Treatment/Comments
	RESPIRATORY DISEASES	
Bacterial rhinitis/ pneumonia (snuffles; pasteurellosis)	Sneezing; nasal and eye discharge; breathing difficulties; head shaking.	Common in stressed rabbits. Treat with antibiotics.
	GASTROINTESTINAL DISEASES	
Malocclusion of teeth ("slobbers")	Excessive salivation; inability to eat; weight loss; lip lacerations.	Trim incisor teeth every 2 weeks.
Hairballs	Loss of appetite; abdominal pain.	Treat using laxatives. Surgical removal sometimes needed. Prevent with brushing, hairball laxative weekly.

Table 47-1   Continued.

Disease	Clinical Signs	Treatment/Comments
Mucoid-enteropathy	Abdominal pain and distension; diarrhea; arched back; dehydration.	Highly fatal in young rabbits; exact cause unknown. Treat with antibiotics to prevent secondary infection; replace fluids. High fiber diet might help.
Coccidiosis	Abdominal pain and distension; loss of appetite; diarrhea; jaundice; weight loss.	Associated with poor sanitary conditions. Treat with sulfa drugs.
Bacterial enteritis	Diarrhea; weight loss; jaundice.	Associated with poor sanitary conditions; also can be associated with improper antibiotic therapy. Treat using a select group of antimicrobial agents.

SKIN AND COAT DISEASES

Disease	Clinical Signs	Treatment/Comments
"Sore Hocks" *(bacterial dermatitis)*	Moist, ulcerated skin lesions on hind feet.	Caused by trauma from wire floors, environmental filth. Treat with antibiotics; change environmental conditions.
Ringworm	Hair loss; crusts on head, ears.	Treat with antifungal medications.
Ear mites	Head shaking; scratching at ears. Crusts and scabs in ears; hair loss on head and neck.	Very common problem in pet rabbits. Treat with ear mite medication; Ivermectin for tough cases.
Mange (Sarcoptes)	Intense itching; hair loss on face, ears, genitalia.	Very contagious to other rabbits. Treat with safe insecticidal shampoo. Ivermectin for tough cases.
Fleas, ticks	Itching; hair loss; anemia.	Treatment same as that for cats.
Pox viruses	Wart-like growths on face, legs, and feet; swollen eyelids; eye discharge; subcutaneous lumps.	Transmitted by biting insects. No treatment; wart-like growths usually regress on their own.

REPRODUCTIVE SYSTEM DISEASES

Disease	Clinical Signs	Treatment/Comments
Pregnancy toxemia	Loss of appetite; depression; seizures in pregnant or lactating does.	Cause unknown. High mortality. Support with antibiotics.
Uterine adenocarcinoma	Infertility; weight loss; loss of appetite; vaginal discharge.	Common in older females. Spay if not metastasized.

URINARY SYSTEM DISEASES

Disease	Clinical Signs	Treatment/Comments
Normal urine	Urine cloudy, thick; often orange or brown in color.	
Nephroma	Loss of appetite, depression; variable signs (associated with kidney disease).	Usually benign, yet affects kidney function.

NEUROLOGICAL DISEASES

Disease	Clinical Signs	Treatment/Comments
Parasitic encephalitis	Tremors; convulsions; incoordination.	Can be caused by exposure to racoon. roundworms or to other infected rabbits.

MUSCULOSKELETAL DISEASES

Disease	Clinical Signs	Treatment/Comments
Splayleg	Inability to walk; support weight; one or all legs can be affected.	Can be genetic or traumatic in origin. Treatment generally unrewarding.
Spinal fractures	Paralysis of hind end and hind legs.	Caused by improper handling or trauma. Treatment generally unrewarding.

48

Ferrets

FERRETS ARE POPULAR as pets in the United States, with tens of thousands of households obtaining one of these curious, rambunctious creatures each year. Ferrets belong to the same family as do minks, skunks, and weasels. Several different species exist, yet *Mustela putorius furo* represents the most common species kept as a pet (FIG. 48-1). This particular ferret is a direct descendent of the European polecat.

For centuries, ferrets have been used by man for a variety of tasks, including pest control and, more popularly, hunting. Only in the past century has their role as house pet been established. Insatiably curious, ferrets love to roam and explore their environment. They also can be quite playful and mischievous with their owners. Ferrets kept in cages or pens should be allowed daily exercise periods in which to expend some of this energy.

Controversy does exist concerning keeping ferrets as pets. This arose from limited reports of ferrets attacking babies and small children. Although the frequency of such attacks by other house pets such as dogs and cats is probably much greater, some cities and states (such as California and Georgia) have laws against keeping ferrets as house pets. It is safe to say that any pet, including ferrets, should never be left unattended with an infant or a small child.

Most ferrets are yellow-brown in color with black faces, tails, and legs. Albino, Siamese, and Silver Mitt ferrets exist as well, yet their appearance is less common. Male ferrets reach weights up to six pounds; females average two to three pounds. Weight increases are common during the fall and winter months, as ferrets store up fat for the winter. This weight is usually lost when spring arrives. The lifespan of an average ferret is seven to nine years.

48-1 *Ferret.*

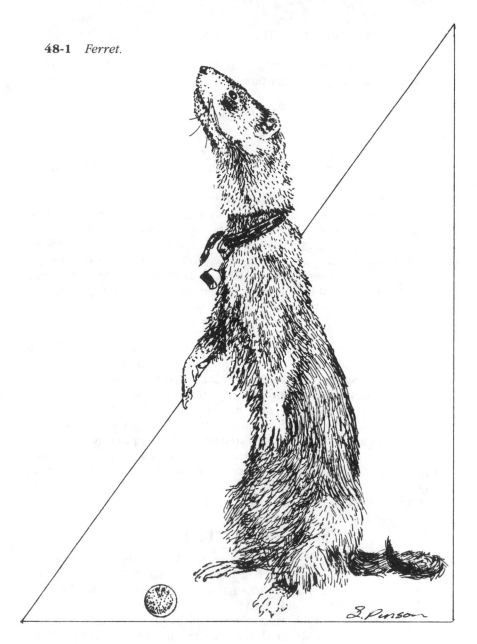

RESTRAINT

Most ferrets are mild-mannered and can be handled with minimal restraint. You can grasp those ferrets resisting capture by the scruff of the neck or tail to impede their movement. Then, one hand can be used to encircle the forequarters, pushing the forelegs together as the ferret is lifted from the cage or carrier. The other hand should support the hind-quarters.

Never *lift* a ferret solely by the scruff of its neck or solely by its tail. Those are two good ways to get bitten!

HOUSING

Ferrets can be housed in any type of enclosure that allows them ample room to move about freely. You can house more than one ferret together, but be aware that males might fight with each other, especially during breeding season.

Wire cages of various sizes are readily available from most pet stores. Choose one with smooth flooring, as wire mesh floor surfaces can be tough on the feet. A small box or hideaway, preferably constructed of plastic, can be placed in one corner of the cage to provide a place for recluse and sleep. Ferrets love blankets to cuddle up and use for hiding.

Ferrets can be trained to use a litterbox; as a result, a litter pan or tray can be placed at the other end of the cage for elimination purposes.

NUTRITION

Ferrets can be fed a commercially available mink or ferret ration. If you have a hard time finding such food, you can use dry cat food can be used as a substitute, but be sure to supplement it with liver or canned-meat baby food to provide added protein. Be sure the food you chose is not high in fiber; ferrets have difficulty digesting fiber.

Ferrets prefer six to eight meals throughout the day rather than one or two large meals. As a result, allow free access to food during the day. Be sure to change the food daily to ensure freshness. Water should be made available free-choice. Choose a water bowl weighted at the bottom to resist spilling. Finally, because of a propensity to develop hairballs, the diet of ferrets should be supplemented with a hairball laxative.

REPRODUCTION

Male ferrets are called hobs; females are referred to as jills. Sexual maturity for both occurs at approximately 8 to 10 months of age. The breeding season for ferrets runs from March to August, the time period in which the reproductive cycle of the jill is active.

Prior to breeding, place a nest box constructed of wood or plastic, complete with bedding material, within the cage or den. It should be large enough to allow the jill to move about freely and lie in it comfortably. As jills come into heat, vulvular discharge and swelling will be noted.

Female ferrets are induced ovulators; that is, the egg from the ovary is ovulated upon copulation. Hobs should be introduced to the jill only long enough for copulation to take place, and then they should be removed. Hobs and jills can inflict serious injury upon one another if left together, and the former can even go so far as kill the offspring when they arrive.

The gestation period for ferrets is approximately 42 days. The average box size ranges from five to eight "kits." They are born blind and hairless. To prevent infant rejection or worse yet, infanticide, try not to disturb or handle a jill and her box unnecessarily during the first three weeks after parturition except for sanitation and feeding purposes. Feline milk replacers should be added to the jill's diet to give an added nutritional boost during the lactation period. Starting at 6 weeks, kits can be gradually weaned off of the jill using canned cat food mixed one to one (1:1) with a commercial feline milk substitute.

Orphaned or abandoned kits can be raised by hand using a feline milk replacement formula. Feedings should be performed at least every two hours for the first week and every four hours for the next three to four weeks. Orphans need to be stimulated to eliminate after each feeding. This can be accomplished using a warm, moist cotton ball and gently massaging the genital region. Starting at 3 weeks of age, the orphan can be slowly weaned onto solid food using the formula mentioned above. As with any orphaned animal, warmth, sanitation, and lots of tender-loving care are needed.

The reproductive cycle of jills is unique in that jills must be bred in order for estrogen levels within their bodies to decline, allowing them to go out of heat. The significance of this lies in the fact that jills that are indeed not bred can develop life-threatening anemia and blood-clotting problems caused by persistently high estrogen levels. As a result, owners must be sure to have their jills bred each breeding season, or have their veterinarian administer a special injection each time to bring them out of heat. Another more preferable alternative is surgical spaying, which can be performed as early as 6 months of age.

HEALTH CARE

Ferrets should receive routine medical checkups just like dogs and cats. For ferrets less than 4 years old, these visits to the veterinarian should be made annually. For ferrets older than 4 years, increase the visits to twice per year.

Preventative care

Ferrets are very susceptible to the canine distemper virus and should be vaccinated against this disease starting at 6 to 8 weeks of age. A booster immunization should be administered at 12 weeks, and then annually. In addition, certain rabies vaccines have recently been approved for use in ferrets, and should be administered on an annual basis.

Interestingly enough, there have been reported cases of clinically ill ferrets testing positive for the feline leukemia virus. This brings up the question of whether or not ferrets should be vaccinated against that disease. While the likelihood of ferrets contracting the actual feline leukemia virus is negligible, it is possible that they are susceptible to a virus very similar to the cat virus—one that cross-reacts with the feline leukemia test. As a result, vaccination against the feline leukemia is not routinely performed.

The same types of intestinal parasites that can affect dogs and cats can infest ferrets. As a result, stool examinations should be performed periodically by your veterinarian, and deworming should be administered if deemed appropriate.

Ear mites are very common in ferrets, hence owners need to be on constant look-out for these pests. Ferrets infested with these mites will shake their heads and have a brown-black discharge in the affected ear(s). The drug ivermectin applied directly to the ears is the most effective method to eliminate an ear mite infestation.

Ferrets are susceptible to canine heartworm disease. As a result, in those areas with large concentrations of this disease, a heartworm preventative medicine should be administered. Contact your veterinarian for his/her recommendations for your particular area.

Routine surgical procedures

Routine surgical procedures performed on ferrets include neutering and de-scenting. Neutering hobs will help reduce their aggressiveness and reduce body odor. If not to be bred, jills should be spayed as well to eliminate the dangers of persistent estrus. Both procedures can be performed at six months of age.

De-scenting can be performed at the same time as neutering to help reduce obnoxious odors emitted from ferrets, especially males. This involves the removal of the anal sacs. De-scenting is a misnomer for this procedure, since it rarely eliminates odor completely. Secretions from glands in the skin beneath the tail also account for the characteristic odor of a ferret. However, de-scenting combined with frequent baths using a hypoallergenic shampoo can make your ferret virtually odor-free.

Because ferrets like to dig, declawing is becoming more popular as a routine surgical procedure in ferrets. The procedure itself is similar to that in the cat. Often, however, it can be avoided simply by keeping the nails trimmed back on a weekly basis.

DISEASES AND DISORDERS OF FERRETS

The following are some selected diseases and disorders seen in ferrets.

Remember that others do exist, which is why definitive diagnosis should only be made by a qualified veterinarian. Identifying and treating diseases in their early stages is the key to successful treatment and cure.

Table 48-1   Diseases & Disorders of Ferrets

Disease	*Clinical Signs*	*Treatment/Comments*
	INFECTIOUS DISEASES	
Canine distemper	Fever; loss of appetite; nasal and eye discharge; convulsions.	No treatment available. Prevent by vaccinating.
Human influenza	Fever; nasal discharge; sneezing; breathing difficulties.	Can be transmitted by humans. Treat with antibiotics and antihistamines.
Retroviral infection	Signs vary with organ involved; can cause cancer; anemia.	Some ill ferrets have tested positive for the feline leukemia virus.
	SKIN DISEASES	
Skin parasites (fleas, mites, ear mites)	Itching; hair loss; inflamed ears.	Treat with pyrethrin-type insecticide.
Mast cell tumors	Itching; hair loss; reddened raised skin lesions.	Can occur along with other tumors. Surgical excision.
	DIGESTIVE SYSTEM DISEASES	
Intestinal parasites (hookworms, roundworms, tapeworms, Giardia, coccidia)	Weight loss; loss of appetite; vomiting; diarrhea.	Treat with dewormer similar to those used in cats.
Proliferative colitis	Green, mucoid diarrhea; weight loss; prolapsed rectum; incoordination.	Age of onset is around 4-6 months. Treat with antibiotics. Might be zoonotic disease.
Hairballs; gastric foreign bodies	Vomiting, loss of appetite.	Treat hairballs as in cats. Foreign bodies might need to be removed surgically.
Insulinoma	Profound weakness; increased salivation; seizures.	This tumor of the pancreas causes low blood sugar. Surgical removal of tumor necessary.
	REPRODUCTIVE SYSTEM DISEASES	
Aplastic anemia	Weakness; loss of appetite; bruising; hemorrhaging; dark, tarry stools.	Caused by persistent heat cycle. Treat with hormones, blood transfusions, bone marrow stimulants. Prevent by spaying at 6 months of age.
	URINARY SYSTEM DISEASES	
Urolithiasis	Blood-tinged urine; straining to urinate; depression	Treatment is the same as for cats.
	CARDIOPULMONARY DISEASES	
Heartworm disease	Weakness; coughing; breathing difficulties.	Treat and prevent the same as in dogs.
Congestive heart failure	Weakness; coughing; breathing difficulties.	Treat as in dogs.
	EYE DISEASES	
Juvenile cataracts	Cloudy eyes; vision difficulties.	Seen in young ferrets. Surgical removal of cataract might be needed to restore vision.

49

Miniature
Pot-Bellied Pigs

MINIATURE POT-BELLIED Pigs (MPBPs) have become the latest craze among the pet-owning population. With origins tracing back to the jungles of Vietnam and China, miniature pigs were first introduced into the United States in 1985. Since then, their popularity has increased to such levels that today there are over 8,000 households containing MPBPs.

Such popularity is attributed to the fact that miniature pigs can make adorable pets. Not only are they relatively clean and odor-free (unlike domestic pigs), miniature pot-bellied pigs are intelligent, easily trainable, and house-broken, and can abound with affection. Their major disadvantage—$$$.

Miniature Pot-bellied pigs represent an investment that can range from $600 to $6,000. In addition, these pigs, like others, like to root, which could pose problems to both carpets and lawns. Certainly those who pride themselves on expensively landscaped lawns should think twice about allowing a miniature pot-bellied pig access to the grounds!

Finally, be sure to check the laws of your particular city or municipality concerning these pets. In some areas, miniature pot-bellied pigs are still considered livestock rather than companion animals, and are not allowed within city limits.

Miniature pot-bellied pigs come in basic black and average anywhere from 30 to 95 pounds in weight and 12 to 18 inches in height when full-grown. The snout of these pigs tends to be longer than those of domestic pigs, and their ears stand erect. Their eyesight is not as keen as that of dogs and cats, yet they have an exceptional sense of smell. The lifespan of a MPBP is comparable to that of a cat or dog (FIG. 49-1).

As with any pet, you will want to be sure the specimen you are

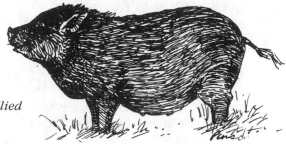

49-1   *Miniature pot-bellied pig.*

choosing is healthy before purchasing it. Health problems to outwardly look for in miniature pot-bellied pigs include obvious skin disorders, malformed snouts, breathing difficulties, retained testicles, lameness, hernias, and *atresia ani*, or incomplete development of the gastrointestinal tract. To be safe, have your veterinarian perform a physical exam on your selection prior to purchase to evaluate your pig's health status.

RESTRAINT

Because of the propensity for musculoskeletal and hip injuries, miniature pot-bellied pigs should be handled with care. When picking one up, be sure to cradle the pig's head and legs end between your own body and forearm/elbow, just as you would with a dog or cat. At the preference of most pigs, place one hand under and support the chin or throat. The legs of the pig should be allowed to hang free. Never grab or pick up a pig by its forelegs or hind legs, as this can quickly lead to joint dislocations. Get ready: Some pigs let out an ear-piercing squeal when restrained or picked up!

HOUSING

Miniature pot-bellied pigs can be housed just like a dog. However, whether kept indoors or outdoors, it is important to remember that the ideal environmental temperature for a miniature pot-bellied pig is around 70 degrees. If too cold, pigs tend to get irritable and stressed, tearing at their bedding and burrowing in order to get warm. On the other hand, if environmental temperatures get too hot, an MPBP can succumb to heat stroke quite rapidly. As a result, if a pig is to be kept outdoors, plenty of shade and fresh water should be provided. In addition, a small wading pool filled with shallow water can provide your pig with hours of wallowing enjoyment!

Finally, pigs love to root and should be provided with a source of dirt and soil in which to satisfy this instinct.

TRAINING

Miniature pot-bellied pigs are intelligent creatures that can be trained just like dogs. Training is most effective when pigs are acquired at a young age (less than 8 weeks of age) and allowed to form an emotional bond with you. Using simple commands, rewards, and praises, you can teach your pig many things: litter-training or house-breaking, leash-training, and even tricks.

NUTRITION

Miniature pot-bellied pigs should be fed commercially available rations designed for miniature pigs. Fruits, vegetables, and vitamins should be added as well to provide supplementation and variety. To avoid the dangers of salt toxicity, be sure a water source is easily accessible at all times.

REPRODUCTION

Miniature pot-bellied pigs reach puberty at 6 to 7 months of age. The heat cycle of female pigs occurs every 21 days and lasts two to three days. Your veterinarian can assist you in timing breedings between the sow and boar to achieve best results. If the breeding is successful, the gestation period for MPBPs is approximately 114 days.

Two weeks prior to parturition (*farrowing*), a noticeable "drop" in the abdomen of the sow will be noted. At this time, a farrowing crate for the sow should be provided. Contact your veterinarian for assistance in crate design and dimensions for your particular pig. Crates should be roomy enough to allow free movement of both sow and offspring. The sow can be kept in this crate until farrowing occurs. Be sure to remove her from the crate three to four times a day for exercise and eliminations.

Litter sizes can range from four to twelve, depending on the maturity of the sow. At birth, piglets weigh about 16 ounces. Because of a propensity for developing anemia, neonatal piglets should receive injections of an iron supplement daily for the first three days of life. The sharp needle teeth that these piglets possess should be clipped back as well to prevent inadvertent injury to the sow and other offspring (FIG. 49-2).

Finally, neonatal piglets are especially susceptible to hypothermia, so be sure temperatures in the environment in which these piglets are kept is maintained at around 75 to 85 degrees Fahrenheit.

HEALTH CARE

Like dogs and cats, miniature pot-bellied pigs kept as pets require routine preventative health care to keep them healthy and happy.

MPBPs should be vaccinated against common diseases seen in domestic pigs, including erysipelas, transmissible gastroenteritis (TGE), atrophic rhinitis, and leptospirosis. Piglets should be vaccinated for these diseases starting at 6 weeks of age, and again at 9 weeks of age. Booster vaccinations should be given at 6 months of age, and then annually thereafter. If you intend to breed your pigs, contact your veterinarian for special vaccination schedules for sows and boars.

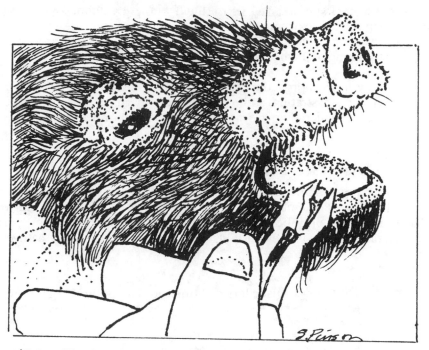

49-2   *Clipping sharp needle teeth on a miniature pot-bellied pig.*

In addition to vaccinations, pigs need to have regular stool checks for intestinal parasites. Roundworms, whipworms, and nodular worms are the most frequent parasites found inhabiting the gastrointestinal tract of these pigs. If any of these are detected, appropriate dewormers can then be administered. (Dewormers usually need to be repeated in three to four weeks.)

Miniature pigs that are to be introduced to households with dogs should be blood tested for the *pseudorabies virus*. This virus is extremely deadly to dogs, which can contract the disease from apparently healthy pigs.

Piglets less than 6 weeks of age are very prone to developing anemia and low blood sugar. Iron supplement and additional sources of glucose may be administered to prevent such problems from arising. Since most piglets are acquired as pets after this age, this is not a concern for most new miniature pig owners.

Miniature pigs should be brushed with a soft bristle brush on a daily basis to help control flaking and dry seborrhea. Hypoallergenic shampoos can be used for periodic bathing, if necessary.

Much to the jealousy of dog and cat owners, fleas have nowhere to hide on miniature pigs, so flea control is usually not an issue! However, the skin of miniature pot-bellied pigs is very sensitive to sunlight and cold, and owners should take care to shield their pig's skin from environmental temperature extremes.

Finally, periodic trimming of tusks (if present) in male pigs and cleaning and trimming of the hooves should be performed on miniature pigs as well.

Routine surgical procedures performed on miniature pot-bellied pigs include spaying, castrating, and removal of the sharp canine teeth. These procedures are generally performed at or before 4 months of age.

DISEASES AND DISORDERS OF MPBPs

The following are some selected diseases and disorders seen in miniature pot-bellied pigs. Remember that others do exist, which is why a definitive diagnosis should only be made by a qualified veterinarian. Identifying and treating diseases in their early stages is the key to successful treatment and cure.

Table 49-1   Diseases & Disorders of Miniature Pot-Bellied Pigs (MPBPs)

Disease	Clinical Signs	Treatment/Comments
	INFECTIOUS DISEASES	
Erysipelas	Characteristic red, diamond-shaped skin lesions; depression; fever; lameness; conjunctivitis.	Can lead to heart disease and arthritis if not treated early. Treat with penicillin antibiotics.
Transmissible gastroenteritis	Diarrhea; vomiting; fever; dehydration.	Caused by a coronavirus (similar to that in dogs and cats). Treat secondary problems with antibiotic and fluid support.
Leptospirosis	Depression; fever; weakness.	Causes anemia and kidney failure in affected pigs. Treatment consists of antibiotics and blood transfusions if needed.
Haemophilus	Breathing difficulties; blood-stained foam from mouth and nose; fever; coughing.	Rapidly fatal if not treated promptly with appropriate antibiotics.
	SKIN DISEASES	
Sunburn/frostbite	Reddening of the skin; ulcerations.	MPBPs quite susceptible to environmental insults.
Seborrhea	Dry, flaky skin.	Caused by nutritional deficiencies intestinal parasites, mange, environmental conditions. Treat according to cause.
Mange (mites)	Itching; small red raised bumps on skin.	Oral Ivermectin and topical dips used to treat.
Greasy pig disease	Greasy skin surface; reddened wrinkled skin; scabs; dehydration.	Caused by bacteria; highly fatal in young pigs. Treat with antibiotics.
	MUSCULOSKELETAL DISEASES	
Posterior weakness/ stiffness	Stiff gait; lameness; can't support weight on hind legs.	Conformation of MPBP and improper restraint techniques makes them prone to muscle pulls, ligament tears, hip dislocation, other musculoskeletal injuries. Treat depending on problem.

Table 49-1   Continued.

Disease	Clinical Signs	Treatment/Comments
Infectious arthritis	Stiffness; lameness; fever.	Can be caused by a variety of organisms. Treat with appropriate antibiotics.
Osteomalacia	Weakness; inability to stand.	Caused by calcium deficiency; seen in nursing or post-nursing sows.

NERVOUS SYSTEM DISEASE

Bacterial encephalitis	Depression; circling; seizures; abnormal gait and posture; blindness; aggressiveness.	Can be caused by a variety of organisms. Treat with appropriate antibiotics.
Shaker pig disease	Tremors, convulsions; shaking.	No treatment needed. Most recover spontaneously.
Salt poisoning	Depression; circling; seizures; abnormal gait and posture; blindness; aggressiveness.	Caused by water deprivation, then allowing free access to water. Treatment generally unrewarding.

RESPIRATORY SYSTEM DISEASES

Atrophic Rhinitis	Snout deformity; sneezing; bloody nasal discharge.	Associated with bacterial infections of the nasal passages in neonatal or newly weaned pigs. Infection can be treated with antibiotics, yet clinical signs often persist.
Pneumonia	Mouth breathing; bluish hue to skin.	MPBP very susceptible to pneumonia. Stress often leads to secondary bacterial infections; other causes include pseudorabies virus, roundworms, lungworms, cleft palate. Treat depending on cause.

DIGESTIVE SYSTEM DISEASES

Motion sickness, excitement, overeating	Vomiting	No treatment needed.
Neonatal diarrheal disease complex	Severe diarrhea; dehydration; abdominal distension and pain.	Can be caused by bacteria (Colibacillosis), parasites (coccidia), viruses (Transmissible Gastroenteritis virus). Treat with antibiotics, fluids.
Intestinal parasites	Bloody diarrhea; dehydration.	Can include roundworms, whipworms, nodular worms, tapeworms. Treat using appropriate dewormer.
Rectal prolapse	Prolapsed rectum; diarrhea; abdominal distension.	Caused by parasitism, chronic diarrhea and straining, coughing. Treatment involves replacing prolapse and antibiotic therapy. Treat underlying cause.
Atresia ani	Inability to defecate due to lack of external anal opening.	Congenital disease. No effective surgical treatment.

URINARY SYSTEM DISEASES

Cystitis/nephritis	Increased urination; straining to urinate; bloody urine.	Can be caused by bacterial infections, kidneyworms, toxins. Treat depending upon cause.
Prepucial diverticulum	Urine dribbling in male MPBPs.	Small pocket in prepuce traps urine and leads to clinical signs. Manually empty pocket, surgical correction of diverticulum.
Urinary calculi	Straining to urinate; bloody urine.	Surgical removal of calculi usually required.

Table 49-1 Continued.

Disease	*Clinical Signs*	*Treatment/Comments*
	REPRODUCTIVE SYSTEM DISEASES	
Cryptorchidism	One or both testicles retained within the abdomen.	Quite common; castration recommended.
Vaginitis/ uterine infections	Vaginal discharge; increased urinations; fever; depression.	Bacteria usual source of the problem. Treat with medicated douches; antibiotics.
	OTHER DISEASES	
Hernias (umbilical, inguinal, scrotal)	Soft tissue swelling or lump on belly; swollen scrotum; diarrhea; painful abdomen.	Surgical repair of hernia required.

50

Reptiles

WHILE THE THOUGHT of keeping a snake or lizard as a pet might send shivers up the spine of some, most fanciers agree that reptiles can be enjoyable and fascinating alternatives to the more conventional pet species. The husbandry involved in keeping these scaly companions healthy is not difficult. In fact, just by knowing the proper nutritional and environmental requirements for the particular reptile species in question, most health problems can be avoided.

Before obtaining a reptile as a pet, visit your local library or pet shop to read up on your particular selection. Also, you can contact your local zoo and talk to an expert on reptiles. Finally, your veterinarian should be able to supply you with valuable information concerning husbandry and health of your reptile species.

CARE OF THE PET BOA OR PYTHON

Although thousands of snake varieties exist, our discussion will be limited to the husbandry and care of the two most popular types, the boa constrictor and the python. In essence, both species are cared for in the same manner (FIG. 50-1).

Restraint

Most snakes become accustomed to being handled by their owners without any special restraint techniques. If special restraint is indicated, start by first gripping the snake just behind its head with one hand, offering you control of this region. The body should be supported with the other hand (FIG. 50-2). To be safe, never handle a very large constrictor snake if no one else is around.

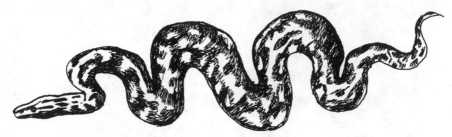

50-1   *Snakes are becoming more popular as pets.*

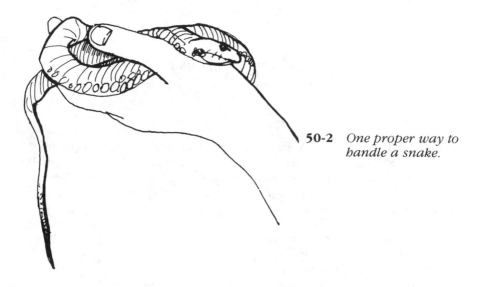

50-2   *One proper way to handle a snake.*

Shedding

Shedding is a process whereby a new skin is formed underneath an old one, with the latter discarded accordingly. It usually occurs every one to three months depending on the age and size of snake involved. Snakes that are about to shed their skin will turn "opaque" for a few days, then turn back to their normal appearance. After several days, the old skin comes off. Owners should keep careful records of the shedding activity of their snake. Any disruption in the normal shedding pattern could indicate illness and warrants the attention of a veterinarian.

To prevent inadvertent damage to the new skin, do not handle snakes undergoing the shedding process until shedding is completed. If an incomplete shed occurs, place your snake in a shallow water bowl and soak the non-shed regions for one to two hours. This should help the shedding to completion.

Occasionally, the skin covering the eyes of a snake will fail to be shed with the rest of the skin. These retained eyecaps might need to be manually removed. However, this should only be performed with the help of a qualified veterinarian, since, if done incorrectly, this procedure can permanently damage your snake's eyes.

Housing

Pet boas and pythons can be housed in ordinary glass aquariums with a secured wire-mesh top to prevent inadvertent escape. Just keep in mind that the most crucial factor in providing a proper artificial environment for any reptile is temperature. In the wild, reptiles regulate their body temperatures (as necessary for various physiological functions) by changing their position in accordance with changes in environmental temperatures. As a result, snakes might choose to bask in the sun on a branch or rock to raise their body temperature, or to crawl into the shade to lower their body temperature. In captivity, these options should remain. For this reason, the cage you keep your snake in should provide both warmer and cooler regions.

An incandescent light bulb with a reflector can be positioned over one end of the cage containing a basking branch or rock. Temperatures in this region should remain between 78 and 85 degrees Fahrenheit. An aquarium thermometer placed on the aquarium glass can be used to monitor this temperature. This light and heat source should be kept on at least 10 hours a day. Commercially available "hot rocks" should not be used to supplement warmth since these could burn the underside of your snake.

Artificial turf, which is non-abrasive and easy to clean, is an ideal substrate to use on the floor of your snake's aquarium. Excretions should be picked up daily, and the flooring should be removed, cleaned, and disinfected at least three times a week for sanitary purposes. Chlorhexidine diluted 1:10 with water is an ideal disinfectant for this purpose. After cleaning, be sure to dry the turf completely before placing it back into the cage. Failure to do so could predispose your snake to skin disease.

Other items needed for your snake's cage include a water bowl big enough for the snake to crawl into and some type of hiding place or small enclosure to be placed at the cool end of the aquarium.

Nutrition

Young, growing snakes should be fed at least twice weekly. As snakes mature, their feedings can be dropped to once a week, and then every two to three weeks. Standard food items for snakes include mice, rats, chicks, and rabbits, depending upon the size of the snake. If at all possible, do not serve live prey to your snake. Even the smallest of prey, if hostile enough, can cause serious, even life-threatening injuries to a snake. Instead, offer prey that is already dead (and harmless) prior to feeding. If live prey can't be avoided, stay with your snake until the kill has been made.

Handling your snake during and within two days following a meal should be avoided to avoid undo stress during the digestive process. In addition, many snakes might become irritable during this time, and might bite!

Owners should keep careful records of the feeding activity of their snake. In this way, loss of appetite or any disruption in the normal feeding habits caused by illness can be noticed and addressed promptly.

CARE OF THE PET IGUANA

Iguanas belong to the family of reptiles called, not surprisingly, *Iguanidae*. Out of this family, the most popular member to be kept as a pet is the green iguana. Fascinating creatures to watch and handle, iguanas as pets are hardy and fairly easy to care for. This is assuming, of course, that the owner is well-versed in the environmental and nutritional needs of these special reptiles (FIG. 50-3).

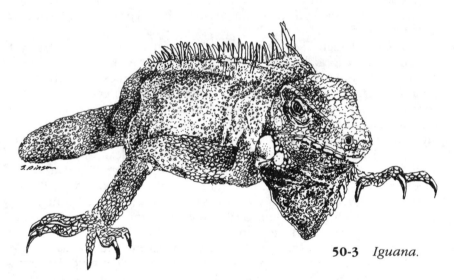

50-3 *Iguana.*

Restraint

Green iguanas are incredibly strong for their size and can be difficult to handle if they have other ideas! When restraining iguanas, grasp the neck area and control the forelegs all with one hand; the other hand should encircle the belly of the lizard and be used to control the back feet as well. Never pick up an iguana by its tail. If you do, you might find yourself holding the tail and your iguana scurrying off in the other direction!

Housing

Like the snake, the green iguana may be kept in an aquarium or other similar enclosure. Again, remember that the most important factor in a proper artificial environment for any reptile is temperature. See the section on snakes in this chapter for more details.

Another item needed to keep your iguana happy and healthy is an ultraviolet (UV) black light. These can be ordered through most pet stores or hardware stores. Since a green iguana kept in captivity is deprived of natural sunlight, it requires this artificial means of ultraviolet rays in order to synthesize vitamin D in its skin. If not enough of this vitamin D is synthesized, nutritional bone disease can result. Contrary to popular belief, placing your pet's enclosure next to a sunny window is not sufficient, since glass can interfere with the effective transmission and absorption of the sun's ultraviolet rays.

The black light should be mounted next to the incandescent light source, about 12 inches above the iguana's basking site. As with the latter, approximately 10 hours of this light should be provided on a daily basis. Black lights should be replaced every six months for maximum effectiveness.

Nutrition

Nutritionally related bone disease due to poor feeding practices is common in green iguanas kept in captivity. Contrary to popular belief, iguanas can't survive on just lettuce alone! They should receive a varied diet consisting of:

○ 70% vegetables, such as dark green lettuce, spinach, broccoli, squash, carrots, tomatoes, etc.

○ 15% fruit, such as bananas and pears

○ 15% canned dog food

○ a calcium supplement such as bone meal (for pets, not plants); ground oyster shell, or a similar substance; sprinkled on the vegetables for added protection against nutritional bone disease.

CARE OF THE PET TURTLE

Turtles are another popular type of reptilian pet. They belong to the reptilian order *Chelonia*, with hundreds of different species existing. The most common turtles kept as pets include box turtles, water turtles, and snapping turtles (FIG. 50-4).

Restraint

Most turtles can be easily and safely handled by grasping the edges of the shell with one hand and supporting the underside of the turtle, or plastron, with the other. Note, however, that snapping turtles and certain other species of turtles do require special precautions when lifting or handling to avoid being bitten and/or scratched. For instance, the only way that snapping turtles should be picked up is by the base of the tail. Since turtles can't reach around and bite too easily because of their shell, this approach is the safest. Other less friendly turtles can be handled safely by grasping the sides of the shell near the hind end.

50-4 *Turtle.*

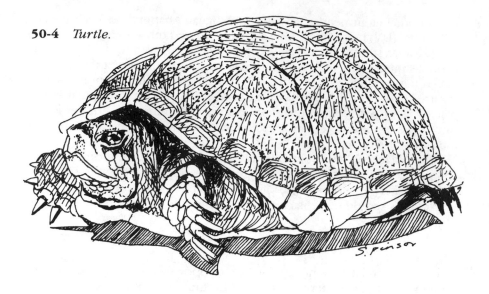

Housing

Turtles can be kept in an aquarium or other similar enclosure. Aquatic turtles obviously need water in which to swim and feed. It needn't be deep; just enough for the turtle to be able to submerge itself. Branches or ledges suitable for climbing and basking should be provided for both aquatic and land turtles. Enclosures should be thoroughly cleaned and, if applicable, the water should be changed, on a weekly basis.

Turtles, like other reptiles, regulate body temperature according to physiological needs. As a result, a simple setup including an incandescent light bulb and reflector over one end of the cage or aquarium should be used to create a "hot spot" of around 80-85 degrees in that area, preferably over a branch for basking. The other end of the enclosure should be kept cooler.

The light-heat source might be attached to a timing device to automatically turn it on and off. In addition to the heat source, a source of ultraviolet light, such as a black light, should be provided to enable the turtle to synthesize its own vitamin D within its body, thereby preventing nutritionally related bone disease (see Green Iguana).

Nutrition

The diet of aquatic turtles, or those with webbed feet, should consist of a variety of foodstuffs—fish, worms, fruits, and vegetables. If desired, a solid or semisolid high-quality dog food can be fed in place of or supplemented with the first two ingredients.

Aquatic turtles like to eat their meals while in the water. Box turtles, on the other hand, prefer to eat on land. They, too, enjoy and need the same type of well-balanced diet as do their aquatic cousins. Just remember: The key to a nutritional diet is variety. Turtles fed just meat items or just vegetable items are prone to nutritional deficiencies and disease.

DISEASES AND DISORDERS OF REPTILES

The vast majority of diseases and disorders seen in reptiles kept as pets are caused by improper living environments (i.e., improper temperatures) and poor nutrition. If your pet is exhibiting clinical signs or any type of strange behavior, take it to your veterinarian immediately for a checkup. If your veterinarian does not work on reptiles, ask him or her to refer you to one in your area who does. Identifying and treating diseases in their early stages is the key to successful treatment and cure. Below are some of the more common diseases and disorders seen in reptiles. Others do exist, which is why a definitive diagnosis should only be made by a veterinarian.

Table 50-1   Diseases & Disorders of Reptiles

Disease	*Reptiles affected* *	*Clinical Signs*	*Treatment/Comments*
Vitamin D deficiency	I, T	"Rubber jaw;" limb and spine deformities; fractures; paralysis.	Review and correct diet—vitamin/ mineral supplement. Provide source of ultraviolet light.
Vitamin D excess	I	General malaise; bone abnormalities.	Over-use of vitamin D supplement. Treat by discontinuing supplement.
Nutritional secondary hyperparathyroidism	I, T	Same as above.	Caused by calcium/phosphorus imbalances. Treatment same as above.
Gout	I	Lameness; general malaise.	Caused by improper diet, water deprivation, kidney disease. No treatment.
Vitamin A deficiency	T	Swollen eyelids; eye and nose discharge; breathing difficulties.	Seen in turtles fed all-meat or all-vegetable diets. Treat by changing diet, vitamin A supplement, antibiotics.
Pneumonia	I, T, S	Gaping and breathing difficulties; nasal discharge; swollen eyelids.	Can be caused by bacteria, fungi, or parasites. Treatment depends on cause.
Skin parasites (mites, ticks, etc.)	I, T, S	Variable, including weakness, loss of appetite.	Can cause anemia. Treat locally with safe insecticide.
Retained eye cap	S	Eye opacity, irritation.	May be retained after shedding. Moisten, then peel off gently.
Mouth rot (infectious stomatitis)	S	Loss of appetite; open-mouth gaping; white discharge within the mouth.	Occurs secondarily to mouth trauma and other diseases. Treatment involves local flushing and antibiotics.
Amoebiasis	I, T, S	Loss of appetite; regurgitation; loose, abnormal stool; weight loss.	Seen in reptiles kept in groups; can be spread by cockroaches. Treat with amoebicide and antibiotics.
Septicemia	I, T, S	Loss of appetite; weakness; lack of muscle tone.	Often secondary to stress and other diseases. Treat using antibiotics and correcting underlying cause.
Lumps and bumps	I, T, S	Abnormal body shape; lumps and bumps.	Suspect food ingestion, eggs, abscesses, tumors.

* I = Iguana
 T = Turtle
 S = Snake

51

Aquariums and Tropical Fish

LOOKING FOR A RELATIVELY low-maintenance pet that doesn't eat much, requires no training whatsoever, and will not bring fleas into your house? Welcome to the world of tropical fish. More and more, these fascinating aquatic creatures are finding their way into the hearts of pet lovers all across the country. In fact, it is estimated that, at some time or another, aquariums have adorned approximately one out of three households in the United States alone.

Another key indicator of the popularity of tropical fish in this country is the amount of money spent on them each year. Retail sales of tropical fish and supplies are well over $500 million per year, with no signs of stopping. So what makes these scaly creatures so fashionable as pets? What's the attraction to owning an aquarium filled with tropical fish?

To begin, aquariums, especially the fresh-water variety, are really quite easy to care for, regardless of what some people might say. With a basic knowledge of aquarium management and tropical fish husbandry, anyone can successfully create and propagate a self-contained aquatic environment. Tropical fish themselves are virtually maintenance-free, requiring only food and a clean, suitable environment in which to live. Unlike man's best friend, they don't require lots of attention on your part, yet you'll find that once you have your aquarium started they'll receive loads of it nonetheless (FIG. 51-1).

Maintaining an aquarium filled with tropical fish is a relatively inexpensive endeavor when compared to other types of pet ownership. Aside from initial start-up costs needed for equipment and supplies—which can run you anywhere from $30 to $500, depending on the size and quality of set-up that you buy—the yearly cost of food, maintenance, and fish

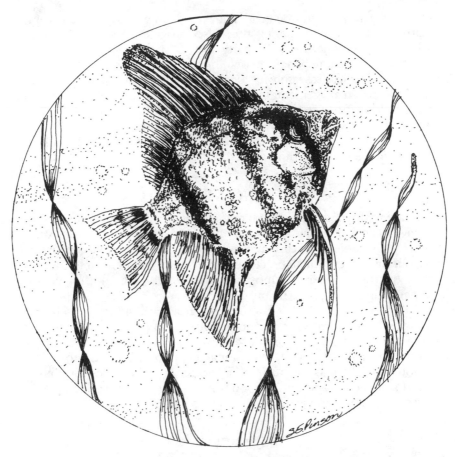

51-1 *Aquariums and tropical fish can provide hours of enjoyment and relaxation.*

replacements place little strain on the average household's budget. Sure, some tropical fish can cost hundreds, even thousands of dollars a piece! But on the average, the hobbyist can expect to pay anywhere from 50 cents to $10 a piece for tropical fish, depending, of course, on species.

Fish do not require yearly vaccinations and checkups by veterinarians to keep them healthy—which, as any responsible dog or cat owner knows, can add considerably to the owners yearly pet expense account. (Researchers are currently working on vaccines for tropical fish, especially for one against the dreaded fish disease commonly known as *Ich*.)

Finally, people who own tropical fish as pets can plan on reaping the same benefits and sharing in the same joy and satisfaction that come with owning a pet. Aquariums can provide their caretakers with entertainment for hours on end and can contribute to our knowledge of an environmental ecosystem so very different from our own. As educational tools for children, aquariums can't be beat. They are a fun way to teach kids about aquatic life and environments; they also provide a means of teaching responsible pet ownership at an early age.

There is one more benefit to owning an aquarium that you might find fascinating. Medical research has actually shown that aquariums can be effective stress-management tools. That is, reduced anxiety levels and lowered blood pressure can result from spending just a few minutes each day observing the steady, flowing movement of aquarium life. Considering today's hectic world, this benefit alone is a good enough reason to rush out and get an aquarium started right away!

GETTING STARTED

There are two types of aquarium environments that tropical fish hobbyists have to choose from: freshwater and saltwater. Since the latter variety require a greater level of care and expertise (and expense) to ensure success, our discussion, for all practical purposes, will limit itself to the freshwater aquarium. This is the most popular type by far, and, for children and beginning hobbyists, the most practical.

In order to create a first-rate freshwater aquarium for yourself or for your kids, you'll need to spend some money on proper equipment and supplies. Of course, the foremost piece of equipment you'll need to obtain is the tank itself, along with ancillary supplies such as substrate for the bottom of the tank, plants (real or artificial), and fixtures for your fish to use for shelter. In addition, a good water-quality control system, including water filtration and aeration devices, is a must.

Aquarium tanks

Aquarium tanks themselves come in all shapes and sizes, from small goldfish bowls to 200-gallon reservoirs. Obviously, the size of the aquarium will dictate how many fish will be allowed to cohabit within, as well as the amount of time necessary for care and cleaning. Regardless of the gallon capacity that you choose (the 10- and 20-gallon varieties are the most popular), it's best to select a tank that is rectangular in shape instead of one that is round or one that is tall and narrow, since the amount of oxygen exchange that occurs between the outside air and the water in the tank is directly proportional to the size of the air-water interface dictated by the shape of the tank (FIG. 51-2). Tropical fish thrive much better in tanks with large surface areas on top, simply because the oxygen levels in these tanks are greater. If a bowl-type aquarium is to be used, be sure to fill it only to the half-way mark with water, in order to achieve the greatest possible surface area for this exchange of oxygen between the air and the water to take place.

Try to avoid aquarium tanks that use metal in their frame construction. Metal, exposed to water over a period of time, could corrode and become a major source of contamination of your tank water. The more

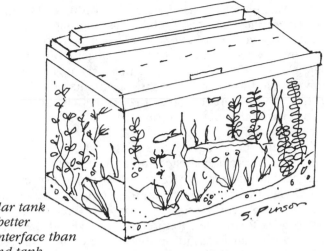

51-2 *A rectangular tank allows for better air-water interface than does a round tank.*

glass in the tank, the better. In fact, aquarium tanks composed entirely of glass with silicone-adhesed edges and corners are preferred over others. Some enthusiasts prefer plexiglass over glass, simply because of its durability, but the biggest disadvantage to plexiglass is that it tends to scratch easily and can become quite unsightly over time. This can be especially true after a number of abrasive cleanings.

Your aquarium tank should come with a cover—again, preferably made of glass—with a hinged access door. The purpose of aquarium covers is to keep dust, silt, and other airborne contaminants out of the water, and to keep the fish in! Some of the fancier models come equipped with light sources and reflectors, which not only can play a useful role in the temperature regulation within the tank, but are also desirable if you so choose to propagate live plants and vegetation within the aquarium setting.

Ancillary supplies

Two inches of gravel, stone, pebble, or sand can be used as a bottom liner for your tank to provide an anchoring substrate for plants and shelters and to serve as anchoring points for the tank's biological filter (explained later). The choice between real and artificial plants is entirely up to you. The main advantage of artificial over natural is ease of maintenance and durability. However, for a more aesthetic and natural look to your aquarium environment, live flora can't be beat.

If you'll recall Biology 101, live plants can act as a source of oxygen for your fish through the process called photosynthesis. They also provide a source of food to some fish, as well as a place to lay their eggs. If you desire real vegetation over the artificial kind, you'll need to be sure to match it with the type of fish you want to keep in the aquarium. For more information about proper matching, ask a local tropical fish dealer or aquarium shop, or consult your local library or bookstore.

Using live plants also means that you'll need to provide a light source for them; these can be purchased as one with your aquarium cover. It's best to use artificial light sources such as fluorescent lighting (approximately 3 watts per gallon of water) instead of natural lighting, since the latter can be difficult to regulate properly. Eight to ten hours of light each day should be enough to allow your plants to thrive in their watery environment. Be aware, however, that too much lighting is not good and can cause harmful temperature fluctuations within the tank, not to mention excessive algae growth.

Finally, every aquarium needs a variety of fixtures and structures designed to provide shelter and security for its finned inhabitants. You can certainly be creative in this department; however, you must also use some caution. If the object you're placing in the aquarium is made of plastic instead of glass, be sure it is nontoxic (including artificial plants!). The same goes for painted fixtures. To be safe, these items should be purchased from an aquarium supply house or store instead of trying to supply them yourself from everyday household items.

WATER QUALITY CONTROL

Before you introduce any fish into your new aquarium, you must make certain that the water you're going to be putting them in is of the highest quality possible. Now this doesn't mean that you'll need to invest in any expensive purification systems or purchase stock in a bottled water company. On the contrary, ordinary tap water from the kitchen faucet works just fine as a water source for your aquarium. However, there are some measures you need to take to ensure that this water is (and, once in the aquarium, remains) of satisfactory quality to ensure success.

Using tap water

Ordinary tap water is often classified as being either "hard" or "soft," depending on the amounts of minerals dissolved within. Test kits are available from aquarium shops that can tell you whether your water supply is hard or soft. Most tropical fish prefer water that is on the soft end (about 40-60 ppm); therefore, if you live in an area with hard water, make sure it is softened before being introduced into the tank. There are several ways to do this. First, the most efficient way (and the most expensive way) is to purchase a water softener that can be hooked into to your house's water supply, and will provide a continuous supply of softened water. Other alternatives to purchasing one of these machines or filters include boiling the water first to remove the mineral deposits, and adding distilled water to your untreated water to effectively dilute out the hardness.

In addition to correcting water hardness, you must also neutralize or remove the chlorine normally found in most water supplies before introducing fish. You can add store-bought tablets or powders designed specifically for chlorine removal, or you can simply let the tap water to be used set out exposed to the air for 24 to 36 hours. Doing so allows the chlorine content of the exposed water to evaporate into the surrounding air.

Water temperature

Water temperature is a vital parameter that warrants a fish owner's special attention. In fact, improper maintenance of water temperature is one of the more common causes of failure that amateurs encounter. Just because fish are called tropical fish doesn't necessarily mean that they automatically thrive in warmer temperatures. In fact, warmer water carries less oxygen, and some of the more sensitive species of tropical fish will do quite poorly in excessively warm water. As a general rule, most tropical fish do well with water temperatures maintained around 74 to 78 degrees Fahrenheit. However, before purchasing many different types of fish for your tank, it would be wise to find out at what temperature is each species most at home. If the temperature ranges differ significantly, then one is going to suffer at the expense of the other.

Marked or rapid temperature fluctuations should be avoided at all costs, since these can be quite harmful to fish. Keep this in mind when replacing water within the aquarium; be sure the water you add is at the same temperature as the existing tank water. And don't worry about the natural thermal layers associated with water; your aerator pump will keep the water circulating enough to prevent significant temperature gradients from being established.

The best way to maintain narrow temperature margins within your tank is to invest in an aquarium water heater and a good, quality thermometer. If possible, avoid mercury thermometers. Though they are quite accurate, should the thermometer break and the mercury enter the water, your entire fish population could be fatally poisoned within a matter of minutes.

Oxygen supply

Fish, like people, rely on oxygen to sustain life. And since fish rely on their water supply for this source of oxygen, it stands to reason that the aquarium enthusiast be sure that the oxygen supply remains adequate. The most common method of ensuring well-oxygenated aquarium water is to install an aerator pump within the tank. These water aerators draw in air from the outside and "bubble" it into the water, helping to stimulate oxygen exchange. The circulating action of these pumps also helps to increase total water contact with the outside air at the surface of the tank, thereby allowing greater amounts of oxygen to be absorbed into the system. An efficient aerator pump should exchange about 2 liters of air per 1 liter of water every hour.

One interesting point to remember is that the fish are literally breathing the air you breathe; nicotine, fumes, and other pollutants in the air being pumped into the aquarium can have adverse effects on the health of some fish. As a result, take care to shelter your aquarium away from those obvious sources of air contaminants.

Live plants, which release oxygen into their surrounding environment through photosynthesis, can also make a significant contribution to the oxygen levels within the aquarium. Also, keeping water temperatures from becoming warmer than the desired ranges and preventing fish overcrowding can both have a positive impact on this aspect of water quality.

Again, the very shape you choose for your aquarium tank (remember the air-water interface?) can directly affect the oxygen content of the water, and hence, its overall quality.

Filter systems

In addition to water aeration pumps, a filter system is needed within the aquarium to remove solid and chemical contaminates from the water before they build up to harmful levels. These filters can be classified as either mechanical filters or biological filters. Mechanical filters hook on to the outside (or sometimes inside) of the aquarium and actively pump water through a filtering substance, such as filter wool or activated charcoal. Ideally, the capacity of the filter should be such that the entire water content of the tank can pass through it and be filtered about every two hours. If mechanical filters are used, its important to replace the filter material on a regular basis, preferably every three weeks.

The other type of filter is the biological filter. Compared with a good mechanical filter, which can run you anywhere from $30 to $100 (or more!), the cost of a biological filter is negligible. Yet they can be an even more effective weapon at waste control than their mechanical, more expensive counterparts. These filters consist of nothing more than a porous tray that is placed beneath the gravel or substrate lining the bottom of the aquarium and serves as a gathering site for bacteria normally found within the tank. These bacteria are ''biological garbage gobblers'' and break down organic wastes that are passively carried through the filter by normal water circulation within the tank. In this way, Nature does the cleaning for you, the natural way!

Aquarium filters function to keep levels of ammonia and nitrites, two highly toxic substances derived from organic waste, within acceptable ranges. Ideally, the pH of the water should be kept somewhere around 6.8 to 7.5, and nitrite levels should be kept to an absolute minimum. Special test kits are available from aquarium shops and should be used to monitor these parameters. Unhealthy rises in pH and nitrite levels in newly established aquariums can often be traced back to an underdeveloped biological filter. Overcrowding and overfeeding can play a significant role as well and should be corrected if indeed present.

Because new biological filters can take three to six weeks to become fully established and functional, daily water rotations (explained below) might be required to dilute out the offending substances.

Regardless of whether you use a mechanical filter, a biological filter, or both, you should still plan on replacing 20% of the water within the tank with seasoned tap water (hardness and chlorine removed) every six weeks or so. This will help eliminate impurities that can't be filtered properly, as well as help ease the burden on the filters themselves. Remember: Change only 20% at a time, not the entire tank, to prevent from upsetting the environmental equilibrium that has already been established in the aquarium.

Cleaning your aquarium

How often does an aquarium need to be cleaned? The answer to this is almost never, assuming of course that the water quality control measures above are kept in force. Aeration, filtration, periodic partial water changes, and scavenger fish (explained below) should do the cleaning for you on a continual basis. Keeping the cover closed on your aquarium will prevent dust and dirt from the outside from scumming up the water.

Finally, algae growth is best kept under control by avoiding excessive lighting, and by preventing overcrowding and overfeeding. If you don't mind getting your hands wet, abrasive, soap-free cleaning pads are quite useful for scraping off any algae that may accumulate on the aquarium glass, artificial plants, or stationary fixtures within your tank.

SELECTING FISH FOR YOUR AQUARIUM

Once you've ensured the quality of the aquarium water, only then are you ready to stock your tank with fish. Now how do you pick between the hundreds of different tropical fish available on the market? The choice is really a matter of your preference and taste. Some people prefer ones with exotic coloring or patterns; others prefer larger varieties over the smaller ones. In addition, some species are more sensitive and delicate than others, and might require greater attention and maintenance than you are willing to devote.

One thing you'll want to be very careful of is not to overstock your aquarium with fish. Tank overcrowding is right up there with poor water quality and temperature fluctuations as a major cause of aquarium failures. As a general rule, you should have no more than 1 inch of fish per 1 gallon of water. Exceed this ratio, and oxygen content and water quality will noticeably suffer.

The various tropical fish species are often classified into groups according to their aggressiveness. For instance, goldfish, guppies, mollies, and platies are all known for their mild-mannered temperaments, whereas red-tailed sharks and Siamese fighting fish can be group-categorized as semiaggressive. Cichlids are highly aggressive fish and won't hesitate to pick a fight with any fish in the tank. Regardless of which species you prefer, don't mix aggressive or semiaggressive fish with nonaggressive fish in the same aquarium settings, for obvious reasons. In fact, if you decide to stock your tank with more aggressive varieties, you'll need to watch individual personalities closely, to prevent your serene, peaceful aquarium setting from becoming a battleground!

Besides the more ornamental varieties, you'll want to stock your aquarium with, for lack of a better word, a *scavenger* species. These fish tend to inhabit the bottom of the tank or cling to its sides, and they feed on the algae and unused food particles that float to the bottom of the aquarium. Scavenger fish play an important role in helping to maintain water quality and should not be overlooked when selecting stock. Some of the more popular names include the *Corydorus* genus of catfish, the suckermouth cats, and the coolie loach. Large, freshwater snails can also be introduced into an aquarium setting and are effective scavenger tools as well.

What to look for

When picking out your fish at the aquarium shop or pet store, there are a few items to look for to ensure that you receive healthy specimens. First, observe the way a particular fish behaves in its current aquarium setting. It should be active and alert and glide smoothly through the water when swimming. Fish that act lethargic or swim in a crooked or sideways pattern should be avoided.

Anatomically, all fins should be erect and intact, and the fish's belly should be slightly rounded versus sunken. Look for blotchy, discolored skin, ulcerations, or any other obvious signs of disease or parasitism. If one fish in a particular tank is showing signs of illness, assume all within that tank have been exposed to the disease, and avoid selecting fish from that tank altogether (FIG. 51-3).

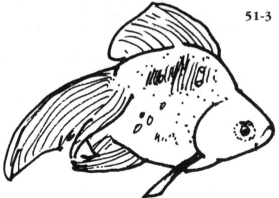

51-3   *Skin diseases can spread rapidly through an aquarium.*

Your fish's new home

Once you've purchased your new friends, you'll want to slowly introduce them to their new home. Again, be sure all pumps and filters are in place and in working order. The transport container with fish inside should be lowered into the tank water, which should already be at the desired temperature (check your thermometer). Leave the container suspended like this for a good 15 to 20 minutes to allow for a gradual temperature equalization between the separated waters. Once this is accomplished, open the container and allow the fish, at their leisure, to enter into their new domain.

Aquarium owners should make it point to keep handling and disturbances to a minimum once the fish are in—and this includes that common urge among beginners to tap on the aquarium glass to get a particular fish's attention! Suppressing this type of behavior will help keep stress levels low and make for a much healthier, happier environment.

If for some reason a fish needs to be removed from the tank, small nets are commercially available for this purpose. Or, as an alternative, a plastic storage bag with small holes punched in its bottom makes an excellent fish-catcher. Regardless of which you use, be as slow, deliberate, and patient as possible when trying to capture one; again, to keep stress to an absolute minimum.

Feeding your fish

Pre-packaged fish food is readily available, and comes in all forms and fashions, such as processed, frozen, or freeze-dried. As a general rule, you should feed only that amount of food that will be consumed within a three to four minute period. Leftovers are not good, and will eventually build up to such levels at the bottom as to start adversely affecting the water quality within the tank. Finally, two feedings, one in the morning and one in the afternoon, should suffice to satisfy even the heartiest of appetites!

DISEASES AND DISORDERS OF TROPICAL FISH

Below are selected diseases and disorders seen in tropical fish. Healthy fish should have smooth, glistening skin surfaces and should exhibit steady, controlled movement within the aquarium. Diseased fish, aside from exhibiting obvious external signs, will exhibit unusual swimming and behavioral patterns. For instance, excessive drifting, circling, hiding, curling, or bottom-sitting are all signs of disease and should alert you to a potential problem.

Poor water quality and failure to quarantine new additions to the aquarium are the two leading factors in diseases of aquarium fish. If you suffer from a disease outbreak in your aquarium, it is important that you quickly identify the problem and institute treatment proceedings immediately. Treatment for disease outbreaks generally consists of isolation of infected fish, partial or complete (including that beneath the gravel layers) water changes performed on a periodic basis, and/or the addition of medications to the water supply.

If you are having problems keeping your fish healthy, contact your local veterinarian for advice. If he/she is not versed in aquarium management and fish diseases, he/she can direct you to the proper resources you need to answer questions and lead to a solution.

Table 51-1   Diseases & Disorders of Tropical Fish

Disease	Clinical Signs	Treatment/Comments
	DISEASES RELATED TO WATER QUALITY	
Ammonia/nitrite toxicity	Death of existing fish; inability to keep new additions alive.	Caused by improper biological filters. Treat by establishing filter; daily water change for 2-3 weeks to keep ammonia/nitrite concentrations low.
	PARASITIC DISEASES	
Ich (Ichthyophthirius)	White spots or pustules on skin.	Known as "White Spot Disease." Treat by complete water changes daily for one week.
Chilodenella; other protozoans; flukes	Excessive body mucus production; damaged gills; irritable behavior; gill rubbing.	Treat by adding formalin to water (1 ml/10 gallons of water), then changing water 8 hours later. Fish in terminal stages of illness could die from treatment.
Hexamita	General unthriftiness; white, stringy feces; thinning.	Common in Angelfish. Treat with metronidazole (250mg/10 gallons of water).
"Hole in the Head"	Ulcerations on head and sides of body.	May be associated with Hexamita. Treat with frequent water changes, metronidazole. Rarely causes death.
Tapeworms	General unthriftiness; thinning.	Treat by adding the drug praziquantel to water (90mg/10 gallons of water).
	BACTERIAL DISEASES	
Aeromonas Pseudomonas	Ulcerations on skin; unthriftiness.	Often occur secondary to parasites or other diseases. Treat with antibiotics added to water.
Columnaris disease	Gray-white patches on skin; fraying/loss of fins and tail.	Treat with frequent water changes and antibiotics to the water.
Septicemia	Reddish hue to skin; lethargy; unthriftiness; bulging eyes.	Treat with antibiotics generally unrewarding; improve water quality.
	VIRAL DISEASES	
Lymphocystis disease	White, raised plaques on surface of skin and tail.	No treatment available. Isolate infected fish; sanitize aquarium.

HEALTH & LONGEVITY OF DOGS & CATS

52

Increasing
Your Pet's Longevity

BY NOW, MOST OF US realize that eating a proper diet, getting plenty of exercise, and avoiding cigarettes can add years to our lives. Well, believe it or not, the same also holds true for our canine and feline friends. Because of recent advancements in veterinary medicine and a growing public awareness about responsible pet ownership, dogs and cats are living longer today than they were ten years ago. Want to find the fountain of youth for your pet? The following tips can lead you down the right path (FIG. 52-1).

Longevity Tip #1:
DON'T LET YOUR PET GET OVERWEIGHT

Obesity causes the same ill effects in pets as it does in people. Pets pushing the scales to their maximums are more prone to, among other things, heart disease, kidney disease, liver disease, and diabetes. They also tend to become sluggish, easily tired, and seem to just crave more and more food (sounds familiar, doesn't it?).

The two biggest culprits underlying obesity in dogs and cats are indiscriminate feeding practices and lack of exercise. Feeding table scraps is probably the worst thing you could do for your pet. Not only do these snacks upset the nutritional balance, but they're often the cause of gastrointestinal disturbances in these pets. Not only that, you're going to create a pet that constantly begs for food, which always goes over big when you're entertaining the neighbors for dinner.

If your pet is indeed fat, simply cutting back on snacks and the amount of food you feed might not be enough. However, there are some

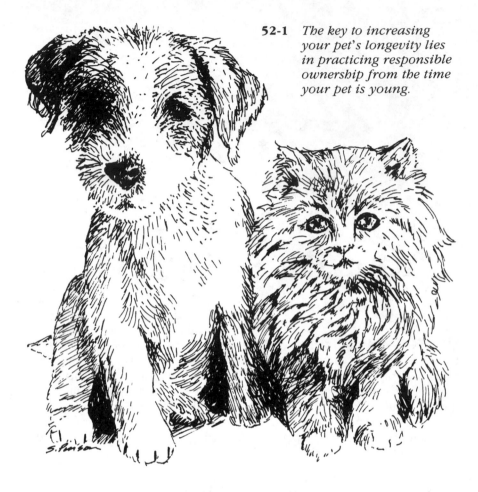

52-1 *The key to increasing your pet's longevity lies in practicing responsible ownership from the time your pet is young.*

great weight-loss diets available that can help your pet lose the added poundage while at the same time satisfying its appetite. Ask your veterinarian for a recommendation on such a diet, since requirements could vary depending upon the age of your pet.

Longevity Tip #2:
FEED YOUR PET A QUALITY DIET

No matter what the pet food companies tell you, you can't beat the new premium-type pet foods on the market today. Lots of research and little filler go into these products, making them popular recommendations of veterinarians across the country. You have many types and brands to choose from; adult formulas, growth formulas, geriatric formulas, and light formulas. The choice is yours. However, when in doubt as to which would be best for your pet, don't hesitate to ask your veterinarian. And though the expense of such rations seems inflated at first, most dog and cat owners find that the amounts consumed per feeding are much less than those for the non-premium foods used previously, making the actual per-feeding cost for the two about the same.

Longevity Tip #3:
KEEP THOSE TEETH CLEANED

Excessive dental tartar and gingivitis play important roles in heart and kidney disease in pets. To make matters worse, most pets show signs of periodontal (tooth and gum) disease by the time they're only 3 years of age! This is why its so important to keep your pet's dental tartar under control.

Simply feeding your pets hard food or biscuits won't do the trick. In fact, foodstuffs such as these actually promote plaque and tartar formation, and subsequent periodontal disease. Surprised? You shouldn't be. Just think about what your teeth would be like if you never brushed your teeth or had a dental cleaning performed, and I think you'll get the picture.

You should have a dental checkup performed on your pet every time you visit your veterinarian (at least annually). If necessary, have your pet's teeth professionally cleaned and polished while you're there. Afterwards, when you get your pet home, make it a point to incorporate some type of dental care into its daily routine, be it brushing with toothpastes formulated for pets or using special pet mouthwashes. These and other dental items can be purchased at your favorite pet store or veterinary office.

Longevity Tip #4:
OFFER YOUR PET PLENTY OF EXERCISE

Exercise affords the same benefits to dogs and cats as it does to us, namely cardiovascular fitness and weight control. Twenty to thirty minutes of moderate exercise daily (walking, chasing the frisbee or toy mouse, etc.) will help keep your pet slim, trim, and healthy (FIG. 52-2).

Jogging with your dog is fine also. Just remember that unless you own a Russian Wolfhound, stride-for-stride, your dog is going to have to work harder than you do, so be sure you don't over-do it. Heat-stroke and/or musculoskeletal injuries can be unfortunate sequelas to such marathon running sessions.

Cats that are leash-trained from the start can have their weights also regulated through exercise. For those that are not, a designated daily play session will help fulfill this role.

As a corollary to this longevity tip: Give your dog or cat plenty of attention each day. The easiest way to stress-out your pet is to ignore it. So keep this in mind the next time you come home from work, and be sure to devote just five minutes to saying hello to your furry companion.

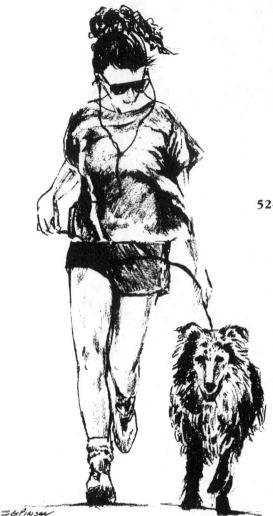

52-2 *Daily exercise can help your pet live longer.*

Longevity Tip #5:
TRAIN YOUR PET PROPERLY

If you do this, it'll help keep your dog off of the street—literally. Dogs that dart off despite their owner's commands to the contrary, or dig escape tunnels out of their backyards, are prime candidates for being hit by a car.

Pet owners need to teach their dogs to respond to the basic commands of stop, sit, stay, and heel. No dog is too old to be taught these commands, yet for those old, crusty canines set firmly in their ways, a good obedience school might be just what the doctor ordered.

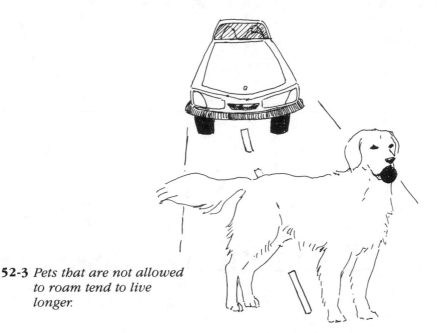

52-3 *Pets that are not allowed to roam tend to live longer.*

Longevity Tip #6:
MAKE YOUR PET AN INDOOR PET

Make no mistake about it: Pets kept indoors are healthier overall than those kept outdoors. For instance, indoor dogs are psychologically healthier owing to an increased contact with their owners. In addition, they are much less prone to physical illnesses such as infectious diseases, skin disorders, gastroenteritis induced by dietary indiscretions, and environmentally induced afflictions such as heat stroke.

Along the same lines, making your cat an indoor pet will significantly reduce its risk of contracting deadly diseases such as feline leukemia, feline infectious peritonitis, and the newest scourge, feline AIDS.

Finally, confining your dog or cat to the house will also reduce the risks that hostile car fenders pose as well (FIG. 52-3).

Longevity Tip #7:
PRACTICE PREVENTATIVE HEALTH CARE

Preventative health care includes keeping your dog or cat current on its vaccinations, parasite checks, and routine checkups, as well as heeding those longevity tips previously mentioned.

Also, if you haven't already done so, consider having your pet neutered. Besides the benefit of population control, there are health benefits as well. For females, the risks of mammary cancer are reduced with neutering. For males, neutering reduces aggressiveness and anxiety, making them better house pets!

53

Zoonotic Diseases

"DOCTOR, I THINK MY DOG has a cold. Can I catch it?" In veterinary practices across the country, questions such as this one are not at all unusual. And though the answer to this particular question is no, there are numerous other diseases that can indeed be transmitted from family pets to unsuspecting owners. Such diseases are properly termed *zoonotic diseases*.

Children are probably at greatest risk of contracting a disease from the family pet, primarily because of their inherent curiosity and often less-than-desirable hygiene habits (FIG. 53-1). However, adults are susceptible as well. Furthermore, failing to provide adequate preventative health care for pets in the household greatly increases the chance of exposure to one of these diseases.

RABIES

Certainly the most infamous of all *zoonoses*, rabies is an incurable, fatal, viral disease that attacks the nervous system of its unfortunate host. Excreted in the saliva of infected animals, transmission to other animals and to people can occur via bite wounds and through contamination of open wounds or sores. Although rabies is primarily restricted to wild or feral carnivores, cases occasionally spill over into the domestic and stray dog and cat population, thus providing the important link between wildlife and human rabies. For more information regarding rabies, see chapter 6 (dogs) and chapter 24 (cats).

Because rabies cannot be cured, the key here is prevention. Obviously it's very important to have all pet dogs and cats vaccinated annually.

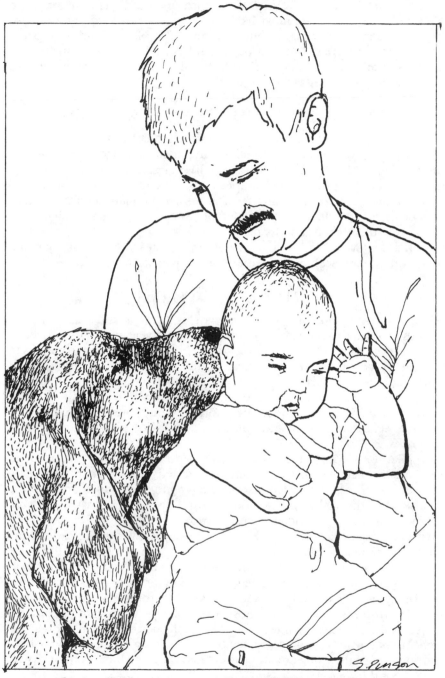

53-1   *Children are especially susceptible to zoonoses.*

In addition, don't allow your pets to roam free outdoors at night, since this is the time they are most likely to interact with wild animals. Use common sense: Discourage your children from playing with or petting stray animals that might come around. And don't keep wild animals, such as de-scented skunks, as pets. Because of their high susceptibility to rabies, doing so is just asking for trouble!

ANIMAL BITE AND SCRATCH WOUNDS

Besides the potential for rabies transmission, a bite from a dog or cat can also lead to severe bacterial infections and tissue damage in the affected individual. Likewise, scratches, especially cat scratches, can be just as bad, if not worse, than those injuries caused by teeth. For instance, *cat-scratch fever*, a disease causing fever and swollen, painful lymph nodes, can be transmitted to an unsuspecting person by the mere scratch of a cat harboring the organism on its nails.

If a dog or cat (even if it's your own pet) bites you or a family member, don't delay! Seek medical attention immediately.

INTESTINAL WORMS

Hookworms, roundworms, and tapeworms of dogs and cats can pose health problems to humans if exposure to infective eggs or larvae occurs. For example, certain types of hookworms can be transmitted from pets to people by contact with soil or sand contaminated with infective larvae. Although these worms will not infest the digestive system of humans, the larvae do have the ability to penetrate and burrow into the outer layer of exposed skin, usually the feet, legs, and/or hands, and cause an intense itching sensation. The name of this condition is *cutaneous larval migrans*.

Like hookworms, roundworms can be transmitted by contact with soil contaminated with feces from an infested dog or cat. The disease caused by these larvae, called *visceral larval migrans*, can be much more serious than that caused by the hookworm. This is especially true for children, or in those individuals with compromised immune systems. For instance, if accidentally ingested by a child, roundworm larvae can migrate and wander aimlessly throughout the organs and tissues of the body, leading to, among other disorders, blindness and nervous-system disorders. As a result, if there was one good reason for having your family pet routinely dewormed and checked for parasites, this is it!

Dipylidium caninum, the most common tapeworm seen in dogs and cats, could conceivably infest the intestinal tract of human individuals who accidentally consume a tapeworm-containing flea that might have hopped off of their dog or cat. Owners can avoid such exposure by practicing good flea control measures.

More seriously though, *hydatid cyst disease*, caused by the tapeworm *Echinococcus*, can be contracted by man through contact with tapeworm eggs shed by a dog harboring the adult form of these worms (FIG. 53-2). Upon ingestion, the tapeworm larvae emerge from the eggs and can migrate throughout all tissues and organs of the body, including the brain. The resulting damage caused by the cysts formed invariably leads to death if not detected soon enough.

Dogs can become infested with adult *Echinococcus* tapeworms by ingesting meat from cattle, sheep, or pigs infected with the larval form of the disease. As a result, prohibiting the consumption of raw meat and offal by dogs is the surest way to keep the risk of this disease low.

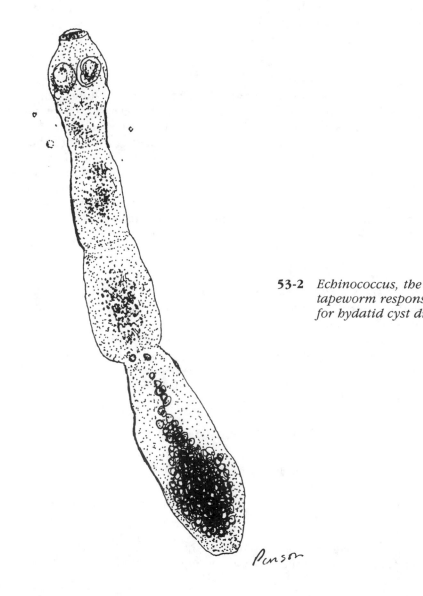

53-2 *Echinococcus, the tapeworm responsible for hydatid cyst disease.*

HEARTWORMS

Rarely, man can be infected by *Dirofilaria immitis*, the canine and feline heartworm. The heartworm larvae, which gain entrance into the body via a mosquito bite, do not migrate to the heart as they do in pets, but rather to the lungs. Here, they can form coin-like lesions that have been mistaken on human chest radiographs for tuberculosis lesions or for cancer. Fortunately, the actual inflammation and disease caused by these lesions is rarely severe.

Besides employing mosquito repellents and environmental control measures, you can reduce the chances of exposure to heartworm-carrying mosquitoes by keeping your dog current on its heartworm preventative medication and encouraging other pet owners to do the same as well.

RINGWORM

Ringworm (*dermatophytosis*) is not a worm at all; it is a fungus that attacks the skin, hair, and nails of both humans and animals (see chapters 6 and 24). In humans, it causes red, itchy skin lesions. Dogs and cats can transmit this disease to owners by direct contact of the latter with the infected skin and coat. Often, an outbreak of ringworm within a household can be traced back to the family cat, since felines are a common carrier of this disease.

Because of its zoonotic potential, ringworm must always be ruled out as the cause of distinct hair loss in the family pet. An exam and/or fungal culture performed by your veterinarian can verify such suspicions.

INFECTIOUS DIARRHEA

Campylobacteriosis, salmonellosis, and *giardiasis*, three diseases often implicated in cases of diarrhea in dogs and cats, also happen to be three major infectious causes of diarrhea recognized in people. Transmitted via infected feces, these organisms have the ability to cause severe cramping, nausea, and diarrhea in exposed individuals. As a result, protect yourself and your family from such diseases by observing good hygiene practices when handling pets. In addition, always seek prompt veterinary care for any diarrheic animal.

TOXOPLASMOSIS

Shed in the feces of infected cats, *toxoplasmosis* is one of the most common zoonotic diseases around. In the United States alone, up to 40 percent of the adult population is believed to have been exposed to this disease at one time or another. The majority of cases occurring in people are *subclinical* in nature (don't show any signs) and often pass undetected.

However, if pregnant women who have never been exposed to toxoplasmosis contract the parasite, serious consequences to the health of the fetus could result. If infection occurs early enough in pregnancy, mental retardation in the unborn child is not uncommon. For this reason, if you are pregnant, avoid activities that involve working with soil or sand (your garden might serve as a litter box for a neighborhood cat), and avoid changing or cleaning cat litter boxes. Contact your obstetrician for more detailed information regarding this disease.

LEPTOSPIROSIS

The leptospirosis organism that infects dogs can infect humans as well, causing, among other things, severe chills, fever, anemia, kidney damage, eye damage, and occasionally brain damage. Exposure to infected urine and other secretions or tissues is the primary method of transmission to people. Keeping dogs current on their vaccinations and reducing their exposure to potential sources of the disease, such as livestock and farm tanks or water pools are the best ways to protect against this disease.

FLEA AND TICK-BORNE ILLNESSES

Fleas and ticks have proven to be effective vehicles for a variety of diseases that infect man. Because dogs and cats can prove to be effective reservoirs for fleas and ticks within households, owners who fail to undertake adequate external parasite control measures could be placing the health of themselves and that of their family in jeopardy (FIG. 53-3).

As mentioned previously, fleas are an important vector for tapeworms in dogs and cats. The chances of a person developing tapeworms following ingestion of tapeworm-infested feces is low; nonetheless, it can occur, especially in children. As a result, minimizing exposure to fleas is a must.

53-3 *Ticks can carry a variety of diseases harmful to man.*

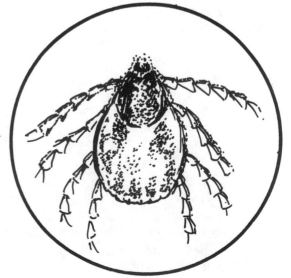

Fleas are also the primary mode of transmission of the plague organism *Yersinia pestis*, the same disease that achieved historical infamy throughout the medieval world. In the Southwestern portions of the United States, plague still occasionally rears its ugly head from time to time. Cats carrying plague-laden fleas pose the greatest threat to human health in these areas. In humans, signs of plague include sore, swollen lymph nodes, fever, seizures, and/or coughing due to pneumonia. Fortunately, if detected early enough, plague can be treated quite effectively with modern medicine. Again, an ounce of prevention is worth a pound of cure, and flea control is the key to protecting your family against this serious disease.

Three of the more infamous tick-borne illnesses that can affect people include *Rocky Mountain Spotted Fever, Ehrlichiosis*, and *Lyme Disease*. Again, dogs and cats can act as reservoirs for ticks carrying the causative organisms. Clinical signs of these diseases in humans can include malaise, headaches, chills, painful muscles and joints, and others. Owners wishing to reduce their chances of exposure to these diseases should practice staunch tick control, and **never** remove a tick from a dog or cat with bare hands.

MITES

The *Sarcoptes Notoedres* and *Cheyletiella* mange mites that normally infest dogs and cats can also cause self-limiting disease in people. As in pets, these mites can cause itchy, irritated skin in exposed individuals. Fortunately, however, these infestations rarely last long and will usually clear up after a short while. Pet owners can help shield themselves from such infestations by having all skin lesions involving itching and/or hair loss that might appear on a pet properly diagnosed and treated by a veterinarian.

CONTROL SUMMARY

The above represent some of the more important zoonotic diseases that parents and pet owners should be aware of. The following list reiterates and expands upon some of those preventative measures previously mentioned to help protect you and your family from zoonotic diseases. Be sure your children understand why these measures are important. By doing so, you can ensure that your relationship with your pet will remain a healthy one (FIG. 53-4).

- ○ Parents and children alike should always wash their hands thoroughly after handling family pets, especially before eating.
- ○ You should discourage "kissing" pets or being licked by pets. After all, you don't know where their mouths have been!
- ○ Have pets routinely examined, vaccinated, and checked for worms by your veterinarian. New puppies and kittens should be routinely

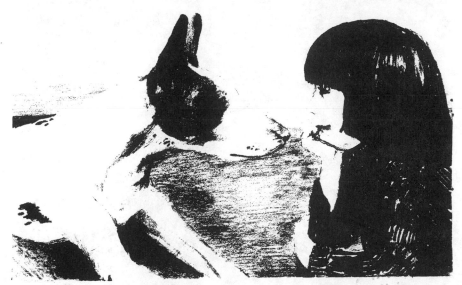

53-4 *Preventative steps can help ensure your relationship with your pet stays healthy and happy.*

dewormed starting at 3 weeks of age. Be sure your dog is on heartworm preventative medication.

○ Control fleas and ticks on your pet.

○ If a pet becomes ill, minimize handling and seek veterinary help immediately. Always separate ill animals from young children.

○ Insist on a veterinary checkup before purchasing any pet.

○ Avoid interactions with stray animals and impress this point upon your children.

○ Clean up and dispose of all animal waste promptly.

○ Keep children's sandboxes covered when not in use, and keep other play areas free of animal excrement.

54

Cancer in Companion Animals

IN THE PAST 20 YEARS, veterinary medicine has made tremendous advances in the diagnosis, treatment, and prevention of disease in the dog. For instance, because of an educated public and readily available vaccines, the incidence of viral disease in companion animals has decreased greatly. Another frequent cause of death, bacterial disease, is now usually arrested comparatively easily with the wide spectrum of antibiotics available. In addition, veterinarians and breeders alike have learned much about the control and elimination of genetic defects through selective breeding, and leash laws and responsible owners have greatly decreased the incidence of pets killed by trauma. Pets, like their owners, are living longer and longer (FIG. 54-1).

It is not at all unusual for veterinarians to be presented with a pet that is 10 to 20 years old whose health has been preserved relatively well through preventative health care (see chapters 3 and 21). Many of these older pets, however, are presented with a disease that we still know little about—cancer. Of course, veterinarians know a great deal more about the diagnosis and therapy of malignant disease in the small animal than they did 20 years ago; in fact, it has only been recently that veterinarian practitioners have focused on cancer therapy for pets.

WHAT ARE TUMORS?

A *tumor* or *neoplasm* is an abnormal growth of tissue whose cells proliferate more rapidly than the tissue from which they came. These cells are not subject to the same control mechanisms that keep normal cells in check. Normal cells grown in a tissue culture medium in a laboratory will

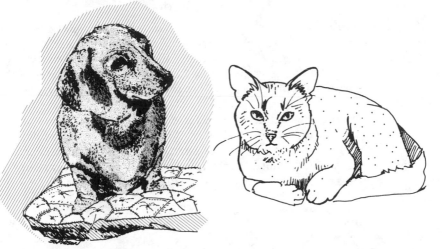

54-1   *Pets, like their owners, are living longer and longer.*

cease growing when they have touched each other and filled their container. This is called *contact inhibition*, and it explains, for instance, why our liver grows to a certain size and doesn't keep growing until we burst. Tumor cells, however, don't display the same respect for boundaries. Instead, they grow relentlessly, tumbling over each other and spilling over the edges of their containers.

Benign tumors

There is a difference between benign tumor cells and malignant tumor cells. *Benign tumors* are "well differentiated"; in other words, they differ only slightly in appearance and behavior from their tissue of origin. These tumors are slow-growing and noninvasive, do not spread throughout the body, and will often have a fibrous tissue capsule around them.

All these characteristics make benign tumors easy to surgically remove completely in most cases. Unless allowed to grow to a huge size, they are seldom a threat to life. However, they might cause significant problems if they are located in a vital organ, such as the brain or intestines. In fact, the most significant alteration that a benign tumor can make in its host organism is that of encroachment on surrounding normal tissue, leading to obstruction or replacement of the normal tissue by tumor.

To identify a benign tumor, the suffix *-oma* is used. For example, a benign tumor of osseous tissue (bone) would be an *osteoma,* and a benign tumor of fibrous tissue would be a *fibroma*. The term *adenoma* is used to suggest a benign tumor of a glandular structure, such as a mammary adenoma or a thyroid adenoma. The term *papilloma* or *polyp* is applied to wart-like projections from epithelial surfaces like skin or intestine.

Malignant tumors

Malignant tumors, on the other hand, grow rapidly. Malignant cells send spreading fingers into the surrounding normal tissue, making it difficult to surgically remove the entire tumor; thus, they frequently regrow even after radical surgery. The cells show marked *de-differentiation* or *anaplasia*; in other words, they do not look like the cells from which they originated.

Generally, malignant tumors are referred to as cancer. Cancers of epithelial or glandular structures are referred to as *carcinomas,* while cancers of other tissues are referred to as *sarcomas.* The major danger of a malignant tumor is its ability to *metastasize,* or spread throughout the body. Vital organs can be invaded, and death can soon occur (FIG. 54-2).

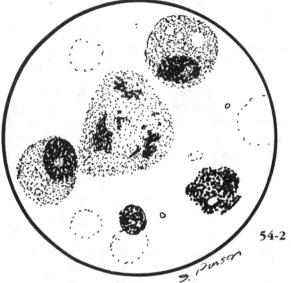

54-2   *Cancer cell undergoing division.*

Carcinomas, as a rule, spread via the lymph vessels, though some can "skip" the lymph nodes and go directly to blood vessels. An example of a carcinoma in dogs which can metastasize either by lymphatics or blood is the mammary carcinoma.

Sarcomas usually metastasize via the bloodstream. Organs that are frequent sites of blood-borne metastasis include the liver and lungs, both of which can be rapidly comprised of tumors.

We have all seen or heard of people who have been seriously debilitated by cancer, and pets are affected similarly. A malignant tumor can cause what is called the *cachexia of cancer*: The animal gradually starves to death as the tumor grows and steals the body's nutrition. Hemorrhage, pain, fever, and infection are frequent secondary effects of cancer.

Some (usually benign) tumors produce side-effects on the host through the production and release of hormones. Normally, these hormones are essential, in small quantities, for life in a healthy pet. However, the tumor typically "goes overboard," and elaborates dangerously excessive quantities. For example, an *insuloma* of the pancreas produces excessive insulin, and animals with this tumor will have very low blood sugar levels with resulting weakness or seizures. *Thyroid adenomas* in the cat can produce excessive thyroid hormone, leading to nervousness and hyperexcitability, weight loss, and diarrhea.

OCCURRENCE OF CANCER IN PETS

What do we know about the occurrence of cancer in pets? Most people are very surprised to learn that dogs and cats have a higher incidence of many tumors than do humans. Dogs have 35 times as much skin cancer as do humans, four times as many breast tumors, eight times as much bone cancer, and twice as high an incidence of leukemia.

The only types of cancer that are more frequently seen in humans than in small animals are not surprising. Lung cancer is seven times higher in humans, and stomach and intestinal malignancies are 13 times more frequent in man than in dogs and cats. This would suggest that the pollutants we take into our bodies do have significant adverse effects on our health.

Breed predilections (dogs)

Through careful statistical evaluation by veterinary researchers, some breed predilections for cancer have been noted. If a veterinarian were to be asked the breed of dog with the highest incidence of cancer, he or she would undoubtedly reply, "the boxer." When a sick, aged boxer turns up at the hospital, the attending veterinarian suspects a tumor almost immediately.

Dog breeds with an extremely *high* incidence of cancer include:

○ Boxer
○ Boston terrier
○ Cocker spaniel
○ Wire-haired fox terrier

Breeds with a very *low* incidence of cancer are the following:

○ Beagle
○ Poodle
○ Collie
○ Dachshund

Why do some breeds have a high incidence of cancer while some are rarely affected with it? The answer to that question is still elusive. One hypothesis deals with the immune system of these pets. The boxer's immune system is thought to be less able to mobilize resistance to cancer than are the immune systems of many other breeds. It is hypothesized that the high incidence of cancer in the cocker spaniel and boxer is related to their great popularity and heavy breeding in the 1940s and 50s. If this is true, we should be seeing a rise in the incidence of cancer in the now-popular poodle over the next decade or so, and the "mixed breeds" should have one of the lowest incidence of cancer. Yet, ironically, the dog of mixed ancestry has only an average incidence, along with the Irish Setter, schnauzer, Labrador retreiver, and many other breeds.

Some types of tumors are more prone to develop in one type of dog than in others. For example, the giant breeds, such as the St. Bernard and the Great Dane, have a much higher incidence *osteosarcoma* (a very malignant bone tumor) than does the general canine population. Collies with lightly pigmented noses are prone to develop carcinomas in that area, probably due to long-term exposure to the ultraviolet rays of the sun. Black dogs have a comparatively high incidence of *melanomas*, or pigmented malignant tumors. The female dog who is not spayed has seven times the chance of developing mammary tumors as does the dog who is ovariohysterectomized early in life. This would seem to indicate that the sex hormones can be potent stimulators of breast cancer in dogs.

Age predilection

The effect of a pet's age on the incidence of cancer is not well understood. In general, cancer is thought of as a disease of advancing age. It is hypothesized that as cells continually divide through the progression of life, there is an increased chance of genetic mutation due to cell division "accidents" and to the effect of *carcinogens*, or cancer-causing agents. Also, depression of the normal immune response in the older animal might play a part in the increased incidence of cancer seen with advancing ages.

WHAT CAUSES CANCER IN PETS?

What is the etiology of cancer in pets? Unfortunately, human tumor research is little more advanced than is veterinary research in this area. The causes of a select number of tumors are known. For instance, the transmissible venearal tumor in the dog is spread by implantation during breeding, and the canine oral papilloma of young dogs is known to be caused by a virus. In cats, cattle, mice, and poultry, lymphosarcoma has been shown to be caused by a virus, but no virus has as yet been recovered from the lymphosarcoma of canines or humans. Squamous cell carcinoma in white dogs, white cats, and in Hereford cattle has been shown to be caused by the ultraviolet radiation of sunlight.

Undoubtedly, many types of tumors have an etiological cause or causes which are as yet to be determined. This is an area in which more research in both human and animal cancer is desperately needed. Until medical and veterinary professionals know the cause of a disease, attempts at "shotgun" treatment will be symptomatic at best and will seldom afford a cure.

What is the risk to an owner from a pet's malignant disease? At this time, researchers can only give a very guarded answer: There seems to be no risk to humans from animal cancer.

Several approaches have been used to evaluate the possibility of transmission. First, animal and human cancers that occurred in the same household were studied to determine whether this simultaneous phenomenon occurred more often than would be expected due to mere chance. However, there was no increased incidence of cancer in humans who had lived closely with a pet with tumors.

Secondly, no viruses that are known to cause cancer in animals infect humans, at least as far as research can determine. The virus that causes feline leukemia can be made to grow in human tissue culture in the laboratory, but no evidence of any infection in man has ever been found. Therefore, although knowledge on the subject is limited, there is currently no known transmission of cancer from animals to humans—or from humans to animals, for that matter.

DIAGNOSING CANCER IN PETS

The diagnosis of cancer is not always as straightforward as it would seem. People have been known to show clinical signs for months before their doctors finally discovered cancer somewhere in their bodies.

Several methods can be used to diagnose neoplastic disease in pets:

1. Physical examination   Sometimes a tumor is readily seen on the pet's skin, in its mouth, or palpated in its abdomen.

2. Endoscopy or laparoscopy   The use of fiber-optic endoscopes is becoming increasingly more common in veterinary medicine. With these instruments, tumors in the esophagus, stomach, bronchi, liver, spleen, and other organs can be visualized without dangerous surgery. Biopsies of tumors can also be obtained with these instruments.

3. Radiography (X-rays)   Both plain films and contrast techniques can be used to demonstrate tumors of the lung, gastrointestinal tract, bladder, and other internal organs. Sometimes a radiograph can be *pathogonomic* (completely typical) for a particular type of tumor, as in the case of bone tumors. Multiple nodular masses in the lung would suggest blood-borne metastasis of a malignant tumor somewhere else in the body. However, in most cases, a tumor visualized on a radiograph must be biopsied to rule in or rule out malignancy.

4. Nuclear medicine   Scans of the liver, thyroid, lung, spleen, kidney, and bone are now used commonly in veterinary colleges and institutions to diagnose cancer. Radioisotopes with short half-lives are used, and anesthesia of the pet is almost never required. These scans cause no adverse effects on the pet.

5. Cytology   Examination of cells pulled from body cavities, mammary gland secretions, nasal exudates, respiratory secretions, bone marrow, lymph nodes, and various "lumps and bumps" has come into increasing popularity in recent years for the diagnosis of neoplastic disease. Sometimes the cytologic diagnosis is certain, whereas other times cytologic examination is used to rule out other causes of swelling, such as bacterial infection or fungal disease.

6. *Biopsy*   Biopsy is the most common and the most certain way to make the diagnosis of cancer in both animals and humans. Gross and microscopic examination of a neoplasm by a competent (preferably veterinary) pathologist can be expected to yield an accurate diagnosis about 90% of the time. Misdiagnosis can occur if too small a sample is submitted or if an area of the tumor is selected for biopsy that does not contain tumor cells. For example, osteosarcoma is frequently misdiagnosed because these tumors contain a great deal of dead tissue and reactive fibrous tissue; if these "benign" areas of the tumor are inadvertently biopsied, the pathologist will not find malignant cells.

7. *Other methods*   Neoplastic disease can be suggested by results obtained in a microscopic and biochemical analysis of a pet's blood. An increase in serum cholesterol and the enzyme alkaline phosphatase is typically found in canine Cushing's disease, which can be caused by an adrenal gland or pituitary gland tumor. A bone marrow cancer can be diagnosed by finding tumor cells in the blood (leukemia).

Prognosis

When cancer has been diagnosed in a pet, the prognosis for survival with treatment versus without treatment must be considered. One factor to consider is that these pets will frequently be older, and other diseases, such as heart and kidney disease, might be present. Therefore, one of the first objectives in deciding whether to treat a pet with cancer should be to identify all of the problems present.

If a pet has progressive kidney or heart disease, it is unlikely that it will live through major surgery. Even small secondary problems can become major primary problems once cancer treatment has begun. For example, a pet might be coping well with hookworm infestation until chemotherapy depresses its immune system. At this point, a raging bloody diarrhea might develop. As a result, before initiating treatment, other problems must be taken care of first, if possible.

Another factor that figures into a prognosis is the behavior of the particular tumor that the pet has. Obviously, biopsies should be done on all tumors to determine information about growth patterns and likelihood of metastasis.

Finally, if the tumor is malignant, the extent of disease must be determined. In most sarcomas, chest radiographs are necessary because the lung is a frequent site of blood-borne metastasis. In carcinomas, both lymph nodes and lungs should be evaluated closely, since either or both sites can be involved at the time of presentation to the veterinarian. In tumors affecting the oral and nasal cavity, skull radiographs are necessary, since prognosis is not as good if there is bone destruction and invasion. If a lymph node is enlarged, cytology should be performed on it to determine whether it is involved with tumor.

TREATING CANCER IN PETS

Treatment of cancer in the dog and cat has been extremely limited until the last few years. In the old days, a pet with a small tumor received surgery; if that tumor grew back or spread to other organs, the pet was probably put to sleep. However, other options are now available. A combination of therapies including surgery, radiation, and chemotherapy is now the optimum protocol to achieve control of a malignancy, whether in animal or man.

Surgery

If the tumor is small, of course, surgery is still the best method to effect a cure. Hopefully, all malignant cells can be removed by this method before any spread occurs to regional lymph nodes. With some tumors, however, regrowth either occurs rapidly, or surgical resection is impossible due to the location or the extensiveness of the cancer. In these instances, radiation therapy is the best option.

Radiation

Many tumors of the dog and cat have been shown to be controllable, if not curable, by the use of radiation. Radiation can be administered with a radioactive implant (*brachytherapy*), or externally, using a radiation beam (*teletherapy*). With either method, radiation will destroy the DNA of cells so that they can no longer reproduce. To be ideal for cure by radiotherapy, a tumor should:

1. Be of a radiosensitive cell type
2. Involve no vital radiosensitive organs, such as the gastrointestinal tract
3. Have readily definable borders
4. Be invasive non-invasive- or late-metastasizing

Frequently, radiotherapy is combined with surgery to cure residual microscopic foci of disease that might have been left by the surgeon.

Chemotherapy

In the past, the expense of chemotherapy has prohibited its widespread use in veterinary medicine. However, today, many of the commonly used anticancer drugs are readily available and are inexpensive enough to make their use a feasible part of treatment. The effect of these drugs is to kill the tumor cells by several mechanisms; some drugs fragment chromosome strands within the cells, while others stop the dividing of cells.

Of course, these effects against tumor cells also cause changes in normal cells, with resultant deleterious side effects in the animal (or human) being treated. These side effects include severe bone marrow depression, nausea, vomiting, hair loss, and hemorrhage. The objective of the veterinarian is to achieve a drug dosage that is enough to control or cure the tumor without causing any severe side effects. This is often very difficult to do, and some nausea is to be expected with chemotherapy.

Some types of tumors are very responsive to chemotherapy. The average expected lifespan after diagnosis of a lymphosarcoma in a dog is 56 days; with chemotherapy, the life expectancy can be increased to about a year.

On the other hand, tumors such as fibrosarcomas and osteosarcomas are notoriously resistant. Human oncology is obtaining some control of these highly malignant tumors with expensive drugs that cost hundreds of dollars per treatment, but these agents have had (understandably) very limited use in dogs and cats.

One disadvantage of chemotherapy is that it is relatively ineffective against large tumors. The number of neoplastic cells must be reduced first by either surgery or radiation therapy before chemotherapy can be effective. This stresses again the point that tumors might be curable at an early stage; when they have metastasized, the prognosis is very poor for a cure.

Immunotherapy

Immunotherapy of cancer is a form of therapy that is still in its very early stages. The assumption is made that the growth of a cancer occurs because of a defect in the pet's immune system. Had immunity been normal, the tumor growth should have been suppressed very early. For this reason, stimulation of the pet's immune system through the use of drugs and vaccines is being researched. It is still too early to make a preliminary evaluation of the efficacy of this mode of therapy in dogs and cats.

Summary

It must be recognized that both surgery and radiation therapy are local treatments for cancer; even if only a few tumor cells have escaped beyond this local area, the treatment will fail. This is the justification for using chemotherapy in combination with surgery and/or radiation therapy. This chemotherapy can be used to destroy microscopic foci of tumor cells that might have already escaped to lymph nodes or blood vessels beyond the radius of the treatment area. Generally, it is recommended in the treatment of tumors that are likely to metastasize early. A combination of surgery, radiation therapy, and chemotherapy is most likely to produce a cure for cancer with today's (limited) therapeutic capabilities.

Obviously, the means of treatment discussed here are not the answers to the control of cancer. Those answers will only be forthcoming when the reasons for the transformation of a cell from normal to cancer-ous are determined. This objective will take extensive research and a great deal more money than has been devoted to cancer study in any human or veterinary medical institution to this point.

Human and veterinary cancer specialists are both striving to reach the same goal—a knowledge of cancer so complete that we are able simply to administer a vaccine against neoplastic disease. Perhaps 30 years from now, veterinarians and pet owners alike will be able to look with amazement (and a little disdain) at the primitive methods now used to control cancer in pets.

55

The Euthanasia Decision

INEVITABLY, EVERY PET OWNER is faced with the difficult decision concerning the euthanasia of a beloved pet. *Euthanasia*, the purposeful humane induction of unconsciousness and death, is certainly an act not to be taken lightly or performed without extensive forethought. When does euthanasia become a consideration or option when dealing with a pet?

Certainly owners with pets suffering from terminal illnesses or irreparable, painful injuries must address euthanasia as a viable option as compared to continued discomfort and pain for their pet. Other pets might have a quality of life that has decreased and become unacceptable due to the effects of aging. For instance, pets that are totally blind, mentally disoriented, or incontinent fall into this category. Often, the quality of life of the owner of these pets has decreased proportionally, owing to time and monetary commitments towards the continual care of their beloved friend. In these instances, euthanasia might be the only humane decision not only for the pet, but for the owner as well.

Finally, euthanasia is a real consideration for those excessively aggressive pets that pose a hazard to human health or may have even bitten someone already. Not only do owners of these fierce pets put the health of themselves and others at risk, but place themselves at an incredibly high liability risk as well.

GRIEVING FOR A LOST PET

Although many might try to deny its existence, a psychological "bonding" does occur between people and their pets. Researchers have even given it a name, referring to this phenomenon as the *Human-Companion Animal Bond*. In fact, veterinary colleges across the country teach courses devoted only to this subject. It certainly makes sense that such a bonding exists. Pets are nothing more than bundles of love and friendship that add that much touch of happiness and companionship to our some-times unfriendly and hectic world (FIG. 55-1). Pets are always ready to lis-ten to our problems, never interjecting their own problems or opinions along the way. Instead, we receive a responsive wag of the tail or a friendly purr.

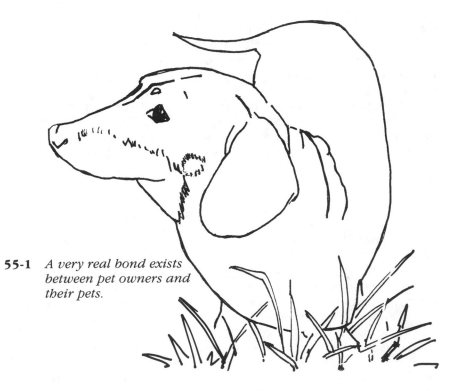

55-1 *A very real bond exists between pet owners and their pets.*

So why is this so important? The proven existence of the human-companion animal bond should help pet owners realize that grieving for a lost pet is perfectly natural. There is a stigma in our society about grieving openly for a pet that has died or has been put to sleep. Failure to do so only causes a strong build-up of emotion and sometimes confusion within the pet owner. This is not only psychologically unhealthy, but also—and most doctors will point this out—physically unhealthy as well.

Stages of grieving

With the loss or impending loss of a loved one, be they animal or human, there are stages of grief that we all experience. Some will experience all four stages sequentially; others might find that one or two stages predominate. Understanding that these stages are natural and should not be suppressed can help you better cope with the impending death of a pet.

The first stage of grieving is the **denial stage**. In this stage, a pet owner has yet to come to grips with the fact that their pet is going to die. In terms of the euthanasia decision, some pet owners find themselves refusing to believe that making such a serious decision should even be presented as an option. This can lead into the second stage of grief, the **anger stage**. Anger can be vented at a veterinarian for even suggesting euthanasia as an option. In other instances, an owner will be angry at himself for considering euthanasia in the first place. The third stage of grief is **depression**—the thought of losing a loved one and how life afterwards will be. Finally, in the **resolution stage**, an owner finally comes to the acceptance of a pet's death, and has learned to cope with it. It is usually in this stage that the burden of the euthanasia decision is finally, and correctly, lifted.

When the grief is just too overwhelming, don't be afraid to contact a psychologist or doctor specializing in grief counseling for help. Support groups do exist which can help pet owners overcome the loss of their loved one. Again, what you are experiencing is very real and very natural, and a trained, understanding ear can be great comfort and relief at times of such emotional distress.

THE PROCESS

The administration of euthanasia itself is painless. Medications designed to induce unconsciousness followed by immediate death are injected into a vein of the dog or cat using either a needle or an intravenous catheter. Depending on the behavior of the pet, and on the degree of pain existing from the injury or illness, some veterinarians will administer a sedative before euthanasia. This helps to calm and relax the patient.

Once the euthanasia agent is given, death takes only seconds to ensue. In some instances, a vocalization or heavy breathing might occur as the agent is administered. In addition, evacuation of the bowels and urinary bladder might occur as well. Pet owners who insist on being present during the euthanasia procedure must realize that these occurrences are not associated with pain or discomfort in any way. Those portions of the brain responsible for conscious perception and pain are shut down long before these other brain centers are stimulated by the euthanasia drug. Pets indeed die peacefully and painlessly this way.

The decision to be with your pet at the time of euthanasia is strictly up to you. Many people prefer to remember their pet as it was during happier times; others need to be present to be able to enter into the resolution stage of grieving (FIG. 55-2). One alternative for pet owners is to have the procedure performed while they are not physically in the room with their pet, with a viewing of the body afterwards. Still others prefer saying goodbye to their pet at home the evening before, allowing a neighbor or

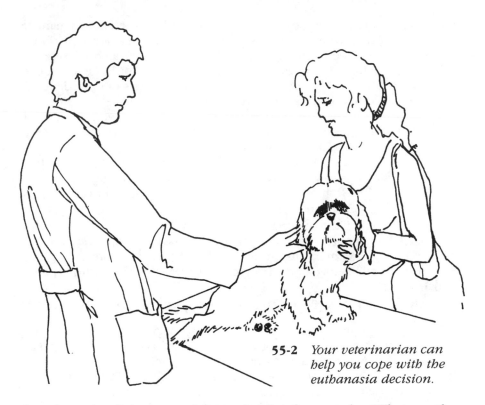

55-2 *Your veterinarian can help you cope with the euthanasia decision.*

friend to take their pet to the veterinarian the next day. Whatever the choice, be sure you feel comfortable with the decision. Don't hesitate to contact your veterinarian if you are having trouble with it.

If you do decide to stay with your pet while it is being put to sleep, try to stay as calm as possible so you do not upset your pet. Gently stroke its head or body, giving comfort and reassurance that its suffering will soon be over. Just one more thing: Remember, too, that it is a very stressful and emotional time for your veterinarian as well. After all, he/she is the one that must physically put this living, loving creature to sleep. There is not a veterinarian alive that I know that takes pleasure in this task. Don't hesitate to ask questions and solicit his/her input once the procedure is completed.

AFTERMATH

Following the euthanasia procedure, the decision as to the disposition of the body must be made. By far, the majority of pet owners choose to have their veterinarian transfer the body for communal burial at a site designated by the city or municipality. Other owners want to bury their pet in a more personal manner, either on their own property or in a pet memorial park.

Realize that most cities have laws restricting the burial of animals within city limits; be sure to check with yours. Pets buried in this manner should be placed within two plastic bags, and then enclosed within a sturdy, sealed wooden crate. It should be buried deep enough as to ensure its protection from scavengers. Pet memorial parks or cemeteries can range anywhere from hundreds to thousands of dollars in cost, depending on location and extent of ground maintenance. Be sure to scrutinize and check into all such cemeteries very closely. After all, you don't want an office building going in over your pet's grave years down the line if the right offer is made to the landowner!

Cremation is another alternative afforded the pet owner. Depending on whether you want your pet's ashes saved, costs can range anywhere from $50 to $500. If this is the desirable option for you, your veterinarian can direct you to the appropriate sources.

If you would like to make a donation in memory of your pet, contact your local humane society, veterinary medical association, or nearest veterinary college. Memoriums are a wonderful means of preserving the memory of your beloved pet. They can also provide aid to those living pets in need.

ALTERNATIVES TO EUTHANASIA

Often, veterinarians are presented with pets for euthanasia that are perfectly healthy, except usually for personality defects (other than aggressiveness) that make them "inconvenient" to their owners. Others are brought in by relatives of a deceased person or someone who has moved away. They claim that the pet would not be happy with anyone else and therefore should be put to sleep. It must be realized that these pets are not candidates for euthanasia and veterinarians should not be expected to honor such requests. Other alternatives do exist, assuming an owner is willing to honor his pet ownership responsibility. It might cost money and time, but that is all part of the responsibility.

For instance, if a pet exhibits a destructive behavior (as with the yard-digging dog or furniture-clawing cat), a visit to your veterinarian is warranted. Often, problem behaviors stem from underlying medical disorders, many of which can be effectively treated. Still others that have a true psychological component can be effectively cured through counter-training or by way of special drug therapy, depending upon the particular case. For instance, a few dollars spent on command training classes might turn that obnoxious, hyperactive pet into the affectionate and fun house pet you were looking for in the first place.

Finding a new home for a pet that needs to leave the household for one reason or another is a much more acceptable option than is euthanasia. Post flyers at your veterinarian's office and ask him/her for help. He/she will be more than happy to help. Also, ask friends and neighbors for leads into a potential home for your pet. Finally, consider running an advertisement in the local newspapers. Remember: Fulfilling your responsibility as a pet owner means undertaking such efforts in order to do what is best for your four-legged companion!

Appendix
FIRST AID FOR DOGS & CATS

THIS SECTION IS DESIGNED to instruct the pet owner on first aid for dogs and cats, and on the recognition of clinical signs and true emergency situations that involve his/her pet. By no means is this chapter intended to replace professional veterinary care. On the contrary, it simply provides a reference source for temporary management of minor and major emergencies until the pet can be seen by a veterinarian.

All drugs, medications, and dosages contained herein are based on the author's recommendation, and are not necessarily the recommendation of the product's manufacturer or distributor.

Would you know the correct way to perform CPR on your cat, how to administer first aid to your dog if it is hit by a car, or what to do if your pet swallows a poisonous substance? If not, here is your opportunity to learn. The ultimate goal of any first aid is simple: To treat and/or stabilize the patient's condition until professional medical care can be obtained.

WHAT TO DO IN AN EMERGENCY SITUATION

If you do encounter a sudden injury or illness in your pet, don't panic! This will only hinder your first aid efforts. The first thing you need to do is determine whether or not a life-threatening situation exists. Cessation of breathing or heartbeat, severe bleeding, poisoning, and shock all demand immediate attention. Once the pet's condition has been stabilized, you can then direct your attention toward other, less serious problems.

Always approach injured or ill animals slowly and with caution. Use a

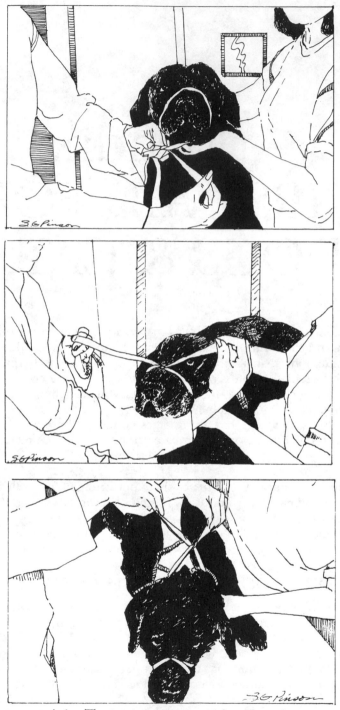

A-1   *The proper way to apply a muzzle.*

calm, reassuring voice and move slowly. Remember that animals that are frightened or in pain might bite. For dogs, you should apply a muzzle made out of sturdy gauze roll or another suitable item or material (such as a necktie, leash, belt, etc.) in order to protect yourself (see FIG. A-1). Note: never use a muzzle on an animal that is vomiting, choking, convulsing, or having breathing difficulties.

For cats and those dogs that have facial conformations that render a muzzle useless, use heavy-duty gloves or a thick blanket or towel to handle the animal. Keep in mind at all times that sharp teeth and claws can penetrate even the most durable of materials.

Don't forget to telephone your veterinarian concerning your pet's injury or illness, no matter how trivial it seems. Not only will you receive helpful advice, but it will also give the veterinarian time to prepare for the arrival of the patient, if necessary. If your veterinarian refers after-hours emergencies to an emergency clinic, be certain to have that telephone number handy at all times.

Never delay in seeking professional help after you have initiated first aid. Sadly enough, many people choose to postpone further treatment of their pet, whether it be for convenience or for monetary reasons. Often, these delays only serve to increase treatment costs and decrease treatment success rates. Remember: With pet ownership comes the responsibility of taking care of that pet's medical needs. Therefore, for your pet's sake, don't delay in seeking veterinary assistance.

Finally, it is important to minimize stress and handling as much as possible once first aid has been rendered. To help keep cats calm, try to transport them to the veterinary clinic in a box or in a pillowcase. If you suspect head or spinal injury, use a board, taut blanket, window screen, or a similar item on which to move the injured pet (FIG. A-2).

Keeping these general first aid principles in mind, we can now focus our attention on specific emergencies commonly seen in dogs and cats, and on the first aid steps that can be applied to each situation. Ready? Let's get started!

A-2 *Using a blanket to move an injured pet.*

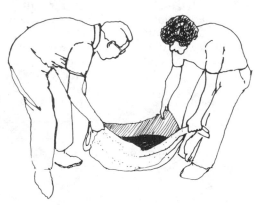

FIRST AID KIT AND HOME REMEDIES

Figure A-3 illustrates some supplies that would come in handy in the event of either a minor or a major emergency involving your pet. Most of these items can be obtained at your local pharmacy or grocery; others can be purchased through your veterinarian. TABLE A-1 provides a quick-conversion chart for metric and English measurement standards. TABLE A-3 lists over-the-counter medications that can be used in the event of an emergency. Please note that the usages and dosages here are those the author recommends and not necessarily those of the product's manufacturer or distributor. Finally, TABLE A-2 lists some important physiological data that you need to know in order to correctly assess the status of an injured or ill pet.

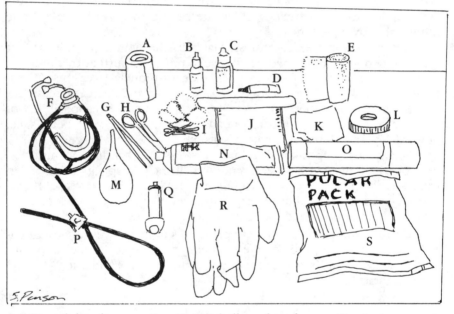

A.	Stretch bandage	I.	Cotton balls and swabs
B.	Tamed iodine	J.	Nonstick wound dressings
C.	Saline solution	K.	Guaze pads
D.	Sterile eye ointment	L.	Tape
E.	Adhesive bandage	M.	Bulb syringe
F.	Stethoscope	N.	Sterile lubricating jelly
G.	Forceps	O.	Silver nitrate sticks
H.	Scissors	P.	Tourniquet

Q. Syringe
R. Latex gloves
S. Thermal pack

A-3 *Items for a first aid kit.*

Table A-1   Useful Conversions

1 milliliters (ml)	= 1 cubic centimeter (cc)
1 teaspoon (tsp)	= 5 milliliters (ml)
1 tablespoon (Tbs)	= 15 milliliters (ml)
1 ounce (oz)	= 30 milliliters (ml)
1 pound (lb)	= 454 grams (gm)
1 kilogram (kg)	= 2.2 pounds (lbs)

Table A-2   Normal Values

Species	Temperature (Fahrenheit)	Pulse (beats per minute)	Respirations (per minute)
Dog	99.5 − 102.5	60 − 120	14 − 22
Cat	100 − 103.2	80 − 140	20 − 30
Small bird	108 − 112	600 − 800	75 − 100
Large bird	108 − 112	200 − 300	30 − 50
Guinea pig	100 − 102.5	250 − 300	80 − 90
Hamster	97 − 100	350 − 425	50 − 125
Gerbil	95 − 100	375 − 400	80 − 125
Rat	95 − 101	375 − 400	80 − 115
Mouse	96 − 100	500 − 600	90 − 150
Rabbit	102 − 103.5	175 − 210	50 − 75
Ferrets	100 − 103	200 − 250	80 − 100
Pot−bellied pigs	100.5 − 103	80 − 100	15 − 30

In addition to keeping your first aid kit well equipped, you should write down the number of your veterinary clinic and the nearest animal emergency clinic for quick reference in case of a problem.

FIRST AID TECHNIQUES FOR DOGS AND CATS

The pages that follow include information for some of the more common emergencies and first aid needs that pet owners are likely to encounter. Priorities for each situation are clearly spelled out to render the first aid more effective.

Table A-3   Over-the-Counter Oral Medications

If possible, always consult your veterinarian before giving anything orally to your pet.

Medication	Indication	Dosage
3% hydrogen peroxide	To induce vomiting General wound cleanser	1 teaspoon per 10 lbs
Pepto-Bismol (do not use in cats unless directed by your veterinarian)	Vomiting Mild diarrhea	1 teaspoon per 15 lbs or 1 tablet per 40 lbs
Aspirin (dogs only)	Fever & inflammation Mild to moderate pain Arthritis	1 adult tablet (5 grain) or 4 baby aspirin per 20 lbs
Acetaminophen (dogs only)	Same as aspirin	1 adult tablet per 25 lbs
Antihistamines (dogs only)	Mild cough Allergic reactions	Use only under the direction of a veterinarian
Kaolin and Pectin	Mild diarrhea	1 tablespoon per 10 lbs.
Syrup of Ipecac	To induce vomiting	1/2 ml per lb
Vegetable oil	Constipation Hairballs	1 teaspoon per 5 lbs mixed in food
Epsom Salts	Constipation (dogs only); as a soak to reduce swelling and inflammation	For constipation, 1 teaspoon per 10 lbs, dissolved in water & given orally; same dilution for soaks
Milk of Magnesia	Vomiting Constipation Deactivate poisons	1 to 2 teaspoons mixed with water
Activated charcoal	Deactivate poisons	5 to 50 grams of powder mixed with water to form a soup-like slurry
Petroleum jelly	Hairballs Constipation	1/2 teaspoon per 10 lbs

Artificial respiration/cardiopulmonary resuscitation

Priorities: • Ensure a patent airway.
 • Perform artificial respiration, if needed.
 • Perform external heart massage, if needed.
 • Obtain veterinary assistance.

The combination of artificial respiration and external heart massage is termed *cardiopulmonary resuscitation* (CPR). You should perform artificial respiration if your pet has stopped breathing. In addition, if the heart has stopped beating, you must institute external heart massage in conjunction with the artificial respiration. [NOTE: Never apply heart massage if the heart is still beating. To do so could actually lead to heart failure.] The purpose of CPR is to supply oxygen to the lungs and to keep the blood circulating unit the pet resumes these functions.

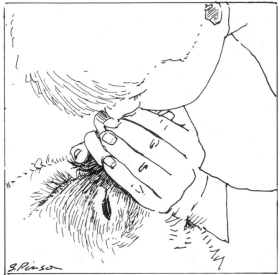

A-4 *Administering artificial respiration to a dog.*

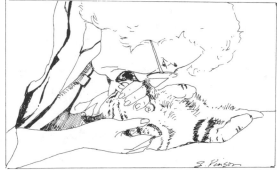

A-5 *Giving artificial respiration to a cat.*

CPR

Is your pet breathing? ──────────► YES ──────► Direct your attention to specific problems. ▲

↓

NO

↓

Use your finger to clear the mouth of any blood, mucus, vomitus, or other debris.

↓

Tilt the head back to straighten the airway, then clasp the mouth shut with your hand and place your mouth over the animal's nose and mouth, forming a tight seal.

↓

Blow into the nose until you see the chest expand. (If a neonate is involved, deliver gentle puffs of breath to prevent over-inflation of the lungs.) If you don't see the chest expand, repeat the first two steps, then try again.

↓

Did the chest expand? ──────────► NO ──────► (See Choke pg. 648)

↓

YES

↓

Release the seal, allowing your pet to fully exhale.

↓

Repeat this sequence once every five seconds until normal breathing resumes or until veterinary assistance is obtained.

↓

Is a heartbeat or pulse ──────────► YES ──────────
detectable?

↓

NO

↓

Perform another artificial respiration

↓

CPR, cont. _____

Does your pet weigh less ——————➤ No ——————————————┐
than 20 lbs?

↓

Yᴇs

↓

If a cat or small dog (< 20 lbs) is involved:

↓

Grasp the animal's chest just behind the elbows with your hand (thumb on one side, fingers on the other). The animal should be lying on its right side.

↓

In a smooth, rhythmic fashion, firmly compress the chest at a rate of 2 compressions per second. Each compression should last approximately one-half second. Remember to release your grip after each compression. Do not use excessive force when performing this procedure, for to do so could damage ribs or internal organs. As a general rule of thumb, the chest should be compressed about 2 inches on each side. For small puppies and kittens, compress the chest no more than one inch per side.

↓

After every 10 compressions, perform another artificial respiration. Remember to use gentle puffs of breath for neonatal puppies and kittens.

If a larger dog (> 20 lbs.) is involved:

↓

Lay the dog on its right side.

↓

Place the heel of your hand on the ribcage just behind the elbow, then place your other hand on top of the first hand.

↓

Firmly and smoothly compress the chest 3 to 4 inches using both hands. Each compression should last approximately one-half second.

↓

Perform these chest compressions at a rate of one per second. After every 10 compressions, perform an artificial respiration.

↓

Continue this sequence until the heartbeat resumes or until veterinary care is obtained.

A-6 *Performing chest compressions on a critical patient.*

Breathing difficulties/choking

Signs of breathing difficulties or choking: coughing, gagging, wide-base stance with head and neck extended, open-mouth breathing, pale or purple gums and mucous membranes, forceful expansion and contraction of the ribcage.

Priorities: • **Ensure a patent airway; relieve choke if present.**
             • **Give artificial respiration or CPR if needed.**

CHOKING _____

Has your pet been coughing ———→ YES ———→ Transport to your
violently or spitting up blood   veterinarian at once.
or mucus?
                                              Give CPR if needed (See CPR
No   pg. 646)

Does your pet have a chest ———→ YES ———→ (See Chest Wounds pg. 661)
wound?

No

Does your pet appear to be ———→ No ———→ Take your pet to your
choking?   veterinarian for
                                          determination of breathing
                                          problem.

YES

Carefully open the mouth
using a tongue depressor or
similar object. Do not use
your finger.

Is an obstruction visible? ———→ YES ———→ If you see a foreign object,
                                          attempt to dislodge and
                                          remove it with the depressor
                                          or tweezers.

No

Does your pet weigh over 20 ———→ No ———→ Place a hand on each side of
pounds?   the chest near the last three
                                          ribs.

YES

Choking, cont. _____

Straddle the pet with your legs, and interlock your hands underneath the chest.

↓

Apply a forceful, upwards-and-inwards motion, actually lifting the pet off of the ground. The objective is to create a forceful expulsion of air from the lungs. A sharp blow to the back might also be useful dislodging the obstruction.

Apply a quick, forceful squeeze inwards and forwards. CAUTION: Too much force can fracture ribs and cause internal injuries.

↓

Repeat until the foreign object is dislodged.

↓

Institute CPR if necessary.

↓

Rush pet to your veterinarian.

Shock (circulatory shock)

Signs of Shock: rapid heart rate; weak, thready pulse; cold, pale mucous membranes; dry, shriveled tongue; weakness; stupor or unconsciousness; panting; subnormal temperature.

Priorities: • **Determine if shock exists.**
              • **Prevent progression of shock.**

Circulatory shock is a life-threatening situation often associated with trauma and other medical disorders in animals. Prompt attention to this condition is vital. In shock, the blood fails to circulate properly throughout the body; as a result, the tissues and organs do not get enough oxygen to maintain their normal functions. Causes of shock can include excessive bleeding, heart disease, infection, and severe stress and pain due to trauma or any major illness. Shock needs to be treated with intravenous fluids and medications administered by a veterinarian; therefore, the sooner you get your pet to your veterinarian, the better its chances of survival are.

SHOCK _____

Are any signs of shock present? ——————→ NO ——————→ For other problems, see appropriate sections.

↓

YES

↓

Be sure the mouth and airway are clear of obstructions.

↓

Shock, cont. _____

Control bleeding using direct
pressure, pressure points, or
a tourniquet (see Deep
Wounds and Punctures
pg. 655).

↓

Obtain a temperature using a
rectal thermometer. Leave the
thermometer in place for
three minutes before taking a
reading.

↓

Is the body temperature ————————→ YES ————→ Use blankets, towels soaked
below normal (see Normal   in warm water, or hot water
Values pg. 643)?   bottles to attempt to raise the
                                                      body temperature to within
                                                      normal limits.

↓   ↓

NO   Monitor the temperature
                                                      every five minutes.

↓   ↓

Attempt to maintain the body
temperature by covering your
pet with a blanket or towel.

                                                      Once the lower end of
←————————————————————————————   normal body temperature is
                                                      achieved, remove all heat
                                                      sources.

↓

Minimize stress. Talk to your
pet using a calm, reassuring
voice.

↓

Institute proper first aid for
severe injuries or infection
(see appropriate sections).

↓

Seek immediate veterinary
help.

Dehydration

Signs of Dehydration: weight loss, loss of skin elasticity, dry mucous membranes,
sunken eyeballs, depression.

Priorities: • **Treat the underlying cause**
             • **Manage shock**

A state of dehydration can occur in dogs and cats whenever there is excessive fluid loss from the body. Conditions that predispose the animal to dehydration include water and food deprivation, burns, large wounds, increased frequency of urination, vomiting, diarrhea, bleeding, increased salivation, and excessive panting. When a pet becomes dehydrated, its blood becomes very thick. As a result, the heart is required to work extra hard in order to pump blood through the blood vessels to the organs throughout the body. In severe cases of dehydration, circulatory shock and subsequent organ failure can result (see Shock pg. 649).

Skin elasticity can be tested by gently lifting the skin along your pet's back, then releasing it. If it fails to return to its normal position, then your pet is dehydrated.

All suspected cases of dehydration should receive prompt veterinary care. Simply allowing the animal unlimited access to water will not correct the condition. On the contrary, intravenous fluids administered by your veterinarian will be needed to rehydrate your pet while the underlying cause of the dehydration is being determined.

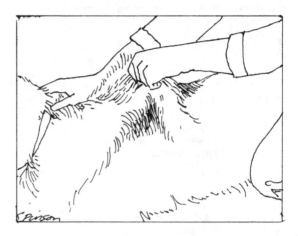

A-7 *Determining hydration status.*

Trauma

Priorities: • Give CPR if needed.
 • Control bleeding and shock.
 • Assess specific injuries and render appropriate first aid.

Table A-4
Common Injuries Resulting From Hit-By-Car

Fractures
Lung bruises/swelling
Internal bleeding
Diaphragmatic hernia
Concussion
Ruptured internal organ

Frequent sources of trauma encountered in small animals include automobiles (including fan belts), gunshot wounds, fights with other animals, falls or jumps from elevations, and blows from blunt objects. Whatever the source of trauma, you should follow these first aid steps:

TRAUMA

Is your pet conscious? ──────→ No ──────→ (See Unconsciousness pg. 653)

↓

YES

↓

Handle all injured animals with caution. If possible, apply a muzzle (see pg. 640)

↓

Are wounds or active ──────→ YES ──────→ (See Deep Wounds and Punctures pg. 655)
bleeding present?

↓

No

↓

Is your pet showing signs of ──────→ YES ──────→ (See Shock pg. 649)
shock, including pale, dry mucous membranes, a dry, shriveled tongue, panting, a weak, thready pulse, and/or a subnormal temperature?

↓

No

↓

Do you suspect any broken ──────→ YES ──────→ (See Lameness pg. 669)
bones as evident by lameness, localized swelling or pain, abnormal limb position or mobility, and/or crepitation (a crackling feel made when two edges of bone rub together)?

↓

No

↓

Are signs of spinal or head ──────→ No ──────→ Transport to your
injury present, including veterinarian for follow-up
paralysis and inability to evaluation.
move, loss of pain sensation, incoordination, unequal pupil size, convulsions, and/or bloody or clear discharges from the mouth, nose, or ears?

↓

Trauma, cont.

YES
↓
Are convulsions occurring?————▶ YES ————▶ (See Convulsions pg. 679)
↓
NO
↓
Slide your pet onto a board,
stiff piece of cardboard,
window screen, or taut
blanket.
↓
Transport to your
veterinarian.

Unconsciousness

Priorities: • **Ensure patent airway.**
• **Institute CPR if needed.**
• **Prevent or control shock.**
• **Transport to your veterinarian.**

If you find a pet unconscious, you must first determine whether or not cardiopulmonary resuscitation is necessary.

UNCONSCIOUSNESS

Is a heartbeat or pulse————▶ NO ————▶(See CPR pg. 646)
detectable?
↓
YES
↓
Is your pet breathing?————▶ NO ————▶(See Artificial Respiration
                                            pg. 646)
↓
YES
↓
Be sure the mouth and
airway are clear of
obstructions.
↓
Control any bleeding using
direct pressure, pressure
points, or a tourniquet (see
Bleeding pg. 654). Institute
proper first aid for severe
injuries or infection.
↓
Cover the pet with a blanket
or towel. DO NOT use heaters
or electric blankets. To do so
could aggravate shock.

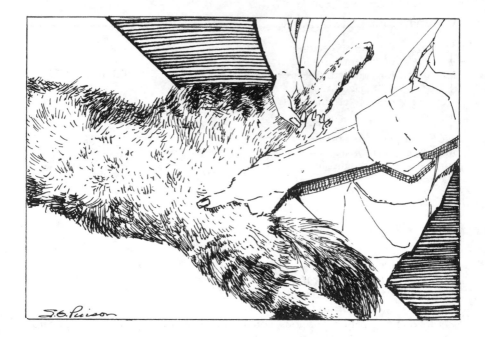

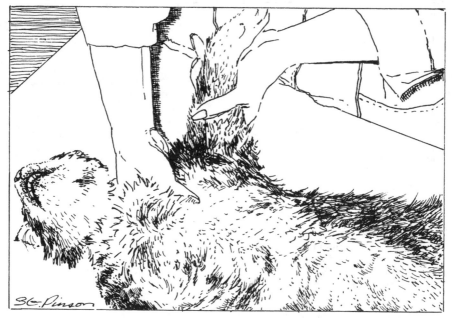

A-8   *Check for a pulse in any unconscious pet.*

Deep wounds and punctures/bleeding

Priorities: • Control bleeding
• Prevent further contamination
• Institute CPR if needed
• Manage shock
• Seek veterinary attention

DEEP WOUNDS

Is there a foreign body within or protruding from the wound? ————→ YES ———→ Do not attempt to remove it unless it is very loose.

↓

NO

↓

Is there active bleeding from the wound? ———— NO ———— Use CPR if needed (see CPR pg. 646)

↓

If the wound involves the chest, (see Chest Wounds pg. 661).

↓

If the wound is penetrating the abdomen, (see Abdominal Injuries pg. 662)

↓

Do not attempt to clean or scrub the wound.

↓

Apply a dressing and bandage to the wound (see pg. 658).

↓

Manage shock (see Shock pg. 649).

↓

Transport to your veterinarian.

YES

↓

Is the wound on an extremity? ————————→ NO ———→ Apply direct pressure to the wound using a sterile gauze, clean cloth, or your hand.

↓

YES

↓

Deep wounds cont. _____

Do you suspect a limb ————————→ YES ————→ Apply direct pressure to the
fracture, characterized by   wound using sterile gauze, a
crepitation, abnormal limb   clean cloth, or, as a last
position or mobility,   resort, your hand.
swelling, pain, and/or loss of
function?

                                                   See Fractures pg. 669.

NO

Elevate the wound if
possible.

Apply direct pressure to the
site of bleeding for five
minutes using a sterile gauze
pad, clean cloth, or other
form of compress.

Is the wound still bleeding? ————→ NO ————→ Apply a dressing and
                                                   bandage (see Dressings &
                                                   Bandages, pg. 658).

                                                   Use CPR as needed (see CPR
                                                   pg. 646).

                                                   Manage shock (see Shock
                                                   pg. 649).

                                                   Transport to your
                                                   veterinarian.

YES

Apply pressure to the
appropriate pressure points
located in the armpit and/or
groin (see FIG. A-8) to reduce
the blood flow to the wound.
Attempt to maintain direct
pressure at the same time.

Deep wounds cont. _____

Apply a tourniquet only if the bleeding cannot be controlled by the aforementioned procedures. Position the tourniquet just above the wound and tie a half knot. Use a stick, pencil, or similar object to twist and tighten the tourniquet down until the bleeding is minimized. You should still be able to slip a finger between the tourniquet and the skin. If you can't, then it is on too tight. Gauze, rubber tubing, belts, neckties, and pantyhose all make useful tourniquets.

↓

Institute CPR if needed (see CPR pg. 646).

↓

Manage shock (see Shock pg. 649).

↓

Transport pet to your veterinarian immediately. NOTE: Prolonged application of a tourniquet could lead to loss of the limb.

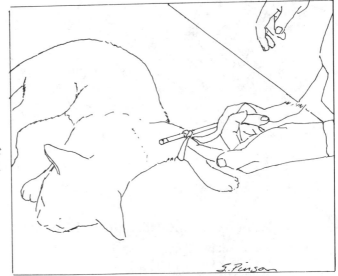

A-9   *Proper tourniquet placement.*

Application of dressings and bandages

A dressing is a protective covering that is placed directly over a wound. It can be made of any material; ideally it should be sterile or at least very clean. It is used to control bleeding, to absorb blood and other fluids, and to minimize wound contamination.

Dressings are held in place by bandages. The most useful bandages are gauze bandages and elastic bandages. Both types can be secured with tape, safety pins, or clips. A bandage should be tight enough to keep the dressing in place, not so tight that it interferes with circulation. Swelling and discoloration at the affected site should prompt you to loosen the bandage.

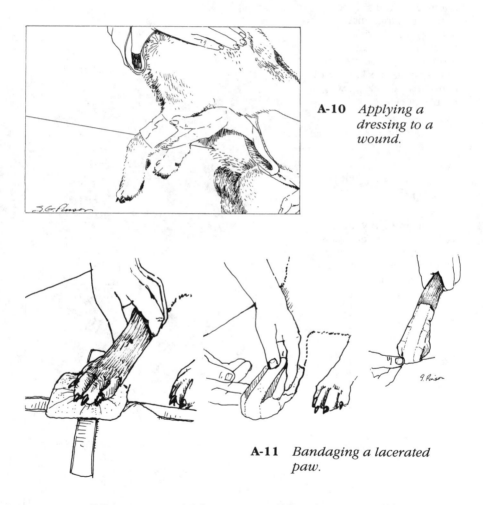

A-10 *Applying a dressing to a wound.*

A-11 *Bandaging a lacerated paw.*

Minor cuts and lacerations/bleeding toenails

Priorities: • Control bleeding.
            • Clean wound.
            • Prevent infection.

MINOR CUTS _____

Is the wound a puncture, is it —————— YES ——————— (see Deep Wounds and
greater than 1/4 inch deep, Punctures pg. 655)
and/or is it bleeding
profusely?

↓

NO

↓

Is a toenail involved? ———————— YES ————→ Apply direct pressure to the
nail for 5 – 10 minutes.

↓

NO

↓

If minor bleeding is   Apply a styptic pencil,
occurring, apply direct   clotting powder, or a silver
pressure to the wound, using   nitrate stick to the exposed
a sterile gauze or clean cloth,   end of the nail. (CAUTION:
for 5 minutes.   Silver nitrate stings!)

↓

Use a mild hand soap and
water or hydrogen peroxide
to clean the wound. (If
clippers are available, clip the
hair from around the wound
before cleaning.)

↓

Rinse thoroughly with tap
water. Gently blot the wound
dry, preferably with a sterile
gauze.

↓

Apply an antibiotic ointment
or cream to the wound three
times a day for 5 to 7 days to
help prevent infection.
Bandaging is optional, yet it
might help prevent excessive
licking or chewing by the
animal (see Bandaging
pg. 658).

↓

Are signs of infection, ————————→ YES ————→ Seek immediate veterinary
including swelling, heat, care.
pain, redness, and/or pus,
present?

↓

NO ——————————————————————————→ If healing is not occurring
within 5 – 7 days, consult
your veterinarian.

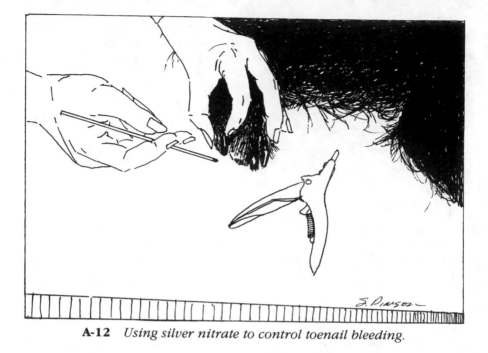

A-12   *Using silver nitrate to control toenail bleeding.*

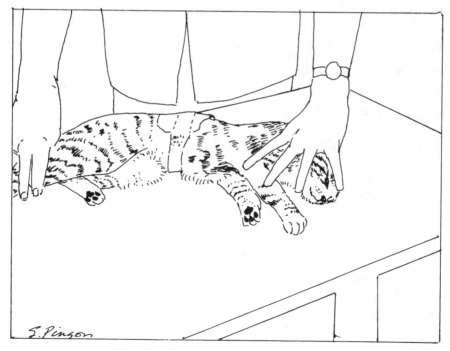

A-13   *Bandaging a chest wound in a cat.*

Chest wounds

Priorities: • Prevent air leakage from the lungs.
   • Control bleeding.
   • Give artificial respiration and/or CPR if needed.
   • Obtain veterinary assistance.

CHEST WOUNDS

Does the wound appear to be ——→ NO ——→ If a minor cut or laceration is
a sucking chest wound,   involved (see Minor Cuts
characterized by a rush of air   pg. 659)
from the wound opening and
breathing difficulties?

If a deep wound or puncture
is involved, (see Deep
Wounds and Punctures
pg. 655).

YES

With a piece of gauze, a clean
cloth, or your hand, seal the
wound by applying firm
pressure. This will also help
control bleeding.

Apply a bandage around the
chest to secure the seal
material (see Bandaging
pg. 658). Be sure the bandage
does not interfere with
normal chest expansion.

Give artificial respiration
and/or CPR if needed (see
CPR pg. 646).

Transport to your
veterinarian as soon as
possible.

Abdominal injuries and pain

Signs of internal abdominal injury and pain: lethargy, weakness, abdominal tenderness, blood in urine or feces, panting, arched back, shock.

Priorities: • Control bleeding.
   • Minimize contamination in the case of an open wound.
   • Manage shock and give CPR if needed.
   • Seek veterinary attention.

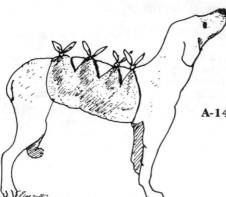

A-14   *Support sling for abdominal wound.*

ABDOMINAL INJURIES

Has a wound occurred whereby abdominal contents or intestines are exposed? ——→ YES ——→ Gently rinse the exposed organs with tap water.

Carefully place the organs back into the abdominal cavity.

NO

If a wound is involved, (see Deep Wounds and Punctures pg. 655).

In all cases of suspected abdominal injury or pain, consult your veterinarian at once, even if no signs of internal injuries are present. These signs might not show up for 12 to 24 hours after an injury occurs.

Pack the wound with a moist towel.

Apply a bandage encircling the abdomen to keep the pack in place.

Give CPR if needed (see CPR pg. 646) and manage shock (see Shock pg. 649).

Give CPR if needed (see CPR pg. 646) and manage shock (see Shock pg. 649).

Seek immediate veterinary help.

Thermal burns

Signs of thermal burns: redness, blisters, charred skin, singed haircoat.

Priorities: • Relieve pain.
• Reduce contamination and prevent infection.
• Prevent or treat shock.

THERMAL BURNS _____

Was the burn caused by ⟶ No ⟶ (See Chemical burns pg. 663)
exposure to flame or heat?

↓

YES

↓

Is the skin blistered or ————— No ⟶ Apply cold water or a cold
broken?   pack to the affected area.

↓   ↓

YES   Apply a small amount of
                                 topical anesthetic cream to
                                 help reduce the pain.

↓

Do not immerse the burned
region in water or apply any
medication to the burned
surface.

↓

Apply a sterile, nonadherent
dressing and bandage (see
Bandaging pg. 658).

↓

Manage shock if present (see
Shock pg. 649).

↓

Seek veterinary attention. ◄————————————————————

Chemical burns

Signs of chemical burns: redness, blisters, charred skin, moist skin and haircoat
(where chemical contact was made).

Priorities: • Neutralize or remove offending chemical.
• Relieve pain.
• Reduce contamination and prevent infection.
• Prevent or treat shock.

CHEMICAL BURNS _____

Flush the affected site
thoroughly with water for 5
minutes, even if the skin is
blistered or broken.

↓

Chemical burns, cont.

Do not apply any topical medication to the burn site.

↓

Is the nature (acid or base) of → NO → Apply a sterile dressing and the chemical involved bandage (see Bandaging known? pg. 658).

↓

YES

↓

If an *acid* is involved, mix 1 tsp. baking soda into 1 cup of water and apply to the affected region.

↓

Prevent your pet from licking or chewing at the affected region.

↓

If a *base* is involved, mix 1 tsp. vinegar into 1 cup of water and apply to the affected region.

↓

Transport to your veterinarian for further treatment. Manage shock if present (see Shock pg. 649).

↓

Flush with water for 5 minutes.

Poisoning

Signs of poisoning: vomiting, diarrhea, depression, unconsciousness, convulsions, muscle tremors, abdominal pain, drooling, panting, shock.

Priorities:
 • **Determine the type of poison involved.**
 • **Dilute or neutralize the poison.**
 • **Give CPR if needed and control shock.**
 • **Rush to veterinarian for specific antidote (if available).**

Poisoning, whether accidental or malicious in nature, is a common emergency situation in small animals. Prompt management is essential to ensure the health of the pet.

Any chemical, drug, or plant found within and around the home should be regarded as a potential poison to the household pet. For instance, antifreeze can quickly cause kidney failure in a pet that consumes only a small portion of the liquid (which, by the way, has a pleasing taste to animals). Aspirin and acetaminophen are very poisonous to cats due to this animal's limited ability to metabolize or break down those drugs.

Other causes of poisoning in pets can include the consumption of rat, snail, roach, and predator poisons; food items such as chocolate and salt; and living creatures such as salamanders and toads. Ingestion or application of flea sprays and other insecticides also account for numerous reported cases of poisonings.

Finally, many household plants can cause nausea, vomiting, diarrhea, heart problems, convulsions, coma, and/or death if eaten by dogs or cats. See TABLE A-6 for a list of house and ornamental plants that can be hazardous to your pet.

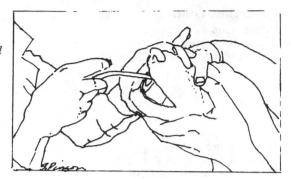

A-15 *Activated charcoal can be placed directly into the stomach (using a stomach tube) to neutralize poisonings.*

Table A-5 Drugs & Medications That Can Be Toxic To Cats

Aspirin
Acetaminophen
Ibuprofin
Iodine
Coal tar shampoos
Organophosphates
Phosphate enemas
Primidone

POISONING

Was the poison swallowed? ──────► No ──────► If the poison was absorbed through the skin (e.g., flea dip toxicity), flush the affected area with copious amounts of water. If the entire body is involved, wash the entire body with soap and water, rinsing well.

Yes
↓

Try to identify the poison. If present, read the label on the container and follow its directions pertaining to accidental poisoning.
↓

Contact a veterinarian immediately and explain what the poison was and how much was consumed.
↓

Is the poison a caustic ──────► Yes ──────► Do not induce vomiting!
substance, or
petroleum-based (see TABLE
A-7)? Does the label specify (cont.)

Poisoning, cont.

"Do not induce vomiting"?
Is your pet severely
depressed, unconscious, or
convulsing?

↓

No

↓

Induce vomiting using
hydrogen peroxide (1
teaspoon), salty water (1 to 2
tablespoons of salt per 1 cup
of water), or syrup of ipecac
(1/2 ml per pound).

↓

Dilute the remaining poison
by giving 2 to 3 cups of   ←
water orally.

↓

Try to deactivate the poison
by giving activated charcoal
(mix 25–50 grams of powder
with water to form a
soup-like slurry, then
administer 1 ml per pound of
this mixture), milk (1 to 2
cups), egg whites (2 per pint
of water), and/or milk of
magnesia (1 to 2 teaspoons
mixed with water).

↓

If necessary, administer CPR
(see CPR pg. 646), and
manage shock (see Shock
pg. 649).

↓

Transport your pet to your
veterinarian as soon as
possible for further
treatment. Be sure to save the   ←
label or container that the
poison was in, and take it
with you to the veterinary
clinic.

Table A-6   Ornamental Plants That Are Hazardous To Pets

Aconite	Hydrangea
Amaryllis	Iris
Azalea	Jerusalem Cherry
Bittersweet	Jonquil
Caladium	Larkspur
Castor Bean	Laurel
Common Box	Lily-of-the-Valley
Crown-of-Thorns	Narcissus
Daffodils	Nightshades
Daphne	Oleander
Dumbcane	Philodendron
Elephant Ear	Pine Needles
English Holly	Poinsettia
English Ivy	Precatory Bean
Euonymus	Rhododendron
Foxglove	Rose Bay
Honeysuckle	Skunk Cabbage
Hyacinth	Wisteria
	Yew

Table A-7   Poisonings In Which Vomiting Should Not Be Induced

Bathroom cleaners
Drain cleaners
Dry-cleaning fluids
Fire extinguisher fluid
Fuels (gasoline, oils, etc.)
Furniture polish
Glues and adhesives
Laundry bleach
Metal cleaners
Oven cleaners
Paint and varnish removers
Rust removers

Lameness and fractures

Priorities:
- Determine if a fracture exists.
- Control bleeding if present.
- Prevent further injury or contamination.
- Stabilize the fracture if possible.

Causes of lameness in dogs and cats can include, among other things, muscle strains, tendon and ligament sprains, abscesses, foreign bodies, tumors, arthritis, bruises, dislocations, and fractures. In all instances, however, the cause of the lameness should be determined by your veterinarian.

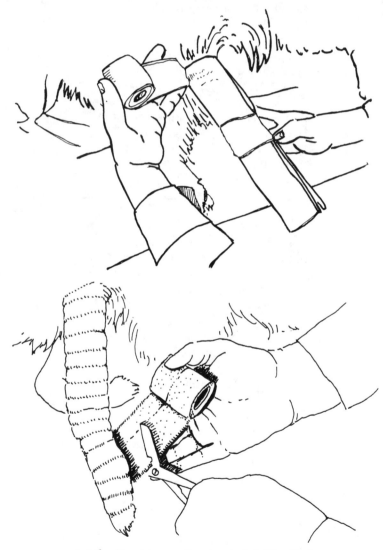

A-16 *Temporary fracture stabilization.*

LAMENESS

Are signs of potential fracture ——► NO ——► Have your pet's lameness
present, including abnormal   evaluated by your
limb position or mobility,   veterinarian.
localized pain, bruising
and/or swelling, or
crepitation (the crackling feel
made when two ends of
bone rub together)?

↓

YES

↓

Is the fracture open, with ——► YES ——► Do not attempt to replace the
ends of bone protruding   exposed ends of bone or to
through the skin?   clean the wound.

↓   ↓

NO   Control bleeding (see
                                              Bleeding pg. 655).

                                              ↓

                                              Apply a sterile or clean
                                              dressing and bandage (see
                                              Bandaging pg. 658).

↓

Is the fracture below your ——► NO
pet's elbow or knee?

↓

YES

↓

Immobilize the fracture by
applying a splint to the
affected region (fractures
above the elbow and knee
are difficult to stabilize with a
conventional splint). A
rolled-up magazine affixed to
the limb with adhesive tape
or cloth (see FIG. A-16) makes
an excellent splint. Other
materials that can be used as
splints include sticks, rulers,
yardsticks, tongue
depressors, etc. Avoid taping
or tying directly over the
fracture site.

↓

Seek veterinary assistance at ◄
once.

Nosebleeds

Priorities: • **Control bleeding.**
             • **Determine cause.**

NOSEBLEEDS

Elevate your pet's nose by pointing it straight up into the air.

↓

Squeeze both nostrils shut with your thumb and forefinger for 5 minutes. Depending on the size or the nostrils, gauze may be packed within the nostrils to control the bleeding.

↓

Is the nosebleed due to ——————→ YES ———→ (See Trauma pg. 652).
trauma?

↓

NO (or unknown)

↓

Have your veterinarian examine your pet.

Fishhooks

Priorities: • **Remove fishhook if possible.**
             • **Control bleeding.**
             • **Prevent infection.**

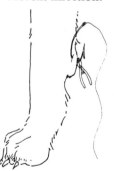

A-17   *Removal of a fishhook from the leg of a dog.*

FISHHOOKS

Is the fishhook embedded in ——→ YES ———→ Do not attempt to remove
the mouth or eye?   the hook.

↓   ↓

NO   Try to minimize movement
                                                 and prevent self-trauma.

↓   ↓

Fishhooks cont.

Advance the hook until the barbed end is exposed.

↓

Snip off the end of the barb with scissors.

↓

Remove the remaining portion of the hook by gently backing it out of the entry site.

↓

All puncture wounds should be seen by your veterinarian to help prevent infection.

Seek veterinary help.

Eye injuries and disorders

Signs of eye injury or irritation: redness, drainage or discharge, cloudiness, protrusion of third eyelid, squinting, pawing at the eye(s).

Any injury to the eye(s) must be regarded as a medical emergency. The same is true for any redness or irritation you note in the eye(s). Prompt first aid administered at home, followed by immediate veterinary care, will help reduce the chances of partial or permanent blindness. With any eye injury, consider taping the animal's front paws or front legs together to help prevent the pet from scratching at and further traumatizing the eye.

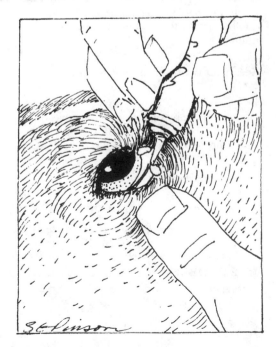

A-18 *Use sterile ointment to help protect injured eyes from further insult.*

Eye prolapse (eye out of socket)

Priorities: • Keep the eyeball moist.
• Prevent further trauma to the eye.
• Treat shock if necessary.

EYE PROLAPSE _____

Apply sterile ophthalmic solution (such as contact lens solution), ophthalmic ointment (if available), or plain tap water in order to keep the eyeball moist.

↓

Do not attempt to push the eye back into its socket.

↓

Prevent your pet from rubbing or further traumatizing the eye.

↓

Watch for signs of shock and treat accordingly (see Shock pg. 649).

↓

Seek immediate veterinary assistance.

Chemical burns of the eye

Priorities: • Dilute the offending chemical.
• Prevent self-trauma to the eye.

CHEMICAL BURNS OF THE EYE _____

Flush the affected eye(s) thoroughly with copious amounts of water for 5 to 10 minutes.

↓

Keep your pet from rubbing the affected eye(s).

↓

Do not apply any ointments to the eye(s). To do so could seal in the caustic agent and cause further damage.

↓

Seek immediate veterinary assistance.

Eye foreign bodies, scratches, and/or bleeding

Priorities: • Remove any foreign matter, if possible.
• Control bleeding if present.
• Prevent self-trauma.

EYE PROBLEMS _____

Is there a foreign body ──────────→YES────────→Do not attempt to dislodge
penetrating the eye?   the object.

↓   ↓

Eye problems, cont.

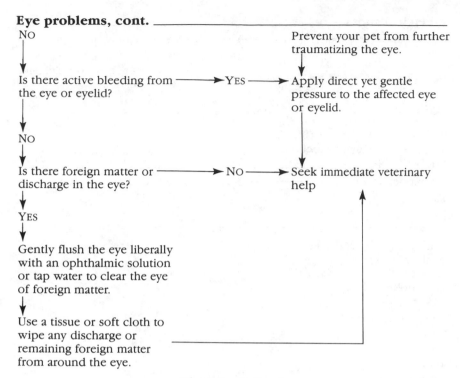

No

Is there active bleeding from ———►YES———► the eye or eyelid?

No

Is there foreign matter or ———► No ———► discharge in the eye?

YES

Gently flush the eye liberally with an ophthalmic solution or tap water to clear the eye of foreign matter.

Use a tissue or soft cloth to wipe any discharge or remaining foreign matter from around the eye.

Prevent your pet from further traumatizing the eye.

Apply direct yet gentle pressure to the affected eye or eyelid.

Seek immediate veterinary help

Electrical shock

Signs of electrical shock: breathing difficulties, unconsciousness, burns noted on the lips, tongue, and corners of the mouth.

Priorities: • **Give CPR if needed.**
  • **Manage circulatory shock.**
  • **Obtain veterinary help as quickly as possible.**

ELECTRICAL SHOCK

Before proceeding, remember that your safety comes first. Disconnect the power supply to the source or turn off the main electrical switch. Use a long pole or similar item to move the pet away from the electrical source.

Is your pet conscious? ————————► No———► (See Unconsciousness pg. 653)

YES

Is your pet having breathing ———► YES———► Give CPR (see CPR pg. 646) difficulties?   if needed.

Rush to your veterinarian.

No

Electrical shock, cont. _____

Does your pet have burns? ───────►YES─────── (See Thermal Burns pg. 663)

↓

Take pet to your veterinarian
for evaluation.

Drowning

Priorities: • **Administer CPR.**
• **Manage shock.**

DROWNING _____

Is your pet unconscious? ───────►YES───────►(See Unconsciousness

↓   pg. 653)

No

↓ ◄───

↓

Hold your pet upside-down
by the hind legs for 20
seconds to allow the water to
drain from the lungs.

↓

Wrap your pet in a blanket or
towel.

↓

Transport to your
veterinarian, watching for
signs of shock (see Shock
pg. 649) or cessation of
breathing (see CPR pg. 646).

Ingestion of a foreign object

Signs: abdominal pain, vomiting, diarrhea, gagging, excessive salivation.

Priorities: • **Induce vomiting if warranted.**
• **Observe for signs of illness.**

INGESTION OF A FOREIGN OBJECT _____

   Ingestion of a foreign object must be considered any time a pet shows sudden abdominal pain, vomiting, and/or diarrhea. Also, this possibility must be ruled out in those animals with a history of chronic vomiting. Due to their inherent curiosity, puppies and kittens are the ones most likely to swallow foreign objects.

Is the ingested object or   ───────► YES───────►(See Poisoning pg. 664)
substance a potential poison?

↓

No

↓

Did the ingested object have ───────►YES───────►Do not induce vomiting.
pointed or potentially sharp
edges?   ↓

↓

Ingestion of foreign object, cont. _____

NO

↓

Is your pet vomiting, or ————————→ YES ——→ Obtain veterinary assistance
showing other signs of   as soon as possible.
illness?

↓

NO

↓

Feed your pet a piece of
bread to help coat and bind
the object.

↓

Induce vomiting (see
Poisoning pg. 664).

↓

If the object is not
regurgitated, has not passed
within 24 hours after
ingestion, or if your pet
shows any signs of illness or
pain in that time, veterinary
intervention is required.

Allergic reactions

Signs of allergic reaction: intense itching, swelling, hives, vomiting, lethargy,
breathing difficulties, fever, shock.

Priorities: • Determine the severity of the reaction.
              • Give CPR if needed.
              • Manage shock if present.

A-19   *Facial swelling caused
by an allergic reaction.*

Allergic reactions can occur following administration of medications, vaccinations, exposure to chemicals and environmental irritants or to snake and insect bites. The degree of reaction can vary considerably with each incident.

Mild to moderate allergic reactions are often accompanied by intense scratching, hives, soreness, vomiting, swelling, fever, and lethargy. Signs, can show up minutes to hours (usually no more than 6 hours) following exposure to the offending substance.

A severe allergic reaction (called *anaphylactic shock*) constitutes a medical emergency. This type of reaction most often appears seconds to minutes after exposure to the offending agent. Signs of this type of reaction include breathing difficulties, shock, collapse, and unconsciousness.

ALLERGIC REACTIONS

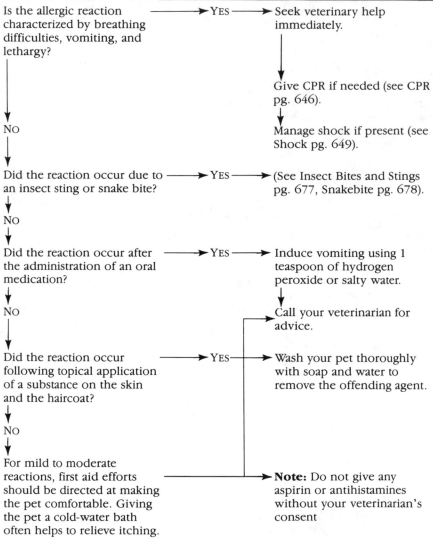

Is the allergic reaction characterized by breathing difficulties, vomiting, and lethargy? ——→ YES ——→ Seek veterinary help immediately.

Give CPR if needed (see CPR pg. 646).

Manage shock if present (see Shock pg. 649).

NO

Did the reaction occur due to an insect sting or snake bite? ——→ YES ——→ (See Insect Bites and Stings pg. 677, Snakebite pg. 678).

NO

Did the reaction occur after the administration of an oral medication? ——→ YES ——→ Induce vomiting using 1 teaspoon of hydrogen peroxide or salty water.

Call your veterinarian for advice.

NO

Did the reaction occur following topical application of a substance on the skin and the haircoat? ——→ YES ——→ Wash your pet thoroughly with soap and water to remove the offending agent.

NO

For mild to moderate reactions, first aid efforts should be directed at making the pet comfortable. Giving the pet a cold-water bath often helps to relieve itching. ——→ **Note:** Do not give any aspirin or antihistamines without your veterinarian's consent

Insect and spider bites and stings

Signs associated with a bite or sting: localized redness, swelling, pain, lameness, salivation, breathing difficulties, shock.

Priorities: • Determine severity of signs.
  • Prevent infection.
  • Treat shock.

INSECT BITES & STINGS _____

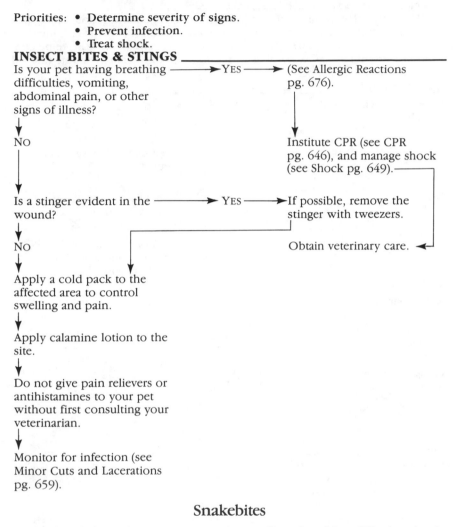

Is your pet having breathing ———►YES———► (See Allergic Reactions difficulties, vomiting, abdominal pain, or other signs of illness?

pg. 676).

No

Institute CPR (see CPR pg. 646), and manage shock (see Shock pg. 649).

Is a stinger evident in the ———► YES———►If possible, remove the wound?

stinger with tweezers.

No

Obtain veterinary care.

Apply a cold pack to the affected area to control swelling and pain.

Apply calamine lotion to the site.

Do not give pain relievers or antihistamines to your pet without first consulting your veterinarian.

Monitor for infection (see Minor Cuts and Lacerations pg. 659).

Snakebites

Signs of snakebite: Fang punctures, pain, swelling, breathing difficulty, shock, paralysis.

Priorities: • Reduce spread of venom.
  • Manage shock.
  • Give CPR if needed.

Consequences associated with snakebite are related to the type of snake involved, the amount of venom injected into the animal, and the location of the bite wound. The venom of pit vipers, such as rattlesnakes and water moccasins, causes tissue damage and destroys red blood cells. On the contrary, coral snake venom often causes little pain or swelling; however, it does affect the animal's nervous system, and difficulty swallowing, depression, paralysis, and death are common sequela to the bite of this snake.

Snakebites that occur on the head and neck can be more serious since they can cause direct damage to many vital structures in these regions and interfere with breathing. Furthermore, bites in these areas are difficult to manage by conventional first aid means. Regardless of the location of the bite, institute first aid immediately and do the best you can.

SNAKEBITES

Is veterinary care readily available? ———————→ YES ———→ Keep your pet as calm as possible.

See Deep Wounds and Punctures pg. 655).

NO

Apply a cold pack to the affected area.

Manage shock (see Shock pg. 649) and give CPR (see CPR pg. 646) if needed.

Keep your pet calm to prevent the rapid spread of venom throughout the bloodstream.

Obtain veterinary care.

Is the bite on an extremity? ———————→ NO

YES

Apply a tourniquet 2 to 3 inches above the bite wound if possible. Roll gauze, rubber tubing, belts, neckties, and pantyhose all make good tourniquets. Tighten the tourniquet using a stick, pencil, or similar object. The tourniquet should be tight, yet you should be able to easily slip a finger between it and the skin.

Is the limb starting to swell below the tourniquet? ———————→ YES ———→ Loosen the tourniquet slightly, but don't remove it.

Snakebites, cont. _____

No
↓
Apply a muzzle. ◄─────────────────────────────────┐
↓

Make a ¹/4-inch-deep incision
over each fang mark (be sure
the animal is muzzled and
restrained) and allow the
wound to bleed for 1 to 2
minutes. Apply suction with
a bulb syringe or syringe, if
available. Do not use your
mouth!
↓

Clean the wound with soap
and water, and apply a first
aid ointment or cream to the
wound (if available).
↓

Apply a sterile or clean
dressing to the wound and
bandage (see Bandaging
pg. 658).
↓

Loosen the tourniquet for 30
seconds every 15 minutes
until veterinary care is
obtained. Prolonged
application of the tourniquet
can result in loss of the limb.

Seizures (convulsions)

Signs of seizures: uncontrollable, involuntary muscle activity; altered behavior.

Priorities: • **Prevent self-inflicted injury.**
• **Prevent injury to owner.**

    A seizure should be suspected any time an animal's behavior is altered or involuntary muscle activity is noted. Some possible causes of seizural activity include epilepsy, poisoning, liver and kidney disease, infections, tumors, hypocalcemia (low blood calcium seen in pregnant and nursing mothers), and low blood sugar (sometimes seen in hunting dogs and young puppies and kittens—see chapters 17 and 35). A thorough physical exam and tests performed by your veterinarian might be necessary to identify the actual cause. There is not much you as the owner can do for a convulsing pet except prevent the animal from hurting itself and others.

SEIZURES _____

Restrain your pet by wrapping it in a blanket
or towel.
↓

Seizures, cont. _____

Do not apply a muzzle.

↓

Do not attempt to give anything orally to
the animal.

↓

Transport the pet to your veterinarian
immediately for diagnosis and treatment.

↓

If your pet becomes unconscious, see
Unconsciousness pg. 653).

Vomiting

Signs of impending vomiting: increased drooling, vocalization, violent contractions of the abdominal muscles.

Priorities: • **Prevent further vomiting and dehydration.**
            • **Obtain veterinary help for persistent vomiting.**

Vomiting, the forceful expulsion of food or stomach secretions through the
mouth, is actually a symptom of some underlying disorder. Dietary indiscretions,
infections, worms, foreign bodies, metabolic diseases (such as kidney disease),
and poisonings are just a few of the many disorders that can be characterized by
vomiting.

Remember that puppies and kittens can dehydrate seven times faster than
adult animals. As a result, any case of persistent vomiting in a young animal
should be especially regarded as a medical emergency.

Vomiting should be differentiated from regurgitation, which can be defined as
the effortless expulsion of food or saliva from the mouth due to a disorder of the
esophagus. This distinction is important since the causes of the two are different.

VOMITING _____

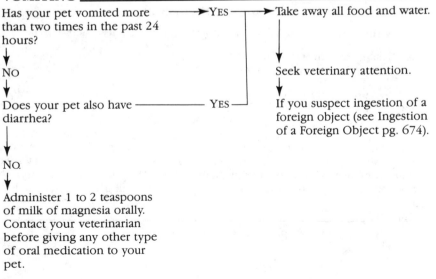

Has your pet vomited more ——→YES——→ Take away all food and water.
than two times in the past 24
hours?

↓   ↓

NO   Seek veterinary attention.

↓   ↓

Does your pet also have ———————— YES┘   If you suspect ingestion of a
diarrhea?   foreign object (see Ingestion
                                                 of a Foreign Object pg. 674).

↓

NO.

↓

Administer 1 to 2 teaspoons
of milk of magnesia orally.
Contact your veterinarian
before giving any other type
of oral medication to your
pet.

Vomiting, cont. _____

↓

Offer only small amounts of
water to prevent
over-drinking and
subsequent stomach upset.

↓

Feed your pet a bland diet
for the next 24 to 48 hours.
Such a diet is available from
your veterinarian or can be
prepared at home using 4
parts boiled rice and 1 part
boiled lean meat, chicken, or
egg.

Diarrhea

Priorities: • **Prevent further diarrhea and dehydration.**

Like vomiting, the danger of diarrhea lies in its ability to rapidly dehydrate
the animal. Because the potential causes of diarrhea are so numerous, any case
that lasts more than 48 hours should be seen by a veterinarian. If, however, the
animal appears markedly depressed, dehydrated (see Dehydration pg. 650), or
exhibits vomiting or blood in the stool at any time, don't delay. Take the pet to
your veterinarian at once. Intravenous fluids and medications may be required
until a diagnosis can be made.

DIARRHEA _____

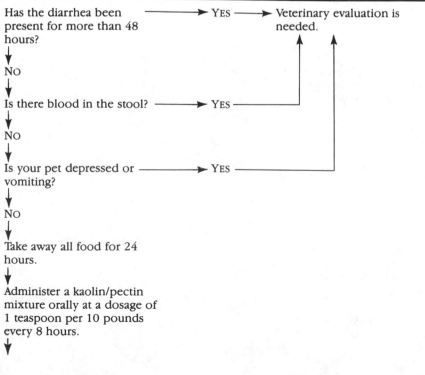

Has the diarrhea been ⟶ YES ⟶ Veterinary evaluation is
present for more than 48   needed.
hours?

↓

NO

↓

Is there blood in the stool? ⟶ YES ⟶

↓

NO

↓

Is your pet depressed or ⟶ YES ⟶
vomiting?

↓

NO

↓

Take away all food for 24
hours.

↓

Administer a kaolin/pectin
mixture orally at a dosage of
1 teaspoon per 10 pounds
every 8 hours.

↓

Diarrhea, cont. _____

↓

After 24 hours, resume feeding using a bland diet (see Vomiting pg. 680) for the next two to three days.

Constipation

Signs of constipation: straining to defecate, passage of dry, hard feces, painful abdomen.

Priorities: • **Differentiate constipation from urination difficulties.**
            • **Relieve constipation.**

If your pet appears to be having difficulty with a bowel movement, constipation might be to blame. Isolated incidents can be treated at home initially, yet if the problem persists, recurs frequently, or is accompanied by lethargy, abdominal pain, or vomiting, a medical exam is warranted. Remember: Many people mistake urinary problems for constipation (see Straining to Urinate pg. 683). If you are in doubt, contact your veterinarian.

CONSTIPATION _____

Has your pet been urinating ——→ No ——→ Seek veterinary assistance.
normally?

↓

YES

↓

Has constipation been a ———→ YES ———
problem for more than 48
hours?

↓

NO

↓

Is your pet exhibiting ———→ YES ———
abdominal pain, lethargy,
and/or vomiting?

↓

NO

↓

Administer hairball laxative
or petroleum jelly orally at 1
teaspoon per 10 pounds
every four hours.

↓

Vegetable oil may also be
used to relieve constipation.
The dosage is 1 teaspoon per
10 pounds (mixed with
food).

↓

Do not attempt to give an
enema at home.

Excessive salivation (drooling)

Priorities: • Seek veterinary help to determine the cause of the salivation if it is not known.

Excessive drooling can indicate excitement, nausea, or some disorder involving the mouth or facial muscles. These disorders can include dental disease, jaw fractures, mouth infections, rabies and other diseases that affect the nervous system, mouth tumors, throat obstructions, and foreign bodies.

If an obstruction or foreign body is involved, carefully attempt to dislodge and/or remove it with tweezers, keeping your safety in mind at all times.

Another cause of excess salivation in dogs and cats is mouth irritation due to the consumption of medications, poisons, plants, insects, or reptiles (especially toads). In these instances, thoroughly rinse the pet's mouth out with copious amounts of water, taking care not to force any water down the animal's windpipe. Follow appropriate first aid measures if poisoning is suspected (see Poisoning pg. 665). In all cases of excessive salivation, consult your veterinarian.

Straining to urinate (urinary obstruction)

Signs of urinary problems: attempts to urinate with minimal to no results, bloody urine, enlarged, painful abdomen, panting, shock.

Priorities: • Seek veterinary attention at once.
  • Manage shock if present.

Both cats and dogs can suffer from a condition in which crystals composed of certain minerals form within the urinary tract and irritate the lining of the tract. In dogs, these crystals can coalesce into actual stones within the bladder, ranging from the size of a small B-B to the size of a softball. In male dogs, stones can prevent the animal from urinating properly, a condition that can prove to be fatal if not treated promptly.

Bladder stones are not as common in the cat, yet the crystals themselves are large enough to create a life-threatening obstruction to urine outflow in male cats.

The reason that obstructions are more likely to occur in males than in females is that the urethra (that portion of the urinary tract that transports urine from the bladder to the outside) of the male is much narrower than that of the female. Consequently, stones and crystals are more likely to become lodged within the male urethra.

If a urinary obstruction is not relieved promptly, death can result due to toxin buildup within the bloodstream, kidney failure, and/or ruptured bladder. As a result, seek veterinary care at once. Don't delay!

Heat stroke

Signs of heat stroke: rapid, noisy panting; bright red mucous membranes; thick, stringy saliva; vomiting; diarrhea; recumbancy; unconsciousness.

Priorities: • Reduce body temperature.
  • Manage shock if present.
  • Give CPR if needed.

Unfortunately, most cases of heat stroke seen in dogs and cats are due to nothing more than owner neglect. As most people know, leaving a pet in a car on a hot day can lead to heat stroke and death in a relatively short period of time. This conditon is also seen in animals left outdoors, restrained on chains or ropes, without adequate shelter, shade, or water. Under these conditions, dogs and cats are very susceptible to over-heating because of their limited ability to "sweat." Panting is the only way they can effectively get rid of excess body heat, and it is easy to see how this mechanism can be overwhelmed by high temperatures. Other predisposing factors to heat stroke include high environmental humidity, exercise, and obesity.

In a case of heat stroke, the animal's temperature often exceeds 106 degrees and if left untreated, can result in permanent brain damage or death. Your prompt action is essential.

HEAT STROKE

Is your pet unconscious? ──────→YES────→(See Unconsciousness pg. 653).

NO
↓

Take your pet's temperature using a lubricated rectal thermometer. Leave it in place at least three minutes before taking a reading.

Does the temperature exceed ────→ No ────→ Move your pet to a cool, shady area.
103 degrees F?

YES   Offer plenty of water, in small portions only.

Move the animal to a cool, shady area.

Immerse your pet in cool water; spray with water from a hose. Use of cold packs is also acceptable.

Monitor rectal temperature every 5 minutes. When the temperature reaches 103 degrees or if more than 20 minutes elapses from the time first aid is instituted (whichever comes first), discontinue the cooling procedure.

Seek immediate veterinary care. Manage shock (see Shock pg. 649) and administer CPR (see CPR pg. 646) if needed.

Offer small amounts of water.

Hypothermia and frostbite

Signs of hypothermia: lethargy, drowsiness, unconsciousness, weak pulse, shallow breathing, shivering, low body temperature.

Signs of frostbite: pale skin, blisters, hair loss.

Priorities: • **Raise and stabilize body temperature.**
   • **Prevent or treat frostbite.**
   • **Manage shock and give CPR if needed.**

Hypothermia and frostbite can occur in any animal exposed to cold temperatures for extended periods of time. Hypothermia is often found in newborns and young puppies and kittens that are not properly kept warm by their mother. Frostbite, when it occurs, usually affects the tips of the ears, tail, and/or scrotum. Blisters might be present.

HYPOTHERMIA AND FROSTBITE

Is your pet conscious? ———————→ No ———→ (See Unconsciousness
                                                                  pg. 653).

↓

YES

Obtain a rectal temperature
using a lubricated
thermometer. Leave it in
place for at least three
minutes before taking a
reading.

Is the body temperature ————→ No—
below 99 degrees F?

YES

Cover your pet with a
blanket or towel and apply
hot water bottles (if
available), or use a heating
pad (low setting).

Monitor rectal temperature
every 15 minutes. When it
reaches the normal range (see
Normal Values pg. 643),
discontinue the reheating
process. The idea is to elevate
the body temperature slowly.

Hypothermia and frostbite, cont. _____

Is there evidence of possible ———→ No ———→ Obtain veterinary care as
frostbite?   soon as possible.

↓

YES

↓

If a portion of the body is
suffering from frostbite, try
to quickly re-warm the
affected area by immersing it
in warm water. *DO NOT RUB
THE AFFECTED PART.*

↓

Keep the injured part
elevated if possible.

↓

Apply a clean or sterile
dressing and bandage to the
region (see Bandaging pg.
658).

Index

So that you will find it easier to use, the index for this book is divided into four sections: *General, Birds, Cats,* and *Dogs.* Please note that those entries in **bold** are emergency/first aid terms. The special emphasis on these words should make it easier for you to find the crucial information you would need in the event of an emergency.

GENERAL INDEX

BIRDS INDEX, 480-555

DOGS INDEX, 1-300

E

ear mites, 257
ears, 83-86, 252-260
  anatomy and physiology, 252-253
  bacterial infection, 256-257
  cleaning the ears, 83-85
  congenital disorders, 59
  cropping ears, 112-113
  deafness and hearing loss, 94, 259-260
  discharge or odor, 18, 57, 255, 256
  ear mites, 257
  hair in ears, 57, 85-86
  head shaking, 55-57, 255, 258
  hematomas, trauma to ear, 260
  inflammation of ear, 253-255, 257-258
  loud noises, 49-50
  odor or discharge, 18, 57, 255, 256
  otitis externa, 253-255
  otitis media and interna, 257-258
  ruptured ear drum, 258-259
  tilting of head, 55-57, 258
  yeast infections, 255-256
eclampsia, 217-218
ectropion, 251
ehrlichiosis, 156-157, 172
elective surgery, 107-114
  administering pills/medications, 113-114
  anesthesia, 107-108
  castration, 110-111
  dewclaw removal, 111-112
  ear trimming, 112-113
  post-surgical care, 113-114
  spaying or ovariohysterectomy, 108-110
  tail docking, 111-112
electrical shock, 673-674
electrocardiogram (ECG) test, 170
enamel hypoplasia (*see* distemper, dogs)
endocrine system, 287-300
  adrenal glands, 288
  anatomy and physiology, 287-289
  diabetes insipidus, 299-300
  diabetes mellitus, 289, 296-299
  glucagon production, 289
  glucocorticosteriods, 289-291
  hormonal imbalances, 231, 287, 295-296, 626-627
  hyperadrenocorticism (Cushing's disease), 292-294
  hypoadrenocorticism (Addison's disease), 294-295
  hypothalamus, 288
  hypothyroidism, 291-292
  insulin production, 289, 298
  older dogs, 94
  parathyroid glands, 288
  pituitary gland, 288
  steroids, 287-291
  thyroid gland, 288
entropion, 249-251
epidermis, 223

epilepsy, 278-280
erythrocytes, 166
esophageal disorders, 191-193
esophageal worms, 140
esophagitis, 192-193
estrous cycle, 97-98
euthanasia for pets, 634-638
exercise, 613-614
excitability, 13
external parasites (*see* fleas and ticks; mites)
eye injuries, cat and dog, 671-673
eyes, 56-57, 240-251
  anatomy and physiology, 240-242
  blindness, 94, 116, 132, 246
  blue-eye, infectious canine hepatitis (ICH), 122-124, 202-204
  cataracts, 247-248
  cherry eye, 240, 248-249
  cloudiness, 18, 56, 246, 247
  congenital disorders, 59
  conjunctivitis, 240, 244
  corneal ulcers and scratches, 242-244
  discharge, 18, 56, 116, 123, 130, 156, 242, 244, 249, 251
  dry eye (keratoconjunctivitis sicca), 248
  ectropion, 251
  entropion, 249-251
  eyelid/eyelash irritation, 57
  glaucoma, 244-247
  masses or tumors on eyelids, 251
  nictitating membrane, third eyelid, 240
  older dogs and vision problems, 94
  redness, 18, 56, 57, 242, 245, 249, 251
  squinting, 56, 249
  ulcerations and scratches, 293
  unequal pupil size, 56
  yellow-tinged whites, 57, 122, 203

F

false pregnancy, 217
feet and legs, dogs
  dewclaw removal, 111-112
  nail trimming, 90-91
  reddened or bleeding pads, 145
fever, 56, 122, 129, 156, 157, 158, 178, 203
fibrinogen, 166
first-aid kits, 642
first-aid procedures, 639-686
fleas and ticks (*see also* external parasites), 17-18, 58, 63-68, 134-136, 225, 621-622
  collar insecticides, 66
  dips, 65-66
  electronic flea collars, 67
  flea-bite hypersensitivity, 227-228
  internal (systemic) insecticides, 66-67
  natural remedies, 67
  powdered insecticides, 65
  shampoos, 65
  spray insecticides, 63-64